ANAC's
Core Curriculum for
HIV/AIDS Nursing
SECOND EDITION

To Kathleen McMahon Casey, Felissa R. Lashley and Anne M. Hughes—
without them, none of this would have been possible

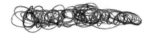

ANAC's
Core Curriculum for
HIV/AIDS Nursing

SECOND EDITION

Edited by
Carl Kirton
The Mount Sinai Hospital, New York, NY

Association of Nurses in AIDS Care

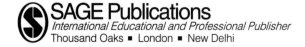

SAGE Publications
International Educational and Professional Publisher
Thousand Oaks ■ London ■ New Delhi

For information:

 Sage Publications, Inc.
2455 Teller Road
Thousand Oaks, California 91320
E-mail: order@sagepub.com

Sage Publications Ltd.
6 Bonhill Street
London EC2A 4PU
United Kingdom

Sage Publications India Pvt. Ltd.
B-42, Panchsheel Enclave
Post Box 4109
New Delhi 110 017 India

Printed in the United States of America

ISBN 0-7619-2777-8 [Special Edition]

03   04   05   06   10   9   8   7   6   5   4   3   2   1

Acquisitions Editor:	Dan Ruth
Editorial Assistant:	Cati Connell
Production Editor:	Melanie Birdsall
Copy Editor:	Cheryl Duksta
Typesetter:	C&M Digitals (P) Ltd.
Proofreader:	Kathrine Pollock
Indexer:	Julie Grayson
Cover Designer:	Michelle Lee
Production Artist:	Sandra Ng Sauvajot

Contents

Introduction   xv

Preface   xvii

Acknowledgments   xix

About the Editors   xxi

Contributing Authors   xxv

Section I: HIV Infection, Transmission, and Prevention   1

1.1   Historical Overview of the HIV Pandemic   2
Jo Anne Bennett, RN, PhD, CS, ACRN

1.2   Epidemiology of HIV Infection and AIDS   4
Jo Anne Bennett, RN, PhD, CS, ACRN

1.3   Prevention of HIV Infection   18
Valery Hughes, RN, MS, FNP

1.4   Pathophysiology of HIV Infection   22
Joseph P. Colagreco, MS, APRN, BC, NP-C

1.5   HIV Testing   29
Jane Schulz, MPH, RN, CNP, ACRN

Section II: Clinical Management of the HIV-Infected Adolescent and Adult   35

2.1   Baseline Assessment   36
Thomas P. Young, MS, RN, APRN, BC, ACRN

2.2   Immunizations   40
Carl A. Kirton, MA, RN, APRN, BC

2.3   Teaching for Health Promotion, Wellness, and Prevention of Transmission   43
Valery Hughes, RN, MS, FNP

2.4   Health Care Follow-Up   49
Kristin Grage, MA, RN, CNP, ACRN

2.5   Managing Antiretroviral Therapy   51
Brian K. Goodroad, PhD, CNP, ACRN

**Section III: Symptomatic Conditions in
Adolescents and Adults With Advancing Disease**   65

A. Symptomatic Conditions in Advanced Disease   66

     3.1   Bartonellosis   66
Hopkins D. Stanley, RN, MS, ACRN, CNS &
Lawrence Marsco, RN, BSN &
Ian R. McNicholl, Pharm.D., BCPS (I.D.)

     3.2   Herpes Zoster   66
Hopkins D. Stanley, RN, MS, ACRN, CNS &
Lawrence Marsco, RN, BSN &
Ian R. McNicholl, Pharm.D., BCPS (I.D.)

     3.3   Human Papillomavirus Infection   68
Doris Carroll, BSN, RN, CCRC & Pamela Dole,
EdD, MPH, MSN, FNP, ACRN

     3.4   Idiopathic Thrombocytopenia Purpura   71
Kristin K. Ownby, PhD, RN, ACRN, AOCN, CHPN

     3.5   Listeriosis   72
Hopkins D. Stanley, RN, MS, ACRN, CNS &
Lawrence Marsco, RN, BSN &
Ian R. McNicholl, Pharm.D., BCPS (I.D.)

     3.6   Oral Hairy Leukoplakia   73
Joyce Keithley, DNSc, RN, FAAN

     3.7   Peripheral Neuropathy   73
Janice M. Zeller, PhD, RN, FAAN &
Young-Me Lee, MSN, RN, DNSc (c)

B. AIDS Indicator Diseases   75

Bacterial Infections

     3.8   Bacterial Pneumonia   75
Kelly Fugate, ND, RN

     3.9   Mycobacterium Avium Complex (MAC)   76
Demetrius Porche, DNS, RN, FNP, CS

     3.10   Mycobacterium Tuberculosis   77
Demetrius Porche, DNS, RN, FNP, CS

     3.11   Salmonellosis   78
Hopkins D. Stanley, RN, MS, ACRN, CNS &
Lawrence Marsco, RN, BSN &
Ian R. McNicholl, Pharm.D., BCPS (I.D.)   79

Fungal Infections

     3.12   Candidiasis   79
Patrick Robinson, PhD, RN, ACRN

     3.13   Coccidioidomycosis   81
Hopkins D. Stanley, RN, MS, ACRN, CNS &
Lawrence Marsco, RN, BSN &
Ian R. McNicholl, Pharm.D., BCPS (I.D.)

3.14 Cryptococcosis 82
Hopkins D. Stanley, RN, MS, ACRN, CNS &
Lawrence Marsco, RN, BSN &
Ian R. McNicholl, Pharm.D., BCPS (I.D.)

3.15 Histoplasmosis 84
Hopkins D. Stanley, RN, MS, ACRN, CNS &
Lawrence Marsco, RN, BSN &
Ian R. McNicholl, Pharm.D., BCPS (I.D.)

Protozoal Infections

3.16 Cryptosporidiosis 85
Kristin K. Ownby, PhD, RN, ACRN, AOCN, CHPN

3.17 Isosporiasis 86
Kristin K. Ownby, PhD, RN, ACRN, AOCN, CHPN

3.18 Pneumocystosis 86
Kelly Fugate, ND, RN

3.19 Toxoplasmosis 87
Hopkins D. Stanley, RN, MS, ACRN, CNS &
Lawrence Marsco, RN, BSN &
Ian R. McNicholl, Pharm.D., BCPS (I.D.)

Viral Infections

3.20 Cytomegalovirus (CMV) 89
Demetrius Porche, DNS, RN, FNP, CS

3.21 Herpes Simplex Virus (HSV) 90
Patrick Robinson, PhD, RN, ACRN

3.22 Progressive Multifocal Leukoencephalopathy (PML) 91
Craig R. Sellers, MS, RN, APRN, BC, ANP, ACRN

Neoplasms

3.23 Cervical Neoplasia 93
Theresa Moran, RN, MS, FNP &
Pamela Dole, EdD, MPH, MSN, FNP, ACRN

3.24 Kaposi's Sarcoma (KS) 94
Theresa Moran, RN, MS, FNP

3.25 Non-Hodgkin's Lymphoma (NHL) 96
Theresa Moran, RN, MS, FNP

3.26 HIV-Related Wasting Syndrome 97
Joyce Keithley, DNSc, RN, FAAN &
S. K. Glenda Winson, MS, RN, ACRN

3.27 HIV Encephalopathy 98
Janice M. Zeller, PhD, RN, FAAN &
Young-Me Lee, MSN, RN, DNSc (c)

C. Comorbid Complications 99

3.28 Fat Redistribution Syndrome 99
Joyce Keithley, DNSc, RN, FAAN &
S. K. Glenda Winson, MS, RN, ACRN

3.29   Impaired Glucose Tolerance (IGT)   100
       Debra E. Lyon, PhD, RN

3.30   Dyslipidemia   101
       Debra E. Lyon, PhD, RN

3.31   Anemia   102
       Richard Ferri, PhD, ANP, ACRN, FAAN

3.32   Leukopenia   103
       Barbara Swanson, DNSc, RN, ACRN

3.33   Thrombocytopenia   103
       Kristin K. Ownby, PhD, RN, ACRN, AOCN, CHPN

3.34   Cardiomyopathy   104
       Carl A. Kirton, MA, RN, APRN, BC

3.35   Psoriasis   105
       Michelle Agnoli, BSN, RN, ACRN

3.36   Arthritis, Reiter's Syndrome   106
       Michelle Agnoli, BSN, RN, ACRN

3.37   Osteopenia, Osteoporosis, Avascular Necrosis   107
       Barbara Swanson, DNSc, RN, ACRN

3.38   Nephropathy   108
       Wade Leon, RN, MA, ANP-CS, CRRN

3.39   Lactic Acidosis   109
       Barbara Swanson, DNSc, RN, ACRN

3.40   Hepatitis A   110
       Kathleen Barrett, MSN, RN

3.41   Hepatitis B   111
       Kathleen Barrett, MSN, RN

3.42   Hepatitis C   112
       Kathleen Barrett, MSN, RN

Section IV: Symptom Management of
the HIV-Infected Adolescent and Adult   123

4.1   Anorexia and Weight Loss   124
       Joyce Keithley, DNSc, RN, FAAN

4.2   Cognitive Impairment   125
       Debra Topham, PhD, RN, CNS, ACRN

4.3   Cough   128
       Kelly Fugate, ND, RN

4.4   Dyspnea   129
       Kelly Fugate, ND, RN

4.5   Dysphagia and Odynophagia   130
       Joyce Keithley, DNSc, RN, FAAN`

4.6   Oral Lesions   132
       Barbara Swanson, DNSc, RN, ACRN

| 4.7 | Fatigue
Julie Barroso, PhD, ANP, CS | 133 |

4.8 Fever | 135 |
Barbara Holtzclaw, PhD, RN, FAAN

4.9 Sleep Disturbances | 137 |
Kathleen M. Nokes, PhD, RN, FAAN

4.10 Mobility Impairment | 139 |
Tracy A. Riley, PhD, RN, CS &
Yvonne Smith, MSN, RN, CNS

4.11 Nausea and Vomiting | 140 |
Bernadette Capili, NP-C, APRN, DNSc

4.12 Diarrhea | 142 |
S. K. Glenda Winson, MS, RN, ACRN

4.13 Pain | 143 |
Gayle Newshan, PhD, RN, NP

4.14 Female Sexual Dysfunction | 146 |
Rebekah Shephard, MS, RN, ANP

4.15 Male Sexual Dysfunction | 148 |
Rebekah Shephard, MS, RN, ANP

4.16 Vision Loss | 150 |
Tracy A. Riley, PhD, RN, CS &
Yvonne Smith, MSN, RN, CNS

**Section V: Psychosocial Concerns
of the HIV-Infected Adolescent and
Adult and Their Significant Others** | 157 |

A. Responses to HIV Diagnosis

5.1 Response to an HIV Diagnosis: Infected Person | 158 |
Rebekah Shephard, MS, RN, ANP

5.2 Response to HIV Diagnosis:
Family and Significant Other | 158 |
Rebekah Shephard, MS, RN, ANP

5.3 Caregiver Burden/Strain | 159 |
Rebekah Shephard, MS, RN, ANP

5.4 Spiritual and Religious Concerns of HIV-Infected Persons | 161 |
Patricia M. O'Kane, MA, RN

B. Selected Psychiatric Disorders in HIV Disease | 164 |

5.5 Depression | 164 |
Wade Leon, RN, MA, ANP-CS, CRRN &
Pamela Dole, EdD, MPH, MSN, FNP, ACRN

5.6 Primary Anxiety-Spectrum Disorders | 168 |
Pamela Dole, EdD, MPH, MSN, FNP, ACRN &
Wade Leon, RN, MA, ANP-CS, CRRN

5.7	Delirium	171
	Rebekah Shephard, MS, RN, ANP &	
	Pamela Dole, EdD, MPH, MSN, FNP, ACRN	

| 5.8 | Mental Illness and Substance Use | 172 |
| | *Carl A. Kirton, MA, RN, APRN, BC* | |

Section VI: Concerns of Special Populations — 175

| 6.1 | Adolescents | 176 |
| | *Mary Geiger, MPH, RN* | |

| 6.2 | The Blind and Visually Impaired Community | 179 |
| | *Nora Merriam, RN, MSN, MPH* | |

| 6.3 | Commercial Sex Workers | 181 |
| | *Margaret Dykeman, RN, PhD, FNP, APRN, BC, ACRN* | |

| 6.4 | Gay and Bisexual Men | 183 |
| | *R. Kevin Mallinson, PhD, RN, ACRN* | |

| 6.5 | HIV-Infected Health Care Workers | 186 |
| | *Craig E. Nielsen, MS, NP, BC, ACRN* | |

| 6.6 | The Deaf and Hearing-Impaired Community | 188 |
| | *R. Kevin Mallinson, PhD, RN, ACRN* | |

| 6.7 | People With Hemophilia | 191 |
| | *Beverly Christie, RN, BSN* | |

| 6.8 | Homeless Persons | 193 |
| | *Margaret Dykeman, RN, PhD, FNP, APRN, BC, ACRN* | |

| 6.9 | Incarcerated Persons | 197 |
| | *Pamela Dole, EdD, MPH, MSN, FNP, ACRN* | |

| 6.10 | Lesbians and Bisexual Women | 202 |
| | *Christine A. Balt, MS, RN, ACRN, APRN, BC* | |

| 6.11 | Migrant and Seasonal Farm Workers | 205 |
| | *Susan Gaskin, MPH, DSN, ACRN* | |

| 6.12 | Older Persons | 206 |
| | *Kathleen M. Nokes, PhD, RN, FAAN* | |

| 6.13 | Rural Communities | 209 |
| | *Susan Gaskin, MPH, DSN, ACRN* | |

| 6.14 | The African American Community | 211 |
| | *Carl A. Kirton, MA, RN, APRN, BC* | |

| 6.15 | Pregnant Women | 214 |
| | *Pamela Dole, EdD, MPH, MSN, FNP, ACRN* | |

| 6.16 | Recent Immigrants | 219 |
| | *Susanne Rendiro, MSN, FNP, BC* | |

6.17	Substance Users	221
	Donna Taliaferro, RN, PhD &	
	Gail B. Williams, RN, PhD	

6.18 Transgender/Transsexual Persons 226
Eric G. Leach, MSN, RN, NP

6.19 Women 229
Pamela Dole, EdD, MPH, MSN, FNP, ACRN

**Section VII: Clinical Management of
the HIV-Infected Infant and Child** 241

7.1 Perinatal Transmission of HIV Infection 242
*Carolyn Keith Burr, EdD, RN &
Dawn D'Orlando, RN, MSN, MPH*

7.2 Clinical Manifestations and Management of
the HIV-Infected Infant and Child 247
*Carolyn Keith Burr, EdD, RN &
Dawn D'Orlando, RN, MSN, MPH*

7.3 Managing Antiretroviral Therapy in
HIV-Infected Infants and Children 257
*Carolyn Keith Burr, EdD, RN &
Dawn D'Orlando, RN, MSN, MPH*

7.4 Adherence to Medical Regimens 261
Elaine Gross, RN, MS, CNS-C

**Section VIII: Symptomatic Conditions
in Infants and Children With Advancing Disease** 267

A. **Symptomatic Conditions in HIV Disease** 268

8.1 Anemia 268
Dawn D'Orlando, RN, MSN, MPH

8.2 Cardiomyopathy 268
Dawn D'Orlando, RN, MSN, MPH

8.3 Dermatitis 269
Dawn D'Orlando, RN, MSN, MPH

8.4 Diarrhea, Recurrent or Chronic 269
Dawn D'Orlando, RN, MSN, MPH

8.5 Hepatitis 270
Dawn D'Orlando, RN, MSN, MPH

8.6 Hepatomegaly 271
Dawn D'Orlando, RN, MSN, MPH

8.7 Herpes Virus 271
Dawn D'Orlando, RN, MSN, MPH

8.8 Leiomyosarcoma 272
Dawn D'Orlando, RN, MSN, MPH

8.9 Lymphadenopathy 273
Dawn D'Orlando, RN, MSN, MPH

8.10   Lymphoid Interstitial Pneumonitis (LIP)   273
       Dawn D'Orlando, RN, MSN, MPH

8.11   Nephropathy   274
       Dawn D'Orlando, RN, MSN, MPH

8.12   Neutropenia   274
       Dawn D'Orlando, RN, MSN, MPH

8.13   Nocardiosis   275
       Dawn D'Orlando, RN, MSN, MPH

8.14   Otitis Media, Recurrent   275
       Dawn D'Orlando, RN, MSN, MPH

8.15   Parotitis   276
       Dawn D'Orlando, RN, MSN, MPH

8.16   Sinusitis, Recurrent   276
       Dawn D'Orlando, RN, MSN, MPH

8.17   Splenomegaly   277
       Dawn D'Orlando, RN, MSN, MPH

8.18   Thrombocytopenia   277
       Dawn D'Orlando, RN, MSN, MPH

8.19   Upper Respiratory Infection, Recurrent   278
       Dawn D'Orlando, RN, MSN, MPH

8.20   Varicella, Disseminated (Complicated Chickenpox)   279
       Dawn D'Orlando, RN, MSN, MPH

**B.   AIDS-Defining Conditions
       in Children With HIV Infection**   279

Bacterial Infections

8.21   Bacterial Infections, Recurrent   279
       Dawn D'Orlando, RN, MSN, MPH

8.22   Mycobacterial Avium Complex (MAC)   280
       Dawn D'Orlando, RN, MSN, MPH

8.23   Mycobacterial Tuberculosis   281
       Dawn D'Orlando, RN, MSN, MPH

8.24   Salmonellosis   281
       Dawn D'Orlando, RN, MSN, MPH

Fungal Infections

8.25   Candidiasis   282
       Dawn D'Orlando, RN, MSN, MPH

8.26   Coccidioidomycosis   283
       Dawn D'Orlando, RN, MSN, MPH

8.27   Cryptococcosis   283
       Dawn D'Orlando, RN, MSN, MPH

8.28   Histoplasmosis   284
       Dawn D'Orlando, RN, MSN, MPH

Protozoal Infections

8.29 Cryptosporidiosis 285
Dawn D'Orlando, RN, MSN, MPH

8.30 Isosporiasis 285
Dawn D'Orlando, RN, MSN, MPH

8.31 *Pneumocystis Carinii* Pneumonia (PCP) 286
Dawn D'Orlando, RN, MSN, MPH

8.32 *Toxoplasma Gondii* 287
Dawn D'Orlando, RN, MSN, MPH

Viral Infections

8.33 Cytomegalovirus Disease (CMV) 288
Dawn D'Orlando, RN, MSN, MPH

8.34 Progressive Multifocal Leukoencephalopathy (PML) 288
Dawn D'Orlando, RN, MSN, MPH

Neoplasms

8.35 Malignancies 289
Dawn D'Orlando, RN, MSN, MPH

8.36 HIV-Related Wasting Syndrome 289
Dawn D'Orlando, RN, MSN, MPH

8.37 HIV-Related Encephalopathy 290
Dawn D'Orlando, RN, MSN, MPH

**Section IX: Symptom Management of
the HIV-Infected Infant and Child** 293

9.1 Pain 294
Lynn Czarniecki, RNC, MSN, CNS-C

9.2 Anorexia 298
Rachel Davis, RN, ACRN

9.3 Weight Loss 299
Rachel Davis, RN, ACRN

9.4 Cognitive Impairment and Developmental Delay 300
Pamela J. Bachanas, PhD, RN, MSN, ARNP

9.5 Fever 303
David J. Sterken, MN, CNS, CPNP

9.6 Skin Lesions 305
David J. Sterken, MN, CNS, CPNP

**Section X: Psychosocial Concerns of the
HIV-Infected Infant and Child and Their Significant Others** 311

10.1 Decision Making and Family Autonomy 312
*Lisa Perry, MSW, LCSW &
Catherine R. Bataille, MSW, LCSW*

10.2   Stress Reduction and Pediatric HIV Infection   316
David J. Sterken, MN, CNS, CPNP &
Rhys VanDemark, BA, CCLS &
Brooke Vanburen-Hay, PhD

10.3   Isolation and Stigmatization   318
Barbara E. Berger, PhD, RN, ACRN

10.4   Surrogate Caregivers   320
Catherine R. Bataille, MSW, LCSW

10.5   Disclosure to the Child   323
Marion Donohoe, RN, MSN, CPNP

10.6   Multiple Hospitalizations   326
Lisa Perry, MSW, LCSW

10.7   Community-Based Care Issues   329
Marion Donohoe, RN, MSN, CPNP

10.8   End of Life Issues   332
Heidi J. Haiken, MSW, MPH

Section XI: Nursing Management Issues   337

11.1   Case Management   338
Tom Emanuele, BSN, RNC, ACRN &
Connie Highsmith, RN, BSN, ACRN

11.2   Ethical and Legal Concerns   340
Craig R. Sellers, MS, RN, APRN, BC, ANP, ACRN &
Richard MacIntyre, RN, PhD

11.3   Preventing Transmission of HIV in Patient Care Settings   345
Leslie Schor, RN, MSN, ACRN

Appendixes

Appendix A: Public Health Service Revised Classification
System for HIV Infection (Adolescents & Adults), 1993 Revised   351

Appendix B: Selected Laboratory Values   355
Martin Lewis, M.Ed, MSN, ANP, ACRN

Appendix C: Treatment of Tuberculosis (TB in Adult and Adolescent
Patients Coinfected With the Human Immunodeficiency Virus [HIV])   363
New Jersey Medical School National Tuberculosis Center

Appendix D: Medications   369
Sande Gracia Jones, PhD, ARNP, ACRN, C, CS, BC

Index   419

Introduction

The Association of Nurses in Aids Care

The Association of Nurses in AIDS Care (ANAC) is a nonprofit professional nursing organization committed to fostering the individual and collective professional development of nurses involved in the delivery of health care to persons infected or affected by the human immunodeficiency virus (HIV) and to promoting the health, welfare, and rights of all HIV-infected persons.

The members of ANAC strive to achieve the mission by:

- Creating an effective network among nurses in HIV/AIDS care
- Studying, researching, and exchanging information, experiences, and ideas leading to improved care for persons with HIV/AIDS infection
- Providing leadership to the nursing community in matters related to HIV/AIDS infection
- Advocating for HIV-infected persons
- Promoting social awareness concerning issues related to HIV/AIDS

Inherent in these goals is an abiding commitment to the prevention of further HIV infection.

Preface

In 1996, the first edition of the *Core Curriculum for HIV/AIDS Nursing* appeared in print and quickly became a significant and valuable compendium of the knowledge of nurses working in HIV/AIDS. That work, the vision of ANAC President James Halloran (1991–1992), represented the voluntary efforts of more than 90 contributors and editors and was well received by clinicians, educators, researchers, and nursing certification boards. Shortly after the printing of the first edition, however, dramatic changes in the epidemic began to emerge, and along with that the nursing care for patients with HIV/AIDS expanded. Throughout this edition, there is much that has been refined and embellished in the light of new nursing and medical knowledge that has been developed since the last edition.

What has not changed is the original intent of the *Core Curriculum for HIV/AIDS Nursing* (or the CORE, as it has come to be known within the nursing community):

- To identify the essential information required by nurses to care for people with HIV/AIDS, regardless of practice setting or role responsibilities
- To serve as a foundation for the ANAC certification process for HIV/AIDS specialty nursing
- To provide a framework for core curriculum content that may be used in undergraduate, graduate, staff development, and continuing education programs related to HIV/AIDS nursing care

To meet these goals the editors have assembled 70 clinicians, researchers, educators, and administrators to document the work they do with persons with HIV/AIDS. Some of the authors are returning, but many are new to this edition. We have made every effort to contact those who contributed to the original edition but were not successful in every instance. It is important that we acknowledge the important contributions that first-edition authors made to the body of knowledge of HIV/AIDS nursing.

The editors and I feel that we selected the best contributors possible, and we strived to ensure that the information contained within this edition is current, accurate, scientifically based, and culturally accurate. We maintained the standardized, outline format of the first edition to enable the reader to quickly find topics of interest. Our intent is to assemble a text that will be important to your practice and be used frequently to guide your decision making in patient care. I welcome your comments and feedback.

Carl Kirton
carl.kirton@msnyuhealth.org

Acknowledgments

The editors and I want to thank all of the authors for their important and informative contributions to this second edition; without them, this project would not exist. We would especially like to thank Dan Ruth at Sage who was instrumental in bringing this project to Sage and nurtured it to its completion. Our special thanks to Melanie Birdsall, assistant production editor, whose oversight, suggestions, and vision for this project were invaluable. We are grateful to Cheryl Duksta, who provided precise and thoughtful copyediting of the manuscripts and to Michelle Lee, thanks for a great cover! It's quite impressive and amazing how you have captured the essence of this organization when the only words you had to work with were "make it pretty."

There are many persons at Sage whom we do not know but who certainly have played an important role in the development of this project. We thank them all.

Carl Kirton

I wish to acknowledge the nurses who have been my mentors throughout this epidemic, the patients who keep me challenged and keep my work rewarding, and Barbara and my parents for all their love and support.

Christine Balt

To all the patients who taught me about their disease and to Carl Kirton, whose quest for excellence, in a compassionate and patient manner, made this edition possible.

Pamela Dole

I want to acknowledge the nurses in Ryan White Title IV and PACTG programs who provide care for children, youth, and families living with HIV/AIDS. They are a very special group.

Elaine Gross

I would like to acknowledge my sun and my moon: husband John, for mornings at the kitchen table watching day break over the ocean, and daughter Kim, for late-night phone calls, "adventures," bus rides, and dinners enjoyed around the world discussing life, art, and literature; my wonderfully diverse family in Massachusetts and Florida, who have shared kids, homes, holidays, showers, travel, and love; Miami and Ft. Lauderdale ANAC chapter friends; and all my ANAC colleagues who have helped me fulfill my dreams innumerable times when I have said "Hey, I have an idea. . . ."

Sande Gracia Jones

To my mother Jayne Swanson, for her selfless love and support.

Barbara Swanson

About the Editors

Carl Kirton, MA, RN, APRN, BC

Carl Kirton received his Bachelor of Science degree in Nursing at Lehman College, NYC and holds a graduate degree in nursing education and a postmaster's certificate in advanced practice nursing from New York University, NYC. Mr. Kirton began his nursing career as a critical care nurse and progressed to the critical care nurse manager at New York University Medical Center. He began his advanced practice career in 1996 and has held a variety of positions in substance abuse, internal medicine, cardiology, and HIV. Mr. Kirton joined the nursing faculty at New York University in 1993 and has taught in both the undergraduate and graduate programs in nursing. During his tenure at NYU, he was promoted to clinical associate professor and coordinator of the acute care advanced practice program. While on faculty at NYU, he maintained a joint appointment to the advanced practice staff at Mount Sinai Medical Center and Hospital in the AIDS Center. Today, he is a nurse practitioner and the clinical manager of the AIDS Center at Mount Sinai Medical Center. He continues to teach in the advanced practice program at NYU as part of its adjunct faculty.

Mr. Kirton is the author of *Handbook of HIV/AIDS Nursing* and has authored or coauthored more than 30 publications. He has held a variety of leadership positions in the professional nursing community, notably, president of the Greater New York Chapter of the Association of Nurses in AIDS Care and board member of the National Association of Nurses in AIDS. In 2001 he was awarded the President's Award from the National Association of Nurses in AIDS Care for exceptional leadership in accomplishing committee work and dedication to the mission and goals of the association.

Christine A. Balt, MS, RN, ACRN, APRN, BC

Christine Balt received an Associate's Degree in Nursing from Purdue University in 1982 and a Bachelor of Science degree in Nursing from Indiana University in 1986. Ms. Balt has worked at hospitals in Indianapolis, Northwest Indiana, and Chicago in pediatrics, emergency rooms, and medical-surgical units. She spent more than 9 years at the VA Medical Center in Indianapolis. During that time, she provided care for patients with and without HIV infection in a primary care setting, and she was instrumental in establishing the HIV program at the VA. Ms. Balt is certified in AIDS nursing care. Ms. Balt expanded her expertise and advanced her nursing skills when she received a Master's in Primary Care Nursing and completed family nurse practitioner training from Indiana Wesleyan University, Marion, Indiana, in December 1996. She began her advanced practice career providing primary care and HIV care in a private family and internal medicine practice. In January 1999, Ms. Balt joined the Indiana University School of Medicine Division of Infectious Diseases as a family nurse practitioner with the HIV team of Wishard Memorial Hospital and Health Services' Infectious Disease Clinic. In addition to her advanced practice role, she is the clinical manager of the HIV team.

Ms. Balt has held a variety of leadership positions in the professional nursing and local HIV communities, such as secretary of the National Association of Nurses in AIDS Care, Board of Directors member and founding member of the Central Indiana Chapter of the

Association of Nurses in AIDS Care, and secretary/treasurer of the Indy Thrift for AIDS. She has authored and coauthored several articles about the various issues of HIV and is a Distinguished Lecturer for the Association of Nurses in AIDS Care.

Pamela J. Dole, EdD, MPH, MSN, FNP, ACRN

Pamela Dole received her Bachelor of Science degree in Nursing at the University of Connecticut. She has several graduate degrees, including a master's in public health and a master's in nursing from Hunter College in New York City, where she currently is an assistant professor. She also holds a doctorate in education from the Institute of Advanced Study in Human Sexuality in San Francisco. She attended one of the first nurse practitioner programs at the University of Massachusetts at Amherst and has practiced for two decades as an adult nurse practitioner. Her clinical practice in the last decade has been dedicated to women with HIV infection. Dr. Dole is an expert colposcopist, managing cervical disease for the last 10 years, including for those individuals living behind bars. She is currently affiliated with St. Vincent's HIV Clinic in NYC. Pamela has been HIV certified by ANAC since its inception in 1997. For the last 3 years she has taught therapeutic touch (TT) for the Theosophical Society and Nurse Healer's Professional Association and is recognized as a Qualified Therapeutic Touch Teacher, Mentor, and Practitioner by the latter.

Dr. Dole has authored or coauthored numerous publications, including the first edition of *ANAC's Core Curriculum for HIV/AIDS Nursing*. She is a contributing author for *Numedx* and is on the editorial board of *HIV Inside* (which provides continuing education for correctional health care professionals on the management of HIV). She has participated in several HIV women's research projects, including projects funded by the Centers for Disease Control and Prevention and is currently a member of the University of California San Francisco International HIV/AIDS Nursing Research Network. Dr. Dole has been active professionally, recently serving as a national board member for the Association of Nurses in AIDS Care and the Association of Nurse Practitioners of New York. In 1996, she was awarded the ANAC fellowship award and is a member of Sigma Theta Tau.

Sande Gracia Jones, PhD, ARNP, ACRN, C, CS, BC

Sande Gracia Jones received her diploma in nursing from St. Luke's Hospital, New Bedford, Massachusetts, and her Bachelor of Science in Nursing from the University of Massachusetts at Dartmouth. She received her MSN at University of Miami and her master's in adult education and postmaster's certificate as an adult nurse practitioner at Florida International University in Miami. Her PhD in nursing is from Barry University in Miami. Dr. Jones has three decades of experience in hospital-based nursing. At Mount Sinai Medical Center in Miami Beach, Florida, she served in a variety of positions, including education coordinator for staff development, nurse manager of the Surgical Special Care Unit, and coordinator of the hospital's Basic and Advanced Cardiac Life Support Program. Dr. Jones served as Mount Sinai's HIV/TB clinical nurse specialist and as the care manager for the HIV Critical Pathways Program. She joined the faculty at Barry University in 1999, teaching in the undergraduate and graduate programs and was also employed as an adult nurse practitioner in a private HIV service. Dr. Jones is currently an assistant professor at Florida International University in Miami. Dr. Jones has authored or coauthored more than 100 articles in clinical, scholarly, and Internet publications. She has held leadership positions in nursing organizations and the community, including president of the Miami Chapter of the Association of Nurses in AIDS Care, director at large and secretary of the National Association of Nurses in AIDS Care, director at large for the Florida Nurses Association, and commissioner for the Commission on Certification, American Nurses Credentialing Center. She has been recognized for her clinical practice and research in HIV/AIDS care through receipt of several awards, including Excellence in Clinical Nursing, Mount Sinai Medical Center; Advanced Practice Nurse of the Year, Florida Nurses Association; inaugural Advanced Practice Nurse Award, American Nurses Credentialing Center; HIV Doctoral Fellowship Award, Association of Nurses in AIDS Care; Melba Cather Award, Lambda Chi chapter of Sigma Theta Tau International; and the inaugural HIV/AIDS Nursing Leadership Award from the Florida Department of Health, Bureau of HIV/AIDS, Patient Care Division. In 2002, she received the Research Article-of-the-Year Award from Sage Publications and JANAC (*Journal of the Association of Nurses in AIDS Care*) for her study of HIV-positive nurses and their experience taking HIV combination drug therapy. Dr. Jones has been designated an HIV/AIDS nurse expert by the American Nurses Association for the International Council of Nurses' Bank of Nurse Experts and was selected as a distinguished lecturer for the Association of Nurses in AIDS Care.

Elaine Gross, RN, MS, CNS-C

Elaine Gross received a diploma in nursing from Geisinger Medical Center School of Nursing, Danville, Pennsylvania in 1967, a Bachelor of Arts in Philosophy from Upsala College in 1983, a Bachelor of Science in Nursing from the State University of New York, Regents College in 1984, and a Master of Science in Parent-Child Nursing from Rutgers University in 1988. Ms Gross is certified as an advance practice nurse/clinical specialist in pediatric nursing.

Ms. Gross has worked in a variety of positions in perinatal and pediatric nursing in Boston, Toronto, and New Jersey, including almost 15 years as clinical and outreach educator of the NICU at the Children's Hospital of New Jersey. In 1987, Ms. Gross joined the Children's Hospital AIDS Program (now the FXB Center) and the National Pediatric and Family HIV Resource Center in Newark. Ms. Gross developed an HIV education program about care of mothers, infants, and children with HIV infection for pediatric and perinatal nurses. This program and its second-generation train-the-trainer curricula for pediatric/perinatal nurses and school nurses have been offered throughout the United States. In addition to developing educational materials for pregnant women living with HIV, she participated in the development of a train-the-trainer program for women's health care providers for reducing perinatal HIV infection, also offered nationally. In addition, Ms. Gross has presented at national and international meetings and has published book chapters and journal articles in the professional literature. She participated in the MATEP Treatment Adherence Initiative and developed the Pediatric and Family Adherence Module for the AETC Provider Curriculum. She has served on the Board of Directors of the Association of Nurses in AIDS Care and, in 2002, received the ANAC Lifetime Achievement Award.

Barbara Swanson, DNSc, RN, ACRN

Barbara Swanson received her Bachelor of Science in Nursing from Elmhurst College and graduate degrees from Loyola University of Chicago and Rush University College of Nursing. She did postdoctoral work in psychoneuroimmunology and HIV at Rush-Presbyterian-St. Luke's Medical Center in Chicago. Dr. Swanson is currently an assistant professor of Adult Health Nursing at Rush College of Nursing where she conducts research on the use of complementary and alternative therapies to manage symptoms and to augment immunity in HIV-infected persons. She has published more than 30 articles and book chapters.

The editors acknowledge and appreciate the contributions Brian K. Goodroad, PhD, CNP, ACRN, made in the preparation of several of the manuscripts in Section I.

Contributing Authors

Michelle Agnoli, BSN, RN, ACRN, Training Specialist, Midwest AIDS Training and Education Center, Jane Addams College of Social Work, University of Illinois at Chicago.
Psoriasis, Arthritis, Reiter's Syndrome

Pamela J. Bachanas, PhD, Clinical Psychologist and Director, Pediatric Mental Health Service, Emory/Grady Pediatric Infectious Disease Program; Assistant Professor, Departments of Psychiatry and Pediatrics, Emory University School of Medicine, Atlanta, Georgia.
Cognitive Impairment and Developmental Delay

Christine A. Balt, MS, RN, ACRN, APRN, BC, Indiana University School of Medicine, Division of Infectious Diseases, Wishard Health Services Infectious Disease Clinic/Indy Core Care.
Lesbians and Bisexual Women

Kathleen Barrett, MSN, RN, Chicago, Illinois.
Hepatitis A, Hepatitis B, Hepatitis C

Julie Barroso, PhD, ANP, CS, Assistant Professor, School of Nursing, University of North Carolina at Chapel Hill.
Fatigue

Catherine R. Bataille, MSW, LCSW, Social Worker, FXB Center for Children (Pediatric Infectious Disease Clinic), University of Medicine and Dentistry of New Jersey, Newark.
Decision Making and Family Autonomy, Surrogate Caregivers

Jo Anne Bennett, RN, PhD, CS, ACRN, Director, Integrated Surveillance, New York City Department of Health & Mental Hygiene.
Historical Overview, Epidemiology of HIV Infection and AIDS

Barbara E. Berger, PhD, RN, ACRN, Clinical Assistant Professor, University of Illinois at Chicago College of Nursing, Chicago.
Isolation and Stigmatization

Carolyn Keith Burr, EdD, RN, Associate Director, National Pediatric & Family HIV Resource Center, FXB Center, University of Medicine and Dentistry of New Jersey.
Perinatal Transmission of HIV Infection, Clinical Manifestations and Management of the HIV Infected Infant and Child, Managing Antiretroviral Therapy in HIV-Infected Infants and Children

Bernadette Capili, NP-C, APRN, DNSc, Clinical Nurse Manger, General Clinical Research Center, Mt. Sinai Medical Center, New York.
Nausea and Vomiting

Doris Carroll, BSN, RN, CCRC, Women's Interagency HIV Study (WIHS) Site Coordinator, University of Illinois at Chicago.
Human Papillomavirus Infection

Beverly Christie, RN, BSN, Program Manager, Hemophilia & Thrombosis Center, University of Minnesota.
Hemophilia

Joseph P. Colagreco, MS, APRN, BC, NP-C, Clinical Assistant Professor of Nursing, New York University, the Steinhardt School of Education, Division of Nursing, New York.
Pathophysiology of HIV Infection

Lynn Czarniecki, RNC, MSN, CNS- C, Former Clinical Nurse Specialist, Francois-Xavier Bagnoud Program, University of Medicine and Dentistry, Newark, New Jersey.
Pain (Section 9.1)

Rachel Davis, RN, ACRN, Clinic Coordinator, South Texas Family AIDS Network, University of Texas Health Science Center at San Antonio, Texas.
Anorexia, Weight Loss

Pamela Dole, EdD, MPH, MSN, FNP, ACRN, Assistant Professor, Hunter College and HIV, Nurse Practitioner, St. Vincent's Hospital, New York.
Human Papillomavirus Infection, Cervical Neoplasia, Depression, Primary Anxiety-Spectrum Disorders, Delirium, Incarcerated Persons, Pregnant Women, Women

Dawn D'Orlando, RN, MSN, MPH, Nurse Practitioner, Francois-Xavier Bagnoud Program, University of Medicine and Dentistry, Newark, New Jersey.
Perinatal Transmission of HIV Infection, Clinical Manifestations and Management of the HIV-Infected Infant and Child, Managing Antiretroviral Therapy in HIV-Infected Infants and Children, Anemia, Cardiomyopathy, Dermatitis, Diarrhea, Hepatitis, Hepatomegaly, Herpes Virus, Leiomyosarcoma, Lymphadenopathy, Lymphoid Interstitial Pneumonitis (LIP), Nephropathy, Neutropenia, Nocardiosis, Otitis Media, Parotitis, Sinusitis, Splenomegaly, Thrombocytopenia, Upper Respiratory Infection, Disseminated Varicella, Recurrent Bacterial Infections, Mycobacterial Avium Complex, Mycobacterial Tuberculosis, Salmonellosis, Candidiasis, Coccidioidomycosis, Crytpococcosis, Histoplasmosis, Cryptosporidiosis, Isosporiasis, Pneumocystis Carinii Pneumonia, Toxoplasmosis, Cytomegalovirus Disease, Progressive Multifocal Leukoencephalopathy (PML), Malignancies, HIV-Related Wasting Syndrome, HIV-Related Encephalopathy

Marion Donohoe, RN, MSN, CPNP, Pediatric Nurse Practitioner, St. Jude Children's Research Hospital, Memphis, Tennessee.
Disclosure to the Child, Community-Based Care Issues

Margaret Dykeman, RN, PhD, FNP, APRN, BC, ACRN, Associate Professor, University of New Brunswick, Canada.
Commercial Sex Workers, Homeless Persons

Tom Emanuele, BSN, RN, C, ACRN, HIV Case Management Supervisor, Amelia Court Clinic Parkland Health & Hospital System, Dallas, Texas.
Case Management

Richard Ferri, PhD, ANP, ACRN, FAAN, Managing Editor, *NUMEDX;* HIV/AIDS Nurse Practitioner, Provincetown, Massachusetts.
Anemia

Kelly Fugate, ND, RN, Clinician II, Critical Care Nursing, Alexian Brothers Medical Center, Elk Grove Village, Illinois.
Bacterial Pneumonia, Pneumocystosis, Cough, Dyspnea

Susan Gaskin, MPH, DSN, ACRN, Professor, Capstone College of Nursing, University of Alabama, Tuscaloosa.
Migrant and Seasonal Farm Workers, Rural Communities

Mary Geiger, MPH, RN, Research Nurse/Study Coordinator, Adolescent Medicine Trials Unit, Mount Sinai Adolescent Health Center, New York.
Adolescents

Brian K. Goodroad, PhD, CNP, ACRN
Managing Antiretroviral Therapy

Sande Gracia Jones, PhD, ARNP, ACRN, C, CS, BC, Assistant Professor, School of Nursing, College of Health and Urban Affairs, Florida International University, Miami.
Medications

Kristin Grage, MA, RN, CNP, ACRN, Nurse Practitioner, Allina Medical Clinic, The Doctors.
Health Care Follow-Up

Heidi J. Haiken, MSW, MPH, Coordinator of Social Work, François-Xavier Bagnoud Center at the University of Medicine and Dentistry of New Jersey.
End of Life Issues

Connie Highsmith, RN, BSN, ACRN, Nurse Consultant, Roche Pharmaceuticals.
Case Management

Barbara Holtzclaw, PhD, RN, FAAN, Professor Emeritus, University of Texas Health Science Center at San Antonio; Graduate Faculty & Research Consultant, University of Oklahoma Health Science Center, Oklahoma City.
Fever

Valery Hughes, RN, MS, FNP, Research Nurse Practitioner and Study Coordinator, Cornell Clinical Trials Unit.
Prevention of HIV Infection, Teaching for Health Promotion, Wellness, and Prevention of Transmission

Joyce Keithley, DNSc, RN, FAAN, Professor, Rush University College of Nursing, Chicago.
Oral Hairy Leukoplakia, HIV-Related Wasting Syndrome, Fat Redistribution Syndrome, Anorexia and Weight Loss, Dysphagia and Odynophagia

Carl A. Kirton, MA, RN, APRN, BC, Nurse Practitioner and Nurse Manager, Infectious Disease Clinic, Mt. Sinai-NYU Health, New York; Adjunct Clinical Associate Professor, New York University, Steinhardt School of Education, Division of Nursing, New York.
Immunizations, Cardiomyopathy, African American Community, Mental Illness and Substance Abuse

Eric G. Leach, MSN, RN, NP, Nurse Practitioner and Primary Care Provider, Michael Callen-Audre Lorde Community Health Center, New York.
Transgender/Transsexual Persons

Wade Leon, MA, RN, CS-ANP, Saint Vincent's Hospital—Saint Vincent Catholic Medical Center, New York Medical College, New York.
Nephropathy, Depression, Primary Anxiety-Spectrum Disorders

Martin Lewis, MEd, MSN, ANP, ACRN, Associate Director, Patient and Community Affairs, Bristol-Myers Squibb Virology.
Selected Laboratory Values

Debra E. Lyon, PhD, RN, Assistant Professor, University of Virginia School of Nursing; Center for the Study of Complementary and Alternative Therapy, School of Nursing, University of Virginia
Impaired Glucose Tolerance, Dyslipidemia

Richard MacIntyre, RN, PhD, Professor and Chairman, Division of the Health Professions and Department of Nursing, Mercy College, New York; Adjunct Associate Professor, New York Medical College.
Ethical and Legal Concerns

R. Kevin Mallinson, PhD, RN, ACRN, Assistant Professor, Virginia Commonwealth University School of Nursing, Richmond.
Gay and Bisexual Men, The Deaf and Hearing-Impaired Community

Lawrence Marsco, RN, BSN, Administrative Nurse Manager, UCSF Positive Health Program at San Francisco General Hospital Ward 84, San Francisco General Hospital.
Bartonellosis, Herpes Zoster, Listeriosis, Salmonellosis, Coccidioidomycosis, Cryptococcosis, Histoplasmosis, Toxoplasmosis

Ian R. McNicholl, Pharm. D., BCPS (I.D.), Clinical Pharmacy Specialist, UCSF Positive Health Program at SFGHMC, Assistant Clinical Professor, UCSF School of Pharmacy, Bldg 80, Ward 86, San Francisco.
Bartonellosis, Herpes Zoster, Listeriosis, Salmonellosis, Coccidioidomycosis, Cryptococcosis, Histoplasmosis, Toxoplasmosis

Young-Me Lee, MSN, RN, DNSc (c), Rush University College of Nursing, Chicago.
Peripheral Neuropathy, HIV-Related Encephalopathy

Nora Merriam, RN, MSN, MPH
Blind and Visually Impaired Community

Theresa Moran, RN, MS, FNP, Hematology/Oncology/Bone Marrow Transplant Nurse Practitioner, Division of Hematology/Oncology/Bone Marrow Transplant, Assistant Clinical Professor, Department of Physiological Nursing, School of Nursing, University of California, San Francisco.
Cervical Neoplasia, Kaposi's Sarcoma, Non-Hodgkin's Lymphoma

Gail Newshan, PhD, RN, NP, Director, Holistic Care Services Department, St. John's Riverside Hospital, Yonkers, New York.
Pain (Section 4.13)

Craig E. Nielsen, MS, NP, BC, ACRN, Instructor-Nurse Practitioner, School of Medicine, Division of Infectious Diseases, University of Colorado Health Sciences Center, Denver.
HIV-Infected Health Care Workers

Kathleen M. Nokes, PhD, RN, FAAN, Professor, Hunter College, CUNY Hunter-Bellevue School of Nursing, New York.
Sleep Disturbances, Older Persons

Patti O'Kane, MA, RN, Department of Psychiatry, Brookdale University Hospital and Medical Center, Brooklyn, New York.
Spiritual and Religious Concerns

Kristin K. Ownby, PhD, RN, ACRN, AOCN, CHPN, University of Texas Health Science Center–Houston, School of Nursing.
Idiopathic Thrombocytopenia Purpura, Cryptosporidiosis, Isosporiasis, Thrombocytopenia

Lisa Perry, MSW, LCSW, Perinatal HIV Social Worker and Case Manager, François-Xavier Bagnoud Center, UMDNJ, Newark, New Jersey.
Decision Making and Family Autonomy, Multiple Hospitalizations

Demetrius Porche, DNS, RN, FNP, CS, Professor and Associate Dean for Nursing Research and Evaluation, Louisiana State University Health Sciences Center School of Nursing–New Orleans, Louisiana.
Mycobaterium Avium Complex, Mycobacterium Tuberculosis, Cytomegalovirus

Susanne Rendiro, MSN, FNP, BC, Family Nurse Practitioner, Betances Health Center, New York.
Recent Immigrants

Tracy A. Riley, PhD, RN, CS, Assistant Professor of Nursing, University of Akron College of Nursing
Mobility Impairment, Vision Loss

Patrick Robinson, PhD, RN, ACRN, Biobehavioral Research Fellow, College of Nursing, University of Illinois at Chicago.
Candidiasis, Herpes Simplex Virus

Leslie Schor, RN, MSN, ACRN, HIV and Blood-Borne Exposure Control Coordinator, Jackson Memorial Hospital, Miami, Florida.
Preventing Transmission of HIV in Patient Care Settings

Jane Schulz, MPH, RN, CNP, ACRN, HIV Clinical Research, Hennepin County Medical Center, Minneapolis, Minnesota.
HIV Testing

Craig R. Sellers, MS, RN, APRN, BC, ANP, ACRN, Fellow, Predoctoral NRSA, NINR/NIH; Director, Adult Nurse Practitioner Program, Senior Teaching Associate, University of Rochester School of Nursing, Rochester, New York.
Progressive Multifocal Leukoencephalopathy, Ethical and Legal Concerns

Rebekah Shephard, MS, RN, ANP, Psychiatric Nurse Practitioner, Core Center, Chicago; Instructor, Rush University College of Nursing, Chicago.
Responses to an HIV Diagnosis: Infected Person, Response to HIV Diagnosis: Family and Significant Other, Caregiver Burden/Strain, Delirium, Female Sexual Dysfunction, Male Sexual Dysfunction

Yvonne Smith, MSN, RN, CNS, Programs Coordinator, University of Akron College of Nursing, Wayne College Campus, Akron, Ohio.
Mobility Impairment, Vision Loss

Hopkins D. Stanley, RN, MS, ACRN, CNS, Clinical Nurse Specialist, UCSF Positive Health Program at San Francisco General Hospital and Medical Center, Ward 84, San Francisco General Hospital.
Bartonellosis, Herpes Zoster, Listeriosis, Salmonellosis, Coccidioidomycosis, Cryptococcosis, Histoplasmosis, Toxoplasmosis

David J. Sterken, MN, CNS, CPNP, Pediatric Infectious Disease Nurse Practitioner, DeVos Children's Hospital, Grand Rapids, Michigan.
Fever, Skin Lesions, Stress Reduction, and Pediatric HIV Infection

Barbara Swanson, DNSc, RN, ACRN, Assistant Professor, Adult Health Nursing, Rush College of Nursing, Chicago.
Leukopenia, Osteopenia, Osteoporosis, Avascular Necrosis, Lactic Acidosis, Oral Lesions

Donna Taliaferro, RN, PhD, Associate Professor, Virginia Commonwealth University, Richmond.
Substance Users

Debra Topham, PhD, RN, CNS, ACRN, Oregon Health Sciences University, Portland Campus.
Cognitive Impairment

Brooke Vanburen-Hay, PhD, Pediatric Psychologist, Spectrum Health-DeVos Children's Hospital, Grand Rapids, Michigan.
Stress Reduction and Pediatric HIV Infection

Rhys VanDemark, BA, CCLS, Certified Child Life Specialist, DeVos Children's Hospital, Grand Rapids, Michigan.
Stress Reduction and Pediatric HIV Infection

Gail B. Williams, RN, PhD, Associate Professor, The University of Texas Health Science Center at San Antonio.
Substance Users

S. K. Glenda Winson, MS, RN, ACRN, Research Nurse, G.I. Immunology, St. Luke's Roosevelt Hospital, New York.
HIV-Related Wasting Syndrome, Fat Redistribution Syndrome, Diarrhea

Thomas P. Young, MS, RN, APRN, BC, ACRN, Medical Science Liaison, ViroLogic, Inc., South San Francisco; Nurse Practitioner, Kaiser Permanente Medical Group, San Francisco; Assistant Clinical Professor of Nursing, University of California, San Francisco, School of Nursing.
Baseline Assessment

Janice M. Zeller PhD, RN, FAAN, Professor, Department of Adult Health Nursing and Associate Professor, Department of Immunology/Microbiology, Rush University, Chicago.
Peripheral Neuropathy, HIV-Related Encephalopathy

Section I

HIV Infection, Transmission, and Prevention

The 1980s witnessed the discovery of a new disease, acquired immunodeficiency syndrome (AIDS). AIDS developed into a pandemic whose impact has had multiple effects on health care, culture, and society in the United States and around the world. It has called attention to everyday practices in science and the health professions, current and past paradigms of healing and disease, public health and preventative policies, and the important role that those infected and affected by HIV have in policy and decision making. Section 1 tells this fascinating story through the eyes of public health experts, clinicians, and researchers.

Worldwide, 15,000 individuals are infected with HIV each day, which speaks to the overwhelming challenges posed by the infection, such as the limitations of public health initiatives, access to care and antiretroviral therapies, and HIV's ability to mutate and develop resistance to antiretroviral drugs. At the same time, opportunities abound for innovative preventive efforts, for the development of new therapies, and, most important, for making medications and care available to the vast majority of people with AIDS who currently have no access to such life-extending measures.

1.1 Historical Overview of the HIV Pandemic

1. The world first became aware of the clinical entity that would become known as acquired immunodeficiency syndrome (AIDS) with the mid-1981 reports of clusters of fatal *Pneumocystis carinii* pneumonia (PCP) and Kaposi's sarcoma cases in relatively young men in California and New York.

2. The commonality among these cases was homosexuality. Within a year, published case reports had described additional opportunistic complications and cases of AIDS in women, infants, and recipients of blood and other blood products.

3. By 1982, it was recognized that AIDS represented only the severe end of a clinical spectrum that comprised a broad range of constitutional symptoms, opportunistic illness, and hematological and neurological impairment.

4. Naming the disease
   a. The syndrome seen in the United States was initially called gay cancer, then labeled GRID (gay-related immunodeficiency), followed by other diverse acronyms, such as CAIDS (community acquired immunodeficiency syndrome), because immunodeficiencies were diagnosed in people with diverse backgrounds, including women and men with no history of homosexual activity.
   b. The label AIDS (acquired immunodeficiency syndrome) was adopted by the Centers for Disease Control and Prevention (CDC) in July of 1982.
   c. In Africa, it was called slim disease because of the profound wasting manifested and the association of death with the progressive weight loss and diarrhea associated with the gastrointestinal pathogens that distinguished AIDS in Africa from the distinctive AIDS-related respiratory infections and neoplasms seen in North America and Europe.
   d. Virus recovered from people with the syndromes were labeled differently by the scientists involved, until it was verified that all the isolates were in fact the same virus, and its molecular-genetic pedigree was clarified: lymphadenopathy-associated virus (LAV); human T-lymphotropic virus type 3 (HTLV-III; the AIDS-related retrovirus (ARV); and immunodeficiency-associated virus (IDAV). An international subcommittee for nomenclature officially named the etiologic virus human immunodeficiency type 1 (HIV-1) in 1986.
   e. A second virus with similar molecular structure, life cycle, and (less virulent) pathogenic capacity that had not spread so widely around the globe was isolated and identified in 1986. It was called HIV-2.

5. Tracking the disease
   a. The CDC established the Kaposi's Sarcoma and Opportunistic Infections (KSOI) Task Force, subsequently renamed KS/AIDS Task Force and, in June of 1981, began systematic surveillance for PCP and KS, publishing weekly surveillance reports.
   b. In October of 1981, the CDC declared the new syndrome an epidemic and state-mandated reporting of cases and their characteristics to public health authorities began in accord with CDC guidelines. The CDC tracked U.S. incidence by gender, race, age, and mode of exposure, using a hierarchically constructed schema that reflected the respective proportion of cumulative cases in each category at the time it was developed. Initially, there were also categories for people from Haiti and for people who had traveled to or from an area of high prevalence, such as Haiti or sub-Saharan Africa.
   c. In September of 1982, the CDC published the first surveillance case definition of AIDS, which has been revised multiple times since then, broadening the list of AIDS-defining conditions and incorporating the development of laboratory tests for both infection and immunodeficiency (see Appendix A for the case definition).
   d. U.S. public health law officially designated AIDS to be reportable in

October of 1983 (i.e., it became mandatory to report the diagnosis to state/territorial health departments, who then report cases, without names, to the CDC).

e. Some states—typically those with relatively low prevalence—began HIV surveillance in 1985, but standardized active (vs. passive) HIV surveillance did not begin until 1991.

f. In December of 1999, the CDC expanded mandatory national case surveillance to include cases of both HIV infection and AIDS to better monitor and characterize the epidemiology of the full spectrum of HIV disease.

6. Searching for the cause of HIV

a. Several theories about causation were proposed. The epidemiologic profile soon made blood-borne infection the strongest hypothesis. The chief competing theories until the infectious etiology was confirmed were immune exhaustion from repeated antigenic challenge or antigenic overload and exposure to an immunotoxic drug.

b. The possibility of a novel agent was considered in 1981, but a number of pathogens known to be immunosuppressive were also suggested as likely etiologic agents.

c. In 1983, French scientists (Luc Montagnier and colleagues at the Pasteur Institute) isolated a virus, which was subsequently shown to be the causal pathogen, from a man with lymphadenopathy who later exhibited AIDS. HIV-2 was discovered in 1986. The two viruses have similar genetic structures and are transmitted by the same mode but display some differences in transmissibility (efficiency of transmission) and natural history (see Section 1.4, Pathophysiology of HIV Infection).

7. Responses to the AIDS epidemic

a. AIDS is a communal phenomenon, and community dynamics have affected individuals' experiences. Entire families, social networks, and neighborhoods confronted devastating tolls of suffering and death. While some communities in the United States were quickly

overwhelmed by the epidemic, in other communities no one even knew anyone who knew someone who had been affected, even in the 1990s. The latter experience, along with epidemiologic distinctions between "groups at risk" and "the general population," often provided a "them and us" connotation that implied that AIDS is a disease of "others." The theme of otherness framed social and political discourse on AIDS, both suggesting and explaining individual and group responses to people with AIDS (PWAs) and to the epidemic.

b. Terminology referring to risk groups inadvertently focused attention on the people affected rather than the modes of transmission of the infectious etiologic agent. This focus had the effect of both stigmatizing those affected and confusing people's perceptions of the nature of the risk. This persistent misperception continues to support denial of the risk associated with heterosexual intercourse, resulting in heightened risk for adolescents, young adults, and, frequently, married couples, while deterring prevention efforts that target them. A corollary term, general population, used to refer to those not identified as particularly affected or at particular risk, further accentuated this misperceived distinction.

c. In addition, recognizing behavioral risk factors served to make distinctions between those who had become infected as a result of their own actions and those who had become infected passively by receiving blood or blood products or by vertical transmission. People infected by the latter two modes were then referred to as innocent victims of AIDS, with the implication that others may have been responsible for, and thus deserving of, their illness.

d. Community mobilization, self-help, and advocacy efforts

i. The epidemic galvanized gay consciousness and pride, community spirit, political activism, volunteerism, and (eventually) coalition building with other disenfranchised groups. The gay community's unprecedented response to the urgent needs brought by the epidemic shaped an entirely new social service network and invigorated health care consumer activism.

ii. Grassroots AIDS organizations spread across the country, and around the globe, as quickly as the epidemic itself, including groups founded by and for drug injectors, PWAs' family members, and commercial sex workers. Groups also formed to address the affected population by age, ethnicity or racial background, and segments or subpopulations of risk groups (e.g., runaway youth, transgendered people, homeless people, people with mental illness, the hearing impaired).

iii. The range of services offered by these community-based organizations (CBOs), also called AIDS-service organizations (ASOs), was broad. Some agencies were created to provide specific services, whereas others maintained mixed agendas. Some emphasized prevention and education; others focused solely on political activism.

e. Governmental responses to the epidemic

i. The HIV pandemic has been a defining political event of the time, nationally and globally, challenging both medical authority and government decision making about health care research and delivery. Many governments were slow to respond, in large part through failure to recognize the magnitude of the problem and its potential impact, along with, many believe, a lack of concern for the disenfranchised groups that were most affected through the first decade. Some U.S. government officials held the view that it was not a broad societal threat and suggested that the public health community and others were exaggerating its magnitude. Many people believed that a cure would be developed quickly.

ii. AIDS emerged in the United States during a decade of reduced federal funding for numerous government programs, including public health programs, leaving cities to cope on their own. Some officials opposed government spending to fund gay organizations or to address sexuality in any way other than extramarital abstinence and heterosexual monogamy.

iii. The Ryan White Comprehensive AIDS Resources Emergency (CARE) Act was passed by Congress in 1990 and was subsequently reauthorized in 1996 and 2000 to provide federal funds to states and territories to improve the quality and availability of primary care and support services to low-income, uninsured, and underinsured HIV-infected persons. Allocation of funds to community-based providers is determined by state and local health planning bodies, whose membership must include proportionate representation of those affected as well as service providers (not just policymakers). Congress earmarks a certain proportion of Ryan White funds to states for AIDS Drug Assistance Programs (ADAPs).

1.2 Epidemiology of HIV Infection and AIDS

1. The HIV pandemic today comprises multiple epidemics that differ in scale, timing, and etiologic determinants. As the epidemiology evolved in magnitude and character, the pandemic grew in complexity. HIV distribution is characterized by a marked heterogeneity across continents, and even within single countries there are mixed low- and high-prevalence populations.

2. Because a basic understanding of epidemiology is essential to interpreting current and changing data about the continuing spread of HIV and its impact in different areas and populations around the world, this overview of HIV epidemiology begins with a review of the fundamental concepts of epidemiology.

3. Epidemiology is the systematic collection and study of the distribution, within and among populations, of diverse health states and health-related events (viz., information about the associated characteristics of time, place, and person and the interactions among these characteristics). Health-related events include behaviors that may be health protective, health damaging, or health threatening.

4. Epidemiologic information comes from systematic surveillance, which is the routine, ongoing collection and analysis of epidemiologic data to detect changes in the trend or distribution of all aspects of the natural history of disease occurrence and spread, including the use of resources to alter them. Sources of surveillance information include the following:

- Mandatory reporting systems
- Vital records (births, deaths)
- Sentinel hospital and laboratory networks
- Hospital admission and discharge data
- Aggregate insurance records
- Disease outbreak investigation: focused intensive study to delineate the causes of a specific outbreak or of changes in trends within a local population group or geographic area
- Case finding: concerted search efforts to identify previously unidentified cases
- Contact tracing: efforts to identify individuals who have been exposed to an infection
- Partner notification
- Network analysis
- Screening: efforts to detect previously unrecognized disease by offering testing to population segments undertaken both to collect information and to facilitate early secondary prevention

- Registry: a system of keeping a file of data about all cases of a particular condition or experience to facilitate follow-up so that sequelae can be monitored, including disease course and interventions. The specific information collected and maintained in a registry will depend on the condition and the purpose of the registry.
- Research

5. Epidemiological terms
   a. Etiology: the origins of a disease
   b. Risk: the likelihood or chance of something happening. By definition, risk is not absolute. The risk that a particular risk factor poses at any given time will depend on the presence, absence, or relative state of other relevant factors. An individual's risk of exposure to an infectious agent at any given time depends on the size of the reservoir (local prevalence) and behavior.
   c. Cause: a stimulus that brings about the occurrence of an event or that changes the amount or frequency of an occurrence
   d. Risk factor: an attribute or occurrence associated with an increased probability of a specified outcome, such as disease exposure, disease onset, disease progression, and disease outcomes.
   e. Risk groups: population segments that have a risk factor in common. It must be remembered that risk groups are usually quite heterogeneous. They include individuals with diverse other risks. Moreover, individuals in a risk group come from multiple diverse social and cultural groups, so no single prevention strategy can address everyone who has a particular risk.
   f. Natural history of disease: the process of disease development and progression in the absence of any intervention to alter its course from prepathogenesis (the period in a disease process before any cellular changes begin that encompasses susceptibility) to cure or death

6. Epidemiologic measurements
   a. Absolute counts of events occurring during a time period or at a particular

point in time are not very useful for comparisons or for tracking trends but are essential for program development and needs assessment for services and resources.

b. Cumulative numbers of cases and deaths may also be reported. In combination, these measures are useful for estimating prevalence. Prevalence is the number of cases of a disease present in a population during a particular time, including previously diagnosed cases.

c. Percentages or proportions

   i. Denominators are key to interpreting the implications of changes. The higher the percentage *and* denominator, the greater the problem.

     (1) The absolute number represented by a percentage will depend on the size of the population being assessed. Changes in percentages over time may represent changes in the size of the population (denominator), rather than growth or decline in morbidity or mortality.

     (2) The implications of the doubling or tripling of occurrences (morbidity or mortality) over a time period will depend on the starting point of the period being assessed. The lower the starting point (denominator), the fewer the additional cases needed to double that number. Geometric increases are thus more likely to be seen early in an outbreak or epidemic. Likewise, apparently slowing rates of increase may not even reflect plateauing, much less declining, morbidity or mortality. Indeed, there may even be need to expand prevention efforts despite a falling percentage increase in new cases.

   ii. Changes or differences in percentages may not reflect changes in a disease's incidence or mortality per se but, rather, trends in the epidemiologic pattern(s) of other, associated diseases. For example, the percentage of HIV-infected persons who develop tuberculosis (TB) will reflect the prevalence of latent TB infection (LTBI) in the HIV population, which in turn will be determined by historic as well as current prevalence of active TB in the general population (i.e., the reservoir to which HIV-infected persons may be exposed). The percentage of people with active TB who are HIV-infected will not only depend on the prevalence of latent TB infection in the HIV-infected population but will also reflect the progression of immunodeficiency among them, as well as the relative likelihood that HIV-positive and HIV-negative people will have latent TB diagnosed and treated. If latent TB is treated, the incidence of active disease will be less. HIV/AIDS, by enabling activation of LTBI, fuels expansion of the TB reservoir, precipitating further spread of infection.

   iii. Case-fatality rate: the percentage of people with a disease who die as the result of that disease within a specified period, often measured in years (e.g., 1-, 2-, 5-, and 10-year periods). (This calculation requires following all patients in the denominator for an adequate period of time to capture all attributable deaths. In other words, the longer survival, the longer follow-up must be.)

   iv. Proportional mortality rate: the percentage of deaths in a given year and place due to a particular disease. The numerator is the number of deaths from the specific disease, and the denominator is the total number of deaths due to all causes during the time period being measured.

d. Rates: arithmetic expressions of event occurrence or frequency relative to the size of a population (population proportions or fractions) that are multiplied by a constant, such as 1,000 or 100,000 to facilitate comparisons across populations. The numerator is the number of events occurring in a specified time period; the denominator contains all members of the identified population at the same specified time period. Official census counts are usually used to determine the denominators.

  i. Incidence rates: the number of new cases of a specified disease diagnosed or reported during a defined period of time, divided by the number of people in a stated population (gender-specific, age-specific, location-specific, or specific for any other population characteristic or combination of characteristics) in which the cases are being counted. It is usually expressed as cases per 1,000 or 100,000 per year.

  ii. Prevalence rates: the proportion of cases present in a population (including both new occurrences and surviving previous cases), usually expressed as a rate per 100,000 people at a specified point in time (point prevalence) or over a specified period of time (period prevalence).

  iii. Mortality rates: estimations of the proportion of the population that dies in a given time period, usually expressed as a rate per 100,000

   (1) Crude rates describe the experience of the total population (the denominator).

   (2) Specific rates describe the experience for a specified population segment (the denominator), such as men or women, age groups, or men or women in a specific age group.

   (3) Years of potential life lost (YPLL) is a measure of mortality that takes into account the age and anticipated life span of persons dying from a particular disease. In the United States, YPLL may be calculated three ways—using 65 as the projected life span (to track historical trends) or using 75 and 85, respectively, as projected life spans (to provide a more realistic estimate of the impact, given current life expectancy). Deaths that occur after the criterion being used (i.e., > 65, > 75, or > 85) would not be included in the calculation. YPLL is then reported as the number per 1,000 population under the criterion.

  iv. Attributable risk: the proportion of disease occurrences during a given period that may be associated with a risk factor. It is the difference in incidence rates between populations: the population with a risk factor and the population without a risk factor. Calculations of attributable risk will be limited by the accuracy of estimates of prevalence of the risk factor.

 e. Relative risk ratio: a comparison that suggests the excess risk for individuals with a particular factor. It is an estimate of how much individual risk is associated with a particular risk factor (i.e., how much greater the likelihood for disease occurrence). It is calculated by dividing the disease incidence in the population of people who have the risk factor by its incidence in the population without the risk factor. The accuracy of this calculation depends on how well the prevalence of the risk factor can be estimated.

7. Transmission routes and cofactors affecting HIV transmission

 a. The reservoir for HIV is the blood and certain body fluids and tissues of infected humans.

 b. The period of communicability is not known but is presumed to begin early after the onset of infection and continue throughout the life of the host. Clinical latency does not reflect quiescent disease or noninfectiousness.

 c. The mode of transmission is direct host-to-host transmission through sexual, percutaneous, mucocutaneous contact with the blood and body fluids of an infected person, including vertical transmission to fetus and to newborn during intrapartum and breastfeeding. By definition, sexual contact includes vaginal intercourse, oral intercourse (fellatio or cunnilingus), and rectal intercourse between heterosexual or homosexual partners.

d. Factors that may enhance or reduce transmission

   i. Alterations of normal mucosal barriers, including lesions due to trauma or disease (e.g., genital ulcer disease, chancroid, syphilis, herpes), provide access, thereby augmenting the contact during exposure. Genital ulcers on the infected person allow direct exposure to HIV-laden blood.

   ii. Different types of sexual activity carry different risks for transmission, depending on the degree of contact with infected body fluid.

   iii. Sexual activities may traumatize vaginal or rectal mucosa (e.g., fisting [insertion of fist in rectum or vagina], use of sexual toys, sex with little lubrication).

   iv. Mechanical contraceptive barriers may traumatize the vagina or alter the integrity of the uterine cervix.

   v. Circumcised men have reduced risk of being infected by an infected partner.

   vi. Spermicides, such as nonoxynl-9, enhance transmission (contrary to previous recommendations for their use to inhibit transmission).

   vii. Sexually transmitted diseases, including nonulcerative disease, not only alter the integrity of the mucosa but also enhance susceptibility by altering immunocompetence.

   viii. A number of drug-injecting practices increase the likelihood of transmission when needles are shared (e.g., booting, frontloading, and backloading).

e. Infection with HIV-1 or HIV-2 is sufficient for disease to emerge, although diverse factors may influence the host response to infection and the subsequent disease course. Infectivity of HIV is relatively low. For example, comparisons are frequently made to the relatively higher infectivity of hepatitis B virus.

f. Because transmission is dose-dependent, there is a risk differential related to the relative efficiency of different transmission routes: A more efficient route allows a larger amount of infected blood, body fluid, or tissue to be involved in the exposure contact, thereby potentially allowing a larger dose of virus (i.e., a larger inoculum) to be transmitted. Efficiency thus differs among exit portals and among entry portals. (The relative risk associated with more efficient routes will, of course, be heightened or reduced by the viral concentration in the blood, fluid, or tissue involved in an actual exposure.)

   i. The most efficient mode of transmission is transfusion of contaminated blood or components because transfusion provides a direct route for a potentially large inoculum of virus to enter the bloodstream.

   ii. Ejaculation is an efficient means of transmitting the virus from an infected male to a sexual partner. Female-to-male vaginal-penile transmission is less efficient.

   iii. The vagina and rectum are relatively efficient entry portals. The presence of mucosal tears enhances transmission. Anal-receptive intercourse is the most effective mode. Rectal fisting and rectal douching enhance this risk by damaging the integrity of the rectal mucosa.

   iv. The risk of transmission from oral sex is not easily quantifiable and is presumed to be low for both partners.

   v. The efficiency of percutaneous exposure will depend on both the size and depth of the entry portal and also the volume of inoculum. Because the latter also depends on the volume of infected blood, body fluid, or tissue that can exit the source, the risk associated with a needlestick exposure will depend on the size of the needle bore.

vi. Vaginal delivery is more efficient than Cesarean section.

g. Susceptibility to infection is apparently universal, with rare exceptions.

    i. Rarely, women with repeated heterosexual exposure to the same infected partner have not become infected. The mechanism by which infection is averted in these exposures is not understood.

    ii. A woman's susceptibility may differ at different times in the menstrual cycle and during or at the transitions between different life stages (perimenopause, postmenopause). Pregnancy does not appear to alter susceptibility.

    iii. Variable biological factors may influence susceptibility and the body's response to infection, which can, in turn, also affect the rate of disease progression (Buchacz, Wilkinson, Krowka, Koup, & Padian, 1998).

      (1) The presence of the CCR5-Δ 32 homozygous mutation can render people highly resistant to infection by macrophage-tropic HIV strains.

      (2) HIV-specific T-helper cells that proliferate or secrete interleukin-2 in response to HIV antigens may stimulate cytotoxic T-lymphocyte or other potentially protective immune responses.

      (3) Specific human leukocyte antigen (HLA) polymorphisms that affect the strength of immune responses may inhibit HIV virions or destroy infected cells.

      (4) Mucosal HIV-specific IgA and IgG antibodies may inhibit HIV at the mucosal surfaces and prevent or clear HIV infection of cells.

      (5) Increased production of particular β-chemokines may enhance efficiency of viral binding to CCR5 and prevent entry of macrophage-tropic HIV strains into host CD_4 cells.

      (6) HIV-specific cytotoxic T-cell responses by CD_8 or CD_4 cells, or both, may destroy HIV-infected cells.

      (7) CD_8 T-lymphocyte antiviral factor (CAF) may inhibit replication of HIV-1 and HIV-2 in infected CD_4 cells, probably at the level of transcription.

8. Global HIV epidemiology

a. Incidence (UNAIDS, 2002)

    i. In the 20 years since AIDS was first identified, HIV has killed 25 million people, becoming the world's fourth leading cause of death and the leading cause of death in Africa. The most severely affected countries are in sub-Saharan Africa, where about two thirds of AIDS cases have occurred, and infection prevalence is more than 20% in some countries. There are slightly more men infected with HIV than women.

    ii. More than 90% of new infections occur in developing or resource-poor countries. The proportion of HIV-infected persons who in the absence of treatment are expected to develop AIDS is more than 90%, about half within 10 years. In the United States and other Western countries, the annual incidence of AIDS has declined markedly since the mid-1990s, but it has continued unabated at high levels in sub-Saharan Africa. South Africa has the world's highest per capita incidence. Although 90% of European cases have been in

Western Europe, since 1995 the epidemic has been rising sharply in Central and Eastern Europe.

b. Demographics (UNAIDS, 2002)

    i. Fifteen- to 24-year-olds account for more than half of all new infections, and about 10% of new infections occur in children younger than age 15. In sub-Saharan Africa, more than two thirds of new infections are in women and in other areas of Africa, the female-to-male ratio of new infections is even higher: 5:1 to 6:1.

    ii. Adolescent girls are at higher risk of getting infected, in part due to sexual mixing between older men and younger girls, lack of knowledge among adolescents, cultural norms that prevent women from protecting themselves during sexual activity, myths among men that having sex with a virgin can cure HIV, and adolescent female biology (greater risk of vaginal tearing in younger girls).

    iii. About half of HIV-infected girls in Kenya contracted HIV before age 15.

c. Prevalence

    i. WHO/UNAIDS estimated that about 40 million people (adults and children) were living with HIV at the end of 2001, including 3 million children younger than 15 years of age (UNAIDS, 2002).

        (1) Low-prevalence countries are those where no segment of the population has more than 5% prevalence of infection.

        (2) In some countries, the epidemic remains concentrated. That is, HIV prevalence is more than 5% in specific high-risk population groups, while less than 1% of the wider, general population is infected. Concentrated epidemics are seen in the following:

- Selected areas of southern India, particularly among pregnant women.
- Eastern Europe and Central Asia: The epidemic among addicted injecting drug users is spreading rapidly to occasional drug users and their sexual partners, mostly young people. Concentration in drug-using segments of a population is frequently characteristic of the period following the recent introduction of the epidemic to an area.
- United States (Centers for Disease Control and Prevention, 2002): HIV prevalence may be as high as 7% in some urban areas among 15- to-22-year-old men who have sex with men. Even higher prevalence may be seen among African American men who have sex with men (14%). HIV is also more prevalent among Hispanic men who have sex with men (7%) than among White men who have sex with men (3%).

    (3) When HIV prevalence reaches more than 1% of the total population, the epidemic is said to be generalized, and incidence tends to rise rapidly.

        (a) In 12 sub-Saharan countries, at least 10% of people between ages 15 and 49 are estimated to be infected. The highest prevalence (40%) is in Botswana.

        (b) Outside sub-Saharan Africa, high HIV prevalence rates (> 1%) among 15- to 49-year-olds have been noted only in a few countries in the Caribbean (Bahamas, Guyana, and Haiti) and in South and Southeast Asia (Myanmar, Cambodia, and Thailand).

d. Mortality (UNAIDS, 2002)

  i. The case-fatality rate in developed countries in the absence of effective anti-HIV treatment was 80% to 90% within 3 to 5 years after the diagnosis of AIDS. Since the introduction of Highly Active Anti-Retroviral Therapy, (HAART) in the mid-1990s, AIDS deaths have sharply dropped in all developed countries, but they have continued to climb steadily in most developing countries with high HIV prevalence.

  ii. YPLL: In the 20 sub-Saharan African countries with the highest prevalence of AIDS, the YPLL with each AIDS death ranges from 8 years in Burkina Faso (where the expected life span for a person with AIDS is 48 years vs. 56 years for persons without AIDS) to 34 years in Botswana (where life expectancy for a person with AIDS is 36 years vs. 70 years for persons without AIDS). People currently living with AIDS in Botswana alone could bring about a further loss of 16.5 million years of life within the next 5 years.

e. Transmission

  i. Injecting drug use is currently driving HIV transmission in many areas of the world.

  ii. Breast-feeding accounts for one third to one half of the estimated 600,000 mother-to-child transmissions that occur each year.

f. Occupational risk

  i. Whereas barely 4% of the world's HIV-infected population lives in North America and Western Europe, more than 90% of documented occupational HIV transmission cases have been reported from these areas. In other words, documentation of potential and actual occupational exposures is scarce and, because postexposure prophylaxis and worker's compensation is lacking, there is little impetus to undertake surveillance and reporting of these events and their outcomes.

    (1) The risk to health care workers in developing countries is exacerbated by the following:

    - A lack of basic protective equipment (gloves, gowns, masks, goggles) and safe disposal systems for contaminated waste
    - Improper sterilization practices
    - The excessive handling of contaminated needles (including reuse of nonsterile needles and administration of unnecessary injections)
    - The continued use of hazardous equipment (nonretracting finger-stick lancets, glass capillary tubes, and nondisposable needles and syringes)

  ii. In industrialized countries, the cost of protective devices and equipment to reduce blood exposure is expected to be offset by lower expenditures for testing and prophylaxis following exposures, for medical treatment and compensation following infection, and for insurance premiums. But in most developing countries, these economic incentives do not exist.

g. Any loss of health care workers further strains already fragile, understaffed, and overextended health care systems in countries, and their shortened careers robs the country of its investment in their training.

h. Access to anti-HIV treatment: WHO/UNAIDS (UNAIDS, 2002) reports that less than 2% of infected people are receiving antiretroviral therapy, and more than 70% of those with such treatment live in high-income countries where less than 0.1% of AIDS deaths have occurred.

9. HIV in the United States
   a. Incidence (Centers for Disease Control and Prevention, 2002)
      i. Overall, the incidence of HIV infection peaked around 1985. The Centers for Disease Control and Prevention (CDC) estimates HIV prevalence in the range of 650,000 to 900,000. Since 1992, the annual number of HIV infections has been stable around 40,000.
      ii. The incidence of newly diagnosed HIV infection is rising, particularly among youth (13 to 25 years of age). At least half of all new HIV infections are among people under age 25, and almost half (47%) of these are in women. Infections among teenagers are also more frequent among women (61%) than among men (39%).
      iii. Cumulatively, three fourths of infections in women in this age group are in African American and Hispanic women. More than three fourths occurred via heterosexual transmission.
      iv. Seroprevalence surveys suggest that the most vulnerable youth are homeless or runaways, juvenile offenders, and school dropouts.
      v. Before perinatal preventive treatments were available, an estimated 1,000 to 2,000 HIV-infected infants were born each year. After the 1994 Public Health Service recommendations, perinatally acquired pediatric HIV declined. In 2000, 19 states did not report any new pediatric AIDS cases.
   b. AIDS prevalence (Centers for Disease Control and Prevention, 2002)
      i. AIDS prevalence in the United States is currently higher than ever before. As of December 2000, there were about 339,000 persons with AIDS—most (99%) were adults; four fifths (79%) were men.

   (1) In 1996, AIDS incidence and mortality declined for the first time. They continued to decline through 1998, but the rate of decline in both then began to slow. And despite declining overall incidence, AIDS incidence is rising in some population groups. Perinatally acquired AIDS cases declined by 66% in the 5-year period from 1992 to 1997.
   (2) These declines have been primarily attributed to the early use of combination antiretroviral therapy, which delays disease progression to AIDS and death, and to the reduced perinatal transmission resulting from antiretroviral therapy for pregnant women and newborns.
   (3) Differences in the incidence of AIDS-defining illnesses (ADIs) have been seen in the post-HAART era, both in demographic characteristics of who presents with ADIs and also greater proportion of neoplasms than previously reported, perhaps reflecting both a decline in the number of opportunistic infections and longer survival with immunodeficiency.
   c. Mortality (Centers for Disease Control and Prevention, 2002)
      i. Mortality due to HIV infection is tracked via death certificates and includes non-AIDS deaths (i.e., deaths without an AIDS-defining illness). The annual HIV death rate peaked in 1995, declined through 1997, and leveled after 1998. About 70% of HIV-related deaths have occurred in people between 25 and 44 years old.
      (1) HIV no longer ranks among the top 15 causes of death in the United States, as it did in 1995, when it was the leading cause of death for men between 25 and 44 years of

age. In 1998, the age-adjusted death rate dropped to the lowest rate (4.6 deaths per 100,000) since 1987, which was a 70% decline since 1995.

(2) HIV remains the fifth leading cause of death for 25- to 44-year-old Americans and the third leading cause of death among African American and Hispanic women in this age group. These rankings reflect HIV having caused 20% of all deaths in this age group in 1995 and 6% of the deaths in 2000.

(3) HIV disease was the fourth leading cause of YPLL < 75 in 1994 and 1995, when it caused 8% of all deaths in people younger than 75 years of age. In 1999, it was only the ninth leading cause, when it underlay just 2% of the total years of life lost under 75 years of age.

d. Geography (Centers for Disease Control and Prevention, 2002)

i. The initial epicenters were East and West coast cities with relatively large populations of gay men and northeastern and southeastern cities with relatively high prevalence of injecting drug users.

(1) Throughout the first decade, the epidemic spread to an ever-widening circle outside the large coastal cities, and incidence rose in the central region of the country and in smaller cities and rural areas. Currently, the largest proportion (more than 80%) of AIDS cases reported in each region is in larger urban areas.

(2) Almost half (about 42%) of AIDS cases to date have occurred in 10 cities (New York, Los Angeles, San Francisco, Miami, Chicago, Houston, Philadelphia, Newark, Atlanta, and Washington, DC).

(3) Fifteen cities had reported more than 10,000 cases of AIDS through June 2001 (the two decades of AIDS reporting in the United States). Listed according to incidence, they are New York; Los Angeles; San Francisco; Miami; Washington, DC; Chicago; Philadelphia; Houston; Newark; Atlanta; Baltimore; Boston; Fort Lauderdale; Dallas; and San Diego. In addition, San Juan, Puerto Rico, reported almost 16,000 cases. (New York, with more than 122,000 cases, reported more than 4 times more cases than any other city.)

e. Demographics (Centers for Disease Control and Prevention, 2002)

i. About 70% of new infections occur in men, half of whom are African American. Injecting drug use accounts for a larger proportion of the cumulative cases among women (more than half) than among men (less than one third).

(1) The disproportionately high rates of HIV infection, including AIDS, among African American and Hispanic men, women, and children is a pattern that has remained constant throughout the epidemic. This overrepresentation is seen in nearly every transmission category, although it initially reflected the higher prevalence in drug users, their sexual partners, and offspring.

(a) The impact on the African American community has been devastating. In 2000, more African Americans were reported with AIDS than any other racial/ ethnic group: The incidence rate was double that in Hispanics and 8 times greater than that in Whites.

(b) Women of color and their children have always been disproportionately affected by the HIV epidemic.

   (i) Although African American and Hispanic women together represent less than one fourth of women in the United States, they account for more than three fourths of AIDS cases.

   (ii) This disparity is growing: During the latter half of the 1990s, AIDS rates rose among women and minority populations; in 2000, minority women represented 80% of AIDS cases in women.

   (iii) The 2000 AIDS rate for Hispanic women was 7 times higher than that for White non-Hispanic women. The rate for African American non-Hispanic women was 23 times higher than that for White non-Hispanic women.

  ii. Racial and ethnic minority populations are more heavily affected by injecting drug use–associated AIDS (31% of AIDS cases in Hispanics is associated with injecting drug use, compared with 26% of AIDS cases in African Americans and 19% in Whites).

  iii. Cumulatively, 45% of men and 43% of women were in their 30s at the time of diagnosis; 16% of men and 21% of women were in their 20s. However, 33% of nonpediatric male infections and 43% of nonpediatric female infections are reported in people younger than 30.

f. Transmission (Centers for Disease Control and Prevention, 2002)

  i. There has been little change in the modes of HIV transmission since the beginning of the epidemic. Most cases have resulted from sexual contact, but during the last decade the distribution of cases across risk categories and demographic groups has shifted.

   (1) Cumulatively, about 14% of infected adults and adolescents have reported a history of multiple possible modes of exposure.

   (2) Men with male sexual contact still account for the largest number of AIDS cases in the United States. And more than half of new infections in males, including 13- to 24-year-olds, were in men who had had sex with men (MSM). In 2000, 44% of adult AIDS cases were in MSM, 9% of whom also injected drugs. (In other words, 4% of new AIDS cases were in MSM who also injected drugs, and 40% were in MSM with no drug-injecting history.)

   (3) From the beginning of the epidemic, drug abuse has played an important role in HIV transmission. Since then, injection drug use has directly and indirectly accounted for more than one third (36%) of AIDS cases. Injecting drug use–associated AIDS cases include the sexual partners of drug users (13%) and children of injecting drug users or their sexual partners (1%). About 25% of new infections in both men and women are among injection drug users.

    (a) Injecting drug users can acquire and transmit HIV when they share syringes and other paraphernalia for preparing and injecting drugs. More than 86% of AIDS cases associated with injection drug use reported in 2000 were in drug injectors.

(b) Injecting and noninjecting drug users are at greater risk for engaging in unprotected sexual activity, which, in turn, can result in acquiring or transmitting HIV. Indeed, the majority of infection transmitted among injecting drug users themselves may actually occur via sexual exposure. In fact, some researchers have found that high-risk sexual behavior, not sharing needles to inject drugs, is the biggest predictor of HIV infection for both male and female injecting drug users (Mathias, 2002).

(4) Heterosexually transmitted cases are increasing most rapidly.

(5) Female-to-female transmission has not been confirmed. If it occurs, it is rare. Women with AIDS who reported having had sex only with women almost always (98%) also reported another exposure risk, usually injection drug use. However, in half the cases of female AIDS, information about history of sex with women is not known because it was not recorded. Surveys of convenience samples of women who have sex with women (the finding of which may have limited generalizability) have found relatively high rates of injection drug use and unprotected vaginal sex with bisexual men and men who inject drugs.

(6) Perinatal (vertical) transmission: Without

intervention, a 15% to 30% mother-to-infant transmission rate would result in the birth of an estimated 1,700 to 2,000 HIV-infected infants annually in the United States, perhaps growing higher if prevalence rose among childbearing women. Before effective prophylactic intervention became routine in the mid-1990s, AIDS had become the first and second leading cause of death, respectively, in Hispanic and African American children younger than 5 years old, with the majority of deaths occurring in the 1st year of life.

(7) Transfusion-related HIV transmission was effectively halted in the United States following the implementation in 1985 of routine HIV-antibody screening of blood.

(8) Occupational exposure of health care and laboratory workers: Cumulatively, about 5% of adults with reported AIDS diagnoses in the United States for whom occupational information is known have been health care workers; 73% subsequently died. The majority (about 44%) are nurses (more than 5,000 cases) and health aides (more than 5,000 cases).

(a) Most of these persons have also reported other risk factors.

(b) Only 57 cases have documented seroconversion following occupational exposure (i.e., were known to be uninfected at the time of occupational exposure). Half of these cases have progressed to AIDS. These exposures included concentrated virus (N = 2), infected blood

(N = 49), visible bloody fluid (N = 1), and unspecified body fluids (N = 4). Exposure by route includes percutaneous injury (N = 48); mucocutaneous or skin contact, or both, (N = 5); both percutaneous and mucocutaneous contact (N = 2); unknown route (N = 2).

    (c) About 137 cases of HIV infection among health care workers with history of occupational exposure have not reported other risk factors.

  (9) Transmission to patients during invasive procedures is rarely reported. The first reports were in 1990–1991: three cases in patients of a single dentist. The precise risk is not known, but it is very low.

g. Risk factors

    i. The percentage of sexually experienced high school students in the United States dropped slightly (from 54.1% to 49.9%) from 1991 to 1999, whereas condom use rose (from 46.2% to 58%), indicating a reversal in the trend of the previous two decades.

    ii. Many students report using alcohol or drugs when they have sex.

    iii. One in 50 high school students reports having injected an illegal drug.

    iv. Both homosexual male injecting drug users and heterosexual female injecting drug users appear to be at dual risk. Gay male injecting drug users are more likely to visit shooting galleries and share needles.

h. Surveillance

    i. The current case surveillance definition applies to both HIV-1 and HIV-2 infection in adults or children and incorporates the 1993 definitions for AIDS-defining conditions. This definition is accepted for reporting infection in all U.S. states and territories (though it is not intended to guide clinical practice—either diagnostics or therapeutics). (See Appendix A.)

    ii. The CDC categorizes transmission of adult cases of HIV and AIDS in a hierarchical system. Cases are hierarchically classified in a single category according to the person's whole risk history rather than according to either a specific exposure (possible transmission) incident or the most frequent exposures. That is, when a person's history of possible exposures indicates that he or she could have been infected in more than one way, there is no way to know for sure which exposure actually resulted in transmission, but the case is nevertheless counted in only one of the following categories, according to the order listed. (The hierarchy reflects the chronology of each risk factor's recognition following the recognition of AIDS in 1981. In other words, it does not reflect an inherent importance among the risk factors or transmission categories.) The CDC categories are:

- Men who have sex with men (includes men who report sexual contact with both men and women [i.e., bisexual men]).
- Injecting drug use
- Men who have sex with men and also inject drugs
- Received clotting factor for hemophilia/coagulation disorder
- Heterosexual contact

    – With injecting drug user
    – With bisexual male
    – With person with hemophilia/coagulation disorder
    – With HIV-infected transfusion or transplant recipient
    – With an HIV-infected person who has no specified risk

- Recipient of blood transfusion, blood components, or tissue allograph
- Other/risk not reported or identified (The category of no identified risk (NIR) is for persons who report no history of possible exposure; this category also includes cases for whom exposure history is unknown, either when data are unavailable or when epidemiologic follow-up is still ongoing.)

iii. Categories of transmission to children < 13 years are:

- Received clotting factor for hemophilia/coagulation disorder
- Mother with or at risk for HIV infection via:
    - Injecting drug use
    - Sex with injecting drug user
    - Sex with bisexual male
    - Sex with male with hemophilia coagulation disorder
    - Sex with HIV-infected transfusion or transplant recipient
    - Received blood transfusion, blood components, or allographic tissue
    - Other/risk not reported or identified

iv. Registries
    (1) Registries have been maintained for HIV-infected pregnant women who have taken antiretroviral agents to track pregnancy outcomes and long-term sequelae affecting their offspring.
    (2) A registry for health care workers who received prophylaxis following an occupational exposure to HIV was operated from mid-1996 through 1999. CDC continues to maintain a national registry for prospective surveillance following nonoccupational postexposure prophylaxis.
    (3) Tuberculosis registries are used to monitor infectiousness, the organism's drug susceptibility/resistance profile, and patients' completion of an effective regimen.
    (4) Registries are used to track and evaluate cancer outcomes. It was through registries that the changing incidence and mortality of Kaposi's sarcoma was documented in the early 1980s.

v. Cohort studies: With more than 5,500 male enrollees in four cities, the multicenter AIDS cohort study (MACS), begun in 1983, is one of the largest prospective HIV studies in the world. It provides an observational database for the study of disease natural history and treatment outcome in real-world clinical practice (i.e., outside research trials). A women's cohort study was started in 1990, the Women's Interagency Health Study (WIHS).

10. Emerging and future trends in HIV disease epidemiology
    a. The word *epidemic* may convey the wrong message. Epidemics can be stopped, and once dealt with, other issues get attention. This is not the case with HIV, and where it is not halted, its consequences will be around for decades.
    b. Given continuing transmission and the large number of persons already infected, incidence will continue to rise into the foreseeable future. New epidemic waves in different demographic groups can be expected in the United States. In endemic urban areas, such as New York City, changes are unlikely to be as widespread across populations or as dramatic as they were through the first decade. Subtle rises in prevalence in small population segments will not be as easy to recognize because surveillance data may not be sensitive enough either to discern improvements in prevention or to identify those at the

leading edge of the epidemic and describe their demographic characteristics and risk factors.

c. Surveillance efforts are being refocused to ensure ascertainment of new areas of epidemic spread and to facilitate the evaluation of prevention activities and tracking of the changing epidemiology of HIV-associated illness. In the past, surveillance has characterized transmission risks; in years to come its role will be to evaluate and focus attention on success in preventing and caring for HIV infection.

d. The number of HIV cases reported nationally will increase as states implement mandatory reporting. Initially, large boluses of reports of prevalent infection will occur and decline over time. Eventually (in those states that began HIV case reporting sooner), the number of new reported cases will reflect more recently infected persons. Then epidemiologic tracking will more accurately reflect the current transmission dynamics.

e. AIDS morbidity and mortality still remain the most consistent measure of the pattern and volume of HIV in the community because both are visible events, not dependent on whether a person sought or was offered testing.

f. The availability of effective therapies presents new public health challenges and roles for surveillance.

g. However, it is difficult to predict future AIDS incidence, even if current HIV incidence could be accurately known because it will depend on the epidemiology of use of treatment and because the impact of currently available and future treatments on disease progression is not known. Access, adherence, treatment costs, and viral resistance will influence use and efficacy of treatments and, in turn, their effects on AIDS incidence and mortality trends.

h. It is increasingly important to identify all infected individuals, so they can obtain timely, effective antiretroviral treatment, and to focus appropriate preventive measures on those who constitute the reservoir of HIV.

i. The long-term consequences, beneficial and adverse, of prolonged survival with antiretroviral regimens are not yet known. It is not unrealistic to expect that long-term sequelae, such as malignancy and chronic degenerative diseases, may eventually occur.

1.3 Prevention of HIV Infection

1. HIV is a universal risk when individuals are exposed, in any way, to infected body fluids.
2. Risk assessments
   a. Heterosexuals may have increased risk for exposure because of the following:
      i. They believe that safer sex messages are not directed at them.
      ii. The use of alcohol and drugs may lead to disinhibition and increase risky behavior; incidence among heterosexual partners of injection drug users has continued to increase steadily (MMWR, 1996).
      iii. The inequities of power in relationships may make it impossible for a person to demand or negotiate safer sex from a partner.
      iv. HIV is more easily transmitted from man to woman because of the following:
         (1) Concentration of virus is higher in semen than vaginal secretions.
         (2) The vaginal wall is more friable than penile skin.
         (3) The vaginal structure acts as a reservoir, prolonging exposure.
      v. The presence of ulcerative lesions (e.g., herpes, and syphilis) or presence of non-ulcerative infections such as gonorrhea, chlamydia, or nongonococcal urethritis increases risk.
      vi. Absence of knowledge of one's HIV status also increases risk.
   b. Gay and bisexual adults may be at greater risk because of the following:
      i. The use of alcohol and drugs may lead to disinhibition and increase risky behavior.

ii. The inequities of power in relationships may make it impossible for a person to demand or negotiate safer sex from a partner.

iii. The presence of ulcerative lesions (e.g., herpes and syphilis) or the presence of non-ulcerative infections such as gonorrhea, chlamydia, NGU increases risk.

iv. The possible increased number of partners contributes to risk.

v. Absence of knowledge of one's HIV status increases risk.

vi. People who take antiretroviral therapy may feel they cannot transmit the virus; in one study, HIV-infected men who have sex with men (MSM) who were taking protease inhibitors decreased condom use (Diclemente et al., 2002).

c. Adolescents may be a greater risk because of the following:

i. The belief that safer sex messages are not directed at them.

ii. Feelings of omnipotence, which are characteristic of the adolescent stage of development.

iii. The tendency to engage in experimental activities, including alcohol and drug use and sexual activity (Tapert, Aarone, Sedlar, & Brown, 2001).

iv. Additional issues for gay and bisexual adolescents, such as issues of self-esteem and feelings of invisibility in both the adolescent world and the gay/bisexual world.

v. The need for homeless youth to exchange in sex for food or shelter.

vi. The coming-out process, which may include activities of denial, such as heterosexual activity to prove they are straight.

vii. Partners of adolescents, who are often older and more at risk for extant HIV infection.

viii. Absence of knowledge of one's HIV status or the status of one's partner.

ix. The definition of "having sex," which is not universal (e.g., some adolescents feel that anal and oral sex, because it preserves virginity, is not really sex).

3. Primary prevention of HIV infection

a. Abstinence

i. Abstinence only message has proven to be an ineffective risk reduction strategy.

ii. A full discussion of what constitutes risky behavior, along with harm-reduction strategies, is more likely to be effective for people to understand all options for protection.

b. Barrier protection

i. Male latex or polyurethane condoms

(1) Natural membrane condoms are not recommended.

(2) Condoms are more effective if used with water-soluble lubricant.

(3) People should avoid nonoxynol-9 (see discussion later in this section).

ii. Female polyurethane condoms

(1) Advantages

(a) Its use is controlled by the woman.

(b) It protects during cunnilingus.

(c) It is odorless, without systemic side effects, requires no health care provider to fit or prescribe, and is impermeable to oil or water-based lubricants.

(d) Found to be impenetrable by trichomonas, CMV, herpes virus, hepatitis B, and HIV in in vitro testing in one study (Gilbert, 1999).

(2) Disadvantages

(a) It is expensive and not always available.

(b) It is aesthetically unappealing to some men and women.

iii. Dental dams (sheets of latex) can be used to protect against transmission during oral-genital or oral-anal contact.

c. Spermicides/microbicidal gels

    i. The once popular nonoxynol-9 is now not recommended and in fact may actually increase risk of transmission because of genital irritation and ulceration (Roddy, Zekeng, Ryan, Tamoufe, & Tweedy, 2002).

    ii. Microbicidal gels are currently being developed; however, none are yet available.

    iii. Sex toys should not be shared. Condoms may be used to protect toys that are inserted (e.g., dildos), and vibrators that are used externally should be washed with warm, soapy water.

d. Circumcision: Keratinization of the mucosal skin of the glans, which may lead to increased resistance to sexually transmitted diseases (STDs), can occur. The foreskin itself contains Langerhans cells, which express the CD_4 and CCR5 receptors, both critical receptors for HIV acquisition (Cohen & Eron, 2001). Thus circumcision may lead to decreased susceptibility to HIV.

e. Safer sex

    i. How a partner will react to the suggestion of safer sex will vary depending on the circumstances.

    ii. Women may risk abuse or abandonment as a consequence of insisting on safer sex.

    iii. Cultural and religious beliefs figure prominently in acceptance of safer sex practices.

    iv. Prostitutes and others offering sex for money may make more money to engage in riskier behaviors.

    v. Peer education, rather than education from health care providers or teachers was found to be better accepted among African American adolescents in one study (Jemmott, Jemmott, & Fong, 1998). Finding the person who can best reach any given audience is key in having the message heard.

4. Preventing blood to blood transmission

a. Injection drug use

    i. Injection drug use is a major risk for HIV, both for the injecting user and his or her sexual partner.

    ii. Injection drug users are at increased risk for blood borne pathogens, including HIV, hepatitis C, and hepatitis B.

    iii. Sharing of contaminated injection equipment is the main method of transmission among injection drug users, and the sexual partners of injection drug users are among the majority of new cases of HIV transmission.

    iv. One animal model study shows that cocaine use may increase the cell-to-cell spread of the virus (Roth et al., 2002).

b. Cessation of drug use

    i. Methadone treatment for opioid addiction is available. Such treatment is somewhat underused for a variety of reasons, including the following:

        (1) Systems set up to cultivate abstinence may alienate many drug users.

        (2) Slots for new patients are limited.

        (3) Drug users may not be ready to stop using.

        (4) Addiction itself is characterized by recidivism and may be perceived as failure by the injection drug user.

        (5) Limited options for treating cocaine addiction leave such users with fewer alternatives.

        (6) Currently there are studies underway to explore the use of nonopioid replacement medications for heroin users, such as clonidine and lofexidine (Gottheil et al., 2002).

c. Harm reduction

    i. Principal concept of harm reduction is that any step to reduce the negative effects of drug use is valuable.

    ii. Harm reduction views drug use from the medical and public health perspective and eliminates moralizing (Gunn, White, & Srinivasan, 1998).

iii. Harm reduction addresses issue of accessibility to care for a traditionally disenfranchised population (Gunn et al., 1998; Murphy, 2002)

iv. Using the principles of harm reduction, health care providers would encourage injecting drug users to do the following:

(1) Ideally, abstain from using drugs and seek treatment.

(2) Use a new needle and syringe each time drugs are injected.

(3) Clean injection equipment (i.e., container for cooking, needle and syringe, and cotton or "works").

(a) Works may be cleaned by boiling for 15 minutes.

(b) If boiling is not possible, equipment should first be thoroughly rinsed several times with clean water to remove blood. Next, the equipment should be soaked in full-strength household bleach at least once for a minimum of 1 minute, followed by another thorough clean-water rinse.

(4) Have own personal injection equipment that is never shared.

(5) Share only needles and syringes that have been correctly cleaned between use.

(6) Use condoms with sex partners who share injecting equipment.

(7) Health care providers need to recognize that often injection drug users are marginalized and may have difficulty making changes. Confounding this is the often present issue of dual diagnosis. Behavior changes may be slow, but small advances over time can make a difference (Springer, 1996).

(8) Needle exchange

(a) It is generally acknowledged that needle exchange programs lead to a decreased rate of transmission of HIV.

(b) Numerous studies in the United States and in England and Europe (DesJarlais et al., 1995; Hurley, Jolley, & Kaldor, 1997) showed decreased rates of transmission in those communities with established needle exchange. Further, the rate of injection drug use is no higher in cities with needle exchange than in those cities without it.

(c) The implication is that needle exchange will take activism from the grass roots to accomplish a change in local government's response to the needle exchange question.

5. Vertical transmission: the transmission of HIV from an infected woman to her infant during pregnancy, at the time of birth, or in the weeks following birth. For a full discussion of the prevention of perinatal transmission of HIV see Section 7.1.

6. Blood, blood products, and tissue transplantation

a. HIV transmission related to blood transfusion accounts for approximately 3% of HIV infections in developing countries (Family Health International, 2002).

b. In North America the screening of blood, mandated by the Food and Drug Administration (FDA), has decreased the risk of transfusion related viral infections.

c. The FDA proposed new rules to reduce risk of infectious diseases from transplantation of human tissues (American Medical Association, 2001). Nonetheless, two recalls of transplant tissue occurred in August 2002 (Blakeslee, 2002), and one was for lack of screening for HIV and hepatitis C (Rueters Medical News, 2002).

d. In the United States there is no risk of HIV transmission through donated blood.

7. HIV vaccines

a. Response to HIV infection involves both humoral and cellular immunity. The goal of vaccination is the elaboration of neutralizing antibodies and long-lasting anti-HIV cytotoxic T-lymphocyte (CTL) activity (Graham, 2002). Challenges to achieving this goal include the wide variety of viral strains and the ability of the virus to evade immune control.

b. Preventive vaccines hope to stimulate humoral and CTL response to HIV before exposure to the virus. The humoral or antibody response is important to control the initial viral spread. The CTL response is key to remove HIV-infected cells and to control further activation of the virus in latently infected cells.

c. AIDSVAX (VaxGen, Inc.), which is made from a synthetic protein, is the only preventive AIDS vaccine to reach Phase III of human testing. This double-blind study inoculates subjects during a 36-month period: some with the vaccine and some with a placebo. The vaccine's efficacy will be determined by comparing HIV infection between the two groups. The primary components of AIDSVAX are genetically engineered proteins. These synthetic proteins are identical to a protein (gp120) on the surface of HIV, which the virus uses to fuse through and infect healthy cells. The synthetic proteins in AIDSVAX prompt the immune system to produce antibodies to gp120. If the antibodies can successfully attach to gp120 and prevent the virus from entering cells and replicating, the virus cannot survive. Vaccine efficacy data is expected to be released in 2003.

d. Therapeutic vaccines hope to suppress viral replication and decrease the need for antiretroviral therapy by stimulating the CTL response, which will in turn control replication by controlling infected cells. There are currently no therapeutic vaccines being tested in humans.

e. Obstacles to vaccine development include the following (Mitsuyasu, 2001):

i. Severe immune suppression that may prevent the development of CTLs with insufficient T-helper cell function

ii Wide viral diversity that may forestall narrowly targeted vaccines from elaborating a powerful immune response

iii. Immunologic escape by the constant mutation of the virus

iv. Defective antigen presentation by the mutated virus

f. The science of vaccine development is currently rapidly evolving, and at the time of publication there is no definitive data on any of the clinical trials for both preventive and therapeutic vaccines.

1.4. Pathophysiology of HIV Infection

1. Retroviruses, RNA viruses (taxonomy)

a. Retroviruses can be classified into subgroups based on their pathogenic potential.

i. Oncovirus (induces neoplastic disease in vivo)

(1) Human T-lymphotrophic virus-I (HTLV-I)

(a) Etiologic agent of acute T-cell leukemia (ATL) and T-cutaneous lymphoma

(b) Endemic to southern islands of Japan, parts of the United States, most of the Caribbean, northern South America, and Africa

(2) Human T-lymphotrophic virus-II (HTLV-II): associated with hairy-cell leukemia and hemophilia with a peculiar immune deficiency state

(3) Human T-lymphotrophic virus-V (HTLV-V): associated with mycosis fungoides

(4) Feline leukemia virus (FeLV): animal retrovirus found only in cats

(5) Simian T-lymphotrophic virus (STLV): animal retrovirus found in Japanese macaque

and Asian and African monkeys and apes

  ii. Lentivirus (*Lentiviridae*) subgroup or slow virus; lack neoplastic potential

    (1) HIV type 1 (HIV-1)

      (a) HIV-1 is the most prevalent human retrovirus in the world.

      (b) HIV-1 comprises three distinct virus groups: M, N, and O.

      (c) M is the predominant group, and it consists of 11 clades. These subtypes are denoted A through K.

    (2) HIV type 2 (HIV-2)

      (a) HIV-2 is primarily localized to Africa, especially Western Africa.

      (b) There are six subtypes of HIV-2, denoted A through F.

    (3) Simian immunodeficiency virus (SIV) and feline immunodeficiency virus (FIV): animal retroviruses that are linked to AIDS-like disease in Asian macques and domestic cats, respectively.

b. Unique properties of retroviruses

  i. Genes are encoded in two single-stranded RNA (RNA viruses).

  ii. Transcription of genetic message is reversed: RNA to DNA versus DNA to RNA.

  iii. Reverse transcriptase enzyme is responsible for transcribing RNA into DNA.

  iv. Three common genes are *env, pol, gag.*

  v. Able to incorporate viral DNA into host T-cell nuclear genome

    (1) Incorporated retroviral DNA can be activated to produce exogenous budding viruses.

    (2) Internal core proteins are most conserved or common among viruses within the group.

    (3) Envelope glycoproteins are least conserved or more distinct for each virus within the group.

2. Human immunodeficiency virus (HIV)

a. The structure of HIV

  i. Retrovirus is slightly > 100 nm in diameter.

  ii. General appearance is of a dense cylindrical viral core surrounded by a lipid envelope.

  iii. Principle components of the viral core are two strands of HIV RNA, reverse transcriptase (p51), protease (p11), and integrase (p32).

  iv. The lipid envelope contains the glycoproteins gp120 and gp41.

  v. The HIV genome contains three structural genes called *env, pol,* and *gag* and six additional structural genes called *nef, vpr, vpu, vif, tat,* and *rev.*

b. Two phases of HIV life cycle

  i. Establishing infection in a host T-cell

    (1) Attachment

      (a) Attachment is via binding of viral gpl20 to the CD_4 surface molecule of T4 helper/inducer lymphocytes, monocytes, and macrophages.

      (b) HIV uses both the CD_4 cell receptor and the chemokine receptors CCR5 and CXCR4 to gain entry into the cell.

        (i) Different strains of HIV-1 have affinity for different coreceptors.

          1. Non-syncytia-forming variants of HIV (NSI) bind preferentially to cells with the CCR5 chemokine receptors; they are called macrophage tropic strains of HIV.

          2. Syncytia-inducing (SI) T-cell trophic strains of HIV (typically found in late infection)

use the CXCR4 coreceptor.

(2) Entry
 (a) Following fusion, the viral protein core uncoats itself and releases the HIV genome and enzymes into the host T-cell's cytoplasm.

(3) Transcription
 (a) The reverse transcriptase enzyme in the HIV viron transcribes viral RNA to viral DNA in the host T-cell's cytoplasm.
  (i) Two linear strands of DNA are synthesized into a double-helix configuration.
  (ii) Single-stranded RNA template is degraded by viral ribonuclease H.
  (iii) Some of the double-stranded DNA join together to form a closed circle, while other strands remain in linear form.
 (b) HIV entry into nucleus: Circular viral DNA are inserted into the host T-cell's genome by integrase while the proportion of linear viral DNA may remain in the host T-cell's cytoplasm.

(4) Latency
 (a) Host T-cell is in a quiescent state.
 (b) This is a period of nonproductive expression of the integrated proviral DNA

ii. Active productive infection
 (1) Assembly
  (a) The infected host T-cell is activated by antigens, mitogens, or cytokines.
  (b) Proviral DNA is transcribed into mRNA, which is then transported out of the nucleus into the cytoplasm.
  (c) mRNA codons are then translated into amino acid sequences for the polyprotein precursors located in the viral protein core and the virion envelope.
  (d) Protease modifies (cleaves) the larger polyproteins into the active protein subunits, p24, p15, p17, gpl20, gp4l, needed for assembly of new virion.

 (2) Budding
  (a) A virion core with HIV RNA, modified proteins, and enzymes is assembled at the plasma membrane of the host T-cell (now a mature virion).
  (b) The mature virion fuses with the host T-cell's membrane. The HIV virus buds from the cell surface.
  (c) During budding, gpl20 and gp4l are incorporated into the outer lipid membrane of the virion. The budding virion incorporates some of the host T-cell's protein, which aids the virion to infect other host T-cells.

c. Differences between HIV-1 and HIV-2
 i. Absence of *vpu* gene in HIV-2
 ii. Presence of the accessory gene *vpx* in HIV-2 genome
 iii. Amino acid sequence differs in structure of the envelope glyco-proteins for HIV-l and HIV-2.
 iv. HIV-2 appears to be less virulent and possibly has a longer period of clinical latency.

d. Origin of AIDS
 i. HIV-1 (clades M, N, O) is closely related to SIVcpz virus found in the *Pt. troglodytes*, a species of West Central African chimpanzees. HIV-2 is closely related to the SIVsm virus found in the sooty mangabeys, whose geographic boundaries appear to have extended from Gabon to Cameroon

in West Central Africa to an eastern limit in Tanzania (Hahn, Shaw, DeCock, & Sharp, 2000).

ii. The origins of HIV-1 and HIV-2 are considered to be the result of transmission of primate lentiviruses to humans. There are two competing theories regarding the transmission of these primate lentiviruses to humans. The theory for which there is stronger evidence is that the transmission is the result of hunting and dressing of infected chimpanzees and sooty mangabeys. The second theory is that zoonotic transmission is related to the development of oral poliovirus vaccination (OPV) trials carried out in the Belgian Congo in the 1950s. This theory is based on use of sooty mangabey kidneys in the vaccination preparation. The OPV theory is not consistent with current phylogenetic relations of the known simian lentiviruses.

iii. Other primate species are known to be infected with similar lentiviruses that could infect humans (Hahn et al., 2000). They are potential reservoirs for human lentiviruses other than HIV-1 and HIV-2.

3. Normal immunology
   a. Cells of the immune system
      i. Types of leukocytes (white blood cells)
         (1) Neutrophils: Major phagocytic cells in the blood. They represent approximately 60% of circulating leukocytes. Production is mediated by inflammatory cytokines: G-CSF and GM-CSF.
         (2) Eosinophils: Participate in allergic reactions. They represent 5% of circulating leukocytes.
         (3) Basophils: Involved in early inflammatory reactions. They represent approximately 1% of circulating leukocytes.
         (4) Monocytes and macrophages (differentiated monocytes): Functions include phagocytosis, antigen presentation, cytokine secretion, and target T-cell killing. They are found within the blood and represent 5% to 10% of blood leukocytes. Macrophages are large phagocytic cells found in the brain (microglial), skin (Langerhans), spleen, liver, lungs (alveolar), and lymphoid tissues that participate in local immune responses. They may be free (in blood) or fixed (permanently located in specific organs, such as Kupffer cells in the liver).
         (5) Lymphocytes: Major participants in specific immune reactions. They represent 5% to 10% of circulating leukocytes. Postnatal lymphocyte division (prior to antigenic stimulation) takes place in the bone marrow and thymus. Lymphocyte maturation is antigen dependent.
            (a) Types of lymphocytes
               (i) B-cells are the antibody-producing cells, and they are one type of antigen-presenting cells. They represent approximately 10% of lymphocytes in peripheral blood. Lymphocytes are the major lymphoid cell in lymphoid organs outside of the blood.
               (ii) T-cells represent 70% to 90% of all circulating lymphocytes. They are found in lesser amounts in lymphoid tissues. They can serve as either effector cells or regulatory elements of the immune system. They contain

surface markers (e.g., CD_4, CD_8, CD_3). T-helper cells carry the surface marker of CD_4; helper cells secrete lymphokines that help orchestrate antigen-destroying immune responses (e.g., IL-2). CD_4-Th1 cells facilitate cell-mediated responses, whereas CD_4-Th2 cells facilitate humoral immune reactions. T-suppressor cells carry the marker of CD_8; suppressor cells secrete lymphokines that signal the termination of the immune response. Cytotoxic T-cells (CTLs) carry the marker of CD_8; CTLs have the ability to kill antigens by inserting toxic molecules into the cell membrane of the antigen.

(iii) Natural killer (NK) cells are neither B-nor T-lymphocytes. They represent 5% to 15% of circulating lymphocytes and kill virus and tumor targets. NK cells do not require antigen-presenting cells (APCs) to function; they attack either directly or through antibody-dependent T-cell-mediated cytotoxicity.

b. Characteristics of the immune system responses

   i. Nonspecific immunity

     (1) Physical, mechanical, chemical, and microbial barriers: skin, mucous membranes, soluble factors, and natural flora

     (2) Phagocytosis

       (a) Particle uptake by cells of the granulocytic and mononuclear phagocytic lineages

       (b) Protective mechanisms against invading bacteria

     (3) Inflammatory response

       (a) Increased blood flow to site of injury

       (b) Increased capillary permeability

       (c) Accumulation of phagocytic cells

       (d) Complement system: consists of 10 plasma proteins that are primarily involved in the inflammatory and immune response

   ii. Specific immunity

     (1) Humoral immunity (B-cell involvement)

       (a) B-cells secrete antibodies (humors); antibodies are immunoglobulins.

       (b) Basic structure of antibodies: Fab region (recognizes antigenic specificity); Fc region (activates complement and binds to phagocytic cells)

       (c) Immunoglobulins proliferate in response to antigen and secrete a specific antibody.

       (d) Differentiation into plasma cells (clones of original B-cell); requires T-helpers and lymphokines. Opsonization of bacteria (renders the bacteria susceptible to phagocytosis), and complement activation (see later discussion)

       (e) Generation of memory cells

(2) Cell-mediated immunity (T-cell involvement)

  (a) Lymophyctes are processed in the thymus gland to recognize antigens.

  (b) Mature T-cells have surface proteins that determine its function. The major functions of the cell-mediated responses are as follows:

- Cytotoxcicity: direct killing of target T-cells with the help of circulating antigen-presenting cells (dendritic cells, mononuclear phagocytes, and B-cells)
- Delayed hypersensitivity: involved in the inflammatory response and mediators that influence other cells
- Memory: response for the secondary immune response (see later discussion)
- Control: inhibit both humoral and cell-mediated immune responses

(3) NK cells

  (a) Special group of lymphocytes with the surface marker of CD_{16}.

  (b) May become activated by undefined chemical changes on the surface of virally infected or malignant T-cells

  (c) Lyse target T-cells following direct binding to altered cell membrane; antigens bound to Class I MHC alert NK (and CD_8 CTLs) to virus-infected or cancer-transformed cells

  (d) Lyse antibody-coated targets through antibody-dependent T-cell cytotoxicity; binding is at Fc receptor.

4. The immune system response to HIV infection

  a. CD_4 T-helper/inducer cells

    i. Target for infection by HIV (chemokine receptors CCR5 or CXCR4 required)

    ii. CD_4 cells become reservoirs of latency in early HIV infection.

    iii. Progressive decline in CD_4 cell numbers over course of disease by direct and indirect mechanisms

    iv. Progressive loss in proliferation and cytokine secretion by CD_4-Th1 cells that promote cell-mediated immune responses

    v. Excessive activation of CD_4-Th2 cells that promote generation of humoral immune responses

  b. CD_8 CTLs and CD_8 suppressor cells

    i. Increase in cell numbers during acute infection

    ii. Activated CD_8 T-cells are cytotoxic to HIV-infected CD_4 cells, with surface expression of *env, gag,* or *pol* proteins, and cytotoxic to uninfected CD_4 T-cells with surface-bound HIV envelope proteins.

    iii. There is a decline in number of CTLs and suppressor cells at the time of an AIDS diagnosis.

    iv. There is increased expression of activation markers on cell surface that correlates with stage of illness.

    v. There is diminished HIV-specific cytotoxic lymphocyte activity as disease progresses.

  c. NK cells

    i. NK cells produce perforins that bind to the cell membrane and create channels in the membrane. The result is osmotic death.

    ii. NK cells can be reservoirs for latent HIV infection. NK cells have IgG Fc receptors that bind antibody antigen complexes and facilitate viral entry into NK cells.

d. B lymphocytes
  i. There is an expression of activation markers on cell surfaces.
  ii. There are elevated levels of immunoglobulins.
  iii. B-cells produce antibodies against viral proteins. The major target is the viral envelope, especially gp120.
  iv. Some antibodies bind the viral envelope without destroying it, but they facilitate viral entry into macrophages and NK cells by antibody-dependent T-cell-mediated cytotoxicity.
  v. Reduced specific humoral immune response to immunization is associated with late stages of illness.
e. Mononuclear phagocytes
  i. Targets for infection by HIV.
  ii. Macrophages can be reservoirs for latent HIV infection because they have IgG Fc receptors that bind antibody antigen complexes and facilitate viral entry into them.
  iii. There is decreased migration to inflammatory stimuli.
  iv. There is diminished phagocytosis and bacterial killing.
f. Granulocytes: No consistent alterations reported.
g. Lymphoid organs: main anatomical sites of early infection and clinically latent infection
h. Follicular dendritic cells: help establish antibody or complement responses to HIV because they are CD_4 negative cells with Fc or C1 receptors

5. The natural history of HIV infection
a. Primary infection (time 0)
  i. The period immediately after HIV infection where virus infects cells
  ii. Characterized by high levels of viremia and immune system activation. The viral load, if measured, usually exceeds 100,000 copies/mL and often exceeds 1 million copies/mL.
  iii. CD_4 cells and CD_8 cells decrease initially, but the decrease is transient and soon followed by lymphocytosis.

  iv. Clinical manifestations include acute retroviral syndrome.
    (1) Occurs in 30% to 50% of people with primary infection
    (2) Occurs 3 to 6 weeks postprimary infection and lasts approximately 2 to 4 weeks
    (3) Although most symptomatic patients seek medical consultation, the diagnosis is often missed because the symptoms are nonspecific.
    (4) Common symptoms include fever, arthralgias, myalgias, lymphadenopathy, pharyngitis, anorexia, and weight loss.
    (5) Serum antibodies develop and are detectable after 2 to 5 weeks (seroconversion).
b. Chronic infection
  i. Characterized by a decrease in the level of viremia, and the resolution of symptoms associated with acute retroviral syndrome (if present)
  ii. After a period of fluctuation, the plasma level of HIV and CD_4 cell count stabilizes (often called the set point). Once the set point is established, the natural history of HIV progresses is as follows:
    (1) Clinical latency: a period (typically 12 weeks to 8 years) before the development of clinically apparent disease. The length of time of clinical latency is largely influenced by the set point. This period is characterized by the following:

    • Sequestration of HIV, primarily in lymphatic tissue with viral replication
    • Chronic immune system activation
    • Continued viral spread to uninfected tissues and cells
    • CD_4 cell count > 500 cells/mm^3 with a gradual attrition of CD_4 lymphocytes

(2) Symptomatic HIV disease: a period (typically 8 to 10 years) after primary infection in which signs and symptoms of diseases associated with HIV infection begin to emerge. This period is characterized by the following:

- Viral replication with increasing amount of virus detected in circulation
- Deterioration of lymphoid microenvironment
- CD_4 cell count between 200 and 500 cells/mm^3 with a continued attrition of CD_4 lymphocytes

(3) Advanced HIV disease (AIDS): period (typically 10 to 11 years) after primary infection in which the CD_4 cell count is < 200 cells/mm^3 or there is an AIDS indicator condition as defined by the CDC. This period is characterized by the following:

- Failure of the immune system mechanisms to control viral replication; thus, large amounts of virus are detected in the circulation
- Profound immunodeficiency, with CD_4 lymphocyte counts between 0 and 200 cells/mm^3

1.5 HIV Testing

1. HIV tests detect the presence of antibodies or antigens. Currently several methods are available (Bartlett & Gallant, 2001).
   a. Enzyme-linked immunosorbent assay (EIA) with positive findings confirmed by Western blot (WB) is the standard HIV screening test. EIA, sometimes called ELISA, detects the presence of antibodies to HIV. Usually a venipuncture is required. EIAs are very sensitive (picking up nearly all positives) but not so specific (i.e., not able to identify all of the true negative tests in a population). Because of the possibility of false positive results, HIV-positive results should not be given solely on the result of a positive EIA. Some EIAs are able to test for HIV-1 and-2 simultaneously.
   b. Western blot, or sometimes an immunofluorescent assay (IFA), test is done on a repeatedly positive EIA to confirm the findings. These are more complicated, more expensive, and more labor intensive tests than the EIAs. Sensitivity and specificity of these tests combined is greater than 98%. At this time, it is recommended to contact the CDC regarding testing for HIV-2.
   c. Other antibody tests are currently available (Bartlett & Gallant, 2001).
      i. Single Use Diagnostic System (SUDS) is the only FDA-approved rapid test available at this time. It takes 15 to 30 minutes to complete, and it requires a venipuncture. A confirmatory WB is required for positive SUDS. At 99.9%, its sensitivity and specificity are similar to EIA.
      ii. OraSure test system is the FDA-approved HIV test on saliva. The test collects saliva and detects IgG for determining antibody presence through EIA testing. This is a noninvasive test consisting of placement of a specially treated spongelike swab between the cheek and gum tissue, and leaving it in place for 2 min. The swab is placed in the container provided with the kit and mailed to a central lab. The results are faxed or mailed. Sensitivity and specificity are comparable to standard serologic testing.
      iii. Calypte HIV-1 urine test is available to be administered only by a health care provider. Its sensitivity is greater than 99%. It is an EIA-only test, so positive results must be verified by a confirmatory serology test.

iv. Home Access Express test is the only FDA-approved test for home use. It requires an individual to collect a blood sample from a finger stick and mail it to a central lab. Double EIAs and confirmatory IFAs are used. Each kit provides a code number by which results may be obtained. The person phones a central number, and negative results are provided on a prerecorded message; opportunity to talk with a counselor is available. In the case of a positive result, callers talk with a counselor. Sensitivity and specificity of this test approach 100%.

d. Antigen, DNA, or RNA detection tests (Bartlett & Gallant, 2001) include those listed in the following sections.

i. Polymerase chain reaction (PCR) tests use a technique that amplifies HIV DNA or RNA particles to a measurable quantity. It is not dependent on antibody production. It is, however, very expensive. Consequently, an HIV diagnosis is made with this testing method when there is controversy over the results from routine screening testing or when making a diagnosis in infants. Sensitivity is 99% and specificity is 98% for DNA PCR; the sensitivity for RNA PCR is 95–98%. The RNA PCR is dependent on the stage of illness and may report false positives, especially in the low ranges.

ii. PBMC HIV culture isolates the virus and is very expensive, labor intensive, and the reliability can vary from lab to lab. It is used when there is controversy over the confirmatory antibody test or for HIV detection in infants.

2. Interpretation of HIV screening test results (Bartlett & Gallant, 2001)

a. Negative test results mean there is no evidence of HIV antibodies on the day the person was screened. False negatives are usually due to testing during the "window period," a time between infection and the presence of measurable antibodies. This is roughly a 10- to 14-day period with the newer EIA testing methods. Nearly all HIV infection will be detected within 6 months. If a person has had risks within the window period and the test is negative, they should avoid additional risks and retest within 3 months. Additional reasons for false negative test results are infection with HIV-2 and technical error.

b. Positive test results mean there was a repeatedly reactive EIA and the WB result also meets the criteria for positive HIV infection; the client is considered infected with HIV. The requirement for a positive WB is reactivity on bands gp41 plus gp120/160, or p24 plus gp120/160. Some reasons for false positives are experimental HIV vaccination, some autoimmune diseases, or technical failure. Reported HIV-positive tests without written confirmation should always be repeated. Positive tests with low evidence of risk from risk assessment should also be repeated.

c. Indeterminate test results indicate the client's EIA was repeatedly reactive, but the band pattern of the WB does not meet the criteria for positive results. The most common reason for this result is that an infected individual tested during the window period and had not yet produced antibodies. Some other causes are experimental HIV vaccination, cross-reacting nonspecific antibodies, infection with HIV-2, and technical error. People who are in the process of seroconversion usually test positive within a month. Repeat testing is recommended at 1, 2, and 6 months if a positive test result is not obtained.

3. Issues related to testing and counseling

a. Risks and benefits to testing

i. Risks of testing include possible physical injury or infection at the site of venipuncture and bruising and soreness from venipuncture. Anxiety and stress related to possible social, family, and work repercussions of a positive test result may occur.

ii. Benefits of testing include knowledge of one's HIV status—whether HIV-positive or negative. When the test result is negative, safety and risk reduction behaviors can be reinforced. If the result is positive, medical intervention and appropriate health promotion activities can be discussed, and safety and risk-reduction regarding transmission of HIV to others and protecting oneself from diseases may be reviewed with the client.

b. Anonymous versus confidential testing (Centers for Disease Control and Prevention, 1999)

i. Anonymous testing is a CDC-recommended, voluntary system that allows people to test for HIV without having to provide identifying information. It also allows for reporting of HIV infection without breaching confidentiality. The client provides a code number but no other identifying information. Records, specimens, and results are linked only to that person's code number. Anonymous testing is usually provided by state health departments, HIV counseling and testing sites, public health clinics, and STD clinics. One disadvantage is the inability to locate a client for test results.

ii. Confidential testing links clients to their tests by identifying information such as names, medical record numbers, or other identifying information. The counseling information and test results are entered into the client's medical chart. The advantage of this testing system is that test counselors have information by which they are able to locate HIV-positive individuals. Medical planning and follow-up is easier to facilitate.

c. Informed consent (Centers for Disease Control and Prevention, 1999)

i. With few exceptions, informed consent before testing is essential.

Information about informed consent must be presented verbally or in writing and in language understood by the client. Documentation of consent should be in writing, preferably with the person's signature. HIV testing should be voluntary and free of coercion. Refusal of testing should not affect quality of care for that person.

ii. The HIV test counselor must assess the client's capacity to understand and sign an informed consent. If there is question, the test should be deferred until the person is capable (free from effects of medication, intoxication, anxiety that indicates coercion, etc.). Cognitive delay/impairment may also result in deferring consent and must be documented. Contact the person who has legal authority to provide permission. Parents can consent to testing for minor children. Adolescents may consent to their own HIV and STD testing under minor consent laws; these laws may vary from state to state.

iii. HIV testing may be mandatory when the activity that requires an HIV test is, itself, voluntary, such as in blood donation or foreign travel.

d. Disclosure of HIV status (Stein, 2001)

i. Disclosure of HIV status should be discussed with clients before testing and at the results session, especially if the result is positive. Information should be provided regarding the appropriate state reporting laws for HIV infection. In some states reporting HIV-positive status is required, and in others reporting is not required until an AIDS diagnosis is made by a medical provider. Clients must be informed of their legal rights and responsibilities regarding failure-to-disclose laws that may result in criminal apprehension for HIV-positive individuals.

ii. Partner disclosure should be discussed in the session before the test and at the results session. HIV-positive individuals should be encouraged to talk with partners, but they may be unable to do it. State health departments may offer services to assist HIV-positive people with locating and notifying partners.

4. Initial (pretest) HIV-test counseling session (Centers for Disease Control and Prevention, 1999)

a. The goal of HIV-test counseling is to reduce HIV acquisition and transmission by 1) providing accurate and current information about HIV; transmission and acquisition; and the HIV test, including risks and benefits of taking the test, potential test results, and their meanings; 2) assessing the person's individual risk behaviors, discussing methods for risk reduction, the person's knowledge of HIV/AIDS, and his or her capacity to comprehend HIV testing and consent; and 3) seeking a commitment to reduce risk behaviors. This information should be provided even if the person chooses not to test. Typically there is one session prior to testing, but there may be more than one depending on individual need.

b. HIV-test counseling is becoming more common among health care providers as a part of routine preventive care. Questions for all patients might be "What are you doing to prevent HIV and other STDs?" or "What are your risks for HIV and other STDs?" Be sure the client understands that the discussion will include disclosure of personal information that will remain confidential. The responses from the patient will lead to further assessment and the offering of a test at that time, if it is appropriate.

c. Consider the following issues and questions when assessing risk:

i. Keep questions client focused; make no assumptions but keep in mind any cultural, racial, sexual orientation, religious, class, and other differences regarding HIV. Be sure that recognizable and understandable terms are used. Recognize that the greater the number of behavioral risks taken, the greater the risk of HIV acquisition.

ii. Ask open-ended questions about the reasons the client is testing at this time, STD history, IDU (IV drug use) and other drug and alcohol use, numbers of and the gender of sexual partners, use of condoms and other barriers during sexual activities, the client's ability to negotiate safer sex with partners, and so forth. Assess for seroconversion illness and, if appropriate, pregnancy. Ask how the client feels he or she would respond to a positive test result. Reinforce risk reduction behaviors and encourage a personal commitment to HIV prevention.

iii. Provide information about HIV and AIDS, the tests, natural history of HIV transmission (including pregnancy), risk behaviors, prevention behaviors, state reporting laws, and an appointment for receiving results.

iv. Clients should be seen individually for counseling. If they want someone with them, suggest to the client that the person attending would be someone who understands the stress of testing and would be a support if the test were positive.

5. Test-result (posttest) counseling session (Centers for Disease Control and Prevention, 1999)

a. It is preferred that clients return for the test result in person, and the same counselor should provide the result if that is possible. Share the result at the beginning of the session and show the client the lab copy if possible. Allow time for the client to react to the result and to ask questions.

b. If the results are negative, assess the client's feelings about this result. Review the risk assessment that was started in the previous session. Review the meaning of a negative test and reinforce the client's personal risk-reduction behaviors. If the test was done in the window period, encourage the client to avoid risk situations and to return for another test in a time line that is appropriate to the individual's risk experiences.

c. If the results are positive, be very sensitive to the client's reaction. It may be very different from what he or she presented during the initial counseling session when asked about a reaction to a positive result. Follow the client's lead regarding questions and discussion of the results. Be encouraging about HIV treatment and living with HIV, while acknowledging the difficulty of living with a chronic, potentially life-threatening disease. Be aware that all of the information presented may not be comprehended by a person who has just received this diagnosis. Provide resource information for HIV/AIDS help lines, psychosocial services, and medical referral, if necessary. Encourage healthy living and the establishment of early medical care. Review the signs and symptoms of seroconversion disease and assess whether the client may be in this phase of infection. Review the meaning of a positive antibody test and the state's reporting laws.

d. Recognize that an HIV-positive diagnosis may result in discrimination, shameful feelings, fear of losing support of family and friends, fear of job loss, and fear of illness and death. Be prepared to refer the client to mental health services immediately if his or her reaction to the diagnosis is extreme or if there is interest in seeking counseling.

References

American Medical Association. (2001). *New regulations proposed for human tissue transplantation.* Retrieved June 24, 2002, from www.ama-assn.org/ama

Bartlett, J. G., & Gallant, J. E. (2001). *Medical management of HIV infection: 2001–2002 edition.* Baltimore: Johns Hopkins University, Division of Infectious Diseases.

Blakeslee, S. (2002, August 15). Recall is ordered at large supplier of implant tissue [Electronic version]. *New York Times.*

Buchacz, K. A., Wilkinson, D. A., Krowka, J. F., Koup, R. A., & Padian, N. S. (1998). Genetic and immunological host factors associated with susceptibility to HIV-1 infection. *AIDS, 12*(Suppl. A), 87–94.

Centers for Disease Control and Prevention. (1999). *Technical expert panel review of CDC HIV counseling, testing, and referral guidelines. MMWR, 50*(RR19), 1–58.

Centers for Disease Control and Prevention. (2002). U.S. HIV and AIDS cases reported through June 2001. *HIV/AIDS Surveillance Report, 13*(1), 1–41.

Cohen, M. S., & Eron, J. (2001). *Sexual HIV transmission and its prevention.* Retrieved June, 2002, from www.medscape.com/viewprogram/704

DesJarlais, D. C., Hagan, H., Friedman, S. R., Friedmann, P., Goldberg, D., Frischer, M., et al. (1995). Maintaining low HIV seroprevalence in populations of injecting drug users. *Journal of the American Medical Association, 274,* 1226–1231.

Diclemente, R. J., Funkhouser, E., Wingood, G., Fawal, H., Holmberg, S., & Vermund, S. H. (2002). Protease inhibitor combination therapy and decreased use of condoms in gay men. *Southern Medical Journal, 95,* 421–425.

Family Health International. (2002). *Technical services: Blood safety and universal precautions.* Retrieved November 15, 2002, from http://www.fhi.org/en/aids/wwdo/wwd10.html

Gilbert, L. K. (1999). The female condom (FC) in the U.S.: Lessons learned. *American Journal of Public Health, 89*(6), 1–28.

Gottheil, E., Mannelli, P., Collins, E. D., Van Bockstaele, E. J., Ling, W., & Woody, G. E. (2002, April). *Recent developments in opiate detoxification.* Paper presented at the American Society of Addiction Medicine 33rd Annual Meeting & Medical-Scientific Conference, Atlanta, GA.

Graham, B. S. (2002). Clinical trials of HIV vaccines. *Annual Review of Medicine, 53,* 207–221.

Gunn, N., White, C., & Srinivasan, R. (1998). Primary care as harm reduction for injection drug users. *Medical Student JAMA, 280,* 1191–1195.

Hahn, B. H., Shaw, G. M., DeCock, K. M., & Sharp, P. M. (2000). AIDS as zoonosis: Scientific and public health implications. *Science, 287,* 607–614.

Hurley, S. F., Jolley, D. J., & Kaldor, J. M. (1997). Effectiveness of needle-exchange programmes for prevention of HIV infection. *Lancet, 349,* 1797–1800.

Jemmott, J. B., Jemmott, L. S., & Fong, G. T. (1998). Abstinence and safer sex HIV risk-reduction interventions for African American adolescents: A randomized controlled trial. *Journal of the American Medical Association, 279*(19), 1529–1536.

Mathias, R. (2002). High-risk sex is main factor in HIV infection for men and women who inject drugs. *NIDA Notes, 17*(2), 5, 10.

Mitsuyasu, R. (2001). AIDS vaccine 2001: Looking to the future. *Medscape HIV/AIDS eJournal 7*(5). Retrieved May 22, 2002, from www.hiv.medscape.com

MMWR. (1996). *Journal of the American Medical Association, 285,* 2129.

Murphy, N. (2002). *Practicing HIV harm reduction health care.* Unpublished manuscript.

Reuters Medical News. (2002). *Body parts recalled by Texas medical institution.* Retrieved August 15, 2002, from www.medscape.com

Roddy, R. E., Zekeng, L., Ryan, K. A., Tamoufe, U., & Tweedy, K. G. (2002). Effect of nonoxynol-9 gel on urogenital gonorrhea and chlamydial infection: A randomized controlled trial. *Journal of the American Medical Association, 287,* 1117–1122.

Roth, M. D., Tashkin, D. P., Choi, R., Jamieson, B. D., Zack, J. A., & Baldwin, G. C. (2002). Cocaine enhances human immunodeficiency virus replication in a model of severe combined immunodeficient mice implanted with human peripheral blood leukocytes. *Journal of Infectious Diseases, 185,* 701–705

Springer, E. (1996, September). *Effective HIV prevention with marginalized populations: The harm reduction model of behavior change.* Paper presented at the National HIV Prevention Conference, Atlanta, GA.

Stein, G. J. (2001). *AIDS update 2001.* Upper Saddle River, NJ: Prentice Hall.

Tapert, S. F., Aarone, G. A., Sedlar, G. R., & Brown, S. A. (2001). Adolescent substance use and sexual risk taking. *Journal of Adolescent Health, 28*(3), 181–189.

UNAIDS. (2002). *Report on the global HIV/AIDS epidemic: 2002.* New York: World Health Organization.

Section II

Clinical Management of the HIV-Infected Adolescent and Adult

Long-term success in the health of individuals infected with HIV is determined by a variety of factors, including postdiagnosis care. Section II describes many of the major activities crucial to the care of those infected with HIV. The section begins with a description of the baseline assessment, which affords the clinician to see how HIV impacts the life of the affected. This section also serves as an important guide for tailoring health education efforts, which are described in Section 2.3, Teaching for Health Promotion, Wellness, and Prevention of Transmission. This section concludes with an expertly written discussion on the current state of the "when to," "why" and "how" of antiretroviral therapy.

2.1 Baseline Assessment

1. Baseline assessment
   a. Chief complaint: HIV infection—the nurse should assess the patient's knowledge about his or her HIV infection, including risk factors, possible date or timing of infection, and client understanding of treatment options. The nurse should also assess the educational needs of the client and plan educational interventions as appropriate.
   b. The patient's coping mechanisms should be assessed. For example, is the patient having difficulty accepting his or her HIV diagnosis? Does the patient have a significant other, a support system, or both, available, and can these systems be easily accessed?
   c. The nursing team should assess the patient's HIV treatment history and experience with treatments, such as medications, side affects, and comfort level with health care provider, and expectations regarding treatment. The patient's previous records should be obtained when possible. The nurse should assess if the patient has any urgent questions about treatment options and plans.
   d. The nurse should help the patient prepare to discuss the short-term and long-term treatment goals with his or her primary care provider by providing reassurance and privacy during the visit and helping the client to explore his or her own treatment and health care expectations.
2. Health history
   a. Medical history: A complete assessment of the past medical history of the person with HIV is necessary. In addition to the patient's HIV medical history, it is also important to include other health care maintenance needs. This assessment includes exploration of other concomitant medical problems or complaints (Bickley, 2003).
   b. STD history: Because HIV is a sexually transmitted disease (STD), the patient's history of sexually transmitted infections (STIs) should

be noted. The nurse should also assess if appropriate treatment and follow-up was obtained for the condition (Centers for Disease Control and Prevention, 2002c).
   c. Surgical history: The date and outcome of any surgical procedures should be noted. The history should also include any appropriate and related laboratory results and any adverse sequelae.
   d. Medication history: The health history should include a complete list of current medications including doses and frequency. Note any over-the-counter medications and nutritional supplements. Any allergic reactions or adverse symptoms experienced from medication use should be recorded. Details regarding the type of reaction (e.g., hives, rash, shortness of breath) should be noted.
   e. Immunizations: The nurse must ascertain if the patient can recall or has documentation of childhood illnesses and immunizations. The patient's history of completion of all adult immunizations (i.e., diphtheria/tetanus, pneumococcal pneumonia) should be noted. Any allergic or sensitivity reactions to vaccines should be identified. Because hepatitis and HIV coinfection are increasing in prevalence and can contribute to the overall morbidity, careful attention should be paid to obtaining an accurate history of the patient's hepatitis A, B, and C status and the need for vaccinations.
   f. Family history: The nurse should obtain a complete family history if possible. Long-term treatment of HIV infection is associated with many comorbid conditions, and care should be taken to assess for cancer, diabetes, cardiac disease, rheumatoid disease, renal disease, and other metabolic or endocrine conditions. Additionally a complete mental health and psychiatric history of the patient should be obtained. A complete health database is especially important as people with HIV live longer lives. It is important to continue age-appropriate health

maintenance activities, such as colon cancer screening and mammography as appropriate.

g. Social history

i. Sexual history: A thorough sexual history is important to assess for ongoing risk factors of STIs and reexposure to HIV that might confer resistance to current treatment. The nurse should ask if the patient is sexually active and if he or she is having sex with men, women, or both. The patient's understanding of safer sex should be ascertained to determine risk-reduction education needs and to prevent further HIV transmission. Does the patient participate in other high-risk activities, such as sharing needles, tattooing, or sharing of razors? Is the patient in a monogamous relationship or does he or she have multiple sexual partners?

ii. Needle and blood exposure: Although all donor blood is screened for HIV and hepatitis B and C, the patient's history of blood or blood-product transfusions should be documented (the dates and reasons for transfusion should be recorded). The nurse should assess the patient's knowledge and need for education on needle safety and for implementation of any harm-reduction activities, such as needle exchange.

iii. Tobacco use: The patient's history of tobacco use should be discussed, and if the patient is currently smoking cigarettes, the nurse should assess the patient's desire to quit and advise the patient to stop smoking. If the patient wishes to stop smoking, appropriate interventions should be determined. Additional educational needs about the risk of smoking should also be explored.

iv. Alcohol use: The patient's alcohol use should be assessed, and the nurse should ascertain whether there is a history of alcohol abuse.

A useful tool for screening is the CAGE alcohol assessment (Bickley, 2003). The following four questions should be asked: (1) Do you ever feel you should Cut down on drinking? (2) Do you get Angry at others' criticism of your drinking? (3) Do you feel Guilty about your drinking? and (4) Do you ever need an Eye opener to get going? A positive response to two or more questions indicates a need for further assessment.

v. Drug use: The patient's use of mood-altering substances should be assessed. The types of drugs or substances and length of use should be documented. The nurse should explore whether the patient's use of such drugs or substances has altered their ability to perform activities of daily living, interfered with his or her responsibilities, or increased risk-taking behaviors (i.e., unsafe sexual practices). The nurse should also explore and document attempts to stop drug use, including interventions used and reasons for relapse into using behaviors.

vi. Health insurance: The nurse should assess the patient's health insurance resources and coverage. The nurse can assess whether the patient needs assistance with referrals to social services or supplemental programs, such as the AIDS Drug Assistance Program (ADAP), Medicare, or Medicaid.

vii. Travel: The patient's travel history and plans should be explored to assess whether there are risks for exposure to any opportunistic infections or a need for vaccinations or prophylactic medications for communicable disease. The nurse should also explore whether the patient requires any health education related to travel, such as safe drinking water and hygiene precautions.

viii. Exercise and sleep: The patient's sleep pattern and habits should be assessed to ensure that they are getting adequate rest. If the patient is experiencing sleep disturbances, causes of the problem should be explored as well as appropriate interventions. The patient's exercise routine should also be discussed to ensure that they have an appropriate outlet for stress and an adequate amount of activity for their age, gender, and general state of health.

ix. Pets: The nurse should determine whether there are any pets in the patient's environment and if the pets have received recommended vaccinations. The facilities for pet hygiene and the patient's need for education about animal health should be explored (i.e., wearing face mask for cat litter box care).

x. Occupational history: The patient's current and past occupations should be discussed to assess whether there are any occupation-related health problems, (i.e., injuries, risks or problems associated with exposure to occupational hazards). Use of protective equipment and gear should be reviewed.

xi. Nutrition history: The patient's eating habits should be assessed and resources to meet nutritional needs, adequate food storage, preparation facilities, and dietary restrictions, food allergies, or intolerances should be determined. The patient's nutritional concerns or educational needs should also be explored; an HIV-knowledgeable dietician would be an appropriate resource referral.

xii. Women's health: The patient's obstetrics and gynecological history should be discussed. Previous records should be obtained when available to review all pertinent women's health examinations, procedures, and laboratory tests. Additional information should be obtained regarding obstetrics history (e.g., gravida and para status) and any contraceptive needs and education.

3. Review of systems (ROS) is completed at entry to the health care system and at the initial evaluation (Bickley, 2003). Care should be taken to ensure for patient privacy and comfort with the interview. The ROS should include, but is not limited to, a review of the following:

- General appearance, energy level, fatigue, weight changes, and acute complaints
- Skin ulcerations or lesions, itching, healing problems, alopecia, nail changes, and dryness
- Head: injuries, headaches; ears: hearing problems, pain, discharge, vertigo; eyes: blurred vision, floaters, pain, acuity problems, history of eye surgery or other conditions, last eye exam; nose/sinuses: drainage, nosebleeds, stuffiness, pain, injury; throat/mouth: gum sensitivity, bleeding, oral lesions or pain, last dental exam, difficult or painful swallowing
- Respiratory system: shortness of breath, dyspnea at rest or on exertion, sputum (color), wheezing, history of lung infection other disease, last chest X-ray; breast: lumps, pain, nipple discharge, last mammogram
- Cardiovascular system: elevated blood pressure, chest pain, palpitations, murmurs, orthopnea, pedal edema, calf tenderness, paroxsysmal nocturnal dyspnea (PND)
- Gastrointestinal system: nausea, vomiting, diarrhea, constipation, melena, flatulance/bloating, hemorrhoids, rectal bleeding, abdominal pain, irregular bowel habits, mucus in stools, history of gastrointestinal disorders (gallbladder, hepatic, or pancreatic problems), diagnostic work-ups (sigmoidoscopy, occult blood testing, colonoscopy)
- Genitourinary system: dysuria, nocturia, burning, frequency, urgency, incontinence, hematuria, pain, urinary infections or stones, STIs, erectile dysfunction (males), inorgasma (women), sexual interest and practices (safer sex assessment); gynecologic system: menstrual cycle, contraception

history and use, discharge, dysuria, gravida/para status, abortion history

- Musculoskeletal system: myalgias, arthralgias, joint swelling or redness, injury or history of fractures
- Neurological system: syncope, headaches, seizures, weakness, parasthesias, tremors
- Psychiatric and emotional system: depression, mania, insomnia, panic attacks, anxiety, mood changes/swings, history of mental illness
- Endocrine system: increased thirst, hunger or urination, hot flashes, cold spells, skin changes, temperature sensitivity
- Hematopoietic: fatigue, shortness of breath, bruising or bleeding, transfusion history

4. Physical examination should be completed in entirety at baseline. Ensure privacy and comfort as complete disrobing of the patient for a full evaluation is required. The complete exam should include the following:

- General examination: Include weight, height, and vital signs.
- Skin examination: Look for evidence of seborrheic dermatitis, Kaposi's sarcoma, folliculitis, fungal infections, psoriasis, and dermatological manifestations of hepatitis C, such as prurigo nodularis.
- Head, ears, eyes, nose, and throat examination (includes a complete assessment of the mouth and oral cavity): Fundoscopic examination is essential in patient with advanced HIV disease. It may be appropriate to refer to ophthalmologist for a detailed examination. The oropharynx should be examined for evidence of oropharyngeal candidiasis.
- Lymphatic system: Generalized adenopathy may be present in acute HIV infection. Localized adenopathy or splenomegaly may be a sign of infection or malignancy.
- Respiratory/thoracic examination: Include breast exam.
- Cardiovascular examination: Include peripheral vascular assessment.
- Abdominal examination

- Musculoskeletal examination
- Neurological examination includes a general assessment of cognitive function. Emphasis should be placed on gait, motor, vibratory, and sensory examinations because these may be altered in patients with distal sensory polyneuropathy.
- Genitourinary examination male/female: Conduct rectal, prostate, and pelvic examinations at baseline and as indicated/recommended. Carefully examine the anogenital area for evidence of STDs, such as condyloma or herpes lesions.

5. Laboratory and diagnostic evaluation: The following laboratory tests should be obtained at the baseline assessment. Previous results should be obtained to assess for clinically significant changes.

- Immunology profile (CD_4/CD_8 absolute and percent cell counts); HIV viral load testing (HIV polymerase chain reaction or branched DNA); complete blood count (CBC); multichemistry panel (fasting), including lipids, triglycerides, cholesterol, and glucose; urinalysis with microscopic; pregnancy testing and Papanicolaou (Pap) smear, if indicated; venereal disease research laboratory (VDRL) or rapid plasma regain (RPR); gonorrhea/chlamydia cultures, if clinically indicated
- Tuberculin skin testing (TST) should be completed if the patient has not had a positive test in the past. If the patient has a history of a positive TST, an assessment of isoniazid treatment and a baseline chest X-ray should be obtained.
- The following testing should be obtained if not previously done or if records are not available:

  – Hepatitis A antibody; hepatitis B surface antigen, surface antibody, and core antibody; hepatitis C antibody

  – Toxoplasmosis, cytomegalovirus, and varicella antibody testing

  – Glucose-6-phosphate dehydrogenase level (G6PD) to ensure there are no contraindications with medications, such as Septra, which may be used as prophylaxis or treatment for opportunistic infections

- Immunizations as indicated and recommended
- Resistance testing if indicated; consider if newly or recently infected patient.

2.2 Immunizations

1. Vaccine administration and patient education about vaccine preventable diseases (VPDs) are important nursing activities in contemporary HIV/AIDS nursing.
2. Persons with profound immunodeficiency may have impaired humoral response and may not respond to vaccines with the usual adult doses. It may be necessary to require supplemental doses to demonstrate serological evidence of protection from disease (Salvato & Thompson, 1999).
3. Live vaccines are associated with active replication of the bacteria or virus and generally should not be administered to those with severe immune deficiency. MMR (measles-mumps-rubella vaccine) is the only live vaccine recommended for persons with HIV infection who do not have immunity.
4. Vaccine preventable diseases
   a. Measles, mumps, and rubella
      i. Measles, mumps, and rubella are three separate viral conditions that generally result in an acute systemic viral illness. Today, because of the success of childhood vaccination, complications from disease are rare.
      ii. The MMR vaccine is commonly administered in childhood. Immunity is considered lifelong and can be demonstrated by antibody testing. Adults born before 1957 are considered immune.
      iii. One dose is recommended for those born in 1957 or later, if that person has not been previously vaccinated (a second dose of MMR may be required). The vaccine is given as a 0.5 ml subcutaneous (SC) injection.
      iv. The vaccine is relatively contraindicated in patients who are severely immune compromised (CD_4 percentage < 14) or receiving high doses of prednisone.
      v. Fever and rash are the most common side effects associated with this vaccine. Arthralgia and joint symptoms are reported in 25% of women and are attributed to the rubella component. Pregnant women should not receive the vaccine. Persons with a history of anaphylaxis to neomycin should not receive the rubella vaccine.
   b. Haemophilus influenzae type B
      i. Haemophilus influenzae (Hib) is a bacterium that can cause a whole host of diseases that include, but are not limited to, meningitis, sepsis, epiglottis, pneumonia, and osteomyelitis. Bacterial infections with Hib commonly occur in children under the age of 5 and rarely cause disease in adults.
      ii. The role of vaccination for Hib in the HIV-infected adult has not been clearly established and is not currently recommended in routine vaccination. The Advisory Committee on Immunization Practices (ACIP), however, recommends that this vaccine be considered in adults with HIV infection (Centers for Disease Control and Prevention, 1993).
      iii. The following Hib vaccines are available: ProHIBiT, HibTITER, PedvaxHIB, ActHib, and OmniHIB. Unvaccinated adults should receive one dose of one type of vaccine mentioned here. The recommended dosage is 0.5 ml, given as an intramuscular (IM) injection.
      iv. Vaccine is considered safe. Swelling, redness, and pain at the injection site are the most common problems.
   c. Influenza
      i. Influenza is a viral illness contracted by direct contact with or inhalation of droplets. There are

three subtypes of the influenza virus: influenza A, influenza B, and influenza C. Influenza A commonly affects adults and can cause a severe viral illness. Influenza B and C rarely affect adults.

ii. Influenza vaccine should be offered to all HIV-infected adults annually between September and mid-November. It is most effective when it proceeds 2 months prior to the influenza season, which, in the United States, is December. In some cases, the vaccine can be administered up to 4 months after the influenza season.

iii. Patients with severe immune deficiency ($CD_4 < 100$ cell/mm^3) may have a poor antibody response to the vaccine, providing them with little or no protection. A second dose does not improve response (Kroon, van Dissel, de Jong, & Furth, 1994).

iv. There are two types of vaccines available: whole and split vaccines. Whole-virus vaccines are prepared by using chick embryos. HIV patients can receive whole or split vaccines. Dosage is 0.5 ml given by IM injection.

v. Rare allergic reactions can occur in patients allergic to eggs and who receive the whole-virus vaccine; thus, vaccination should be deferred in patients who have a documented or self-identified allergic reaction to eggs. Split-virus vaccines are prepared using organic solvents or detergents, and reaction to one of these components is rare. These vaccines can be used by people with egg allergies.

vi. Local reactions at the injection site, such as erythema, pain, and induration, can occur following vaccine administration. Nonspecific symptoms, including fever, chills, and myalgias, are reported in less than 1% of vaccine recipients and usually occur in individuals with no previous exposure to viral antigens in the vaccine (Centers for Disease Control and Prevention, 2002b).

vii. Vaccines are prepared annually and are formulated based on the suspected circulating strain. Effectiveness of the vaccine is determined by how close the vaccine matches the circulating influenza strains. Therefore, the nurse should inform the recipient that influenza could occur despite vaccination. Because of the potential for a viral illness to occur despite vaccination, the nurse should provide the patient with instructions on how to care for oneself during a viral illness. This includes information regarding the importance of bed rest and hydration, especially when febrile. Gargling with and drinking warm fluids, such as teas, will soothe the sore throat that accompanies illness, and using aspirin or Tylenol, if not contraindicated, will help relieve fever and myalgias.

d. Pneumococcal pneumonia

i. Pneumococcal pneumonia is a disease caused by the *streptococcus pneumonia* bacteria and is a common cause of hospital admission and a major cause of mortality in HIV disease.

ii. Pneumococcal vaccine (Pneumovax 23, Pnu-Immune 23) is administered as a 0.5 ml IM or SC injection. HIV-infected patients should be vaccinated 5 years after their initial dose.

(1) Protection from the vaccine does not occur until 2 to 3 weeks after injection. Inform the patient that illness can occur during this period. Teach the patient how to protect from infection through such techniques as good hand washing.

(2) Inform the patient that vaccination does not confer immunity from pneumococcal disease. At best, the vaccine

has a protective efficacy of approximately 60% (U.S. Department of Health and Human Services, 1998).

(3) The vaccine is considered safe; however, the recipient may complain of some mild pain at the injection site.

e. Hepatitis
   i. Hepatitis is inflammation of the liver. Vaccines exist only for hepatitis A and B.
   ii. Prevaccination serologic testing
   iii. Hepatitis A vaccine
      (1) The two licensed vaccines are HAVRIX and VAQTA. The recommended HAVRIX adult dose is 1,440 EL.U per 0.5 ml. The adult dose of VAQTA is 50 units in 1.0 ml. The recommended schedule for vaccination is at 0 months and then 6–12 months. Both vaccines are given as IM injections. Hepatitis A is also licensed as Twinrix in combination with hepatitis B. When this vaccine is administered, the recommended schedule is 0, 1, and 6 months.
      (2) The vaccine prompts an antibody response in only about 75% of HIV-positive patients, compared with 95% of the general population (Kemper et al., 2001).
      (3) Injection site pain, erythema, or swelling is reported in 20% to 50% of recipients. These symptoms are generally mild and self-limited.
   iv. Hepatitis B vaccine
      (1) There are two licensed vaccines, Recombivax HB and Engerix-B. Both vaccines can be used interchangeably. However, the nurse should be alerted that, for the immune-compromised patient, the recommended Recombivax dose is 40 mcg in 1 ml and the Engerix-B dose is 40 mcg in 2 ml. The recommended schedule for vaccination is at 0, 1, and 6 months. Hepatitis B is also licensed as Twinrix in combination with hepatitis A. When this vaccine is administered, the recommended schedule is 0, 1, and 6 months.
      (2) The vaccine prompts an antibody response in only about 50% of HIV positive patients. Additional doses may be necessary to achieve an adequate antibody response. The vaccine provides protection from hepatitis B for a period of approximately 10 years (Bonacini, 1992).
      (3) Gluteal injections of hepatitis B vaccine should be avoided because immunogenicity is decreased via this route (Dolan, 1997).
      (4) Postvaccination antibody testing should be performed 30 to 60 days after the last vaccine to determine appropriate response.
      (5) The vaccine is considered safe, but fever and myalgias have been reported. The only known effect is some discomfort at the injection site. Teach the patient that application of heat to the affected area may improve vaccine-associated discomfort.

f. Tetanus-diphtheria (Td)
   i. Tetanus is a serious disease caused by endotoxin produced by the bacillus *Clostridium tetani* that can cause painful spasms of the muscles. Diphtheria is a contagious disease caused by the bacillus *Corynebacterium diphtheriae.*
   ii. Childhood vaccination programs generally administer tetanus in combination with diphtheria (DT or Td) or diphtheria and pertussis (DTP or DTaP). If the HIV-infected adult has never been vaccinated,

they should receive the full childhood series of three injections of Td, at 0 months, the second dose 1 to 2 months later, followed by the third dosage at 6 to 12 months.

   iii. Adults who have received the full childhood series may be protected for life; however, in some adults protective immunity may fall over time. As a result, a booster of Td is recommended every 10 years for adults.

   iv. The recommended adult dosage is 0.5 ml given IM, preferably in the deltoid muscle.

   v. Local reactions at the injection site may occur, such as pain, redness, or induration. Inform the patient that a nodule may be palpable at the injection site for several weeks. The nurse must question the recipient about previous immunization. Patients should not receive the vaccine more than every 10 years. Frequent administration can lead to an exaggerated local reaction called Arthus hypersensitivity reaction. This manifests as a painful swelling from the shoulder to the elbow 2 to 8 hours after injection.

g. Other vaccines

   i. Travel to foreign and exotic areas has become an attractive option for some HIV-infected individuals, and thus vaccination for travel is important to maintain the clients' health abroad.

   ii. Inactivated vaccines (e.g., rabies, cholera, plague, anthrax, Japanese encephalitis vaccines) can be safely administered to the HIV-infected person when required.

   iii. Live travel vaccines (e.g., vaccinia, typhoid, yellow fever, polio) are contraindicated for persons with HIV. Persons at risk for exposure to typhoid fever should be administered an inactivated parenteral typhoid vaccine. When a polio vaccine is required for travel, the inactivated polio vaccine (IPV) is recommended.

2.3 Teaching for Health Promotion, Wellness, and Prevention of Transmission

1. Safer sex

   a. Safer sex may be defined as sexual contact that poses the least risk of sharing potentially infectious body fluids. The safest sex is abstinence.

   b. The Public Health Service recommends condom use, citing studies of serodiscordant couples using latex condoms consistently, which indicate that transmission is substantially reduced under those circumstances (Center for AIDS Prevention Studies, University of California, 1995). Studies in California and Italy showed that condom use can result in "an approximately sevenfold decrease in seroconversions" (Johns Hopkins University, Division of Infectious Disease, AIDS Service, 2002). Concerns that arise with condom use include accessibility, ability to negotiate use with a partner, correct application, maintaining use during sexual activity, proper removal, and possible breakage.

   c. The polyurethane female condom has been found to be effective against a variety of sexually transmitted diseases, including HIV. Advantages of the female condom include the lack of side effects, the ability to attain a condom without assistance from a health care provider, minimal partner negotiation, application before starting sexual activity, comfortable fit, and cleanliness (Gilbert, 1999).

   d. The use of nonoxynol-9 is no longer recommended (Richardson, 2002; Roddy, Zekeng, Ryan, Tamoufé, & Tweedy, 2002). Other microbicidal gels are in development, but none are currently on the market.

2. Pregnancy

   a. Two separate issues arise when an HIV-infected woman becomes pregnant: the risk of transmitting HIV to the infant and the risk of the pregnancy to the health of the mother.

   b. In separate studies in Italy and Seattle, Washington, pregnant HIV-positive women had an adjusted relative risk of developing an AIDS-defining illness that was insignificant, compared with nonpregnant HIV-infected women (Buskin, Diamond, Hopkins, 1998).

c. The risk of vertical transmission is discussed in Section 7.

3. Exercise

a. Wasting used to be the most common nutritional problem in people with HIV infection. Wasting consists of loss of lean muscle mass as well as fat. There are increased caloric requirements in patients with a chronically high viral load.

b. Metabolic abnormalities in people with HIV are becoming increasingly prevalent. The most obvious of these is the syndrome commonly called lipodystrophy or fat redistribution, wherein fat is lost from the extremities and often the face and gained in the intraabdominal space, the breasts, and sometimes in the dorsocervical fat pad (often called the buffalo hump).

c. Maintaining a reasonable weight and lean muscle mass in all Americans is increasingly difficult and no less so for those infected with HIV. The protease inhibitors as a class of drugs has proven to cause weight gain though mostly fat (Strawford et al., 1999).

d. Regular aerobic and weight-training exercise can accomplish several things: reduce fat accumulation, promote production of lean muscle mass, provide for cardiac conditioning, and provide an outlet for stress.

4. Stress management

a. Cortisol and epinephrine are two hormones secreted during periods of high stress. These hormones, once adaptive for the flight or fight response, are now maladaptive. Chronic exposure may be linked to atherosclerotic changes, hypertension, and stroke (Carter-Martin, 2002).

b. Daily relaxation and stress management techniques may help decrease the chronic exposure to stress related hormones. Meditation, yoga, biofeedback, and exercise are some techniques useful for stress management.

c. Recognizing stress is not always easy for individuals. Thus it should be part of a routine assessment to ask patients how they perceive their stress levels and how they are coping. Direct questioning about depression (appetite changes, sleeping patterns, and feelings of guilt or hopelessness), relationships, feelings of anxiety, and drug or alcohol use may indicate a need for stress management (National Institute for Occupational Safety and Health, 2002).

5. Nutrition

a. The nutritional complications of antiretroviral therapy are as challenging as the nutritional problems of untreated HIV infection. Problems such as fat atrophy, fat redistribution, insulin resistance, hyperlipidemias, and mitochondrial dysfunction are much more common now.

b. The genesis of lipodystrophy, or fat redistribution, is still not clear. The use of protease inhibitors (PI) was initially thought to be the cause, but other factors may also have an impact. Combining PIs with nucleoside reverse transcriptase inhibitors have been suggested as the etiology of body habitus changes associated with lipodystrophy. Also implicated are older age and chronic disease, CD_4 nadir, immune reconstitution, comorbidities such as hepatitis C infection, and the individual's basic metabolic function (Kotler, 2002). There is still no conclusive case definition and certainly no effective treatment strategy (Kotler, 2001).

c. Insulin resistance is associated with atherosclerosis and coronary heart disease in non-HIV-infected people. Studies are underway to ascertain if the same is true in people infected with HIV. It has been established that protease inhibitors as a class can cause reversible insulin resistance. Increased visceral adipose is known to increase insulin resistance and is associated with the development of Type II diabetes. A registered dietitian should evaluate patients with abnormal blood sugar levels.

d. Mitochondrial dysfunction is thought to be the cause behind lipodystrophy, peripheral neuropathy, avascular necrosis, and lactic acidosis. Treatment with thiamin and riboflavin may be effective in treating patients with lactic acidosis (McComsey & Lederman, 2002). Making the assumption that use of vitamin therapy is preventative for mitochondrial dysfunction is not proven, but a daily multiple vitamin supplement should be used.

e. Hyperlipidemia, or the increase in total cholesterol, LDL cholesterol, and triglycerides, is associated with the use of protease inhibitors. Decreasing fat intake and increasing complex carbohydrates may control hyperlipidemias to some extent, as will increased intake of omega-3 fatty acids. Often treatment with fenofibrates or statins is indicated.

f. Nutrition status is a predictor of survival and plays a role in slowing disease progression. Malnutrition is related to adverse outcomes.

g. Of all people with AIDS, 88% are considered malnourished. Anorexia, malabsorption, infection, or lack of access to food may cause compromised nutrition.

h. Wasting is defined as involuntary weight loss of > 10% of baseline weight, plus chronic diarrhea $\geq$ 2 loose stools/day for $\geq$ 30 days (Fenton, 1999). About 18–20% of people with AIDS are also diagnosed with wasting syndrome.

i. Death may occur when lean body mass (LBM) loss reaches 54% of normal body weight or when weight loss is equivalent to 66% of ideal body weight.

j. Nutritional intervention is indicated at the time of HIV diagnosis.

k. Dietary changes are difficult for patients to make and require repeated teaching sessions. Evaluation by a registered dietitian is key in this process. Evaluation and intervention must include assessment in the context of the patient's ethnic, social, and economic circumstances.

6. Hand washing
   a. Hand washing is the single most important way to stop the spread of infection. Hands should be washed several times a day and before eating, after using the toilet, after cleaning up small children, and after handling pets.
   b. Hand washing technique is simple. Use of any soap is fine, although many prefer liquid soap. Antibacterial soap is not recommended because it may only serve to wipe out normal flora and leave resistant organisms behind. Hands should be wet with water, and lather should be created using friction that contacts all parts of the hand, including between the fingers and on wrists. Jewelry should be left on, so it can be washed as well. Careful and thorough rinsing is key as is thorough drying using a clean towel or paper towel.

7. Food and water safety
   a. Food-borne illness of microbial origin is the most serious food safety problem in the United States (Food and Drug Administration, 1999). The danger is increased if immune suppression from HIV is present.
   b. Food-and water-borne infections include but are not limited to salmonella, campylobacter, listeria, cryptosporidium, E. coli (enteropathogenic and enterotoxigenic, O157:H7/enterohemorrhagic), and shigella.
   c. Patients should be taught basic food safety and be given written instructions or instructed in how to seek teaching materials on the Internet. A useful link with full explanations for consumers is http://www.cfsan.fda.gov/~mow/intro.html.
   d. Basic instructions for food safety include the following:

   - Cook all meat and poultry until no longer pink in the middle. If using a thermometer, cook poultry until it is 185°, other meats until 165°.
   - Cook fish until flaky (not rubbery).
   - Wash hands carefully after touching any raw meat.
   - Thoroughly wash any utensils, knives, countertops and cutting boards after handling raw meat, using hot, soapy water.

- Do not let meat, poultry, or fish stay out of the refrigerator or freezer for more than 15 min. Cook immediately or place in refrigerator.
- Never eat unpasteurized dairy products.
- Never eat raw or undercooked (runny) eggs or food that contains raw eggs (such as classic Caesar salad, hollandaise, or uncooked dough or batters).
- Carefully wash all fruits and vegetables, especially alfalfa sprouts and tomatoes.
- Pay attention to the dates on fresh foods when shopping. Be sure that the sell-by date has not passed.
- Make sure packaging is intact. Bag meat and poultry separately to avoid dripping of juices onto other groceries.

  e. Water-borne illnesses are of concern to people infected with HIV. Because tap water in some areas is not safe, patients may need to boil or filter water or buy bottled water to drink and make ice cubes. Filtration at home is rarely effective enough to remove serious pathogens, and bottled water is often just expensive water that is no more pure than tap water.
  f. To kill possible pathogens, water must be boiled for at least 1 min. To restore some of the taste, filtering may be helpful after the water has cooled.

8. Skin and hair care
   a. The skin is the largest organ in the body, and it is first line of defense. Commonsense approaches to skin care need to be supplemented by the understanding of practices that may be more risky in people with HIV than in those who are not infected.
   b. Body art is becoming more common. The three most common types are tattoos, piercing, and branding. In all populations, tattoos are associated with neoplasms, and piercing is associated with transmission of hepatitis B and C. Branding puts the recipient at great risk for infection. None of these practices is regulated by any governing body, and

there are no assurances that the people who perform these services are trained in aseptic technique or even basic levels of hygiene (Greif & Hewitt, 1998). Therefore, it is wise to caution people with HIV regarding these procedures.

9. Mouth care (New York State Department of Health, 2001)
   a. Oral hygiene is important in reducing possible sources of infection and maintaining the integrity of teeth and gums. Patients should be encouraged to see a dentist at least annually and to have professional scalings at least twice a year. Twice-daily brushing and daily flossing are recommended. For more information about oral health, refer to the section about gum disease and periodontitis.
   b. Oral hairy leukoplakia (OHL) causes a whitish scale to form on the tongue, usually on the sides, and is caused by a virus. Excessive brushing will not help to remove it and may cause pain and bleeding. The same is true of oral candidiasis, commonly called thrush, which is a fungal overgrowth of normal oral flora and must be treated with medication. Oral hygiene has little impact on reducing thrush and can often cause bleeding and pain when mechanically removed.
   c. Angular chelitis, characterized by cracking, pain, and sometimes bleeding from the corners of the mouth, is a fungal infection complicated by inflammation. It can be treated using antifungal creams or antifungal-steroid creams. Any underlying oral candidiasis needs to be treated as well. Prevention includes good oral hygiene and keeping lips (especially the corners) moisturized with an oily barrier lip balm.
   d. Apthous ulcers can be very painful. Rinsing with diluted baking soda solution may be helpful. There are over-the-counter mouth rinses available (e.g., UlcerEase). If apthous ulcers are persistent, multiple, or especially long lasting, the use of Kenalog in orabase (triamcinolone in a thick paste that adheres to mucous membranes) may be prescribed by the patient's provider.

e. Herpes simplex virus (HSV), often called cold sores, causes oral and perioral blisters that rupture and crust over and can be painful. HSV activity is increased in sunlight. Treatment ranges from topical over-the-counter remedies to systemic treatment with acyclovir.

f. Oral Kaposi sarcoma can manifest in varying severities: from a slight shadow on the oral mucosa to a huge space-occupying lesion on the gums, palate, or anywhere else in the mouth. Correction of high-HIV viremia and increasing CD_4 count can cause lesions to recede, but if that is not possible, then chemotherapy (either systemic or by local, intralesional injection) is often an option.

10. Pet care

a. HIV-infected people do not have to give up their pets, but because pets may carry illnesses that affect the immune-compromised person, some caution must be taken when caring for and interacting with pets (USPHS/IDSA, 2001). In general, people with compromised immune systems should avoid caring for sick animals.

b. Pets should be fed pet food or thoroughly cooked meat. Care should be taken to keep pets from eating other animals' feces.

c. Avoidance of animal feces is another caution, so using gloves when scooping feces and proper hand washing afterwards should be taught.

d. Cats may carry toxoplasmosis. Disposable gloves should be worn when changing the litter box, and hands should be properly washed afterwards. Immune-compromised patients should be careful to avoid being scratched to prevent exposure to Bartonella infection, so keeping a cat's claws clipped is important. If scratched or bitten, the wound should be immediately washed with warm water and soap and advice sought from the person's medical provider. A strictly indoor cat is less of a risk than a cat who goes outside and may hunt and eat raw meat.

e. Dogs should not be allowed to drink from the toilet or eat other animals' feces. Control of fleas is key to avoid risk of Bartonella.

f. Birds may carry *mycobacterium avium intracellulare, cryptoccoccus neoforms, psittacosis,* or *histoplasma capsulatum.* Usually healthy birds are not a problem but care must be taken when cleaning cages.

g. Reptiles may carry salmonella. Gloves should be worn when caring for aquariums, which may harbor *mycobacterium marinum,* and proper hand washing should follow.

11. Alcohol

a. The problems associated with alcohol involve its overuse in most cases, although there is some evidence that even moderate alcohol intake can interact with medications and complicate existing liver problems, such as hepatitis B and C.

b. One study from the Johns Hopkins School of Medicine suggests that increased alcohol use was associated with decreased medication adherence, increased HIV ribonucleic acid (RNA) levels and decreased CD_4 counts (Lucas, Gebo, Cahisson, & Moore, 2002).

c. In another study, the use of alcohol in women who were also using drugs resulted in increased incidence of unsafe sex (Rees, Saitz, Hortom, & Samet, 2001).

d. Patients who start antiretroviral therapy may be at risk for liver toxicity if they drink alcohol and have hepatitis C or B (Nunez, Lana, Mendoza, Martin-Carbonero, & Soriano, 2001).

e. Simian models suggest that chronic exposure to alcohol in simian immunodeficiency virus infected animals caused a decrease in production of a pulmonary protective cytokine (Stolz et al., 2002) and a decrease in polymorphonuclear leukocytes (Stolz et al., 1999).

12. Tobacco (Kirton, 2001b)

a. Pre-HAART data suggest that patients with AIDS who smoke are more at risk for oral thrush and an accelerated form of pulmonary emphysema than are HIV-negative people.

b. Data regarding the effect of cigarette smoking on clinical HIV in the post-HAART are lacking.

c. The known association of smoking with respiratory illnesses is enough to promote cessation as part of routine health care.

13. Drug use (including harm reduction)

a. The use of illicit drugs for people infected with HIV is a complicated issue. Most mood-altering substances are disinhibiting and cause people to engage in activity that normally better judgment might prevent. These actions include unprotected sex, which contributes to the spread of HIV and other sexually transmitted diseases. In addition, injection drug use, when injection equipment is shared, increases the risk of transmitting hepatitis and strains of HIV that the patient may not already have.

b. Illicit drugs are also mainly metabolized by the liver, as are most anti-HIV medications, and little is known about the pharmacokinetic interactions of antiretrovirals and street or party drugs (Gerber et al., 2001).

c. People are often unwilling or unable to give up using drugs, and for them the concept of harm reduction is key. Harm reduction includes any activity that makes actions even slightly safer. One of the most important harm reduction ploys is needle exchange. The use of sterile needles has been proven to prevent HIV and hepatitis C and B transmission and to decrease exposure to other pathogens that cause illness in injecting drug users (Gunn et al., 1998).

14. Travel

a. Traveling for people with HIV infection requires planning. Even within the United States, people who take medication need to be prepared to carry all their prescribed medications. It is also a good precaution to have the name of an HIV specialist in the area one plans to visit in case something unexpected arises.

b. Travel to developing countries can be somewhat more complicated. It is best to contact the World Health Organization or the Centers for Disease Control and Prevention (Centers for Disease Control and Prevention, 2002a) to see which vaccinations are required for the area to be visited. Some vaccinations are not safe for people with impaired immunity.

c. Other health maintenance issues are food and water safety. Water safety includes swimming because it is probable that one will swallow a small amount of water when swimming.

d. Mosquitoes can be a great nuisance, but they are also vectors of serious diseases that may be complicated by a compromised immune system. It is important to avoid being stung by using insect repellent containing DEET. The admittedly better-smelling insect repellents such as Avon's Skin So Soft are not effective.

e. While traveling, people should avoid the following:

- Raw vegetables and fruit that one cannot peel, including almost all salads
- Raw or undercooked seafood or meat
- Unpasteurized dairy products
- Tap water
- Drinks with ice made from tap water
- Swimming in water where animals bathe

f. People who travel should remember the following:

- Take a full supply of all medications and put them in carry-on luggage.
- Take a list of medications and a brief health history.
- Take a prescription for an antidiarrhea medication and an antibiotic, such as Ciprofloxin, which is often prescribed for travelers' diarrhea.

15. Adjunctive therapies

a. The use of complementary or alternative forms of treating illness has increased in the general population in the last several years. In people with HIV infection, alternative approaches were virtually the only options for treatment for many years, prior to the development of effective combination antiretrovirals. Thus the use of adjunctive therapy has a long history in the health care of people with HIV. It is estimated that the use of such alternatives in people with HIV ranges from 30–80% (Duggan, Peterson, Schutz, Khuder, & Charkraborty, 2001). Alternative therapies are often recommended for stress management.

b. Alternative or complementary approaches may be defined as anything that is not generally provided in Western medical clinics and hospitals and may include such diverse treatments as chiropractic services, massage therapy, herbs, homeopathics, meditation, traditional Chinese medicine (TCM), and exercise.

c. The goal of alternative and complementary approaches is usually symptom relief. More recently, those wishing to find relief from common side effects of antiretroviral therapy have used alternative therapy. These side effects include fat redistribution, hyperlipidemias, and peripheral neuropathy (Swanson, Keithley, Zeller, & Cronin-Stubbs, 2000). Some of the therapies tried include Cholestin and garlic. There are no randomized studies that prove or disprove the effectiveness of these adjunctive therapies.

d. There is little pharmacokinetics data on the interaction of most antiretroviral medications and herbs. The issue of St. John's Wort (hypericin) and its effect on indinavir (Crixivan) was a problem that did not emerge for some time after the two medications were given together. Herbs are often very active pharmaceutically, and there is less clinical trial data and no Food and Drug Administration regulation to protect the consumer.

e. The cost of alternative therapy needs consideration as well. Most alternative or complementary therapy is not covered by insurance.

f. Consumers of alternatives need to be aware of the importance of getting reliable advice. The Internet, which is often used for looking up the newest information, is not regulated. One pilot study showed that anyone can claim anything and not always what is in the best interest of a person with HIV infection (Schmidt & Ernst, 2002). It may be useful to compile a list of Web sites that contain reliable information.

g. Nurses in HIV/AIDS care are often asked to assist patients to make informed decisions about integrating alternative therapies into their overall health care. Safety, efficacy, and cost are the main issues to be considered when choosing from the wide variety of options. There is more literature emerging about this topic, and it is useful to keep up with the most current information available. Finding practitioners of alternative therapies who are knowledgeable about HIV and common Western treatments may make combining the standard and alternative approaches safer and more effective.

2.4 Health Care Follow-Up

1. Frequency of follow-up visits and laboratory monitoring depends on the patient's overall status and immune function (Bartlett & Gallant, 2001).

   a. Asymptomatic patients with viral load and CD_4 counts that have remained stable can be seen every 3 to 6 months for routine follow-up care.

   b. Individuals who have had a change in antiretroviral therapy, new clinical symptoms, breakthrough in a previously stable viral load, or a CD_4 count trending downward to below 200, or a CD_4 percentage below 14% will need follow-up on a monthly basis until their condition stabilizes.

2. Laboratory parameters evaluated during routine follow-up visits are used to assess immune function, response to antiretroviral treatment, disease progression, drug toxicities, and evidence of opportunistic infections, new infections, or both. Additional laboratory data are collected for routine health care maintenance according to patient's age and risk profile. Frequency will increase in the presence of concerns regarding drug toxicity, viral breakthrough,

adherence, or a change in the patient's status (Bartlett & Gallant, 2001).

a. The CD_4 and CD_8 cell absolute and percentage parameters determine immunologic integrity and are evaluated every 3 to 6 months. They are repeated more frequently (e.g., every 2 to 4 weeks), if results vary from previous trends, during a change in drug therapy, or if levels approach those recommended for initiating or changing treatment (Kirton, 2001a). CD_4 counts < 50 cells/mm^3 do not require more frequent monitoring unless in the presence of monitoring antiretroviral response. The absolute count can vary considerably, even on separate specimens obtained on the same day. The CD_4 percentage is less variable than the absolute count and hence a more stable marker of immune integrity (Bartlett & Gallant, 2001; Kirton, 2001a). It is important to teach patients that the percentage and absolute counts are used when evaluating their results.

b. The viral load (VL) quantifies viral particles in the serum and is used as a measure of antiretroviral effectiveness. Many health care providers and patients have undetectable VL as a therapy goal. Ultrasensitive tests can detect viral particles down to < 50 copies/ml. When ultrasensitive tests are not available, a test that detects viral particles to < 400 copies/ml is performed. VL can be measured using either branched chain DNA (bDNA) or HIV RNA PCR methodologies. Consistency of type of test should be maintained to avoid misinterpretation of level of viremia. Concurrent illness or recent immunization can temporarily increase VL, and results should be interpreted accordingly (Kirton, 2001a).

c. A complete blood count (CBC) with differential is performed along with the CD_4 count. The CBC monitors for anemia, thrombocytopenia, and other blood dyscrasias.

d. Blood chemistry testing includes, but is not limited to, evaluation of the levels of serum creatinine, blood urea nitrogen, bicarbonate, sodium, chloride, and glucose. These measures as well as others evaluate renal, endocrine, and metabolic functions.

e. Monitor liver functions, especially aminotransferases for individuals on hepatotoxic drugs (some protease inhibitors and nonnucleoside reverse transcriptase inhibitors), infected with hepatotrophic viruses, on lipid lowering agents, and those with alcohol abuse.

f. Monitor lipid profiles, such as total cholesterol, triglycerides, high-density lipoproteins (HDL), and low-density lipoproteins (LDL), at least every 3 to 4 months, especially in patients on protease inhibitors and nonnucleoside reverse transcriptase inhibitors. These drugs can cause dangerous increases in lipid levels, leading to pancreatitis and early coronary artery disease (Bartlett & Gallant, 2001).

g. Tuberculin skin testing should be done annually on patients with previous negative results and who are at risk for tuberculosis. Positive results for HIV patients include any induration of 5 mm or greater. False negatives may occur in patients with depressed CD_4 counts (Bartlett & Gallant, 2001; Talotta, 2001b).

h. Annual Papanicolaou (Pap) test from a cervical sample is recommended for routine health care maintenance in HIV-infected women. The CDC recommends a Pap smear every 6 months the 1st year after diagnosis, then annually if results are normal (Centers for Disease Control and Prevention, 2002d). Some women may need more frequent screening (e.g., those with human papilloma virus (HPV) , advanced degree of immune suppression, and risk factors for new acquisition of any sexually transmitted infection). Women with symptomatic HIV or CD_4 < 400 cells/mm^3 should be checked every 6 months. Atypical squamous cells of undetermined significance (ASCUS), or low-grade squamous intraepithelial lesion (LGSIL) results require repeat Pap every 4 to 6 months. Colposcopy is recommended for women with abnormal Paps, with treatment as appropriate. Repeat Pap every 3 to 4 months following treatment of preinvasive lesions (Talotta, 2001a).

i. There is increasing yet insufficient evidence to implement into guidelines the performance of anal Pap smears on men and women who have had evidence of genital HPV or history of anal intercourse (Bartlett & Gallant, 2001; Centers for Disease Control and Prevention, 2002d).

j. Sexually transmitted infection testing is recommended annually or more frequently, depending on risk behaviors (Bartlett & Gallant 2001; Kirton, 2001d). This should include a VDRL (Venereal Disease Research Laboratory)/RPR (rapid plasma reagin) test and gonorrhea and chlamydia screening.

k. Serology testing for *Toxoplasmosis gondii* should occur annually for previously negative patients whose CD_4 drops below 100 cells/mm^3 (Bartlett & Gallant, 2001; Winson, 2001).

l. Additional testing and screening depends on patient history and presentation. Ongoing attention should be paid to age-appropriate routine health maintenance and screening, such as mammography, completion of vaccination series and annual flu shots, flexible sigmoidoscopy or colonoscopy, and prostate specific antigen levels.

3. Return visits for HIV follow-up will be built on the previously established relationships within the clinic setting. A comprehensive approach will facilitate building trust between the patient and the health care provider.

a. Health history taking and physical exam at follow-up visits involves exploration of any new chief complaint and a focused review of systems. Differential diagnosis of chief complaint may be guided by immune function.

b. Behavioral history taking should explore medication adherence, current mood, sexual risk behaviors, and tobacco, alcohol, and drug use. The clinician should pay particular attention to new over-the-counter medications, herbal remedies, vitamin and nutriceutical supplements, and

therapies prescribed outside of their particular clinic setting.

c. Social history taking includes current travel and living arrangements, availability and interest in support networks, employment, and eligibility for assistance.

d. Patient teaching should be built on previous visits and patient's willingness to acquire new knowledge. Because HIV disease is now considered a chronic illness, health promotion remains the emphasis at each health care visit. Health promotion teaching for the HIV-infected patient mirrors that of the non-HIV-infected patient.

e. Regular diet and exercise should be emphasized to minimize long-term metabolic changes often seen with antiretroviral therapy.

f. Food safety information should be reviewed with patients regularly. Food-borne illnesses are preventable and a source of opportunistic infections (e.g., *toxoplasmosis*) for the immune-compromised patient (Centers for Disease Control and Prevention, 2002d; Winson, 2001).

g. Review patient knowledge and practice of safer sex regularly (Kirton, 2001c). Emphasize both minimization of the spread of HIV and the acquisition of new and resistant viral strains. Discussion of family planning should be included as part of general health care follow-up.

h. Recommend annual eye exams with an ophthalmologist. Use Amsler eye tests with patients who have $CD_4 < 100$ cells/mm^3 and those with symptomatic vision changes.

i. Recommend twice yearly dental check-ups for cleaning. Encourage ongoing daily flossing and regular brushing to minimize gingivitis. Gum disease can lead to the acquisition of new infections.

2.5 Managing Antiretroviral Therapy

1. The therapeutic use of antiretroviral (ARV) medications requires a thorough understanding of the classes of currently approved drugs, appropriate combinations of classes and specific medications, and

side-effect management issues. Medication monitoring and side-effect management are important facets of general HIV/AIDS nursing. The advanced practice nurse with prescriptive duties must have an even more thorough understanding of these important medication concepts. This section introduces the currently approved medications and the process through which antiretrovirals may be managed. Remember that this chapter provides general, introductory information and that the use of antiretroviral combinations or "cocktails" is a complex skill acquired through knowledge and practice. The reader is cautioned that a more thorough reading about medications and consultation with an HIV-experienced clinician, as a mentor and resource, are necessary to become an expert HIV/AIDS nurse.

2. HIV drug classes

   a. Nucleoside reverse transcriptase inhibitors (NRTIs): These classes of medications inhibit the reproduction of HIV by binding to the enzyme reverse transcriptase (RT). This binding causes disruption of the enzymes' catalytic site, thereby inhibiting transcription of the viral RNA (Deeks & Volberding, 1999). This action effectively stops the formation of proviral DNA and prevents further infection of the CD_4 cell. The first anti-HIV medication to be approved, zidovudine (Retrovir, AZT), is a member of this class of drugs. Others in this class include zalcitabine (Hivid, ddc), didanosine (Videx, ddI), stavudine (Zerit, d4T), lamivudine (Epivir, 3TC), and abacavir (Ziagen, 1592). Several medications (Combivir, Trizivir) are marketed as combinations of these medications. (See Appendix D, which lists the current FDA-approved HIV medications, usual dosing, and common side effects.) Dietary restrictions are also included. A serious and potentially fatal side effect of hyperlactemia or lactic acidosis has been associated with use of this drug class.

   b. Non-nucleoside reverse transcriptase inhibitors (NNRTIs): This class works similarly to NRTIs in that they bind to and prevent the action of reverse transcriptase. Unlike NRTIs, these drugs do not require intracellular phosphorylation to become active. Although these two antiretroviral classes inhibit the same enzyme, there is no evidence for cross-resistance between the classes (Deeks & Volberding, 1999). Drugs in this class include nevirapine (Viramune), delavirdine (Rescriptor), and efavirenz (Sustiva). Rashes are a common side effect to all three medications in this class as are elevations in serum transaminase levels. Additionally, resistance to this class of medications is quite readily developed. These drugs should only be used in combinations with other classes of medications.

   c. Nucleotide reverse transcriptase inhibitor: The most recently approved new medication for HIV treatment is tenofovir (Viread). Although often included in the NRTI class, this medication is really a nucleotide reverse transcriptase inhibitor. This class of medication requires less processing in the body to reach its active form than do NRTIs. Due to its long half-life, this medication need only be taken once per day. This easier dosing schedule may be beneficial to people for whom adherence is an issue. Data on the use of this medication is limited to clinical trials in which tenofovir has been used in salvage therapy (for people with significant previous history of exposure to multiple ARV medications). The data on the use of this medication in ARV-naive clients is still being collected, and therefore its use as a first-line medication is not yet recommended.

   d. Protease inhibitors (PIs): These medications prevent the enzyme protease from cleaving or cutting up the newly formed viral precursor proteins into viral structural proteins and enzymes. This action prevents the production of mature, infectious new virions from the CD_4 cell. When this class of drugs began to be used in combination with other classes, the HIV life cycle was interrupted in two different sites. This disruption was evidenced by significant virological and clinical improvement for many infected people. Approved drugs in this class include saquinavir (Invirase, Fortovase), indinavir mesylate (Crixivan), ritonavir (Norvir), nelfinavir mesylate (Viracept), agenerase (Amprenavir) and lopinavir/ritonavir (Kaletra). These medications often require many pills and frequent dosing. Also, the food and fluid restrictions can be troubling for people taking the medications, and adherence should be monitored closely. Liver transaminase elevations have been associated with the use of these medications and should be monitored closely.

e. Other agents: There are currently a number of medications in clinical trials that exert their effects in other stages of the HIV life cycle. These include fusion inhibitors (T20) and integrase inhibitors. Fusion inhibitors prevent attachment of HIV to the CD_4 cell by inhibiting the harpooning effect of the viral surface protein gp120. Integrase inhibitors prevent the copied viral DNA from becoming part of the host cell (CD_4) genome.

f. Several side effects of antiretrovirals and especially combinations of these medications have been noted. These side effects include such mild effects as transient nausea, headache, diarrhea, and fatigue. However, more serious side effects have been noted. These effects include lactic acidosis, hepatic steatosis, hepatotoxicity, hyperglycemia, fat maldistribution, hyperlipidemia, increased bleeding episodes in people with hemophilia, osteonecrosis, osteopenia, and osteoporosis (U.S. Department of Health and Human Services, 2002). Additionally, a severe skin rash and even fatal Steven Johnson syndrome have been noted. Examination of these adverse effects in detail is beyond the scope of this section. However, the reader is cautioned to learn more about these potentially harmful conditions and the nursing implications involved.

3. Prescription guidelines
   a. Goals of therapy: The U.S. Department of Health and Human Services (DHHS; 2002) guidelines for the use of antiretroviral medications for adults and adolescents define the goals of therapy as 1) maximal and durable suppression of viral load, 2) restoration or preservation of immunologic function, or both, 3) improvement of quality of life, and 4) reduction of HIV-related morbidity and mortality. Furthermore, tools to help the client reach these goals are offered. These tools include 1) maximization of adherence to the antiretroviral regimen, 2) rational sequencing of drugs, 3) preservation of future treatment options, and 4) use of resistance testing in selected clinical settings. Nurses play vital roles in helping to attain and maintain these treatment goals including interventions aimed at improving and maintaining medication adherence, managing HIV and medication-related symptoms, and helping the client to improve overall health. Nurses may also suggest rational and appropriate drug regimens. Advanced practice nurses have the additional responsibility in prescribing appropriately sequenced drug regimens and ordering resistance testing when appropriate.
   b. Risks and benefits of therapy: Prior to starting antiretroviral therapy, the clinician and the client should perform a thorough risk-benefit assessment. Potential risks that must be considered include adverse effects of the medication on quality of life; inconvenience of most of the suppressive regimens, which may also affect adherence and lead to drug resistance; limitation of future drug options due to resistance; and the risk of transmission of resistant strains of HIV. Benefits to therapy, especially early therapy, include early suppression of the virus, preservation of immune function, longer period of disease-free living, and a decrease in the risk of viral transmission. These risks and benefits must also be considered in relation to

Table 2.5a   Recommendations for Therapy in Asymptomatic Individuals

Clinical Category	CD$_4$ Cell Count	Plasma HIV RNA (VL)	Recommendation
Asymptomatic	< 200 cells/mm^3	Any value	Treat
Asymptomatic	> 200 cells/mm^3 but < 350 cells/mm^3	Any value	Treatment should be offered, although controversial.
Asymptomatic	> 350 cells/mm^3	> 55,000 copies/ml	Therapy may be initiated, given that 3-year risk for progression to AIDS is > 30%; therapy may also be deferred and CD$_4$ and VL monitored closely.
Asymptomatic	> 350 cells/mm^3	< 55,000 copies/ml	Therapy may be deferred and condition monitored closely. Other clinicians may suggest starting therapy.

SOURCE: Department of Health and Human Services (2002).

other factors that may be influencing the choice to start medication. These factors include current level of viral activity and immune dysfunction (measured by HIV viral load and CD$_4$ counts, respectively), presence of any symptoms that indicate immune dysfunction (e.g., thrush, recurrent severe herpetic infections) or opportunistic infections (OI) (e.g., pneumocystis carinii pneumonia or PCP) and the client's willingness or readiness to begin and maintain treatment.

c. Readiness to start treatment: One of the most important assessments prior to initiating therapy is determining the willingness and readiness of the client to begin treatment. Readiness should be established prior to writing the first prescription. Part of this assessment includes determining the client's usual lifestyle, daily schedule, and desires for treatment regimen (i.e., ease of dosing vs. strength of regimen). The medication regimen should have the highest potential for viral suppression and must also be acceptable to the client. Long-term strict adherence is required to maintain durable viral suppression (see later section on adherence).

d. Initiating therapy in asymptomatic disease: HIV clinicians differ in opinion regarding the optimal time for starting therapy in the HIV-infected asymptomatic person. Evidence regarding the most advantageous timing is still being collected. However, guidelines do exist. Table 2.5a outlines the DHHS recommendations for starting the asymptomatic person based on CD$_4$ count and viral load. The regimen used should be expected to achieve sustained suppression of plasma HIV RNA, a sustained increase in CD$_4$ cells, and a favorable clinical outcome (i.e., delayed HIV progression). Most commonly, a combination of two NRTIs and a PI or NNRTI is recommended (U.S. Department of Health and Human Services, 2002). Table 2.5b lists the recommendations for initial combinations of medications. Antiretroviral regimens should contain one choice each from columns A and B. Drugs are listed in alphabetical order, not in order of priority. Using ritonavir in a dual PI regimen to boost the plasma concentration of other HIV medications is also frequently seen. These dual PI regimens may lead to decreased pill burden, decreased side effects, and overall improved adherence. When initiating therapy, all drugs should be started simultaneously at full dose. The

Table 2.5b   Recommended Antiretroviral Agents for Initial Treatment

	Column A	Column B
Strongly recommended	Efavirenz Indinavir Nelfinavir Ritonavir + Indinavir Ritonavir + Lopinavir Ritonavir + Saquinavir (SGC or HGC)*	Didanosine + Lamivudine Stavudine + Didanosine Stavudine + Lamivudine Zidovudine + Didanosine Zidovudine + Lamivudine
Recommended as alternatives	Abacavir Amprenavir Delavirdine Nelfinavir + Saquinavir (SGC) Nevirapine Ritonavir Saquinavir- SGC	Zidovudine + Zalcitabine
No recommendation: insufficient data	Hydroxyurea with any ARV Ritonavir + Amprenavir Ritonavir + Nelfinavir Tenofovir	
Not recommended: should not be offered	All monotherapies Saquinavir-HGC (except with Ritonavir)	Stavudine + Zidovudine Zalcitabine + Didanosine Zalcitabine + Lamivudine Zalcitabine + Stavudine

SOURCE: Department of Health and Human Services (2002).

*SGC = soft gel capsules; HGC = hard gel capsules

exception being dose escalation regimens recommended for ritonavir and nevirapine.

e. Initiating therapy in advanced disease: It is recommended that all persons diagnosed with advanced HIV disease should be treated with antiretroviral agents regardless of HIV plasma viremia levels (U.S. Department of Health and Human Services, 2002). Advanced HIV disease is defined as the presence of or having had any condition meeting the 1993 CDC definition of AIDS. Additionally, HIV-infected persons without a diagnosis of AIDS but with symptomatic evidence of immune dysfunction (e.g., thrush, fever, wasting) should also be treated. When initiating HAART during an acute illness or opportunistic infection, the health care provider must consider all factors affecting ability to take a regimen prior to initiating therapy. These factors

include but are not limited to drug toxicity, potential interaction with other OI therapies or medications, ability to adhere to treatment regimens, and laboratory abnormalities. HAART treatment should continue during the occurrence of an OI or malignancy unless drug toxicity, intolerance, or interactions are of concern (U.S. Department of Health and Human Services, 2002). Again, a maximally suppressive regimen, which is acceptable to the client, should be used. Care must be taken when prescribing HAART for the person with AIDS who is on multiple medications. Close assessment for potential interactions with other medications must be undertaken, and dangerous combinations of medications should be avoided.

f. Interruption of therapy: Therapy might be interrupted because of side effects of

Table 2.5c   Criteria for Changing Antiretroviral Therapy

Less than a 0.5–0.75 log reduction in HIV viral load by 4 weeks following initiation of therapy or less than 1 log reduction by 8 weeks

Failure to suppress viral load to undetectable levels within 4–6 months of initiating therapy

Repeated detection of virus in plasma after initial suppression to undetectable levels (suggests resistance)

Any reproducible significant increase, defined as threefold or greater, from the nadir of HIV viral load not attributable to intercurrent infection

Undetectable viremia in the client receiving double nucleoside therapy

Persistently declining CD_4 cell numbers, as measured on at least two separate occasions

Clinical deterioration

SOURCE: Department of Health and Human Services (2002).

the medication, treatment fatigue, or, under certain circumstances, in what is known as structured or supervised treatment interruptions (STIs). STIs have been studied as part of therapy directed to patients who have developed multiple medication resistance patterns (salvage therapy) in an effort to allow for the reemergence of HIV that is susceptible to ARV therapy. It has also been used to give the HIV-infected person's immune system a jump-start to stimulate the individual's immune function. This process is also known as autoimmunization. Additionally, STIs have been used to allow less total time on antiretrovirals. At this time, there is not enough known about STIs, and their use in general clinical practice is not recommended. Whatever the reason for stopping, it is currently recommended to discontinue all antiretroviral agents simultaneously rather than continuing one or two agents. Stopping all antiretroviral medications at once minimizes the potential for emergence or resistant viral strains (U.S. Department of Health and Human Services, 2002).

g. Changing therapy: There are many factors to assess when considering changing antiretroviral therapy. These factors include recent viral load levels and changes in those levels measured on two separate occasions, CD_4 percentage and absolute count and any recent changes, history and physical findings, remaining treatment options, and potential for resistance already existing in the client. Additionally, similar to initiation of therapy, a thorough assessment of treatment readiness should be undertaken. This assessment is especially essential because any adherence problems that may have led to loss of viral suppression must be addressed. It is also important to determine if this change in therapy is secondary to side effects of the medications or drug failure. Side effects requiring therapy change in the presence of viral suppression allows for substitution of one drug in the treatment regimen. However, when drug failure has occurred, the clinician must rely on a thorough history of previously used medications, adherence issues, and other medications used by the client to help determine recommendations for the next regimen, which will usually include a significant change in medications and classes from those previously used. Table 2.5c offers specific criteria for consideration of treatment change.

h. The use of testing for antiretroviral resistance: Resistance testing has quickly become an invaluable tool in guiding antiretroviral therapy. There are currently two methods for testing, including genotypic and phenotypic assays. Genotype assays measure drug resistance by sequencing the RT and protease genes to determine the drug resistance mutations that are present in the viral genes. This test is usually cheaper and quicker than phenotype testing, but interpretation of results requires an expert clinician. Phenotype assays measures the ability of the virus to grow in differing concentrations of antiretroviral drugs. Recombinant assays are available and have decreased the time for testing to 2 to 3 weeks, but they still are generally more expensive than genotypic tests. Resistance assays should be performed when the person is taking ARV medications, and results need to be interpreted with the client's complete HIV medication history in mind. Currently, it is recommended to proceed with resistance testing when the client experiences virologic failure in the presence of HAART. Also, testing is recommended when the client experiences suboptimal suppression of viral load after initiation of antiretroviral therapy. Resistance testing is to be considered prior to starting therapy during acute HIV infection. Resistance testing is not generally recommended prior to initiation of therapy in people with chronic HIV infection, after discontinuation of drugs, and with plasma viral load less than 1000 copies/mL (U.S. Department of Health and Human Services, 2002).

i. Treating acute infection: Acute infection is defined as the period of time when, after exposure to HIV, the body's normal immune response to an invading pathogen occurs. This period usually occurs 2 to 6 weeks after the initial exposure and is often accompanied by a flulike illness but may be asymptomatic. During this period of time, the screening methods of HIV antibody testing for infection are usually negative. Evidence used for detection of HIV at this time should be HIV viral load testing, or, alternatively, a test for a specific HIV protein known as p24 antigen may be used when viral load testing is not readily available.

During acute infection, there is a high viral production, and then the body's immune system will begin to control the infection and decrease the viral load to a lower level, known as the set point. Early studies indicate that treatment during this acute infection has a positive impact on laboratory markers of disease progression. That is, treatment at this point may decrease the severity of the acute illness and may lower the initial viral set point. This lower set point may ultimately affect the rate of HIV disease progression. Theoretically, there may be less chance of viral mutations and longer preservation of immune function. It is important that a person with high-risk behavior and resultant symptoms be assessed for potential acute HIV infection. This assessment should be guided by an expert HIV clinician, especially when considering medications for treatment.

j. Special considerations
   i. The HIV-infected adolescent: Generally, adolescents infected with HIV through sexual contact or through injecting drugs during adolescence follow a disease course similar to that of adults. Adolescents infected through perinatal transmission or through blood transfusion as a young child have a somewhat different course. Although adolescence is a period of growth and hormonal change, no evidence exists that these factors affect the use of HIV medications. This lack of a difference is especially true for NRTIs; however, there is little experience with PIs and NNRTIs with this population (U.S. Department of Health and Human Services, 2002). Currently, it is recommended that antiretroviral medications used in the adolescent should be dosed on the Tanner staging of puberty and not on any specific age. Adolescents in Tanner stage I–II should be dosed under pediatric guidelines, and those in late puberty (Tanner stage V)

should use adult dosing guidelines. Those adolescents in the midst of growth (Tanner III females and IV males) may use either guideline depending on physical characteristics; however, close monitoring should be undertaken for medication efficacy and toxicity.

ii. The HIV-infected pregnant woman: Generally, a pregnant woman with HIV should have the same considerations for the need for antiretroviral treatment as a nonpregnant woman with HIV. Pregnancy should not preclude the use of optimal therapeutic regimens. If clinical, immunogical, and virological findings indicate that antiretroviral treatment should begin, there should be no delay due to pregnancy. However, a woman with HIV in her 1st trimester who is not already on therapy may wish to delay treatment until after the 10th or 12th week of gestation, assuming that the delay in treatment would not be harmful to the infected woman. Important counseling for the infected pregnant woman should include information regarding the reduction of perinatal transmission through control of HIV in the mother and the administration of antiretrovirals during labor and delivery and to the infant after birth. Treatment of the infected pregnant woman should be monitored by an expert clinician who is familiar with changes in pregnancy that may require dosing alternations and correct medication administration to decrease the potential for perinatal transmission.

4. Adherence to prescribed regimens
   a. Overview of adherence to medication regimens in chronic disease: The concept of adherence was studied in other chronic illnesses before complex HIV therapies came into existence. Research examining adherence to medications for hypertension, asthma, diabetes, and congestive heart failure revealed adherence rates from 20–70%, with an average of approximately 50% (McDermott, Schmitt, & Wallner, 1997; Rand & Wise, 1994; Shaw, Anderson, Maloney, Jay & Fagan, 1995). Typically, these studies defined adherent as correctly taking at least 80% of the prescribed doses. This level of adherence, though appropriate for other chronic illnesses, is clearly not at the 90–95% range required for continued HIV suppression (Paterson, Swindells, Mohr et al., 2000). Studies of self-reported adherence to HIV medication regimens clearly reveal suboptimal self-medicating behavior. Data from the Adult AIDS Clinical Trials Group (AACTG) revealed low adherence in a representative national sample ($n = 75$). Ten centers throughout the United States administered the AACTG self-report adherence questionnaires to patients taking combination antiretroviral therapy, including at least one protease inhibitor (Chesney et al., 2000). Results indicated that 11% of patients reported missing at least one ART dose the day before the interview, and 17% (13) reported missing at least one dose during the prior 2 days. Of those reporting missed doses during the prior 2 days, 11 of 13 noted that their PI was the medication missed. In fact, these 13 nonadherent subjects skipped between 10% and 65% of their pills, with a median of 18% skipped. Clearly, people are having difficulty maintaining adherence to HAART, especially at the level necessary to maintain long-term viral suppression.
   b. Client challenges to adherence: Factors associated with an individual's ability to adhere to a prescribed regimen are multifaceted and multidimensional. Included are client characteristics (e.g., psychosocial factors, substance use, sociodemographics), medication regimen factors (e.g., number of doses, complexity of regimen, medication side effects), client-provider relationship factors (e.g., client perception of

provider communication, client's overall satisfaction with provider), disease factors (e.g., immunologic factors, symptomatology), and setting factors (clinical environment, confidentiality) (Ickovics & Meisler, 1997). More than one factor might be exerting control on adherence at any given time. Additionally, these factors may hold differing levels of importance to any one individual (Crespo-Fierro, 1997). Any assumption on the part of a health care provider regarding a person's potential for adherence based on only one factor is myopic. It is important to remember that although overall factors suggesting problems with adherence may be determined, an assessment of the individual's unique potential for adherence is necessary.

c. The health care provider and adherence: It is important that health care providers do not make recommendations for treatment or withhold treatment based on preconceived notions of what affects an individual's ability to adhere. This is especially true for clients who may have a history or may currently be using illicit or legal drugs. An assessment of the individual nature of adherence for the drug-using client is necessary. Because adherence is multifaceted, a thorough evaluation of all life factors of the drug-using client should be considered in assessing readiness for HAART.

d. Another important aspect for the health care provider's consideration is the development of a relationship of trust with the client. This trusting relationship may be fostered through the provider's use of a harm reduction approach (see later topic in this section). The health care provider may also wish to explore other nonmedical model methods for assisting with adherence, such as the health belief model, transtheoretical model, or the theory of reasoned action (Glanz, Lewis, & Rimer, 1997).

e. Evidence-based strategies to enhance adherence: Although current studies examining strategies to improve adherence specific in HIV disease are underway, the DHHS (2002) does make recommendations based on the current literature regarding HIV medication adherence and adherence in other chronic illnesses. These recommendations include those specific to the client, the medications, and the heath care team. Client and medication specific strategies include 1) informing the patient and anticipating and treating side effects; 2) simplifying food requirements; 3) avoiding adverse drug interactions; 4) reducing dose frequency and number of pills, if possible; and 5) taking time—and often multiple encounters—to negotiate a treatment plan that the client understands and finds acceptable. This process includes education regarding the goals of therapy and the importance of adherence. It is also suggested that family and friends may be helpful in supporting an individual's adherence. An adherence care plan should be developed, including concrete plans for specific regimens in relations to meals, daily activities, side effects, and so forth. Often reminder tools are helpful in assisting with adherence. This may mean assistance with development of a daily written schedule, including pictures of medications and the provision of pillboxes, alarm clocks, pagers, or other mechanical aids to adherence. Trials of medication schedule using jellybeans may also be helpful in identifying adherence issues to prevent the development of resistance if using real medications.

f. Health care providers should consider adherence interventions as a function of a team. Nurses, physicians, pharmacists, case managers, peer educators and other support personnel should all be considered when developing a team approach to adherence education and intervention. The adherence or treatment maintenance message should be provided by the entire health care team. A plan should be developed for what occurs when the client cannot maintain adherence and what efforts will be made to help the person return to treatment maintenance.

g. Theoretical models for behavior change

   i. The transtheoretical model: This model is so named because it incorporates elements from a number of psychotherapy and behavior change theories into its structure (Prochaska & Velicir, 1997). The major premise is that people progress through a series of stages when they attempt to change behavior. The first three stages (precontemplation, contemplation, and preparation) are stages in which the person is not yet ready to take the actual behavior change action but may have begun preparations toward taking the action. The authors of this model suggest that health care providers can intervene even when a person is not yet ready to undergo the actual behavior change by assisting in movement toward that healthier behavior. To put a person in a program or ask the person to undergo a behavior change when they are not in the action phase of the model will doom them to failure. Related to HIV medications, an assessment of the stage of change might help prevent starting a person with HIV on medications when he or she is not ready. Also, interventions should be developed to help the person not yet ready for medications to move toward readiness for action. Interestingly, relapse, or a return to the unhealthy behavior, is addressed in this model as a part of the human change process. This relapse plan would mean that periods of nonadherence to HIV medications would be expected in the human change process and that a plan for return to adherent medication behavior is an important part of this model.

   ii. The harm reduction model: The harm reduction model was developed in Europe and the Netherlands for applications related to intravenous drug use behavior. Harm reduction can be thought of more as a philosophy of care than a true model. In this philosophy, health behaviors are thought of as either beneficial, neutral or harmful. The premise is to decrease the number of harmful behaviors and increase the number of beneficial behaviors. Inherent in this philosophy is the belief that the person might not be able to completely remove all harmful behaviors but that any reduction in these behaviors is beneficial. So a person injecting dugs may not be able to stop the drug behavior but might be able to reduce the potential harm by participating in a needle exchange program that will decrease the potential for other harmful outcomes, such as HIV or hepatitis infection (Riley, 1993). Application of the model to HIV-medication adherence does not mean that it is appropriate to encourage people to take medications when they are able or that taking medications some of the time is more beneficial than taking no medications. In fact, it is known that partial dosing encourages the development of drug resistant viral mutations. However, the model might be applied to other medication-related factors. For example, if the client needs to take dosings with a high-fat meal, but is able to do this only one time a day instead of two, perhaps the addition of a snack at the second dosing may improve absorption without requiring an entire meal. This model allows for the reality of human nature and often times inability to follow the instructions to the exact specifications.

   iii. The Freirean approach: Developed in the 1970s by a Brazilian educator Paulo Freire, this approach stresses the importance of considering racism, sexism, the exploitation of workers, and other forms of oppression in the development of curriculum. Freire suggests that any curriculum that does not consider these important variables supports the status quo or unequal distribution of power. He suggests that practical and expedient interests play a determining role in education (Heaney, 1995). Application of this approach to HIV-medication adherence would mean that power distribution in society affects individual power and the ability to be adherent to medications. Unequal societal distribution of power (i.e., oppression of some) affects an individual's ability to maintain drug adherence. It would be imperative then to consider these larger environmental and social factors when assessing an individual's potential for adherence.

iv. Other models: Other models may be helpful in understanding adherence issues and planning for adherence interventions. These include but are not limited to the health belief model, the theory of reasoned action, and the theory of planned behavior. Additionally, the model of adherence factors offered by Ickovics and Meisler (1997) is specific to HIV-medication-taking behavior and can be especially useful.

References

Bartlett, J. G., & Gallant, J. E. (2001). *2001–2002 medical management of HIV infection.* Baltimore: Johns Hopkins University, Division of Infectious Disease.

Bickley, L. (2003). *Bates' guide to physical examination and history taking.* Philadelphia: Lippincott Williams & Wilkins.

Bonacini, M. (1992). Hepatobiliary complications in patients with human immunodeficiency virus infection. *American Journal of Medicine, 92,* 404–411.

Buskin, S., Diamond, C., & Hopkins, S. (1998). HIV-infected pregnant women and progression of HIV disease. *Archives of Internal Medicine, 158,* 1277–1297.

Carter-Martin, A. (2002). *It's never too late to start: Seven steps toward good health.* Retrieved July 29, 2002, from www.medscape.com

Center for AIDS Prevention Studies, University of California. (1995). *Prevention: Do condoms work?* San Francisco: Author.

Centers for Disease Control and Prevention. (1993). Recommendations of the Advisory Committee on Immunization Practices (ACIP): Use of vaccines and immune globulins in persons with altered immunocompetence. *Morbidity and Mortality Weekly Report, 42*(RR-04).

Centers for Disease Control and Prevention. (2002a). *Food and water precautions and travelers' diarrhea prevention.* Retrieved June 22, 2002, from http://www.cdc.gov/travel

Centers for Disease Control and Prevention. (2002b). Influenza. In *Epidemiology and prevention of vaccine-preventable diseases, pink book* (7th ed.). Washington, DC: Author.

Centers for Disease Control and Prevention. (2002c). Sexually transmitted disease treatment guidelines 2002. *Morbidity and Mortality Weekly Report, 51*(RR-6), 36–52.

Centers for Disease Control and Prevention. (2002d). 2002 USPHS/ISDA guidelines for the prevention of opportunistic infections in persons infected with human immunodeficiency virus. *MMWR, 51,* 1–46. Retrieved June 14, 2002, from http://www.cdc.gov/mmwr/preview/mmwrhtml/rr5108a1.htm

Chesney, M. A., Ickovics, J. R., Chambers, D. B., Gifford, A. L., Neidig, J., Zwickl, B., et al. (2000). Self-reported adherence to antiretroviral medications among participants in HIV clinical trials: The AACTG adherence instruments. Patient Care Committee & Adherence Working Group of the Outcomes Committee of the Adult AIDS Clinical Trials Group (AACTG). *AIDS Care, 12*(3), 255–266.

Crespo-Fierro, M. (1997). Compliance/adherence and care management in HIV disease. *Journal of the Association of Nurses in AIDS Care, 8*(4), 43–54.

Deeks, S. G., & Volberding, P. A. (1999). Antiretroviral therapy for HIV disease. In P. T. Cohen, M. A. Sande, & P. A. Volberding (Eds.), *The AIDS knowledge base* (3rd ed., pp. 241–260). New York: Lippincott William & Wilkins.

Dolan, S. A. (1997). Vaccines for hepatitis A and B. *Postgraduate Medicine, 102*(6), 74–80.

Duggan, J., Peterson, W. S., Schutz, M., Khuder, S., & Charkraborty, J. (2001). Use of complementary and alternative therapy in HIV-infected patients. *AIDS Patient Care and STDs, 15*(3), 159–167.

Fenton, M. (1999). *Guidelines and protocol of care for providing medical nutrition therapy to HIV-infected persons.* Retrieved June 22, 2002, from www.infoweb.org

Food and Drug Administration. (1999). *How can I prevent food-borne illness?* Retrieved June 15, 2002, from www.cfsan.fda.gov

Gerber, J., Rosenkranz, S., Segal, Y., Aberg, J., D'Amico, R., Mildvan, D., et al. (2001). Effect of ritonavir/saquinavir on stereoselective pharmacokinetics of methadone: Result of ACTG 401. *Journal of Acquired Immune Deficiency Syndromes, 27,* 153–160.

Gilbert, L. K. (1999). The female condom in the U.S.: Lessons learned. *American Journal of Public Health, 89*(6), 1–28.

Glanz, K., Lewis, F. M., & Rimer, B. K. (1997). *Health behavior and health education: Theory, research and practice* (2nd ed.). San Francisco: Jossey-Bass.

Greif, J., & Hewitt, W. (1998). The living canvas. *Advance for Nurse Practitioners, 6*(6), 26–31, 82.

Gunn, N., White, C., & Srinivasan, R. (1998). Primary care as harm reduction for injection drug users [Electronic version]. *Medical Student JAMA, 280,* 1191–1195.

Heaney, T. (1995). Issues in Freirean pedagogy. *Thresholds in education.* Retrieved August 1, 2002, from http://nlu.nl.edu/ace/Resources/Documents/Freire Issues.html

Ickovics, J. R., & Meisler, A. W. (1997). Adherence in AIDS clinical trials: A framework for clinical research and clinical care. *Journal of Clinical Epidemiology, 50,* 385–391.

Johns Hopkins University, Division of Infectious Disease, AIDS Service. (2002). *Condoms and HIV prevention.* Retrieved, December 18, 2002, from http://hopkins-aids. edu/prevention/prevention4.html

Kemper, C., Haubrich, R., Frank, I., Buscarino, C., McCutchan, J., Deresinkski, S., et al. (2001, February). *The safety and immunogenicity of hepatitis A vaccine (Havrix) in HIV + patients: A double-blind, randomized, placebo-controlled trial.* Paper presented at the 8th conference on retroviruses and opportunistic infections, Chicago.

Kirton, C. A. (2001a). Clinical application of immunological and virological markers. In C. A. Kirton, D. Talotta, & K. Zwolski (Eds.), *Handbook of HIV/AIDS nursing* (pp. 26–42). St. Louis, MO: Mosby.

Kirton, C. A. (2001b). Promoting healthy behaviors in HIV primary care. *Nurse Practitioner Forum, 12*(4), 223–232.

Kirton, C. A. (2001c). Risk assessment, identification, and HIV counseling. In C. A. Kirton, D. Talotta, & K. Zwolski (Eds.), *Handbook of HIV/AIDS nursing* (pp. 51–64). St. Louis, MO: Mosby.

Kirton, C. A. (2001d). Sexually transmitted diseases. In C. A. Kirton, D. Talotta, & K. Zwolski (Eds.), *Handbook of HIV/AIDS nursing* (pp. 452–465). St. Louis, MO: Mosby.

Kotler, D. P. (2001). *Conference report: Third International Workshop on Adverse Drug Reactions and Lipodystrophy in HIV, Athens, Greece.* Retrieved August 22, 2002, from www.hiv.medscape.com

Kotler, D. P. (2002). *Update on lipodystrophy. Or is it just lipoatrophy? Medscape coverage of XIV International AIDS Conference.* Retrieved August 22, 2002, from www.hiv.medscape.com

Kroon, F. P., van Dissel, J. T., de Jong, J. C., & Furth, R. (1994). Antibody response to influenza, tetanus and pneumococcal vaccines in HIV-seropositive individuals in relation to the number of CD4 + lymphocytes. *AIDS, 8*(4), 469–476.

Lucas, G. M., Gebo, K. A., Cahisson, R. E., & Moore, R. D. (2002). Longitudinal assessment of the effects of drug and alcohol abuse on HIV-1 treatment outcomes in an urban clinic. *AIDS, 16*(5), 767–774.

McComsey, G. A., & Lederman, M. L. (2002). *High doses of riboflavin and thiamine may help in secondary prevention of hyperlactatemia.* Retrieved August 22, 2002, from www.hiv.medscape.com

McDermott, M. M., Schmitt, B., & Wallner, E. (1997). Impact of medication nonadherence on coronary heart disease outcomes. A critical review. *Archives of Internal Medicine, 157*(17), 1921–1929.

National Institute for Occupational Safety and Health. (2002). *Families taking charge: Controlling stress.* Retrieved August 22, 2002, from www.nlm.nih.gov/medlineplus

New York State Department of Health. (2001). *NYSDOH AI booklet—Oral health care for people with HIV infection.* New York: Author.

Nunez, M., Lana, R., Mendoza, J. L., Martin-Carbonero, L., & Soriano, V. (2001). Risk factors for severe hepatic injury after introduction of highly active antiretroviral therapy. *Journal of Acquired Immune Deficiency Syndromes and Human Retrovirology, 27*(5), 426–431.

Paterson D. L., Swindells, S., Mohr, J., Brester, M., Vergis, E. N., Squier, C., et al. (2000). Adherence to protease inhibitor therapy and outcomes in patients with HIV infection. *Annals of Internal Medicine,133*(1), 21–30.

Prochaska, J. O., & Velicer, W. F. (1997). The transtheoretical model of health behavior change. *American Journal of Health Promotion, 12*(1), 38–48.

Rand, C. S., & Wise, R. A. (1994). Measuring adherence to asthma medication regimens. *American Journal of Respiratory and Critical Care Medicine, 149*(2, Pt. 2), 69–76, 77–78.

Rees, V., Saitz, R., Hortom, N. J., & Samet, J. (2001). Association of alcohol consumption with HIV sex- and drug-risk behaviors among drug users. *Journal of Substance Use Treatment, 21*(3), 129–134.

Richardson, B. A. (2002). Nonoxynol-9 as a vaginal microbicide for prevention of sexually transmitted infections: It's time to move on. *Journal of the American Medical Association, 287,* 1171–1172.

Riley, D. (1993). *The harm reduction model: Pragmatic approaches to drug use from the area between intolerance and neglect.* Retrieved August 1, 2002, from http://www.ccsa.ca/docs/harmred.htm

Roddy, R., Zekeng, L., Ryan, K. A., Tamoufé, U., & Tweedy, K. A. (2002). Effect of Nonoxynol-9 gel on urogenital gonorrhea and chlamydial infection: A randomized controlled trial. *Journal of the American Medical Association, 287,* 1117–1122.

Salvato, P. D., & Thompson, C. D. (1999). Clinical, virologic, and immunologic features of influenza vaccination in HIV infection. *AIDS Reader, 9,* 624–629.

Schmidt, K., & Ernst, E. (2002). "Alternative" therapies for HIV/AIDS: How safe is Internet advice? A pilot study. *International Journal of STD and AIDS, 13*(6), 433–435.

Shaw, E., Anderson, J. G., Maloney, M., Jay, S. J., & Fagan, D. (1995). Factors associated with noncompliance of patients taking antihypertensive medications. *Hospital Pharmacy, 30*(3), 201–203, 206–207.

Stolz, D. A., Nelson, S., Kolls, J. K., Zhang, P., Bohm, R. P., Murphey-Corb, M., et al. (1999). Ethanol suppression of the functional state of polymorphonuclear leukocytes obtained from uninfected and Simian immunodeficiency virus infected rhesus macaques. *Alcoholism: Clinical and Experimental Research, 23*(5), 878–884.

Stolz, D. A., Nelson, S., Kolls, J. K., Zhang, P., Bohm, R. P., Murphey-Corb, M., et al. (2002). In vitro ethanol suppresses alveolar macrophage TNF-alpha during Simian immunodeficiency virus infection. *American Journal of Respiratory and Critical Care Medicine, 161*(1), 135–140.

Strawford, A., Barbieri, T., Van Loan, M., Parks, E., Catlin, D., Barton, N., et al. (1999). Resistance exercise and supraphysiologic androgen therapy in eugonadal men with HIV-related weight loss. *Journal of the American Medical Association, 281,* 1282–1290.

Swanson, B. S., Keithley, J. K., Zeller, J. M., & Cronin-Stubbs, D. (2000). Complementary and alternative therapies to manage HIV-related symptoms. *Japan Associate Nurses in AIDS Care, 11*(5), 40–60.

Talotta, D. (2001a). Gynecological and cervical disorders and therapeutics. In C. A. Kirton, D. Talotta, &

K. Zwolski (Eds.), *Handbook of HIV/AIDS nursing* (pp. 121–149). St. Louis, MO: Mosby.

Talotta, D. (2001b). Tuberculosis screening, diagnosis, and infection control. In C. A. Kirton, D. Talotta, & K. Zwolski (Eds.), *Handbook of HIV/AIDS nursing* (pp. 110–120). St. Louis, MO: Mosby.

U.S. Department of Health and Human Services. (1998). *Clinician's handbook of preventive services* (2nd ed.). Washington, DC: U.S. Government Printing Office.

U.S. Department of Health and Human Services. (2002). *Guidelines for the use of antiretroviral agents in HIV-infected adults and adolescents.* Washington, DC: Author.

USPHS/IDSA. (2001). *USPHS/IDSA guidelines for the prevention of opportunistic infections in persons infected with human immunodeficiency virus: A summary.* Retrieved August 22, 2002, from at http://www.hivatis.org/

Winson, G. (2001). HIV/AIDS nutritional management. In C. A. Kirton, D. Talotta, & K. Zwolski (Eds.), *Handbook of HIV/AIDS nursing* (pp. 344–360). St. Louis, MO: Mosby.

Section III

Symptomatic Conditions in Adolescents and Adults with Advancing Disease

This section provides comprehensive information about the common conditions experienced by individuals with HIV/AIDS; the AIDS indicator diseases; and, new to this edition, comorbid conditions seen in HIV. Many of these conditions are seen as a result of patients living longer with the disease. Sometimes the conditions present as a result of the therapies associated with HIV, whereas in some cases the exact etiology remains elusive.

Each section discusses the pathophysiology, clinical presentation, diagnostic work-up, and treatments for a specific disorder. Each section concludes with the most important nursing implications. Nurses should use these implications as a guide when tailoring their interventions to the specific settings, populations, and scope of practice.

A. Symtomatic Conditions in Advanced Disease

3.1 Bartonellosis

1. Etiology/Epidemiology
   a. Etiologic agents are *Bartonella quintana* and *Bartonella henselae*. *Bartonella* is a family of small, slow-growing, gram-negative rods.
   b. Body louse is the only known source of *B. quintana;* ticks and fleas may be vectors for *B. henselae.* Scratches from cat claws contaminated by flea feces has been suggested as a transmission mode.
2. Pathogenesis
   a. *Bartonella* is thought to replicate in erythrocytes and endothelial cells and to stimulate endothelial cell proliferation.
   b. Bacillary angiomatosis (BA) is the anatomic lesion resulting from *Bartonella* infection. Lesions can form in the skin, bone, brain, parenchyma, lymph nodes, bone marrow, and GI and pulmonary tract.
   c. Disseminated disease, with bacteremia and sepsis, or endocarditis can occur.
3. Clinical presentation
   a. Patients usually present with constitutional symptoms of anorexia, vomiting, and weight loss.
   b. Cutaneous BA usually presents as multiple or single reddish, vascular lesions that are difficult to distinguish from KS lesions.
   c. Extracutaneous disease can involve many organ systems: osteolytic lesions of the long bones, GI and pulmonary tract lesions; lymph node involvement resulting in firm, nontender nodules; and bone marrow involvement associated with hepatosplenomegaly and thrombocytopenia.
   d. Bartonellosis has been associated with aseptic meningitis, parenchymal brain masses, and chronic central nervous system dysfunction in HIV-infected patients.
   e. Focal necrotizing infections of the lymph nodes, liver, and spleen are seen in patients with CD_4 counts < 50 cells/mm^3.

4. Diagnosis
   a. Serology for *B. quintana* and *B. henselae* (not available in most locales)
   b. Blood cultures for *Bartonella*
   c. Biopsy and differential diagnosis for cutaneous BA, which resembles KS
   d. Radiographs and biopsies to diagnose extracutaneous BA
5. Prevention/Treatment
   a. Cat fleas are a major vector for *B. henselae.*
      i. Wash hands after petting or handling pets.
      ii. Wash bites and scratches immediately with soap and water.
   b. *B. quintana* infection is associated with head and body lice, and exposure should be avoided.
   c. Minimum of 3-month course of erythromycin or clarithromycin is the current treatment choice for BA (Koehler, 1999; Slater & Welch, 2000). Doxycycline, tetracycline, and minocycline can be used in erythromycin intolerant-patients.
   d. Acutely ill patients require hospitalization and IV therapy initially and a minimum 4-month treatment course.
   e. Patients with recurrent disease may require lifelong maintenance therapy.
6. Nursing implications
   a. Educate about infection control measures to prevent exposure.
   b. Teach about probability of disease relapse and need for suppressive therapy.
   c. Monitor laboratory results and other indices for adverse effects and response to therapy. Patients may initially respond to therapy with fever, myalgia, and constitutional symptoms.
   d. Monitor closely for recurrent disease.

3.2 Herpes Zoster

1. Etiology/Epidemiology
   a. Varicella-zoster virus (VZV) is a member of the herpes family; humans are the only known reservoir for VZV.
   b. Intimate contact is associated with transmission; risk of developing zoster increases with age.

c. Varicella infection is considered a childhood disease, and the majority of cases occur in children younger than age 15. The incidence of varicella has decreased with the use of vaccinations.

d. An estimated 300,000 episodes of zoster occur annually, of which 95% are initial occurrences and 5% are recurrences (Centers for Disease Control and Prevention, 2002b).

2. Pathogenesis

a. VZV infection results in two clinically distinct entities: primary infection or chicken pox and reactivation of latent infection or herpes zoster (shingles).

   i. Primary VZV infection is thought to result from pulmonary inhalation of aerosolized viral particles.

   ii. Epithelial cells undergo degenerative changes characterized by ballooning, resulting in a characteristic vesicular rash that ruptures and releases infected fluid.

   iii. VZV infection characteristically remains latent in the dorsal root ganglia after resolution of the primary infection.

3. Clinical presentation

a. VZV is characterized by a painful, unilateral vesicular eruption with a dermatomal distribution; thoracic and lumbar dermatomes are most frequently involved. VZV can be disseminated with bilateral skin involvement.

b. Onset of dermatomal pain precedes appearance of lesions by 48–72 hours; lesions form over 3–5 days and resolve in 10–15 days. Lesions may be very painful; acute pain (burning, stabbing) frequently occurs. Chronic pain syndrome (postherpetic neuralgia) can be a severe and disabling complication.

c. VZV rarely results in disseminated disease; anorexia, fever, and cough may indicate dissemination, a potentially fatal complication. Retina or the central nervous system (CNS) may be involved, without concomitant skin involvement.

4. Diagnosis

a. Immunofluorescent assay (IFA) or culture can detect virus antigens.

5. Prevention/Treatment

a. Varicella-naive persons (especially those who are older, debilitated, or pregnant) should avoid persons with chicken pox or herpes zoster. Administer varicella zoster immune globulin (VZIG) within 96 hours of exposure to persons with chickenpox or zoster.

b. A high dose of acyclovir can be administered.

   i. Best response occurs if initiated within 72 hours of outbreak.

   ii. Parenteral therapy can occur in severe disseminated skin infection or retinal or CNS disease. A maintenance dose may be required in AIDS patients with recurrent VZV.

c. Famciclovir can be administered.

   i. Famiciclovir is shown to decrease the incidence of postherpetic neuralgia in the elderly; clinical implications in persons with AIDS are unknown.

d. Other treatment options are valacyclovir, foscarnet, and ganciclovir.

6. Nursing implications

a. Monitor laboratory values and other indices to monitor for adverse effects and response to therapy.

b. Maintain strict isolation until all lesions are crusted; hospitalization may be necessary.

c. Local lesion care is required because open lesions can develop superimposed bacterial infections.

d. Teach pain management for both acute illness and postherpetic neuralgia.

e. Provide patient education.

   i. Teach local wound care.

   ii. Emphasize need for strict isolation.

   iii. Counsel varicella-naive visitors or staff not to enter the patient's isolation room.

   iv. Use separate cloth to clean affected areas to prevent autoinoculation and dissemination.

3.3 Human Papillomavirus Infection

1. Epidemiology
   a. Human papillomavirus (HPV) infection is the major risk factor for squamous intraepithelial lesions (SIL), irrespective of the site; cervical intraepithelial neoplasia (CIN); or anal/vulva/vagina intraepithelial neoplasia (AIN, VIN, VAIN; Ellerbrock et al., 2000; Moscicki et al., 2001; Palefsky, 2000; Schlecht et al., 2001).
   b. Sexual intercourse is primary mode of transmission.
      i. Of HIV-infected sexually active gay men 93% are HPV DNA positive (Palefsky, 2000).
      ii. Approximately 50% of women with CD_4 counts < 200 cells/mm^3 are infected with HPV 16.
      iii. HPV DNA was detected in 13% of lesbian women (HIV status not screened) who had never had sex with men (Marrazzo, Koutsky, Kiviat, Kuypers, & Stine, 2001).
   c. Cofactors for HPV disease progression differ among studies and may include genetic predisposition, immune status, HPV subtypes, smoking, injecting drug use, age, presence of both HIV-1 and HIV-2, and possibly nutritional factors.
   d. Characteristics of HPV in HIV-infected individuals include the following:
      i. Prevalence of HPV infection is doubled in HIV-infected individuals (Minkoff, Feldman, DeHovitz, Landesman, & Burk, 1998; Palefsky et al., 1999; Sun et al., 1997).
      ii. There is an increased risk for multiple HPV subtypes (Sun et al., 1997), including oncogenic subtypes in HIV-infected women (Ellerbrock et al., 2000; Minkoff et al., 1998; Uberti-Foppa et al., 1998).
      iii. Rates of SIL are 5 times greater in HIV-infected individuals (Ellerbrock et al., 2000; Massad et al., 1999).
         (1) HIV-infected women show an increased frequency and severity of HPV-associated cervical lesions (Duerr et al., 2001; Jamieson et al., 2002).
         (2) A review of 15 studies comparing the relationship of HIV, HPV, and CIN found that an interaction between HIV and HPV exists (Mandelblatt, Kanetsky, Eggert, & Gold, 1999).
         (3) Increased SIL progression and decreased regression are noted in HIV-infected individuals (Fructher et al., 1996; Mandelblatt et al., 1999). Of 328 HIV-infected women without SIL, 20% developed SIL within 30 months (Ellerbrock et al., 2000). In HIV noninfected women, one third of all grades of SIL regress, 41% persist, and 25% progress.
         (4) Persistence of HPV infection and oncogenic subtypes and disease progression are related to advanced immunosuppression (Luque, Demeter, & Reichman, 1999; Minkoff et al., 2001; Minkoff et al., 1998; Palefsky et al., 1999).
   e. HPV types in SIL disease
      i. Benign HPV types 6/11/42/43/44/54/57/66 are associated with viral condylomata.
      ii. Moderate oncogenic HPV types responsible for dysplasia and some cancers are 26/33/39/45/51/52/55/56/58/59/60/70.
      iii. High oncogenic HPV types 16/18 are responsible for 50% of cervical/anal cancers. Types 31/35 are responsible for about 20% of cervical/anal cancers (Palefsky, 2000; Sun et al., 1997).
2. Pathogenesis
   a. Subepithelial T-cells and Langerhans cells in the cervix can become infected with HIV; HIV and HPV are synergistic.
   b. HPV encodes for two transforming proteins, E6 and E7, which interfere with cellular proteins that suppress

tumor growth (Zwerschke & Jansen-Durr, 2000).

   c. Cytotoxic T-cell lymphocytes (CTLs) necessary for HPV immunity and response to E6 are lacking in HIV-infected individuals (Nakagawa et al., 2000).

3. Clinical presentation

   a. The HPV screening tool is the Papanicolaou (Pap) smear.

   b. Pap smear cytology results are based on the 2001 Bethesda System (see http://bethesda2001.cancer.gov/terminology.pdf).

      i. Squamous cells

         (1) Atypical squamous cells

            (a) of undetermined significance (ASC-US)

            (b) cannot exclude high grade squamous intraepithelial lesion (ASC-H)

         (1) Low-grade squamous intra-epithelial lesion (LSIL; includes HPV, mild dysplasia/CIN-1 [AIN, VIN, VAIN])

         (2) High-grade squamous intra-epithelial lesion (HSIL; includes moderate dysplasia/CIN-2, severe dysplasia/CIN-3, carcinoma-in-situ/CIS [AIN, VIN, VAIN])

      ii. Glandular cells (four categories)

4. Diagnosis

   a. Pap smear is the primary screening tool; associated with low incidence of false-negative results.

   b. Indications for colposcopic exam include cytologic abnormality or history of untreated abnormal Pap smear. Consider colposcopy when there is evidence of HPV infection or after treatment for SIL. Some professionals suggest colposcopy for individuals with $CD_4 < 200$ cells/mm^3 (Abularach & Anderson, 2001).

   c. The use of colposcopy versus Pap smear for screening remains controversial. Due to high incidence of SIL and low sensitivity of a single Pap smear for detecting SIL, some professionals have suggested colposcopy screening. A cost-effectiveness analysis by Goldie, Weinstein, Kuntz, and Freedberg (1999) suggested colposcopy screening alone was not cost effective and that the 1998 Centers for Disease Control and Prevention (CDC) recommended guidelines, which includes two initial Pap smears 6 months apart, then annual screening, is only slightly more expensive.

5. Prevention/Treatment

   a. Prevention measures include targeting safer sex educational efforts toward all individuals who are sexually active and emphasizing the causal links between HPV, HIV, and SIL. Condoms and dental dams may not be effective in preventing HPV shedding, which is increased in HIV-infected individuals and may contribute to the persistence of HPV infections.

   b. Current recommendation from the CDC and the Infectious Diseases Society of America include the following:

      i. HIV-infected women should have two Pap smears during the 1st year after HIV diagnosis; if both are negative, then yearly Pap smears should occur, if there are no risk factors (Centers for Disease Control and Prevention, 1998; United States Public Health Service and Infectious Diseases Society of America, 1999).

      ii. An individual with a history of cervical/anal dysplasia or abnormal Pap smears should continue Pap smears every 6 months at minimum.

   c. HIV-infected men who are at risk for HPV infections also need anal Pap smears with similar management as women.

   d. The impact of HAART on SIL progression and regression is evolving. HAART showed no impact in several studies, and in other studies increased regression of SIL was shown twice as often for those individuals on HAART. A 40% HPV regression was most evident with larger CD_4 cell counts when on HAART and was twice as high in HSIL than LSIL (Heard, Tassie,

Kazatchkine, & Orth, 2002; Minkoff et al., 2001).

e. Experimental approaches include topical vaginal 5 fluorouracil (5-FU), oral difluoromethylornithine (DMFO), and HPV vaccines. 5-FU can reduce recurrence (Maiman et al., 1999) but may enhance transmission of sexually transmitted diseases (STDs) due to mucosal inflammation and toxicity (Andersen, Smereck, Hockman, Ross, & Ground, 1999).

6. Nursing implications
a. Assess and educate individuals regarding risk of HPV infections.
b. Identify and reduce barriers to self-care.
c. Establish relationship with the patient.
d. Assess well-being and address immediate concerns.
e. Assess and address knowledge and skills deficits.
f. Assist the patient in directed positive changes.
g. Provide team approach for HIV care (team may include the provider, nursing staff, pharmacy, social workers, case managers).
h. Provide transportation and child care (Andersen et al., 1999; Leenerts, 1998).
i. Reinforce importance of screening with scheduled Pap smears and follow-up with provider for results (Cejtin et al., 1999).
j. Review treatment modalities and side effects.
    i. Loop electrical excision procedure (LEEP) uses a fine wire loop with electricity to remove abnormal tissue. Allows for both diagnosis and treatment. Requires local anesthesia. Minor risk of infection and bleeding. Vaginal spotting and discharge occurs for 2–3 weeks. Nothing should be inserted into vagina until follow-up appointment.
    ii. Cryotherapy includes freezing of abnormal tissue. The procedure has a high rate of treatment failure and is not routinely performed. Watery, pinkish discharge occurs for 4–6 weeks postprocedure due to sloughing of cells. Nothing

should be inserted into vagina for 4–6 weeks.

iii. Conization includes removal of cone-shaped abnormal tissue. Performed in the operating room with general anesthesia or intravenous sedation. Treatment for dysplasia or carcinoma in situ is indicated. Increased risk for complications, such as bleeding, infection, and cervical scarring. Nothing should be inserted into vagina until follow-up appointment.

iv. 5-FU is an antineoplastic cream applied intravaginally for recurrent CIN. Dosing is variable. Inflammation may occur with frequent dosing (e.g., vaginal itching, burning, ulceration, discharge). Apply at bedtime, wear pad, and use petroleum jelly on labia. Avoid intercourse during application.

v. Laser ablation involves a CO_2 laser directed at abnormal tissue and may be used for larger lesions. The procedure is performed in the operating room with general anesthesia and may be used on an outpatient basis for smaller lesions. It is more effective than cryosurgery. Vaginal spotting and discharge occurs for 2–3 weeks. Nothing should be inserted into vagina until follow-up appointment.

vi. A hysterectomy is an option for recurrent CIN in nonchildbearing women or in cases of CIS. Hysterectomies are a major surgical procedure with significant risks and extended recovery time. Although recurrence rate is low, vaginal dysplasia can occur.

k. Promote health maintenance behaviors and safe sex practices.
    i. Gynecological examinations every 6 months, including Pap smear
    ii. Usage of male/female condoms
    iii. Avoidance or minimization of cigarette, alcohol, and drug use

iv. Notification to provider regarding pain, bleeding, or discharge

l. Provide psychosocial support to patient and family.

    i. Explain all aspects of CIN, including incidence, prevalence, diagnosis, treatment, and follow-up.

    ii. Review diagnostic procedures, expected side effects, and outcomes.

    iii. Reinforce health maintenance of HIV disease and correlate relationship between CIN and HIV.

    iv. Ascertain coping methods and support as needed.

    v. Elicit partner and family support as needed.

3.4 Idiopathic Thrombocytopenia Purpura

1. Etiology/Epidemiology

    a. Idiopathic thrombocytopenia purpura (ITP) occurs in as many as 40% of HIV-infected patients. Severe thombocytopenia (platelet count $< 50,000/mm^3$) is seen in 5% of HIV-associated ITP.

    b. HIV-associated ITP is an early manifestation of HIV infection and occurs before the development of any AIDS-defining condition.

2. Pathogenesis is unknown. Hypotheses include production of platelet-specific autoantibodies and direct HIV infection of megakaryocytes.

3. Clinical presentation

    a. Patient is often asymptomatic, despite low platelet counts.

    b. Symptoms include ecchymosis, petechiae, purpura, abnormal menstrual bleeding, blood in urine or stool, epistaxis, and bleeding from the gums.

    c. Mild splenomegaly may be present.

4. Diagnosis

    a. Complete blood count reveals low platelets.

    b. Bone marrow biopsy may be normal or may show increased megakaryocytes.

    c. Coagulation profiles (e.g. PT/PTT) are normal.

    d. Platelet-associated antibodies may be detected (Nardi, Karpatkin, Hart, Belmont, & Karpartkin, 1999).

5. Prevention/Treatment

    a. Effective prevention is not currently possible because the causes and risk factors are unknown.

    b. Treatment

        i. HAART increases platelet counts (Burbano et al., 2001; Carbonara et al., 2001).

        ii. Zidovudine stimulates thrombopoiesis (Aboulafia, Bundow, Waide, Bennet, & Kerr, 2000).

        iii. Steroid therapy (i.e., prednisone) may lead to short-lasting responses but may increase the risk of developing an opportunistic infection.

        iv. Anti-RhO-(d) IgG (WinRhO) has been shown to produce a response, but it is not usually sustained (Scaradavou et al., 1997).

        v. Splenectomy is indicated if the person does not respond to medication; however, the patient is at increased risk for fulminant infections.

        vi. High-dose gamma globulin injections produce a rapid rise in platelet counts, but the effect is generally temporary. Use is limited to acute episodes of life-threatening bleeding or before a surgical procedure or dental extraction in patients with low platelet counts ($< 30,000/mm^3$).

        vii. Danazol has been used as a second line therapy.

        viii. Immunosuppressive agents (vincristine, vinblastine) can be used for refractory ITP.

        ix. Platelet transfusions are reserved for patients whose platelet counts are $< 10,000$ cells/mm^3 or in emergency cases.

6. Nursing implications

    a. Assess for changes related to bleeding: decreased or loss of consciousness, hematuria, blood in the stool, hemoptysis, and hematemesis.

b. Provide soft toothbrushes or soft swabs for oral hygiene; avoid flossing, hard toothbrushes, or commercial mouthwashes.

c. Instruct patient to avoid blowing or picking the nose, straining at bowel movements, douching, or using tampons. Patient should use electric razors to shave.

d. Do not administer any injections intramuscularly. Do not insert rectal suppositories.

e. Use paper tape and avoid strong adhesives that may traumatize the skin.

f. Instruct patient to avoid medications that inhibit platelet production or function. Nonsteroidal antiinflammatory agents (NSAIDs) or aspirin-containing medications should be avoided.

g. If patient is receiving immune globulin (Gamimune N), monitor vital signs during the infusion and observe for the following adverse reactions: fever; irritability; infusion reaction; headache; nausea; chest tightness; dyspnea; chest, back, or hip pain; aseptic meningitis syndrome; transient renal insufficiency; and anaphylaxis.

3.5 Listeriosis

1. Etiology/Epidemiology
   a. *Listeria monocytogenes* is a gram-positive rod that rarely causes disease in the general population.
   b. The organism is ubiquitous in the environment and is commonly found in soil, decaying vegetation, and mammal fecal flora.
   c. Transmission is via food, and vectors have been traced to unpasteurized milk and contaminated or undercooked meat.
   d. An estimated 2,500 people will become seriously ill with listeriosis in the United States, of which 500 will die (Centers for Disease Control and Prevention, Division of Bacterial and Mycotic Diseases, 2001). Listeriosis is associated with a higher incidence in AIDS populations compared with non-AIDS populations.

2. Pathogenesis
   a. GI tract is infected following ingestion of food-borne organism. *L. monocytogenes* can cross the mucosal barrier, resulting in hematogenous spread.
   b. The disseminated organism tends to seed placental and central nervous system (CNS) tissues. Cerebral infection, meningitis, and brain abscesses may be seen.

3. Clinical presentation
   a. Listeriosis most commonly presents in HIV-infected patients as bacteremia, with or without CNS involvement.
      i. Meningitis may only manifest as a low-grade fever and subtle personality changes.
      ii. Cerebritis may present as headache, fever, and varying degrees of paralysis resembling cerebrovascular accident.
   b. Presentation is generally subacute but may be fulminant.
   c. Although rare, various focal infections have been reported, including ulcerative skin lesions, purulent conjunctivitis, acute anterior uveitis, and lymphadenitis.

4. Diagnosis
   a. Listerosis should be considered as part of CNS or GI diagnostic differentials when working with HIV-infected populations.
   b. Definitive diagnosis requires culture and isolation of the organism from tissue or fluid specimen. The organism grows under aerobic conditions on enrichment media, and specimens should be delivered to the clinical laboratory promptly.

5. Prevention/Treatment
   a. Recommendations for listeriosis prevention in at-risk populations include the following (Centers for Disease Control and Prevention, Division of Bacterial and Mycotic Diseases, 2001):

      - Thoroughly cook all food from animal sources.
      - Thoroughly wash raw vegetables before eating.

- Store vegetables and cooked or ready-to-eat foods separately from uncooked meats.
- Avoid unpasteurized milk, unpasteurized milk products, and soft cheeses.
- Reheat leftover and ready-to-eat foods, such as hot dogs, until steaming hot before eating.

  b. There have been no controlled clinical trials to establish clear therapy guidelines.
  - i. Ampicillin is usually treatment of choice, and trimethoprim-sulfamethoxazole (TMP-SMZ) can be used in penicillin-intolerant patients.
  - ii. All patients should receive minimum of 3 weeks of therapy, even in the absence of CNS or cerebrospinal fluid abnormalities because of high seeding potential.
6. Nursing implications
   a. Monitor laboratory results and other indices for side effects of therapy, adverse effects, and response to therapy.
   b. Provide patient education. Discuss possible sources of infection with HIV-infected patients, particularly with HIV-infected women of childbearing age.

3.6 Oral Hairy Leukoplakia

1. Etiology/Epidemiology
   a. Definition: An oral infection caused by Epstein-Barr virus, which infects and replicates in epithelial cells and is associated with frequent viral recombination (Walling, Flaitz, Nichols, Hudnall, & Adler-Storthz, 2001).
   b. Prevalence: It is present in 20% of men and 6% of women; prevalence increases with disease progression, high viral load, or both (Chapple & Hamburger, 2000; Greenspan et al., 2000).
2. Pathogenesis
   a. It is unclear whether Epstein-Barr virus is reactivated from latent site within tongue epithelial cells or Epstein-Barr virus infects/reinfects tongue epithelium from oral cavity or circulating B lymphocytes (Walling et al., 2001).

3. Clinical presentation
   a. White hairy or smooth areas on lateral, dorsal, or ventral surfaces of tongue; may extend to buccal mucosa
   b. Can occur concurrently with oropharyngeal candidiasis but cannot be scraped off like candidiasis
4. Diagnosis
   a. Presence of nonremovable, nonpainful, white, hairy or smooth tongue lesions
   b. Histopathological evidence of epithelial hyperplasia with little or no inflammation
   c. Evidence of Epstein-Barr virus DNA by polymerase chain reaction (PCR) with in situ hybridization (Mabruk et al., 2000)
   d. Difficulty chewing/swallowing, reduced/altered taste perception
   e. Rule out oropharyngeal candidiasis, squamous cell carcinoma, smoker's leukoplakia, epithelial dysplasia
5. Prevention/Treatment
   a. Condition generally is asymptomatic and not treated.
   b. Acyclovir, ganciclovir, desciclovir, and podophyllum resin (Gowdey, Lee, & Carpenter, 1995) provide temporary symptomatic relief; relapses are common.
   c. Antifungal therapy given to minimize coinfection with oropharyngeal candidiasis.
   d. Meticulous oral hygiene and dental care is recommended.
6. Nursing implications
   a. Instruct patient to perform frequent oral assessments and oral care.
   b. If taking acyclovir, patient should drink adequate fluids to prevent dehydration and renal toxicity.
   c. If taste is altered, recommend eating seasoned, spicy, or pickled foods and avoid smoking before meals.
   d. If difficulty chewing/swallowing, suggest eating soft or moist foods, drinking with a straw, and avoiding sticky foods.

3.7 Peripheral Neuropathy

1. Epidemiology
   a. Peripheral neuropathy (PN) involves damage to nerves outside the brain and

spinal cord. Although generally not life threatening, it causes significant morbidity in persons with HIV infection (Klaus, 1996).

b. Although only a small portion of individuals experience symptoms of PN early in the course of HIV infection, more than 30% of persons with AIDS are symptomatic, and 100% show evidence of PN at autopsy (Singer & Germaniskis, 1995; Verma, 2001).

2. Etiology
   a. There are a number of different HIV-related neuropathies, with varying etiologies (Pardo, McArthur, & Griffin, 2001).
   b. PN may be the result of direct HIV infection of nervous tissue; HIV infection of macrophages and lymphocytes, which results in immune dysregulation and cytokine elaboration; direct damage to mitochondria by antiretroviral drugs; or infection with cytomegalovirus (CMV) or vesicular stomatitis virus (VSV) (Kolson & Gonzalez-Scarano, 2001; Pardo, McArthur, & Griffin, 2001).
   c. The illness can be further complicated by other drugs or ongoing nutritional alterations that exacerbate symptoms (Scherer, 1990).

3. Pathogenesis
   a. Depending on the etiological agent, there are a number of different pathophysiological responses to nerve injury (Poncelet, 1998).
   b. Damage may occur at the axon, the motor neuron or dorsal root ganglion, or the myelin sheath (Poncelet, 1998).

4. Clinical presentation
   a. Patients typically present with sensory loss or pain in the extremities, weakness, or motor dysfunction (Pardo, McArthur, & Griffin, 2001).
   b. Presentation differs depending on the type of PN disorder.
      i. Distal symmetric polyneuropathy (DSP) is the most common HIV-associated PN. It occurs in mid to late HIV infection and presents as pain, tingling, or burning, usually in the lower extremities (Verma, 2001; Wulff, Wang, & Simpson, 2000).

ii. Inflammatory demyelinating polyneuropathy (IDP) may occur acutely at the time of HIV infection or later in the course of the disease. It presents as motor weakness, with only minimal sensory loss (Verma, 2001; Wulff, Wang, & Simpson, 2000).

iii. Mononeuritis multiplex (MM) is a rare complication of either early- or late-stage HIV infection. It presents as multifocal motor or sensory alterations, or both (Verma, 2001; Wulff, Wang, & Simpson, 2000).

iv. Progressive polyradiculopathy (PP) most commonly occurs in the advanced stages of HIV infection. It commonly presents with pain in the sacrogenital area that rapidly progresses to motor loss and urinary and bladder incontinence (Verma, 2001; Wulff, Wang, & Simpson, 2000).

v. Autonomic neuropathy is most likely to present in the later stages of HIV infection and is characterized by symptoms of sympathetic (e.g., syncope, diarrhea) and parasympathetic (e.g., palpitations, tachycardia) dysfunction (Verma, 2001; Wulff, Wang, & Simpson, 2000).

5. Diagnosis
   a. Differential diagnosis of specific PN disorder is critical in choosing the appropriate treatment (Wulff & Simpson, 1999).
   b. Diagnostic work-ups involve a comprehensive history, neurological exam, blood studies, cerebrospinal fluid determinations, nerve conduction tests, and electromyelography (Wulff & Simpson, 1999).

6. Prevention/Treatment
   a. Once the underlying cause of PN is determined, appropriate therapy is to be initiated, including withdrawal of neurotoxic medications, initiation of immunomodulatory therapy, or treatment of opportunistic infections (Wulff & Simpson, 1999).

b. The World Health Organization (WHO) analgesic ladder is used to guide pain management (World Health Organization, 1996).

7. Nursing implications
   a. Educate patients to identify early signs of PN.
   b. Routinely perform neurological assessments.
   c. Recommend good foot care, comfortable shoes, and walking aids.
   d. Assess home for safety hazards.
   e. Recommend exercise or massage to improve circulation to the feet.
   f. Advise regarding pain management strategies (e.g., analgesics, foot cradles to reduce pressure of bedcovers on feet; relaxation techniques).
   g. Refer to community resources for supportive/restorative care (e.g., support groups, podiatry clinics, physical therapists).

B. AIDS INDICATOR DISEASES

Bacterial Infections

3.8 Bacterial Pneumonia

1. Etiology/Epidemiology
   a. The most common etiologic agent in HIV infections is *S. pneumoniae.* Other causative pathogens are *H. influenza, Mycoplasma pneumoniae, C. pneumoniae, S. aureus, Streptococcus pyogenes, N. meningitidis, Moraxella catarrhalis,* and *Klebsiella pneumoniae.*
   b. Population-based studies suggest pneumococcal pneumonia occurs 200 times more frequently in patients with HIV disease than in age-matched populations (Musher, 2000).
   c. Recurrence is relatively common. Thirteen percent of cases recur within 6 months, and the reported mortality rate among HIV-infected persons with bacteremic pneumococcal pneumonia is 5% to 11% (Centers for Disease Control and Prevention, 1999).
2. Pathogenesis
   a. Bacteria are transmitted by respiratory droplets spread by close person-to-person contact.
   b. Bacteria adhere to pharyngeal cells and subsequently colonize.
   c. Complications include otitis media, sinusitis, and bronchitis.
3. Clinical presentation
   a. Symptoms of acute respiratory infection often include several of the following: fever, productive cough, chills, dyspnea, pleuritic chest pain, orthopnea, fatigue, and malaise.
4. Diagnosis
   a. Baseline assessments
      i. Chest radiography is performed to substantiate diagnosis of pneumonia and as a baseline to assess response to treatment.
      ii. Sputum gram stain and culture for conventional bacteria should be considered.
      iii. Complete blood cell and differential counts, serum creatinine, urea nitrogen, and electrolyte, bilirubin, and liver enzyme values are determined.
      iv. Blood cultures from at least two different sites are taken before treatment.
      v. A test is conducted for *Mycobacterium tuberculosis* using an acid-fast bacilli stain and culture for selected patients, especially those with cough or other symptoms suggestive of tuberculosis (TB).
5. Prevention/Treatment
   a. Immunization with 23-valent pneumococcal polysaccharide vaccine should always be offered to all patients with HIV. Vaccination can occur on initial clinical contact, and revaccination should occur every 3 to 5 years thereafter.
   b. The risk of pneumococcal pneumonia is greatly reduced in vaccinated individuals with CD_4 counts > 500 cells/mm^3.
   c. *Pneumocystis carinii* pneumonia (PCP) prophylaxis with trimethoprim-sulfamethoxazole (TMP-SMX) may decrease risk of infection (Musher, 2000).
   d. Cefotaxime or ceftriaxone are the antibiotics of choice; ampicillin is also used. In patients who are allergic to

beta-lactam antibiotics, vancomycin or a quinolone antibiotic may be used. If bacteremia is suspected, treat with IV antipseudomonal beta-lactam (e.g., imipenem) combined with an aminoglycoside (e.g., tobramycin) (Musher, 2000).

6. Nursing implications
   a. Promote optimal gas exchange (e.g., incentive spirometry, oxygen therapy, chest percussion, drainage therapy).
   b. Promote hydration with fluids, 2.5 to 3L/day, and provide nutritional support, such as vitamin and mineral supplements and increased calories.
   c. Monitor laboratory results, such as hemoglobin and hematocrit, white blood cell count, bilirubin, lactate dehydrogenase, and adverse effects, such as empyema and response to therapy.

3.9 Mycobacterium Avium Complex (MAC)

1. Etiology/Epidemiology
   a. MAC consists of two closely related species, *M. avium* and *M. intracellulare,* that are ubiquitous (food, water, soil); *M. avium* is more virulent.
   b. MAC is not considered contagious.
   c. The environment is source of most human infections.
   d. MAC bacteria were found in the blood of 43% of people within two years of their AIDS diagnosis (Project Inform, 2001).
2. Pathogenesis
   a. Infects gastrointestinal or respiratory tracts; asymptomatic colonization is probably an essential step in the disease. *M. avium*–infected macrophages evade host defense by inactivating normal intracellular killing mechanisms. HIV infected monocytes may enhance intracellular replication of *M. avium;* widespread replication results in metastatic seeding.
   b. Disseminated MAC (DMAC) occurs when CD_4 cell counts < 50 cells/mm^3; DMAC is probably a newly acquired infection rather than a reactivation (Bick, 2001; Zwolski & Talotta, 2001).

3. Clinical presentation
   a. GI: chronic diarrhea, abdominal pain, chronic malabsorption, and extrabiliary obstructive disease
   b. DMAC: characterized by constitutional symptoms, such as fatigue, fever, weight loss, night sweats, abdominal pain, diarrhea, lymphadenopathy, organomegaly, and anemia (Centers for Disease Control and Prevention, 2001; Zwolski & Talotta, 2001)
4. Diagnosis
   a. Mycobacterial blood cultures: single positive culture is diagnostic; bone marrow/tissue biopsy can be done but is rarely used.
   b. AFB smears: Since *M. avium, M. intracellulare,* and *M. tuberculosis* are acid-fast bacilli, positive AFB smear is treated as *M. tuberculosis* infection until definitive diagnosis.
   c. MAC cultures in sputum and stools are controversial. Sputum cultures may represent colonization. X-ray or endoscopic procedures may assist in diagnosis (Zwolski & Talotta, 2001).
5. Prevention/Treatment
   a. Prevention: Prophylaxis when CD_4 cell counts < 50 cells/mm^3; preferred regimen—Clarithromycin 500 mg PO BID or Azithromycin 1,200 mg PO once weekly; alternative regimen—Rifabutin 300 mg PO q day or Azithromycin 1,200 mg/week plus Rifabutin 300 mg q day (Bartlett & Gallant, 2000; Centers for Disease Control and Prevention, 2001; Zwolski & Talotta, 2001)
   b. Treatment: preferred regimen—Clarithromycin 500 mg PO BID or Azithromycin 500 to 600 mg PO q day plus Ethambutol 15 mg/kg/day PO with or without Rifabutin 300 mg/day PO; alternative regimen—Ciprofloxacin, Ofloxacin, or Amikacin (Bartlett & Gallant, 2000; Centers for Disease Control and Prevention, 2001; Zwolski & Talotta, 2001)
   c. Maintenance: preferred regimen—Clarithromycin 500 mg PO BID plus Ethambutol 15 mg/kg PO q day with or without Rifabutin 300 mg PO q day; alternative regimen—Azithromycin 500 mg PO q day plus Ethambutol

15 mg/kg PO q day with or without Rifabutin 300 mg PO q day (Bartlett & Gallant, 2000; CDC, 2001; Zwolski & Talotta, 2001)

6. Nursing implications
   a. Monitor laboratory results (CBC with differential) and other indices for side effects, adverse effects, toxicity, and response to therapy.
   b. Perform blood cultures 4 to 8 weeks after initiation of therapy (Bick, 2001; Zwolski & Talotta, 2001).
   c. Provide patient education and monitor for multiple drug interactions, especially rifabutin and rifampin.

3.10 Mycobacterium Tuberculosis

1. Etiology/Epidemiology
   a. *Mycobacterium tuberculosis* (mTB) is caused by acid-fast bacilli that are transmitted through droplet nuclei that become aerosolized via talking, laughing, coughing, or singing; droplets can remain airborne for 48 hours.
   b. Risk of tuberculosis (mTB) activation in an HIV-positive person is 8% to 10% per year versus 7% to 10% lifetime risk for a HIV-negative person (Bick, 2001; Centers for Disease Control and Prevention, 2001).

2. Pathogenesis
   a. *M. tuberculosis* is inhaled and the organisms penetrate the lung parenchyma. The bacilli are transported to hilar lymph nodes by macrophages, and the macrophages disseminate organisms in the blood or wall off infection in granulomas, preventing active disease (latent tuberculosis).
   b. Cell-mediated immunity is activated to halt the infectious process and dissemination. The infection can be detected in 2 to 10 weeks with a tuberculin skin test (TST). A breakdown of cell-mediated immunity (CD_4 cell count < 200 cells/mm^3) results in reactivation of TB and possibly active disease (Zwolski & Talotta, 2001).

3. Clinical presentation
   a. Constitutional symptoms include fever, chills, weight loss, fatigue, and night sweats. Constitutional symptoms of pulmonary tuberculosis include productive cough, hemoptysis, shortness of breath, and pleuritic chest pain. Extrapulmonary tuberculosis includes indistinct symptoms that vary with the system involved (e.g., renal cortex, lymph nodes, bone, meninges, abdomen, pericardium; Zwolski & Talotta, 2001).

4. Diagnosis: TST, using Mantoux method; chest X-ray; acid-fast bacilli smear and culture of sputum or any other body fluids or tissue (Bartlett & Gallant, 2000).

5. Prevention/Treatment
   a. All HIV-infected patients should have an annual TST.
   b. Preventive regimens can be provided to patients who have a positive TST (> 5 mm induration), who had a recent TB contact, or who have a history of inadequate TB treatment that healed.
      i. Preferred regimen: 9 months; isoniazid (INH) plus pyridoxine
      ii. Alternative regimen: rifampin and pyrazinamide for 2 months (clients on HAART should have rifabutin substituted for rifampin)
   c. Treatment of active disease: Several treatment and dosage options exist; consult the most current recommendations (see Appendix 12.2). A typical regimen for clients on antiretrovirals, who are waiting for culture results, includes the following drugs (rifabutin is contraindicated or requires dosage adjustment with some antiretrovirals):

      • 2 months (induction phase): INH, rifabutin, pyrazinamide, ethambutol
      • 4 months: INH and rifabutin
      • Multidrug resistant MTB (MDR-TB): Choice of drugs requires consultation with infectious disease expert.

6. Nursing implications
   a. Teach about and monitor laboratory results (e.g., complete blood count with

differential, liver function test) and other indices to monitor for side effects, adverse effects, toxicity, and response to therapy; test vision for ethambutol-induced optic neuritis.

b. Educate about importance of adherence; consider direct observational therapy (DOT).

3.11 Salmonellosis

1. Etiology/Epidemiology
   a. Causative agents are *Salmonella* bacterial species gram-negative rods.
   b. Humans acquire salmonella by ingesting contaminated food or water.
      i. Salmonella is widely disseminated in the environment and is intimately associated with animals.
      ii. Poultry and poultry products, primarily eggs, constitute the principal reservoir; approximately half of U.S. chickens are culture positive.
   c. Patients with certain types of GI alterations, such as achlorhydria or antacid abuse, alterations in endogenous intestinal flora for unknown reasons, antibiotic use, recent intestinal surgery, and chronic GI disease (e.g., inflammatory bowel disease, malignancies), are at increased risk for salmonellosis. Patients with advanced HIV disease are also at increased risk, especially if they are not receiving AZT or trimethoprim-sulfamethoxazole TMP-SMZ.
2. Pathogenesis
   a. Ingested organisms must pass from the mouth to stomach and small intestine to cause infection.
      i. Mucosal invasion of small bowel and enterotoxin elaboration probably result in diarrhea.
      ii. Infection of macrophages allows for disseminated spread via the blood stream.
   b. A small percentage of infected patients may develop a chronic carrier state (i.e., persistence of salmonella in stool or urine).

3. Clinical presentation
   a. Salmonellosis is divided into the discrete syndromes of enterocolitis, enteric fever, and bacteremia; clinically, however, these syndromes often overlap.
      i. Enterocolitis is indistinguishable from manifestations of other GI pathogens. Onset is usually within 48 hours after ingesting contaminant and symptoms include mild to fulminant diarrhea with vague constitutional symptoms: abdominal cramping, nausea, headache, myalgias, fever, chills, and nonbloody/nonmucoid diarrhea.
      ii. Typhoid, or enteric, fever is a severe systemic illness characterized by abdominal symptoms followed by fever and is caused by the *S. typhi* species.
      iii. Salmonellosis may present as a debilitating, febrile bacteremia without GI symptoms. This is the most common syndrome associated with AIDS.
4. Diagnosis
   a. Definitive diagnosis requires isolating salmonella species from blood. Diagnosis is suggested by isolation of organism from stool.
      i. Stool cultures. If stool cultures are negative or patient has bloody diarrhea, anoscopic or sigmoid exam for direct lesion culture may be indicated; biopsy may or may not be performed.
      ii. Blood cultures. Less than 5% of immunocompetent patients with GI symptoms have positive blood cultures, although blood cultures are indicated in at-risk populations. Draw blood cultures from two separate sites, including a central line if present, before starting antibiotics.
      iii. Bone marrow cultures have a sensitivity of 90% and thus can be used to detect the bacteria.
      iv. Patients with *S. typhi* infection may present with faint, salmon-colored maculopapular rash on

trunk; organisms may be cultured from punch biopsy of lesions.

b. Differential diagnoses include malaria, amoebic liver abscess, visceral leishmaniasis, and viral syndromes.

5. Prevention/Treatment
   a. Avoid obvious sources of salmonellosis: undercooked or raw poultry products, unpasteurized dairy products, and animal feces.
   b. Ciprofloxacin is the optimal therapy for HIV-related salmonella infections.
   c. Chloramphenicol or quinolone antibiotics are treatment of choice for enteric fever. TMP/SMX and ampicillin can be used as alternative therapy.
   d. Neuropsychiatric manifestations of typhoid fever may be treated with high-dose glucocorticoids.

6. Nursing implications
   a. Laboratory results should be reviewed with other indices to monitor for adverse effects and response to therapy.
   b. Monitor patients closely for dehydration and electrolyte imbalance caused by diarrhea and vomiting.
   c. Household contacts of HIV-infected people with salmonellosis should be evaluated for asymptomatic carriage of salmonella.
   d. Travelers to endemic countries should consider typhoid vaccination, although it is generally not recommended.

Fungal Infections

3.12 Candidiasis

1. Etiology/Epidemiology
   a. Candida albicans is the predominant causative agent of candidiasis; other species (*C. glabrata*, *C. parapsilosis*, *C. tropicalis*, *C. kruseii*) can cause candidiasis in HIV disease, but they do so less frequently (Fichtenbaum & Aberg, 1999).
   b. Candida are ubiquitous fungi (yeasts) that grow as single cells and reproduce by budding (Fichtenbaum & Aberg, 1999).
   c. More than 90% of HIV-infected patients will develop oral candidiasis in advanced disease (McCarthy, 1991).

d. Widespread treatment with antifungals (azoles) has led to a decline in the prevalence of mucosal candidiasis, while leading to the emergence of refractory infections that are azole resistant (Hitchcock, 1993).

2. Pathogenesis
   a. Most disease is caused by organisms that are part of the normal flora of the individual; person-to-person transmission is possible but rare (Barchiesi, 1995).
   b. Level of immunosuppression is inversely related to the development of candidiasis in HIV disease (McCarthy, 1991).
   c. Chronic recurrence is common.

3. Clinical presentation
   a. Oropharyngeal candidiasis
      i. Three distinct forms exist: pseudomembranous—removable white plaques that reveal an erythematous or bleeding surface; erythematous—smooth red patches on the palate, buccal mucosa, or tongue; and angular chelitis—erythema, cracks, and fissures at the corners of the mouth (Greenspan & Greenspan, 1995).
      ii. Symptoms include burning pain, altered taste sensation, and dysphagia.
   b. Esophageal candidiasis
      i. Symptoms include dysphagia, odynophagia, substernal chest pain, and feelings of obstruction and heartburn, but patients may be asymptomatic (Tavitian, 1986).
      ii. Usually occurs in the presence of oropharyngeal infection but may occur independently (Tavitian, 1986).
      iii. Considered an AIDS indicator disease.
   c. Vulvovaginal candidiasis
      i. Symptoms include marked itching, watery to cottage-cheese-thick discharge, vaginal erythema with adherent white discharge, dyspareunia, external dysuria, swelling of the labia and vulva with discrete pustulopapular

peripheral lesions (Fichtenbaum & Aberg, 1999).

  ii. Symptoms typically exacerbate the week preceding menses (Fichtenbaum & Aberg, 1999).

d. Disseminated infection is rare in HIV disease.

4. Diagnosis
   a. Oropharyngeal and vulvovaginal candidiasis
      i. Diagnosis is made on its characteristic appearance; recovery of organism is not required.
      ii. Microscopic examination of plaque scraping using Gram's stain or 10% potassium hydroxide (KOH) reveals sheets of hyphae, pseudohyphae, and yeast forms.
      iii. Culture usually not necessary, but it can be helpful if patient is not responding to treatment to rule out other possible etiologies or resistant fungi (Wilcox, 1996).
   b. Esophogeal candidiasis
      i. Presumptive diagnosis made based on characteristic symptoms (Rabeneck, 1994).
      ii. Upper GI endoscopy or blind sweeping of the esophagus can recover organism for microscopic examination to confirm diagnosis (Bonacini, 1990).

5. Prevention/Treatment
   a. Primary prophylaxis is not recommended for candidiasis; however, secondary prophylaxis should be considered for frequent recurrences (Powderly, 1995).
   b. Oropharyngeal candidiasis: Usually responds readily to topical agents, such as nystatin 5 ml suspension to be gargled 5 × daily or clotrimazole troches 10 mg for sucking to dissolution 5 × day, and these should be considered first-line treatment choices because of their ease of administration, low cost, and lack of ability to induce resistance. The azole class of antifungals (fluconazole: 50 to 100 mg PO daily for 10 to 14 days; ketoconazole: 200 to 400 mg PO daily

for 10 to 14 days; itraconazole: 200 mg PO daily for 10 to 14 days) should be used in severe cases (Fichtenbaum & Aberg, 1999).
   c. Esophogeal candidiasis: Systemic treatment with oral azole antifungals in the previous dosages is recommended.
   d. Vulvovaginal candidiasis: Standard treatment consists of topical clotrimazole (about 5 g) intravaginally or miconazole 2% cream for 3 to 7 days (Fichtenbaum & Aberg, 1999). Systemic oral azole therapy should be considered for severe cases.
   e. Refractory cases
      i. Refractory disease is defined as the failure to respond to antifungal treatment with appropriate doses for a standard duration of time (Fichtenbaum & Aberg, 1999).
      ii. Refractory candidiasis tends to occur in advanced disease after chronic exposure to antifungal therapy.
      iii. Fluconazole refractory candidiasis is most common. Increasing dose or switching azoles may be beneficial. Oral amphotericin B is also available for refractory cases (Dewsnup, 1994). *Oral amphotericin is no longer available but can be prepared by a pharmacist.*
      iv. Parenteral amphotericin B 0.3 to 0.8 mg/kg is the drug of choice for severe refractory candidiasis, especially when the esophagus is involved.

6. Nursing implications
   a. Frequent oral hygiene measures should be implemented on patients with oral candidiasis.
   b. Women with vaginal candidiasis should avoid tight-fitting underwear and pantyhose, douching, and foods high in sugar. They should also be encouraged to daily consume yogurt that contains *Lactobacillus acidophilus.*
   c. Nutritional assessment and intervention may be necessary with esophageal candidiasis.

3.13 Coccidioidomycosis

1. Etiology/Epidemiology
   a. Etiologic agent is *C. immitis,* a dimorphic fungus probably related to the ascomycetes. It appears as either a mycelium at room temperature or a spherule at body temperature.
   b. Mycelia grow in the soil during rainy seasons; they become airborne in dry seasons via wind and mechanical soil disruption.
   c. AIDS-associated coccidioidal disease is generally confined to endemic areas (i.e., southwestern United States, northern Mexico, and portions of Central and South America)
2. Pathogenesis
   a. The organism enters pulmonary tract via inhalation. In an immunocompromised host, infection disseminates to the skin, central nervous system (CNS), bones, lymph nodes, and liver.
   b. Disease in HIV-infected populations is generally associated with a CD_4 count < 250 cells/mm^3 and impaired T-cell function. It may reflect reactivation of previously acquired infection or recent exposure.
3. Clinical presentation
   a. Clinical presentation is usually nonspecific and can range from asymptomatic presentation to life-threatening pneumonia or CNS disease.
   b. Constitutional symptoms of malaise, fever, cough, and fatigue are often present.
   c. Pulmonary disease may be indistinguishable from other opportunistic infections. Chest radiographic findings include focal alveolar infiltrates, discrete nodules, hilar adenopathy, or cavitary lesions.
   d. CNS involvement is characterized by the following cerebrospinal fluid (CSF) findings: high cell counts, decreased glucose, and elevated protein.
   e. Other focal findings are related to sites of end-organ disease, such as the skin, CNS, lymph nodes, liver, spleen, kidneys, adrenal glands, and peritoneum.

4. Diagnosis
   a. Diagnosis can be difficult and secondary to nonspecific presentation, especially in nonendemic areas. Review previous living and travel history to prevent diagnostic delay.
   b. Definitive diagnosis established by either culturing organism or by demonstrating spherule presence via histopathologic stains from clinical specimens.
   c. Differential diagnoses include all other pulmonary opportunistic infections.
5. Prevention/Treatment
   a. Routine screening with skin testing has shown no predictive value for disease development; prophylaxis is not currently recommended.
   b. Avoiding endemic areas and excavation or construction sites may reduce risk of infection.
   c. Amphotericin B remains the principal acute therapy for initial and recurrent disease, although precise dose remains unclear. Most investigators recommend 1 mg/kg/day IV for a cumulative total dosage of 500–700 mg before switching to azole maintenance therapy.
   d. Evidence suggests that fluconazole and itraconazole are an effective acute therapy for mild disease.
   e. After completion of acute therapy, HIV-infected people usually require lifelong maintenance therapy with either fluconazole or itraconzole.
6. Nursing implications
   a. Monitor for adverse effects and response to therapy.
      i. For patients treated with amphotericin B consider the following:

      - Concurrent hydration is required to minimize renal toxicity; liposomal form may be used for patients with significant amphotericin B–induced nephrotoxicity.
      - Shivering or rigors can be controlled with narcotics.
      - Monitoring includes the following: twice weekly: serum magnesium and potassium

levels; weekly: complete blood and platelet count; every other day: serum creatinine and BUN while dosage is increased, then at least twice weekly.

   ii. For patients treated with fluconazole, monitor serum creatinine, BUN, and liver function tests as indicated.

   iii. For patients treated with itraconazole, monitor liver function tests and serum potassium as indicated; itraconazole levels may be monitored.

 b. Provide education about importance of maintenance therapy.

   i. Azoles often associated with nausea. Itraconazole capsules must be taken with food to ensure adequate absorption.

   ii. Drug interactions can occur. Concomitant use of rifampin and rifabutin significantly increases itraconazole clearance. Use of these agents as prophylaxis or treatment for mycobacterial infections must be avoided.

   iii. Relapse may occur despite maintenance therapy, and patient should report any symptom of recurrence.

3.14 Cryptococcosis

1. Etiology/Epidemiology
   a. Etiologic agent is *Cryptococcus neoformans,* a yeast characterized by distinctive polysaccharide encapsulations that can be divided into serotypic groups A, B, C, and D.
   b. Organism is ubiquitous in nature and distributed worldwide. Serotypes A and D are found in pigeon droppings and soil; serotype C has been isolated from fruit and fruit juices.
   c. Recurrent disease is thought to involve reactivation of initial infection.
   d. The incidence of cryptococcosis is 0.2 to 0.9 cases per 100,000 in the general population. In persons with AIDS, the annual incidence is 2 to 4 cases per 1,000

(Centers for Disease Control and Prevention, 2002a) and is associated with both advanced HIV disease (CD_4 counts < 100 cells/mm^3) and recrudescence of latent infection. The infection is more commonly seen in IV drug users, ethnic minorities, and south-central areas of the United States for unknown reasons.

2. Pathogenesis
   a. Aerosolized organisms enter pulmonary tract via inhalation. The most common extrapulmonary site of the disease is the central nervous system (CNS), but it can also involve skin, bone, and the genitourinary tract.
   b. *C. neoformans* produces tissue destruction secondary to yeast multiplication and tissue displacement. The infection elicits a variable inflammatory response and well-formed granulomas are generally not seen.

      i. Characteristic lesions are cystic clusters of fungi with minimal inflammatory response (cyptococcoma, cyptococcocal granuloma).

      ii. CNS lesions tend to spread diffusely through the brain to involve basal ganglia, cortical gray matter, and meninges.

3. Clinical presentation
   a. Symptoms are usually insidious in HIV-infected patients but can be acute in advanced AIDS.
   b. Underlying immunodeficiency associated with altered inflammatory response and fever may be either initially absent or low grade.
   c. Pulmonary system can be asymptomatic or have a nonspecific presentation of fever, headache, malaise, cough, dyspnea, and pleuritic-type chest pain.
   d. Symptoms involving the CNS have an insidious or acute onset that can chronically wax or wane with asymptomatic intervals. CNS-specific symptoms include headaches, stiff neck, focal deficits, and seizures. Nonspecific symptoms of CNS infection include nausea, dizziness, irritability, somnolence, clumsiness, confusion or obtundation, and diarrhea.

e. Other numerous sites of end-organ disease have been reported, including skin, bone, renal, oral mucosa, and GU tract.

4. Diagnosis

   a. Diagnosis is not associated with the routine lab abnormalities seen with most infections, and detection of organism by culture or histology is necessary for a definitive diagnosis. Serologic testing for cryptococcal antigen (CRAG) is clinically useful for detecting organisms.

   b. Pulmonary cryptococcosis

      i. Radiographic findings often resemble a tumor with single or multiple circumscribed masses or nodules without hilar involvement. Other patterns include findings of lymphadenopathy or pleural effusions, most often with diffuse mixed interstitial infiltrates.

      ii. Bronchoscopic washings and brushings are usually diagnostic.

      iii. Sputum cultures can be negative with invasive disease; parenchymal and tissue samples are usually necessary for definitive diagnosis.

   c. CNS cryptococcosis

      i. Usually manifests as cerebrospinal fluid (CSF) abnormalities, including increased opening pressure (< 200 mm H_2O), lowered glucose level, increased protein concentration, and leukocyte counts > 20 cells/mm^3

      ii. Positive antigen titers and fungal cultures

      iii. CT scan or MRI findings may be normal or reveal diffuse atrophy, cerebral edema, hydrocephalus, or focal mass lesions.

      iv. Differential diagnosis is focused on ruling out other CNS space-occupying lesions, such as aspergillus, tuberculosis, toxoplamosis, lymphoma, or other neoplasms.

5. Prevention/Treatment

   a. Routine CRAG screening of HIV-infected people is not currently recommended because of limited sensitivity/specificity of the assay.

   b. Avoid sites that are likely to be contaminated with *C. neoformans*; tobacco-smoking cessation may reduce disease risk.

   c. Acute therapy (Aberg & Powderly, 2002; Saag, 2000) for the initial infection or recurrent infection includes the following:

      • Amphotericin B (0.7–1.0 mg/ kg IV daily) for minimum of 2 weeks, with or without 5-flucytosine (100 mg/kg orally QID, adjusted for any renal insufficiency development), followed by consolidation therapy of either fluconazole (400 mg orally daily for 8 to 10 weeks) or itraconazole (200 mg orally twice daily for 8 to 10 weeks).

      • In the absence of obstructive hydrocephalus, CNS disease may require serial lumbar punctures to release increased intracranial pressure. If lumbar puncture is insufficient to manage increased intracranial pressure, lumbar drain, ventriculostomy, or placement of a ventricular-peritoneal shunt may be performed.

   d. Suppressive maintenance therapy is a lifelong process. The usual regimen is fluconazole (200 mg orally daily). Alternative regimens are itraconazole (200 mg orally twice daily) or amphotericin B (1 mg/kg IV once or twice weekly).

6. Nursing implications

   a. See Section 3.13, titled Coccidioidomycosis, for nursing implications relevant to treatment with amphotericin B, fluconazole, and itraconazole.

   b. For patients treated with 5-flucytosine, frequent monitoring of serum alanine aminotransferase (ALT), alkaline phosphatase, aspartate aminotransferase (AST), bilirubin, creatinine, and blood urea nitrogen is indicated.

   c. Ensure lumbar puncture opening pressure is recorded.

d. Educate patient about prevention and importance of maintenance therapy (see Section 3.13 Coccidioidomycosis for specific interventions).

3.15 Histoplasmosis

1. Etiology/Epidemiology
   a. Etiologic agent is *Histoplasma capsulatum,* a fungus deposited in the soil via bird and bat droppings.
   b. *H. capsulatum* is endemic in the southern and midwestern United States from Alabama to southwest Texas and along the Ohio and Missouri river valleys. Hyperendemic areas include Indianapolis, Indiana, and Kansas City, Missouri. It is also found in eastern Mexico, the Caribbean, Central and South America, and parts of Southeast Asia.
   c. In endemic areas, incidence is reported to be approximately 5% of opportunistic infections (OIs), compared with 25% of OIs in hyperendemic areas.
   d. Infections in persons who live outside endemic areas are due to reactivation of previously acquired infection.
2. Pathogenesis
   a. Aerosolized spores enter the pulmonary tract via inhalation. Spores become activated and can spread via reticuloendothelial system to the liver, spleen, and lymph nodes. Infection is characterized by granuloma formation.
   b. Disseminated disease is associated with advanced HIV disease and median CD_4 count of 50 cells/mm^3 at time of diagnosis.
3. Clinical presentation
   a. Constitutional symptoms are present in 95% of cases, and respiratory complaints are seen in 50–60% of cases; hepatosplenomegaly, lymphadenopathy, and septicemia commonly present at time of diagnosis.
   b. Neurologic manifestations, such as meningitis, are reported in 18–20% of cases.
   c. Skin and mucosal ulcers may be present.

4. Diagnosis
   a. Diagnosis can be difficult secondary to nonspecific presentation, especially in nonendemic areas. Review previous living and travel history to prevent diagnostic delay.
   b. Positive culture from blood or tissue specimens is necessary for definitive diagnosis, which can take up to 3 weeks.
      i. Histopathological evaluation of bone marrow or tissue biopsy is useful for establishing diagnosis in 50% of patients.
      ii. Standard antibody serology test is not useful because it does not distinguish current from past infection.
      iii. Histoplasma specific antigen (HAG) can be assayed in both serum and urine specimens, although urine test is more sensitive. Most diagnoses of disseminated histoplasmosis are now made with this test because of its rapid turnaround time, compared with culture.
   c. Differential diagnoses include all other pulmonary opportunistic infections.
   d. Hematologic disturbances are frequently present, primarily anemia.
   e. Diffuse or patchy infiltrates are the most common radiographic abnormality.
5. Prevention/Treatment
   a. Routine skin testing is of little value in endemic areas because most people will test positive. Primary prophylaxis is not currently recommended.
   b. Avoiding endemic areas and excavation or construction sites may reduce risk of infection.
   c. Amphotericin B is the recommended acute therapy for severe initial or recurrent disease (Deepe, 2000; Saag, 2000). Dosage is 0.7–1.0 mg/kg IV daily for 1–2 weeks, followed by itraconazole (200 mg PO BID) consolidation therapy for 10–12 weeks. Itraconazole (200 mg PO BID) for 3 months can be used for treatment of mild disease.
   d. HIV-infected persons usually require lifelong maintenance therapy for suppression after completion of consolidation therapy. Maintenance

therapy is usually itraconazole (200 mg PO QID).

6. Nursing implications: See "Nursing implications" in the Coccidioidomycosis section.

Protozoal Infections

3.16 Cryptosporidiosis

1. Etiology/Epidemiology
   a. The global prevalence of cryptosporidiosis infection is 8%. The prevalence in the United States is estimated to be 6.2%.
   b. Etiologic agent is cryptosporidium, a sporozoa.
2. Pathogenesis
   a. Cryptosporidium exists as an oocyst that releases sporozoites that adhere to the surface of the intestinal mucosa.
   b. Following ingestion and attachment, primarily in the small intestine, it is hypothesized that phagocytes are activated, resulting in the release of soluble factors (i.e., histamine, prostaglandins, leukotrienes) that increase the intestinal secretion of water and chloride and also inhibit absorption.
   c. Intestinal epithelial cells are characterized by villus atrophy and crypt hyperplasia. Histological changes are hypothesized to be the result of either direct viral invasion or inflammatory processes (Goodgame, 1996).
3. Clinical presentation
   a. Diarrhea: may be scant and intermittent or may be cholera-like (up to 20 liters/day)
   b. Other GI symptoms: severe abdominal cramping, nausea, and flatulence
   c. Constitutional symptoms: low-grade fever, malaise, and weight loss
4. Diagnosis
   a. Thorough health history: drinking water that is unfiltered and untreated; involvement in farming practices; sex practices that involve oral/fecal contact; contact with other infected persons or health care employees; living in densely populated urban areas
   b. Stool analyses for ova and parasites using a modified acid-fast stain
   c. Serology: ELISA or antibody immunofluorescence assay for the presence of anticryptosporidial IgM, IgG, and IgA
   d. Small-bowel biopsy is rarely necessary.
5. Prevention/Treatment
   a. Prevention
      i. Hand washing, especially after contact with human or animal feces
         (1) Avoid fecal exposure during sex
         (2) Avoid untreated drinking water and public pools/tubs
         (3) Thoroughly wash fruits and vegetables
   b. Treatment
      i. Antiretroviral therapy improves immune status and will decrease or eliminate symptoms of cryptosporidiosis.
      ii. Paromomycin has been shown to decrease the intensity of the infection and improve intestinal function.
      iii. Spiramycin or dicalzuril may decrease diarrhea and oocyst number.
      iv. Intravenous fluids or oral rehydration with electrolyte solutions can be used.
      v. Medications to slow GI motility, such as opiates, lomotil, somatostatin, might be helpful.
      vi. Diet changes can be suggested. Alternatives include lactose-free, low-fat—using medium chain triglycerides—high-protein, low-residue, and caffeine-free diets.
6. Nursing implications
   a. Teach the patient good hand-washing technique to prevent transmission of organism.
   b. Encourage water safety and food safety: use a 0.1–1.0 micron filter on water faucets, boil untreated water, and avoid unpasteurized foods.
   c. Enteric precautions should be initiated for incontinent patients.
   d. Caregivers should use 5–10% ammonia or full-strength 70% bleach for cleaning contaminated areas.

3.17 Isosporiasis

1. Etiology/Epidemiology
   a. The global prevalence of isosporiasis infection is 4%. The prevalence in the United States is estimated to be 1% to 3%. Isosporiasis is more prevalent in developing countries, such as Africa, South America, and Asia (UNAIDS Technical Update, 1998).
   b. The etiologic agent is *Isospora belli*, a coccidian protozoan.
2. Pathogenesis
   a. Oocytes are ingested and, in the small intestine, mature to sporozoites and then to oocysts.
   b. Oocysts pass into the environment, where they sporulate and become infectious.
3. Clinical presentation
   a. Severe, profuse, watery diarrhea; in some cases, steatorrhea; cramping and abdominal pain
   b. Weight loss
   c. Occasional low-grade fever
   d. Most common in persons with CD_4 cell count below 200; classified as an AIDS-defining illness
4. Diagnosis
   a. Stool studies for ova and parasites; and the presence of oocyst using a modified acid-fast stain; differentiation from cryptosporidiosis important
5. Prevention/Treatment
   a. Prevention
      i. Good hand washing is important to prevent spread of organisms.
      ii. Areas contaminated with infected stool should be cleaned with standard disinfectants.
      iii. All fresh fruits and vegetables should be washed well.
      iv. Persons should drink purified water.
6. Treatment
   a. First-line therapy: trimethoprim-sulfamethoxazole (TMP-SMX) for 10 days, then for 3 weeks
   b. Second-line therapy: ciprofloxacin BID for 7 days for patients who cannot tolerate TMP-SMX

   c. Relapse prevention: chronic suppressive therapy; TMP-SMX or sulfadoxine-pyrimethamine
   d. Symptom management with antidiarrheal agents
7. Nursing implications
   a. Teach patient to practice good hand washing to avoid infection.
   b. Wash all fresh fruits and vegetables before eating.
   c. Avoid fecal contact during sexual contact.

3.18 Pneumocystosis

1. Etiology/Epidemiology
   a. The etiologic agent is the fungus *Pneumocystis carinii* (PCP).
   b. Incidence has decreased in industrialized countries as a result of augmentation of the immune system due to better prophylaxis and HAART.
   c. Survey data suggest pneumocystosis (PCP) infection occurs in approximately 26% of patients with AIDS without prophylaxis (Jones, Hanson, Dworkin, Alderton, et al., 1999).
   d. Data indicate that it remains the most common AIDS-defining illness (Walzer, 2000).
   e. Risk of developing PCP infection has been correlated with a CD_4 count of 200 cells/mm^3 or less (Walzer, 2000).
2. Pathogenesis
   a. Organism attaches to type 1 alveolar cells, replicates, and invades the epithelium of the lung.
   b. The immunocompromised host is unable to mount an alveolar macrophage response, resulting in pneumonia and interfering with the transport of fatty acid substrates, an essential component of lung surfactant. Without surfactant, lung dispensability is diminished.
3. Clinical presentation
   a. Symptoms are insidious and slowly progress over the course of a few weeks; most common symptoms are low-grade fever, nonproductive cough, and dyspnea.

b. Fever, fatigue, and weight loss may precede respiratory symptoms (Kovacs, Gill, Meshnick, & Masur, 2001).

4. Diagnosis

   a. The recovery of the organism from expectorated sputum is difficult. The diagnosis is often made on the presence of classic symptoms, chest radiograph (diffuse, bilateral infiltrates), and pulse oximetry (hypoxemia with activity).

   b. Sputum induction via inhalation of a saline mist performed by specialists is an acceptable, noninvasive diagnostic alternative (Walzer, 2000).

   c. *Pneumocystis carinii* may be identified in bronchoalveolar lavage or transbronchial biopsy but are not required for diagnosis.

   d. Laboratory data, such as arterial blood gases, should be monitored for hypoxemia because prognosis is related to oxygenation at time of presentation (alveolar-arterial oxygen gradient of > 45 mmHg is considered severe disease with a poor prognosis; Walzer, 2000).

5. Prevention/Treatment

   a. Primary prophylactic agents include trimethoprim-sulfamethoxazole (TMP-SMX; preferred therapy), dapsone, aerosolized pentamidine, dapsone/pyrimethamine, atovaquone, trimethoprim, and parenteral pentamidine.

   b. Prophylaxis should be offered to any patient with a CD_4 count less than or equal to 200 cells/mm^3 or less or a patient who has recovered from a previous episode of PCP. Prophylaxis may be discontinued if durable viral suppression is achieved with HAART and a stable CD_4 count > 200 cells/mm^3 for > 3 months (Gottlieb, 1999; Mussini et al., 2000).

   c. The preferred prophylactic regimen is TMP-SMX (Bactrim) DS/day or 1 SS/day.

   d. The treatment duration is 21 days (it may be extended with severe disease). Agents include TMP-SMX, pentamidine, trimetrexate with leucovorin rescue during length of infusion and 3 days beyond last dose, trimethoprim with dapsone, clindamycin with primaquine (especially if TMP-SMX treatment fails), atovaquone, and corticosteroids. The preferred treatment regimen is TMP-SMX (Bactrim) 2 DS tablets TID.

   e. Corticosteroids may be added during the first 72 hours of treatment in patients with an arterial oxygen pressure < 70 mmHg or an alveolar-arterial oxygen gradient > 35mmHg (Walzer, 2000).

6. Nursing implications

   a. Promote optimal gas exchange (e.g., incentive spirometry, oxygen therapy, chest percussion; Flaskerud & Ungvarski, 1999).

   b. Do not place a coughing patient with PCP in a room with an immunocompromised patient until active tuberculosis (TB) is ruled out (Flaskerud & Ungvarski, 1999).

   c. Monitor for side effects or adverse effects of medications, such as rash/photosensitivity, peripheral neuropathy, and liver function abnormalities; extreme caution should be used with desensitization to TMP-SMX; monitor for glucose-6-phosphate dehydrogenase deficiency to prevent hemolysis.

   d. Monitor blood glucose during parenteral pentamidine treatment because hypoglycemia is an adverse effect (Flaskerud & Ungvarski, 1999).

3.19 Toxoplasmosis

1. Etiology/Epidemiology

   a. *Toxoplasma gondii* is a coccidian feline parasite that uses mammals as its intermediate host and exists in three forms:

   - Oocysts, which are shed from the feline GI tract and released as sporozoites (inactive form) from dry feces
   - Tachyzoites (fast-growing, active form), which are found in mammalian tissue prior to mounting an immune response
   - Bradyzoites (slow-growing form), which continue to grow inside tissue cysts that form as part of the immune response

b. Infection occurs via ingestion of oocysts in undercooked contaminated meats or feces-contaminated produce or via inhalation of sporozoites.

c. Toxoplasmosis disease is rare in HIV-seronegative populations and is usually from latent cyst reactivation in HIV-positive populations. Most commonly seen in patients with CD_4 count of < 100 cells/mm^3.

d. The disease is found worldwide, with higher incidence of latent infection in Africa, Haiti, Europe, and Latin America.

    i. Highest incidence in the United States was seen in Florida and may reflect concentration of Haitian and Latin American populations.

    ii. Higher incidence occurs in Hispanic populations in general, particularly in lower socioeconomic classes.

2. Pathogenesis

a. After primary exposure, *T. gondii* can invade and infect contiguous tissue by converting from bradyzoite to tachyzoite form. Cysts can be found in all tissue types.

    i. Most common sites are in brain, heart, and striated muscle.

    ii. There is evidence that cysts rupture and may cause recurrent asymptomatic infections.

3. Clinical presentation

a. Disease is associated with advanced HIV disease, and clinical lab findings generally are too nonspecific to be of diagnostic value.

b. Central nervous system disease is frequently multifocal, with a wide spectrum of clinical findings, including headache, fever, altered level of consciousness, mood changes, seizures, and strokelike symptoms.

c. Extracerebral sites are usually ocular or pulmonary.

    i. Pulmonary symptoms include fever, nonproductive cough, shortness of breath, or a combination of the three, that progresses more rapidly than pneumocystis carinii pneumonia.

    ii. Ocular symptoms include decreased visual acuity and eye pain.

4. Diagnosis

a. Definitive diagnosis of central nervous system disease is based on identification of the organism in tissue via biopsy, although this is rarely done.

    i. Empiric therapy based on typical head CT or MRI findings generally initiated without biopsy given high morbidity and mortality associated with brain biopsies. Serologic test (IgG) for *T. gondii* is also done to document latent infection because the disease is very unusual in AIDS patients with negative *T. gondii* serologic test results.

b. MRI is most sensitive to cerebral lesions. CT is less sensitive but can show characteristic ring enhancing lesions.

c. Differential diagnoses are central nervous system lymphoma, extra-pulmonary *M. tuberculosis,* and cryptococcoma.

5. Prevention/Treatment

a. All HIV-infected individuals should be tested for *T. gondii*-specific IgG antibodies as part of the baseline evaluation.

b. Patients with findings on neuroimaging typical of toxoplasmic encephalitis should receive empiric toxoplasmosis therapy (Montoya & Remington, 2000; Subauste & Remington, 2000):

    i. Pyrimethamine + leucovorin (to prevent pyrimethamine-associated bone marrow toxicity) + sulfadiazine or clindamycin is current standard of therapy.

    ii. Alternative regimens include the following:

- Pyrimethamine + leucovorin + either clarithromycin, atovaquone, azithromycin, or dapsone
- Trimethoprim-sulfamethoxazole (TMP-SMX) as a single agent

c. After completion of acute therapy, HIV-infected persons usually require lifelong maintenance therapy with pyrimethamine, unless their immune system is restored by HAART.

d. Anticonvulsant therapy may be indicated for seizure prevention.

6. Nursing implications
   a. Teach patients to avoid contact with potentially contaminated sources.
      i. Use gloves when handling litter boxes or gardening.
      ii. Disinfect cat litter boxes when changing litter.
      iii. Eat only completely cooked or cured meats.
      iv. Wash hands and kitchen surfaces thoroughly after handling raw meat; avoid touching mucus membranes when handling raw meat.
      v. Wash all fruits and vegetables before eating.
   b. Monitor laboratory results and other indices for adverse drug effects and response to therapy.

Viral Infections

3.20 Cytomegalovirus (CMV)

1. Etiology/Epidemiology
   a. Double-stranded DNA herpes virus that is found in semen, cervical secretions, saliva, urine, blood, and organs.
   b. Transmission modes include perinatal transmission, sexual contact, blood exchange, and transplantation of infected organs or tissues.
   c. In the United States, 60% of the population is CMV seropositive. Seroprevalence can be as high as 100% in IDU and MSM (Bick, 2001; Zwolski, 2001).
2. Pathogenesis
   a. Can cause chorioretinitis, radiculopathy, encephalitis, colitis, esophagitis, and pneumonia (Centers for Disease Control and Prevention, 2001).
3. Clinical presentation
   a. Seen with severe immunosuppression (CD_4 count < 50 cells/mm³).
   b. May be seen with the following: retinitis—decreased visual acuity, floaters, unilateral visual field loss, and scotoma;

radiculopathy—lower extremity weakness, spasticity, areflexia, and urinary retention; encephalitis—personality changes, poor concentration, headaches, and somnolence; colitis—diarrhea, weight loss, and anorexia; esophagitis—odynophagia; pneumonia—dyspnea, dry nonproductive cough, and increased respirations (Centers for Disease Control and Prevention, 2001; Zwolski, 2001)

4. Diagnosis
   a. Retinal exam, which reveals large, creamy to yellow-white granular areas with perivascular exudates and hemorrhages; CSF fluid analysis may be normal. Antigen testing of CMV DNA will be positive and brain biopsy endoscopic examination generally reveals large, white-yellow plaques throughout the esophagus, and colon biopsy reveals ulceration and submucosal hemorrhages; chest X-ray generally reveals diffuse infiltrates and histologic examination of sputum.
   b. Histologic diagnosis is the gold standard; tissue cultures may be positive but are not specific for active disease; urine culture may reveal viral shedding but is not indicative of active disease; CMV serology is necessary to determine active disease (Zwolski, 2001).
5. Prevention/Treatment
   a. Avoid giving CMV-positive blood products to a CMV-negative patient; early detection can be determined by using a visual grid or routine ophthalmology exam to detect vision changes.
   b. Oral ganciclovir 1 gm TID can be used but is not currently recommended for prophylaxis. Side effects outweigh any benefit derived by administration.
   c. Induction with intravenous ganciclovir, 5 mg/kg IV Q12; foscarnet 90 mg/kg IV Q12, or cidofovir 5 mg/kg × 1 week, then reduced to every 2 weeks; intraocular ganciclovir implants every 6 months.
   d. For maintenance, ganciclovir 5 mg/kg IV, or 1 gm PO TID; foscarnet 90–120 mg/kg IV (Bick, 2001; Centers for Disease

Control and Prevention, 2001; Zwolski, 2001).

6. Nursing implications
   a. Arrange for home care if intravenous medications are to be administered in the home. Teach self-administration of oral medications.
   b. Teach high-risk patients use of visual grid; offer visual aid devices if patient suffers visual loss.
   c. Monitor patient for response to therapy and adverse effects; monitor renal function, electrolytes, calcium, magnesium, and CBC with differential.
   d. With advanced immunosuppression, encourage serial ophthalmic exams.

3.21 Herpes Simplex Virus (HSV)

1. Etiology/Epidemiology
   a. Two distinct viruses: HSV-1 and HSV-2
      i. HSV-1
         (1) Initial infection is often during childhood; many initial infections are subclinical.
         (2) Prevalence in those with HIV is approximately 70%, similar to the general population (Safrin, 1991a).
      ii. HSV-2
         (1) Usually acquired via sexual transmission, particularly risky for those with sexually transmitted HIV (O'Farrell, 1994).
         (2) Significant risk factor for acquisition and transmission of HIV.
         (3) Prevalence in those with HIV approximately 75%, much higher than the general population (Safrin, 1991a).
2. Pathogenesis
   a. Primary infection
      i. Transmission occurs by direct contact, during which virus is inoculated onto mucosal surfaces or breaks in the skin.
      ii. Virions travel from the site of inoculation along sensory nerves to the corresponding nerve root

ganglia where infection is permanently established.
      iii. Reactivation/recurrence can occur via a variety of stimuli (i.e., stress, trauma, ultraviolet light).
         (1) The degree of immunosuppression influences the rate and severity of reactivated disease (Augenbraun, 1995).
         (2) During reactivation, the virus replicates in the ganglia, and progeny virions travel peripherally along sensory nerves to the mucosal or epithelial surface innervated by the reactivated ganglion.
         (3) Active viral replication at the cutaneous surface produces lesions and clinical symptoms.
         (4) Frequency of reactivation of HSV-1 is less than reactivation of HSV-2 in HIV disease (Stewart, 1995).
3. Clinical presentation
   a. Manifestations of primary HSV infection include fever, adenopathy, malaise, and painful ulcerative lesions involving mucosal or cutaneous sites.
   b. Subclinical HSV infection usually occurs prior to HIV infection; thus, primary infection in HIV disease is rare (Schacker & Corey, 1997).
      i. Prodromal symptoms of paresthesias, itching, or tingling at the site of impending eruption may precede a recurrence.
      ii. HSV lesions may present as small, localized ulcerations or can spread contiguously to cover large areas (zosteriform). Disease may also present as papules that rapidly evolve into fluid-filled vesicles, painful and palpable.
      iii. Common sites of HSV lesions include orolabial, genital, and anorectal. Involvement of visceral organs can occur in HIV disease (e.g., esophagitis, encephalitis).
4. Diagnosis
   a. Microscopic evaluation with a Tzanck smear reveals giant multinucleated cells characteristic of HSV, but sensitivity and

specificity are low (Schacker & Corey, 1997).

b. Direct virus culture taken from suspected lesions (gold standard). Cultured virus can also be typed (HSV-1 vs. HSV-2), which helps determine possible reactivation rates (Erlich, 1999).

c. Direct antigen detection involves identification of HSV antigens on the surface of cells obtained from suspicious lesion (Erlich, 1999).

d. HSV serology is rarely useful in the clinical setting because level of HSV antibodies is usually high in HIV disease (Safrin, 1991a).

5. Prevention/Treatment

a. Primary infection can be prevented by use of barrier method safer sex (i.e., condoms).

b. Symptomatic HSV infections should be treated aggressively with available antiviral chemotherapy.

c. Antiviral agents used to prevent and treat HSV infection.

i. Acyclovir: Available in oral, intravenous, and topical preparations. Intravenous administration should be considered standard of care and treatment of choice in severe HSV infections (Erlich, 1999). Oral acyclovir can effectively treat mucocutaneous HSV infection (Shepp, 1985) and can be used for secondary prophylaxis against recurrence (Goldberg, 1993). Oral bioavailability of acyclovir is poor and requires frequent dose administration.

ii. Valacyclovir: A prodrug of acyclovir. Administered orally with excellent bioavailability (Spruance, 1996). Effective in the treatment of primary and recurrent infection as well as for long-term suppressive therapy (Centers for Disease Control and Prevenion, 1998). Currently, there are concerns related to its use in the immunocompromised due to the development of blood dyscrasias in clinical trials (Erlich, 1999).

iii. Famciclovir: Analog of panciclovir (another antiviral). Administered orally with excellent bioavailability (Saltzman, 1994). Effective for primary and recurrent therapy as well as suppressive therapy in HIV disease (Sacks, 1996). Topical panciclovir is also available.

iv. Foscarnet: Inorganic pyrophosphate. Administered intravenously, this drug is useful in the management of drug resistant HSV (Safrin, 1991b).

d. Recommended regimens for HSV infection:

i. First clinical episode of genital herpes: acyclovir 400 mg orally TID for 7–10 days, or acyclovir 200 mg orally TID for 7–10 days, or famciclovir 250 mg orally TID for 7–10 days, or valacyclovir 1 g orally BID for 7–10 days

ii. Severe or refractory infections: acyclovir up to 800 mg PO 5x/day or 15–30 mg/kg/day IV at least 7 days or valacyclovir 1 g PO

iii. Recurrent: acyclovir 400 mg PO TID OR 800 mg PO BID or famciclovir 125 mg PO BID or valacyclovir 500 mg PO BID; all given for 5 days

iv. Prophylaxis: acyclovir 400 mg PO BID or famciclovir 125–250 mg PO BID or valacyclovir 500 mg PO BID or 1 g/day

6. Nursing implications

a. Local care of mucocutaneous lesion includes keeping lesions clean and dry, with gentle cleansing using mild soap and water.

b. Pain can be severe and analgesia should be administered as needed.

c. Stool softeners should be considered for patients with anorectal ulcers.

3.22 Progressive Multifocal Leukoencephalopathy (PML)

1. Etiology/Epidemiology

a. PML is a demyelinating disease of cerebral white matter caused by the papovavirus, JCV genus *polyomavirus*; Hou & Major, 2000), which is a neurotropic virus that infects approximately 80% of all adults.

b. Approximately 1–8% of patients with advanced HIV disease will develop PML (Bartlett & Gallant, 2001; Hou & Major, 2000; McGuire & So, 1998).

2. Pathogenesis
   a. JCV is thought to be transmitted by the respiratory route during childhood and remains inactive for life in persons with a healthy immune system.
   b. In immunocompromised hosts, the virus is reactivated. Only patients with a high degree of immunosuppression (e.g., late-stage HIV disease/AIDS, lymphoproliferative diseases, patients treated with immunosuppressive therapies) are likely to develop PML.
   c. JCV causes selective demyelination in the CNS of immunocompromised hosts.

3. Clinical presentation
   a. PML is a subacute or chronic, progressive illness characterized by focal neurologic findings and mental status or personality changes. A protracted clinical course is typical; fever, acutely altered consciousness, or other signs of acute encephalitis are unusual.
   b. Manifestations include weakness (found in most patients); decreased attention and memory; confusion; personality change; dementia; diplopia and other cranial nerve deficits; mono-, hemi-, or quadriplegia; ataxia; bradykinesia; rigidity; sensory deficits (face, arm numbness); headache; vertigo; seizures; coma; and alien hand syndrome (Bartlett & Gallant, 2001; McGuire & So, 1998).
   c. PML may develop as an immune reconstitution syndrome in HAART-treated patients who show rapid improvements in CD_4 T lymphocyte counts and decreased viral loads (DeSimone, Pomerantz, & Babinchak, 2000).
   d. Since the advent of HAART, PML-related deaths appear to be decreasing, although there are conflicting findings on survival rates. Some researchers report a median survival of 545 days after a PML diagnosis (Miralles et al., 1998), whereas others report a median survival of only 3 months (Enting & Portegies, 2000).

4. Diagnosis
   a. Magnetic resonance imaging (MRI) findings suggestive of PML include diffuse, white-matter, nonenhancing lesions without mass effect.
   b. JCV may be demonstrated by polymerase chain reaction (PCR) testing of cerebrospinal fluid (CSF). Peripheral blood PCR for JCV is not clinically useful (De Luca et al., 2000), nor is routine CSF evaluation, which is usually normal (McGuire & So, 1998).
   c. Tissue is acquired from stereotactic brain biopsy; occasionally, direct brain biopsy is required due to the anatomical location of a lesion.

5. Prevention/Treatment
   a. There is currently no known prophylaxis for PML, nor is there an accepted, recommended regimen for its treatment.
   b. A growing body of evidence suggests that HAART has halted or obliterated PML (Bartlett & Gallant, 2001).
   c. Anecdotal evidence supports the use of interferon alpha, or cidofovir, either alone or in combination with HAART.

6. Nursing implications
   a. PML should be considered whenever a person with AIDS presents with unexplained neurological complaints or findings.
   b. In the early years of the HIV epidemic, a diagnosis of PML was uniformly fatal, usually within 2–4 months. Patients were appropriately counseled and plans for comfort and terminal care were made.
   c. Effective treatment regimes specifically against PML remain elusive. Randomized, controlled clinical trials will be required for definitive answers about therapy.
   d. In the meantime, concomitant HAART seems prudent, even though clinical trial evidence of other efficacious agents is currently lacking, and cautious optimism may allow nurses to offer hope to patients and their loved ones where before none existed.

Neoplasms

3.23 Cervical Neoplasia

1. Etiology/Epidemiology
   a. Etiologic agent is human papillomavirus (HPV; see Section 3.3, Human Papillomavirus Infection).
   b. Persistent oncogenic HPV subtypes are the most important risk factor for developing cervical/anal/vaginal/vulvar cancer or dysplasia and is 4.5 times more prevalent in individuals infected with HIV (Ellerbrock et al., 2000; Palefsky, 2000).
   c. Specific HPV subtypes are associated with greater progression from HPV infection to HPV disease (dysplasia), including cancer (neoplasia; see Section 3.3, HPV diseases for oncogenic HPV subtypes).
   d. True incidence of invasive cervical cancer in women is unknown.
   e. In 1993 1.3% of women with AIDS reported to the Centers for Disease Control and Prevention had an initial AIDS diagnosis of invasive cervical cancer (Staats, Sheran, & Herr, 1999).
2. Pathogenesis
   a. Cancer (neoplasia) of the cervix/anus/vagina/vulva is preceded by dysplasia (see Human Papillomavirus Infection, Section 3.3).
   b. Cancer arises at the squamocolumnar junction of the cervix (or anus) in the squamous epithelial cells.
   c. Cancer is invasive when malignant epithelial cells break through the basement membrane and enter the stroma; invasion occurs in 1 to 20 years.
3. Clinical presentation
   a. Pap smear is abnormal; women are asymptomatic in early stages of disease.
   b. Most common symptom is postcoital bleeding. Other more advanced symptoms include metorrhagia and malodorous vaginal discharge.
   c. As the disease progresses, symptoms include abdominal, pelvic, back, or leg pain; weight loss; anemia; and lower extremity edema.
   d. In advanced disease, hematuria and rectal bleeding may be seen.
4. Diagnosis
   a. Colposcopy with directed biopsy is the primary diagnostic tool (see ASCCP for the management of cytologic abnormalities at http://www.asccp.org/).
      i. Biopsies are contraindicated for pregnant women.
      ii. Colposcopy alone without biopsy is not diagnostic (Massad et al., 2001).
   b. Colposcopy is indicated for all HIV-infected women with atypical squamous cells of undetermined significance (ASC-US) or higher pap results (Abularach & Anderson, 2001; Richart, Cox, Twiggs, Wilkenson, & Wright, 2002). Twelve to 56% of HIV-infected individuals with ASC-US have underlying high-grade squamous intraepithelial lesion (HSIL; Holcomb et al., 1999; Solomon, Schiffman, & Tarone, 2001; Wright et al., 1996).
   c. Colposcopy is performed for low-grade squamous intraepithelial lesion/cervical intraepithelial neoplasia 1 (LSIL/CIN 1) biopsy, if indicated; Pap smear is performed q 4–6 months if untreated. Colposcopic exam should occur q 6 months.
   d. For HSIL/CIN 2, 3 or carcinoma in situ (CIS), colposcopy with biopsy, loop electrosurgical excision procedure (LEEP), or conization are procedures of choice. Pap smear is performed q 3–4 months in 1st year, then q 6 months. Consider periodic colposcopy after treatment.
5. Prevention/Treatment
   a. Cervical cancer (neoplasia) and other related HPV neoplasia (anal, vulva, and vagina) are preventable with adequate screening and early treatment of SIL.
   b. Treatment of SIL in HIV-infected individuals includes several options.
      i. Low grade squamous intraepithelial lesion has two practices:
         - Observation with colposcopy-directed biopsy is used because early treatment has not proven to be beneficial with a 39–62%

recurrence posttreatment (Fruchter et al., 1996; Holcomb et al., 1999; Tate & Anderson, 2001). Recurrence rates are also found with positive surgical margins in those women who undergo excisional treatment (Boardman, Piepert, Hogan, & Cooper, 1999).

- Treatment, the second practice, is described below. Treatment choice will often depend on site of disease (i.e., cervical, anal, vulva, or vagina).

   ii. Treatment choices for moderate to HSIL SIL includes LEEP, cryotherapy/cryosurgery, carbon dioxide laser therapy, or cone biopsy.

   iii. Hysterectomy is recommended for cervical cancer greater than carcinoma in situ. Hysterectomies do not alleviate HPV subtypes that often reoccur in the vaginal/vulval/anal area after surgery in HIV-infected women.

c. Optimal therapy for HIV-infected individuals with invasive carcinoma is not yet established.

d. Treatment may include single or combination strategies (e.g., surgery, radiation, or chemotherapy).

e. Response rates in HIV-negative individuals are approximately 70% and have been reported with combination chemotherapy (cisplatin, methotrexate, bleomycin, doxorubicin; Peel, 1995).

f. The National Cancer Institute urges providers to treat metastatic cervical cancer in HIV-negative women with a combination of chemotherapy and radiation; treatment reduces mortality by 30–50%.

g. Experimental approaches include topical 5-FU and oral difluoromethylornithine (DMFO).

6. Nursing implications

a. Relationship with provider is essential; nurses can bridge gaps that may exist within the health care system.

b. Telephone counseling and appointment reminders assist in increasing adherence to medical treatments (Abercrombie, 2000).

c. Advocate for methods that decrease pain during colposcopy such as Hurricane (20% benzocaine) and use of nonsteroidal antiinflammatory agents (NSAIDs) to decrease cramping.

d. Reinforce the need for safer sexual practices after biopsies and treatments because individuals are at increased risk for transmitting HIV and acquiring infections.

e. Assess for posttraumatic stress syndrome related to prior sexual abuse or gynecological treatment, which can affect appointment and treatment adherence (Dole, 2001; Leenerts, 1998).

f. Assess women for signs and symptoms of invasive cervical carcinoma.

g. Educate about the various treatments and management of SIL (see Human Papillomavirus Infection, Section 3.3).

h. Provide brochures, written material, or Web sites related to HPV, such as *http://www.aegis.com/topics/oi/oi-warts. html*.

i. Educate the patient about the specific therapy she will undergo as treatment for either cervical intraepithelial neoplasia or invasive squamous cell carcinoma of the cervix.

3.24 Kaposi's Sarcoma (KS)

1. Etiology/Epidemiology

a. Once thought to be a true malignancy, with rare exception Kaposi's sarcoma (KS) is now known to be a virus-induced cellular proliferation.

b. Ninety to 100% of patients with KS have high antibody titers to human herpes virus 8 (HHV-8).

c. HHV-8 seems to be critical in the development of KS, although the exact mechanism is unknown (Moore & Chang, 1995; O'Brien et al., 1999).

d. Several studies of men who have sex with men (MSM) have shown that HHV-8 may be transmitted sexually. Increasing numbers of sexual partners and history of sexually transmitted disease are risk factors for HHV-8. HHV-8 may also be transmitted by saliva; thus, deep kissing is also seen as a risk factor. The introduction of HAART has significantly impacted the epidemiology of KS. A large international collaborative study that included 47,936 HIV-infected individuals found that the adjusted incidence rate for KS declined from 15.2 per 1,000 person-years in 1992–1996 to 4.9 per 1,000 person-years in 1997–1999, representing a rate ratio of 0.32.

2. Pathogenesis
   a. The cell of origin remains unknown; KS may originate from mesenchymal, smooth muscle cells, or fibroblasts.
   b. HIV-infected cells, HHV-8-infected cells, and KS cells produce cytokines and growth factors that promote the growth of KS cells in vitro.
   c. HIV *tat* genes may initiate the process of cell transformation and increase proliferation of KS-derived spindle cells; interleukin 6 (IL-6) and oncostatin M act synergistically with *tat*.
   d. Uncontrolled growth of these cells with attendant neoangiogenesis and inflammatory cell infiltration results in the characteristic histologic appearance.

3. Clinical presentation
   a. Dermatologic conditions include multicentric skin lesions, which can be localized or disseminated plaques, nodules, or both. Color may vary from brown to red to purple. No characteristic site of involvement is apparent. Conditions may initiate near ears, eyelids, or anywhere on the skin/mucous surface.
   b. Asymptomatic visceral involvement is common, especially in the oral cavity and gastrointestinal (GI) tract; all organs may be involved, including the brain.
   c. Pulmonary involvement is rare.

4. Diagnosis
   a. Diagnosis may be presumptive based on characteristic appearance of lesions, but the Centers for Disease Control and Prevention recommends biopsy prior to starting any therapy.
   b. For pulmonary KS the chest radiograph is not specific but may reveal pulmonary infiltrates or a nodular density. Gallium/thallium scanning may also be included in the evaluation of pulmonary KS. Pulmonary function tests may be helpful in ruling out infectious etiology. Bronchoscopy usually reveals violaceous plaques in the tracheobronchial tree; however, lesions are submucosal and difficult to biopsy.

5. Prevention/Treatment
   a. No proven prevention is available.
   b. HAART may delay onset by reducing HIV RNA viral loads and increasing CD_4 cell count.
   c. No cure is available.
   d. Goals of treatment include palliation, slow progression, and maximization of quality of life.
   e. Highly active antiretroviral therapy (HAART) has affected the incidence of KS, decreasing it by approximately 60% since the advent of HAART (Jones, Hanson, Dworkin, Ward, & Jaffe, 1999).
   f. Radiation therapy
      i. Radiation therapy is used for localized lesions.
      ii. Therapy is less effective when lymphedema of the upper or lower extremities is present, and therapy may cause permanent alterations in lymph drainage.
   g. Cryotherapy
      i. Clinical response rate is as high as 85%.
      ii. Recurrence is likely.
      iii. A hypopigmented area remains.
   h. Intralesional therapy
      i. Low-dose vinblastine can be used to treat lesions.
      ii. Disadvantages to intralesional therapy include multiple office visits, postinjection pain, inflammation, hyperpigmentation, and edema.
   i. Photodynamic therapy is currently under study.
   j. Surgical excision should be reserved for a single problematic lesion; excision is not effective if systemic disease is present.
   k. Topical retinoic acid (Saiag et al., 1998) is available.

l. Chemotherapy
   i. Single agents: Taxol, liposomal doxorubicin, and liposomal daunomycin
   ii. Other agents: vincristine, vinblastine, doxorubicin, bleomycin, and oral etoposide
   iii. Combination therapy: generally not used; single agents: as effective as combination therapy with less morbidity
m. Biologics: subcutaenous interferon (Krown, 1998)
n. Novel approaches: antiangiogenesis compounds, cytokine inhibitors, and anti-human herpes virus-8 inhibitors

6. Nursing implications
   a. Provide education about treatment options, including potential side effects and their management and when to notify a health care provider.
   b. Encourage safer sex techniques (e.g., condoms).
   c. Emphasize the importance of nutrition and rest when undergoing treatments, particularly systemic chemotherapies.
   d. Anticipate body-image changes that can occur as a result of the lesions. Cosmetic interventions (e.g., makeup) should be anticipated.
   e. A negative sequela of KS is social isolation.

3.25 Non-Hodgkin's Lymphoma (NHL)

1. Etiology/Epidemiology
   a. Non-Hodgkin's lymphoma is more likely to occur in persons with substantial immunosuppression (i.e., CD_4 counts < 200 cells/mm^3) and a history of an AIDS-defining illness.
   b. Epstein-Barr virus (EBV) has been implicated in the pathogenesis.
   c. Incidence of AIDS-related lymphoma has declined from 2 cases/100 person years in September of 1995 to 0.4 cases/100 person years in March of 1999 (Levine, 2001).
   d. HAART-associated decline in the incidence of lymphoma has been less than the declines seen for opportunistic infections, suggesting that longer treatment durations are needed to

confer protective effects against lymphoma (Levine, 2001).

2. Pathogenesis
   a. Non-Hodgkin's lymphoma is not completely understood, but it presumably is a multi-step process:

   - Genetic mutations occur.
   - Rearrangement mutations in B cells arrest their maturation, and the proliferation of these immature cells is driven by HIV-induced cytokine dysregulation.
   - Mutations of tumor suppressor genes occur.
   - EBV has been implicated in Burkitt's lymphoma. EBV stimulates B-cell proliferation in the absence of immune regulation and immortalizes B-cell clones.

3. Clinical presentation
   a. Median age at presentation is 35–42 years; 40–60% of people have an AIDS diagnosis (Levine, 2001).
   b. Majority of people have widespread disease at presentation. As many as 70–97% have extranodal disease, often at unusual locations. There is high incidence of central nervous system (CNS) involvement, approximately 20–40%.
   c. Incidence of bone marrow, gastrointestinal (GI), and liver involvement is high.
   d. The patient may present with a primary effusion lymphoma, where there is no discrete mass, only an effusion, such as ascites or pleural effusion; cytology will be positive for lymphoma.
   e. Plasmablastic lymphoma of the oral cavity present, including swollen tonsils and cervical lymphadenopathy.
   f. Signs and symptoms will depend on the location of disease. The patient may present with asymptomatic lymphadenopathy, or if there is involvement of the lungs, the patient may have shortness of breath or dyspnea on exertion. If the GI tract is involved, they may experience abdominal pain, diarrhea, and constipation.

4. Diagnosis
   a. Perform CT scan of chest/abdomen/pelvis.
   b. Gallium-67 nuclear medicine test may help identify areas of NHL involvement.
   c. Positron emission tomography (PET) scan, an imaging modality that provides information based on the biochemical and metabolic activity of tissue, may locate tumors that have higher metabolic/biochemical activity.
   d. Bone marrow biopsy and lumbar puncture looks for disseminated disease.
5. Prevention/Treatment
   a. There is no recommendation for primary prevention.
   b. Survival is possibly improved with early treatment.
   c. Chemotherapy naive patients receive combination chemotherapy with regimen that includes cyclophosphamide, which is the most active agent in NHL.
   d. Therapy with monoclonal antibodies that target cancer cells that express the CD_{20} antigen are used in combination with chemotherapy.
   e. HAART controls viral load, although antiretroviral agents should be carefully selected; saquinivir interferes with the metabolism of some chemotherapeutic agents and may result in unexplained toxicities.
   f. Hematopoietic growth factors are especially important for patients with poor bone marrow reserve.
   g. High-dose methotrexate is used for primary CNS lymphomas.
   h. Radiation therapy is given to areas of bulky disease and large aggregation of tumor.
   i. Few options exist for relapsed or refractory disease.
      i. Mitoguazone has been studied in this population and produced a 20–25% response rate; research is ongoing (Levine, 1998).
      ii. Infusional therapy retreatment with chemotherapy becomes less effective with each course; that is, should the patient relapse after a response to the initial treatment, the chance of inducing a response with the next course of treatment is diminished.
         (1) Monoclonal antibodies may be used in the patient with relapsed disease.
         (2) IL-2 may be used in the patient with relapsed disease.
6. Nursing implications
   a. Provide education about the disease, specific therapies, and potential side effects and their management.
   b. Emphasize the importance of adequate rest and nutrition. In all diseased states the body requires adequate rest and nutrition to heal.
   c. Be alert for tumor lysis syndrome in patients with bulky disease and a high serum uric acid level.
   d. If the patient has CNS lymphoma, address issues of safety and potential for cognitive deficits and motor incoordination.
   e. Provide emotional support for the patient and the family and significant others.

3.26 HIV-Related Wasting Syndrome

1. Etiology/Epidemiology
   a. Definitions include the following:
      i. The Centers for Disease Control and Prevention's (1987) definition of wasting syndrome is involuntary loss of > 10% body weight accompanied by chronic diarrhea, weakness, or fever.
      ii. Proposed new definition is "patient must meet one of the following criteria: 10% unintentional weight loss over 12 months; 7.5% unintentional weight loss over 6 months; 5% body cell mass (BCM) loss within 6 months; in men: BCM < 35% of total body weight (BW) and body mass index (BMI) < 27 kg/m²; in women: BCM < 23% of total BW and BMI < 27 kg/m²; BMI < 20 kg/m²" (Polsky, Kotler, & Steinhart, 2001, p. 413).
   b. Etiologies include reduced food intake, malabsorption with or without diarrhea,

and metabolic abnormalities (Nemechek, Polsky, & Gottlieb, 2000).

c. Prevalence ranges from 33–58% in patients receiving HAART (Wanke, Silva, Knox, Forrester, Speigelman, & Gorbach, 2000).

2. Pathogenesis

a. Suppression of appetite due to elevated IL-1, TNF-alpha, delayed gastric emptying, oropharyngeal lesions, nausea and vomiting, taste alterations, diarrhea, fatigue, secondary infections, depression, and altered cognition

b. Altered absorption resulting from medications, enteric pathogens, and changes in gastrointestinal tract structure and function

c. Activation of abnormal metabolic pathways by IL-l, TNF-alpha, interferon-alpha, testosterone deficiency, and growth hormone resistance/deficiency (Polsky, Kotler, & Steinhart, 2001)

3. Clinical presentation

a. Loss of body weight, skeletal muscle mass, and subcutaneous fat

4. Diagnosis

a. Dietary/clinical history reveals weight loss, inadequate dietary intake, loss of functional status.

b. Body composition measures: weight, lean body mass, body fat mass, and body mass index are less than 95% standard.

c. There is laboratory evidence of anemia, hypoalbuminemia, and hypogonadism.

5. Prevention/Treatment

a. Prevention includes ongoing nutritional assessment and counseling.

b. Treatment includes managing symptoms; treating infections; administering appetite stimulants and testosterone, if indicated; using anabolic agents, recombinant growth hormone, or both; and providing nutrition counseling and support.

6. Nursing implications

a. Educate patient/family/significant other regarding the following:

- Eating foods high in protein and calories
- Using vitamin/mineral and food supplements as needed

- Keeping appetite, weight, and symptom records
- Maintaining appropriate exercise program to increase lean body mass

3.27 HIV Encephalopathy

1. Etiology/Epidemiology

a. HIV-related encephalopathy (also called AIDS dementia complex, subacute encephalitis, HIV dementia, and HIV-related cognitive/motor complex) is an AIDS-defining condition that results from HIV infection of cells in the central nervous system (CNS; Swindells, Zheng, & Gendelman, 1999).

b. HIV-related encephalopathy occurs in 20–30% of persons with advanced disease (Brew, 1999). The effects of HAART on the incidence of HIV-related encephalopathy are unclear. Although HAART has been associated with improvements in neuropsychological functioning (Ferrando et al., 1998), some researchers have failed to find reduced incidence rates of HIV-related encephalopathy in the HAART era (Dore et al., 1999; Sacktor et al., 2002).

2. Pathogenesis

a. HIV-related encephalopathy results from HIV infection of mononuclear phagocytes in the brain. The ensuing inflammatory response results in the generation of neurotoxic substances, including cytokines and nitric oxide, which destroy neurons (Swindells et al., 1999). HIV-induced astrocyte dysfunction leads to decreased neurotransmitter clearance and subsequent accumulation of toxic concentrations of intraneuronal calcium (Brew, 1999). Additionally, viral proteins, such as gp 120, gp 41, *tat*, *rev*, and *nef*, may be directly neurotoxic to primary neurons through activation of N-methyl-D-aspartate (NMDA) receptors (Melton, Kirkwood, & Ghaemi, 1997; Thomas, 2002).

3. Clinical presentation

a. Patients typically present with cognitive, motor, and behavioral symptoms. In the earliest stages, patients manifest attentional deficits, forgetfulness, and motor slowing. In advanced stages, patients show flattened affect, apathy, inability to perform routine mental tasks, and obvious motor dysfunction (Brew, 1999).

4. Diagnosis
   a. Diagnosis of HIV-related encephalopathy is made after excluding other causes. A definitive diagnosis is only possible on autopsy (Melton et al., 1997).
   b. Diagnostic work-up includes MRI, lumbar puncture, and neuropsychological testing.
      i. MRI scans reveal cortical atrophy and white matter pallor.
      ii. Cerebrospinal fluid (CSF) findings include pleocytosis, increased protein, immunoglobulin G, and presence of HIV.
      iii. Findings of neuropsychological testing are consistent with subcortical dementia (i.e., deficits on measures of attention, memory, information processing speed, and motor speed; Thomas, 2002). Because these tests are time-consuming and costly, the HIV Dementia Scale (HDS) is a possible diagnostic alternative. The HDS is an easily administered paper-and-pencil test that can be completed in 10 min and has been shown to be a sensitive measure for detecting HIV-related encephalopathy (Power, Selnes, Grim, & McArthur, 1995).

5. Prevention/Treatment
   a. It remains unclear whether HAART is an effective prophylactic treatment for HIV-related encephalopathy.
   b. There are currently no effective treatments to reverse neurological damage associated with HIV-related encephalopathy; however, initiation of antiretroviral agents that penetrate the CNS is associated with cognitive improvement. Adjunctive therapies include NMDA antagonists and calcium channel blockers (Brew, 1999).

6. Nursing implications
   a. Assess home environment and identify safety hazards.
   b. Identify and reduce barriers to self-care and encourage patients to perform as many activities of daily living as possible.
   c. Refer caregivers to community services as needed (e.g., respite care, support groups, counseling).
   d. Assist with advance directives, home care, and assisted living referrals.

C. COMORBID COMPLICATIONS

3.28 Fat Redistribution Syndrome

1. Etiology/Epidemiology
   a. Definition: HIV-related changes in body fat distribution, also referred to as lipodystrophy syndrome and pseudo-Cushing's syndrome
   b. Etiology: unknown, but proposed etiologies include protease inhibitors (PIs), nucleoside reverse transcriptase inhibitors (NRTIs), immune reconstitution, cytokine activation, abnormal immune or autoimmune responses, and hormonal disturbances (Brinkman, Smeitink, Romijn, & Reiss, 1999; Carr, Miller, Law, & Cooper, 2000; Carr et al., 1999; Kotler, 1999; Saint-Marc & Touraine, 1999)
   c. Prevalence: observed in approximately 50% of patients after 1–2 years of highly active antiretroviral therapy (HAART; Schambelan, 2000)

2. Pathogenesis
   a. Uncertain. Hypotheses include the following:
      i. NRTI-induced mitochondrial depletion in peripheral white fat (Moyle, 2000)
      ii. PI-induced inhibition of insulin-degrading enzymes leading to hyperinsulinemia; because insulin is lipogenic, fat accumulation may result (Martinez & Gatell, 1998)

3. Clinical presentation
   a. Peripheral fat wasting (lipoatrophy): loss of subcutaneous fat in legs, arms, face, and buttocks (men usually have greater fat loss than women); increased prominence of veins in arms and legs; wrinkled skin

b. Central obesity: accumulation of fat in waist and intraabdominal/visceral cavity; dorsocervical fat accumulation ("buffalo hump"); breast enlargement (women usually have greater fat accumulation than men)

c. Risk factors: older age, male, Caucasian, family history, overweight/obesity, high-fat/calorie diet, lack of exercise, extent of immune depletion/reconstitution, type/duration of HAART therapy

4. Diagnosis

a. Waist-to-hip ratio is ≥ 0.95 in men and ≥ 0.9 in women.

b. Single slice CT or MRI at L_4 shows intraabdominal fat deposits.

c. Dual-energy X-ray absorptometry (DXA) and bioelectrical impedance analysis (BIA) to assess body fat amount, but not distribution.

d. Skinfold measures, if reliable, can assess changes over time.

5. Prevention/Treatment

a. Switch from a PI to RTI (Rozenbaum et al., 2000; Saint-Marc & Touraine, 1999)

b. Troglitazone, or metformin, exercise, and resistance training have all demonstrated reduction of total body and abdominal fat (Roubenoff et al., 1999; Saint-Marc & Touraine, 1999; Walli, Michl, Muhlbayer, Brinkmann, & Goebel, 2000)

c. Recombinant human growth hormone can be used to reverse buffalo hump and central adiposity, but growth hormone is costly and associated with adverse effects (Engleson, Glesby, Sheikan, Wang, & Kotler, 2000)

d. Liposuction is contraindicated for visceral fat removal; facial implants have been used to replace facial fat loss

6. Nursing implications

a. Patients may refuse or discontinue HAART due to disfiguring body habitus changes.

b. Assess impact of fat redistribution on patient's treatment decisions, compliance, and psychological and social well-being.

c. Encourage lifestyle changes, such as low-fat/calorie diet, exercise, and resistance training.

3.29 Impaired Glucose Tolerance (IGT)

1. Etiology/epidemiology

a. Insulin resistance, hyperglycemia, and diabetes mellitus have an increased prevalence in patients with HIV.

b. Although new-onset diabetes mellitus is rare, insulin resistance and impaired glucose tolerance (IGT) are common (i.e., 60% of patients treated with protease inhibitors [PIs] have abnormal oral glucose tolerance test results; Walli et al., 1998). IGT is a metabolic stage intermediary between normal glucose homeostasis and diabetes. It is thought to be a risk factor for diabetes and cardiovascular disease.

c. The exact mechanisms are not known. IGT in HIV disease may relate to adverse effects of medications (PIs and non-nucleoside reverse transcriptase inhibitors [NNRTIs]) and metabolic dysfunction secondary to HIV disease itself (Galli, Ridolfo, & Gervasoni, 2001). Coinfections with hepatitis C virus (HCV) may also increase risk for IGT (Duong et al., 2001).

2. Pathogenesis

a. PIs are associated with both increased endogenous glucose production and resistance to multiple effects of insulin (van der Valk et al., 2001). Saquinavir, ritonavir, and indinavir all increase basal glucose transport but decrease insulin-stimulated glucose transport (Germinario et al., 2000).

b. IGT is associated with lipodystrophy, but whether it is caused by or is the cause of lipodystrophy is unclear.

3. Clinical presentation

a. Patients with IGT are generally asymptomatic.

b. Some patients may present with symptoms of frank diabetes (i.e., polyuria, polydipsia, and polyphagia).

c. Morphological changes (i.e., central adiposity, increased waist-to-hip ratio, peripheral fat wasting) may be present and should heighten clinical suspicion.

4. Diagnosis
    a. The fasting plasma glucose (FPG) is the preferred test. With IGT the FPG is greater than or equal to 110 mg/dl (6.1 mmol/1) and less than 126 mg/dl (7.0 mmol/1).
    b. Increased fasting insulin may be seen but is not recommended as a diagnostic test.
    c. Fasting glucose levels may be normal, requiring a 2-hr oral glucose tolerance test. A 2-hr postprandial glucose from 140 to < 200 (7.75 to < 11.1 mmol/L) is considered diagnostic.
5. Prevention/Treatment
    a. The goal is maintenance of normal glycemic control.
    b. Lifestyle modifications, such as dietary moderation, exercise, weight loss, smoking cessation, and limitation of alcohol use, are effective in achieving normal glycemic control.
    c. Metformin (500 mg twice daily) may improve glucose tolerance (Hadigan et al., 2000), but its use has been associated with lactic acidemia. The efficacy of other medications, such as anabolic steroids and growth hormone, are being studied in clinical trials.
    d. Antiretroviral switching may improve glycemic profile.
6. Nursing implications
    a. Assessment of symptoms of diabetes should be a routine part of the nursing assessment.
    b. If appropriate, counsel patients to maintain ideal body weight and encourage exercise, including strength training.
    c. Dietary counseling promoting low-glycemic index foods may be helpful for patients with known glucose intolerance.

3.30 Dyslipidemia

1. Etiology/Epidemiology
    a. Dyslipidemia includes hyperlipidemia, hypercholesterolemia, and hypertriglyceridemia.
    b. The reported prevalence of HIV-related dyslipidemia is very broad, ranging from 5% to 58% (Behrens et al., 1999;

Carr et al., 1998; Keruly, Mehta, Chaisson, & Moore, 1998).
    c. Etiology is unknown though often associated with fat redistribution and glucose intolerance.
2. Pathogenesis
    a. HAART has been implicated. Protease inhibitors (PIs) have been shown to stimulate triglyceride production (Lenhard, Croom, Weiel, & Winegar, 2000). Nucleoside reverse transcriptase inhibitors (NRTIs) have also been implicated because of their toxic effects on mitochondria (Brinkman, 1999).
    b. Dyslipidemia may be a secondary consequence of chronic suppression of HIV replication rather than a primary effect of HAART (Kotler, 1998).
3. Clinical presentation
    a. Lipid abnormalities are likely to be asymptomatic, except in the case of acute atherosclerotic infarction.
4. Diagnosis
    a. A fasting-lipid profile, which includes total cholesterol, low-density lipoproteins (LDL), high-density lipoproteins (HDL), and triglycerides, should be taken. Patients should receive baseline testing prior to starting any type of antiretroviral therapy. Subsequent lipid profiles should be performed every 3 to 6 months.
    b. Also assess cardiovascular risk factors (i.e., hypertension, glucose intolerance, smoking).
5. Prevention/Treatment
    a. Preventive efforts include encouraging appropriate caloric intake and physical activity. Refer overweight persons to a dietitian.
    b. Diet and exercise therapy using combined aerobic and resistance training have demonstrated benefit in reducing subcutaneous body fat, total cholesterol, and triglyceride concentrations (Jones, Doran, Leatt, Maher, & Pirmohamed, 2001).
    c. The potential benefit of switching antiretroviral medications to correct lipid abnormalities remains unclear.
    d. Comorbidities such as alcohol abuse need to be identified due to the increased risk of pancreatitis in patients

with lipid abnormalities, especially hypertriglyceridemia.
6. Nursing implications
   a. Assess patients for cardiovascular symptoms, including chest pain and shortness of breath.
   b. Encourage aerobic exercise and strength training as appropriate.

3.31 Anemia

1. Etiology/Epidemiology
   a. Anemia is a characterized by abnormalities in the hematological system.
   b. It has multiple causes, including decreased erythropoiesis, ineffective erythropoiesis, or increased red blood cell destruction (Levine, 1999).
   c. Anemia is the most common hematological malignancy seen in HIV. Several recent studies have demonstrated a statistically significant relationship between anemia and decreased survival in HIV-infected individuals (Sullivan, Hanson, Chu, Jones, & Ward, 1998)
2. Pathogenesis
   a. Bone marrow damage due to certain cancers, opportunistic infections, or myelosuppressive agents, such as zidovudine, ganciclovir, ribavirin, and vinblastine (Bain, 1999; Coyle, 1997; Levine, 1999), causes decreased erythropoiesis.
   b. Chronic disease is associated with anemia, which is characterized by decreased production of erythropoietin, erythropoietin resistance, abnormalities of iron metabolism, decreased erythrocyte life span, and an increased expression of inflammatory cytokines which may interfere with erythropoietin production (Abramson, Steinhart, & Frascino, 2000; Bain, 1999; Coyle, 1997).
   c. Iron deficiency anemia results from chronic blood loss or a dietary deficiency (Coyle, 1997; Kreuzer & Rockstroh, 1997; Levine, 1999).
   d. Parvovirus B19 can result in aplastic anemia in immune-compromised patients (Sabella & Goldfarb, 1999).

3. Clinical presentation
   a. Symptoms include fatigue, shortness of breath, decrease in cognitive function, impairment of activities of daily living, exercise intolerance, amenorrhea, and pallor.
4. Diagnosis
   a. Severity is based on a graded decrease in hemoglobin: mild = 1–1.9 g/dL below normal range; moderate = 2 g/dL below normal range but > 8.1 g/dL (mild anemia with two or more constitutional symptoms is also considered a moderate anemia); severe = < 8.0 g/dL (Ferri et al., 2002).
   b. Physical signs include weight loss, hepatosplenomegaly, guaiac positive stool, mild peripheral edema, and retinal hemorrhages (Hillman, 1998).
5. Prevention/Treatment
   a. Identify and treat underlying cause.
   b. Substitute or discontinue myelosuppressive agents. Do not reduce dose of antiretroviral agents.
   c. Epoetin alfa is the treatment of choice for mild or moderate anemia. The initial dosage is 40,000 units subcutaneously weekly.
   d. For severe anemia, treatment includes red blood cell transfusions, administration of electrolyte and colloid solutions, and supplemental oxygen (Hillman, 1998). Epoetin alfa should be administered with transfusion to prevent further episodes of anemia (Ferri et al., 2002).
6. Nursing implications
   a. Monitor lab work that is suggestive of anemia: complete blood count (CBC), red blood cell count (RBC), hemoglobin (Hbg), hematocrit (Hct), and reticulocyte count.
   b. Educate patients to recognize and report early signs of anemia, such as fatigue, shortness of breath, and amenorrhea.
   c. Provide dietary counseling and nutritional support as needed. Iron is best absorbed from meat, fish, and poultry. Orange juice doubles the absorption of iron from an entire meal, whereas tea or milk reduces absorption to less than one half.

3.32 Leukopenia

1. Etiology/Epidemiology
   a. Leukopenia is defined as a white blood count < 3,000 cells/mm^3.
   b. Etiology involves ineffective hematopoiesis coupled with peripheral destruction (Doweiko, 1999).
   c. Prevalence increases as disease progresses (Patton, 1999). Disease is found in 40% of patients with acute infection (Kahn, Hecht, Chesney, & Walker, 1999) and 70% of symptomatic patients (Coyle, 1997).
2. Pathogenesis
   a. HIV infection of accessory cells in the bone marrow inhibits production of hematopoietic growth factors (Mitsuyasu, 1999) and induces expression of cytokines that inhibit hematopoiesis (Coyle, 1997).
   b. Myelosuppression may also be related to drugs, concomitant infections, and malignancies (Mitsuyasu, 1999).
   c. HIV may induce apoptosis of lymphocytes (Mitsuyasu, 1999).
3. Clinical presentation
   a. Respiratory tract symptoms, such as cough and sputum production
   b. Urinary tract infection symptoms: frequency, urgency, and burning
   c. Fever
4. Diagnosis
   a. CBC with differential shows decrease in WBCs, including neutrophils, lymphocytes, and sometimes monocytes. Atypical lymphocytes may be seen (Doweiko & Groopman, 1998).
5. Prevention/Treatment
   a. Prevention: through durable suppression of viral replication and judicious use of myelosuppressive medications
   b. Treatment
      i. Antiretroviral therapy to suppress viral replication
      ii. Withdrawal of myelosuppressive therapies, if appropriate
      iii. Administration of hematopoietic growth factors: granulocyte colony-stimulating factor (G-CSF) and granulocyte-macrophage colony-stimulating factor (GM-CSF)

6. Nursing implications
   a. Education of patient, family, and significant other regarding the following:
      i. Strategies to reduce risk for infection (i.e., hand washing, food and water safety, avoidance of contact with infected persons)
      ii. Early detection of infections (i.e., regular monitoring of temperature, prompt reporting of any new signs or symptoms)

3.33 Thrombocytopenia

1. Etiology/Epidemiology
   a. In all risk groups, the prevalence is between 5% and 15% (Mannucci & Gringeri, 2000; Sullivan, Hanson, Chu, Jones, & Ciesielski, 1997).
   b. Medications include hydroxyurea, zidovudine, ganciclovir, trimethoprim-sulfamethoxazole, acetylsalicylic acid (ASA), NSAIDs, and chemotherapeutic agents.
   c. Infiltrative diseases of the bone marrow include MAC, fungal infections (*Coccidioides, Cryptococcus, Histoplasmosis*), neoplasms (non-Hodgkin's lymphoma, KS)
   d. Other causes include chronic alcohol use, liver disease, HIV-associated idiopathic thrombocytopenic purpura (HIV-ITP), and recreational drug use (especially heroin).
2. Pathogenesis
   a. Generally a complication of either an opportunistic infection or opportunistic neoplasm, side effect of a medication, or ITP.
3. Clinical presentation
   a. Bleeding tendencies include epistaxis, bleeding from gums, petechiae, blood in urine or stool, hemoptysis, and vaginal or rectal bleeding.
   b. The potential risk for bleeding is related to the platelet count.
      i. Platelet count < 100,000/mm^3 is clinically significant.
      ii. Platelet count < 50,000/mm^3 indicates mild injury and may result in bleeding.

    iii. Platelet count < 20,000/mm^3 means the patient is at serious risk for a major bleeding episode that may occur spontaneously.

    iv. Platelet count < 10,000/mm^3 means the patient is at risk for a life-threatening bleed. Platelet transfusion must be administered.

4. Diagnosis
   a. Identify certain risk factors, such as recreational drug use, especially heroin.
   b. Obtain a complete blood count CBC with a platelet count. The platelet count will be decreased.
   c. Selenium levels below 145 mcg/l are associated with thrombocytopenia.
   d. Platelet-associated antibodies may be detected with HIV-associated ITP.

5. Prevention/Treatment
   a. Identify and manage the underlying cause.

6. Nursing implications
   a. Prevent bleeding secondary to trauma: use electric razors and soft-bristled toothbrushes or toothettes and avoid flossing teeth.
   b. When platelets are less than 50,000/mm^3, avoid intramuscular injections, rectal temperatures or suppositories, and indwelling catheters.
   c. If venipuncture is performed, the site should have pressure held for at least 5 min.
   d. Teach patient not to take over-the-counter medications that contain aspirin or NSAIDs.
   e. Avoid penetrative anal or vaginal intercourse, vaginal or rectal suppositories, vaginal douching, and rectal enemas or temperatures.
   f. Report any signs of mental status changes, acute pain, nose bleeds, blood in the urine, stool, or sputum.
   g. Teach patient to blow nose gently.
   h. Teach patient not to strain with bowel movements; stool softeners may be initiated.
   i. Teach female patients to avoid tampons and to keep count of the number of pads used during menstruation.

3.34 Cardiomyopathy

1. Etiology/Epidemiology
   a. HIV cardiomyopathy is a complication of HIV-1 infection with high cardiovascular morbidity and mortality.
   b. Dilated cardiomyopathy is the principal type of cardiomyopathy seen in HIV disease and is characterized by echocardiographic findings, including the following:

   - Left ventricular hypokinesis (an ejection fraction of < 45 %)
   - Left ventricular dilation (left ventricular end diastolic volume index > 80 ml per square measure)

   c. The annual incidence of dilated cardiomyopathy in pre-HARRT is estimated to be 15.9 per 1,000 asymptomatic patients (Barbaro, DiLorenzo, Grisorio, & Barbarii, 1998).
   d. The extent of immunodeficiency is most associated with the development of cardiomyopathy.
   e. The benefits of HAART on HIV-associated cardiomyopathy have not been established.

2. Pathogenesis
   a. The pathogenesis of HIV-associated cardiomyopathy is not completely understood. Myocarditis due to viral infections is the most studied mechanism.
      i. HIV appears to infect myocardial cells but is not always found in patients with HIV cardiomyopathy; it appears to involve only a small number of muscle fibers (Barbaro, DiLorenzo, Grisorio, & Barbarii, 1998).
      ii. Coinfection with other cardiotropic viruses (e.g., coxsackievirus group B, cytomegalovirus, Epstein-Barr virus) may cause an autoimmune response to infection but is found in only about 36% of patients with myocarditis (Barbaro et al., 1998).
   b. HIV-infected patients are more likely to have anti-alpha myosin autoantibodies than HIV-negative controls, suggesting

autoimmunity as a cause of cardiomyopathy (Currie et al., 1998).

   c. Nutritional deficiencies of trace elements such as selenium, vitamin B12, and carintine have been associated with cardiomyopathy.

   d. Endocrinopathies, such as growth and thyroid hormone deficiencies, adrenal insufficiency, and hyperinsulinemia, have been found in patients with cardiomyopathy.

3. Clinical presentation

   a. Early in the disease most patients are asymptomatic.

   b. Symptomatic disease occurs when the ejection fraction is < 30%, the left ventricular diastolic dimension is > 60 mm, or both.

   c. Symptomatic disease is similar to symptoms found in left- and right-sided heart failure.

      i. Left-sided symptoms of pulmonary congestion: dyspnea on exertion, orthopnea, and paroxysmal nocturnal dyspnea

      ii. Right-sided symptoms of systemic venous congestion: discomfort on bending, hepatic and abdominal distention, and peripheral edema.

4. Diagnosis

   a. The patient history for gradual exertional intolerance and onset of congestive symptoms, occasionally including chest pain, syncope, or clinical embolic events, is most important to the diagnosis.

   b. The electrocardiogram usually shows left ventricular dilation, with poor R wave progression and higher voltage in V6 than in V5.

   c. The chest radiograph usually shows cardiomegaly.

   d. Two-dimensional and Doppler echocardiogram is essential to diagnosis.

   e. Other laboratory and diagnostic testing is dependent on suspected etiology.

5. Prevention/Treatment

   a. The role of routine screening by echocardiography has not been established.

   b. The prognosis of cardiomyopathy is determined by the stability of the left ventricular ejection fraction and the patient's functional capacity. Patients with an ejection fraction of < 25% have a poor prognosis.

   c. Treatment is directed at contributing factors.

   d. For all patients with symptoms of heart failure, a prescription of angiotensin-converting enzyme inhibitors is indicated. Digitalis glycosides and diuretics may be indicated. Beta-blocking agents improve ventricular function and appear to decrease the progression of the disease in stable heart failure but are not indicated in patients with recent or ongoing decompensation.

6. Nursing implications

   a. Monitor the patient for specific early manifestation of symptoms suggestive of left ventricular failure.

   b. In patients with disease, monitor progression of symptoms.

   c. Educate patient about expected symptoms and what to do if symptoms worsen.

   d. Explain the purpose of pacing and prioritization when symptoms are severe.

   e. Teach the patient energy conservation techniques, such as delegation, work organization, and small, frequent meals.

   f. Evaluate response to prescribed regimens.

3.35 Psoriasis

1. Etiology/Epidemiology

   a. Psoriasis is a chronic inflammatory condition characterized by a rapid turnover of the epidermal layer of the skin, an increase in the number of epidermal cells, and the subsequent formation of scales and well-marginated erythematous plaques.

   b. The etiology is unclear but may involve activity of cytotoxic/suppressor T cells in response to infected or dysfunctional Langerhans cells.

   c. Psoriasis may be exacerbated by stress, sunburn, streptococcal pharyngeal infections, medications, and localized trauma.

   d. Psoriasis is sometimes associated with arthritis.

e. Prevalence of psoriasis in the HIV-infected population is similar to the prevalence in the general population, which is about 1–3% (Maurer & Berger, 1998).

2. Pathogenesis
   a. Psoriasis involves inflammation coupled with alteration of the skin cell cycle leading to chronic scaling of the skin.
   b. High prevalence of HLA-B27 or B7 CREG antigens suggests genetic predisposition (Maurer & Berger, 1998).

3. Clinical presentation
   a. Patient may present with chronic, scaly plaques on elbows, knees, lumbosacral areas, axillae, and groin.
   b. Diffuse dermatitis with thickening may be present; nail dystrophy also may be seen but is not present in many patients.
   c. Involvement is bilateral, rarely symmetrical.

4. Diagnosis
   a. The diagnosis of psoriasis is often made based on clinical presentation, the distribution and appearance of the lesions, and the response to therapy.
   b. It is important to exclude secondary infection by culture and stains.
   c. The only way to definitively diagnose the disease is by taking a biopsy of the lesion.

5. Prevention/Treatment
   a. Treatment is variable, depending on the stage of disease and the site, extent, and degree of disability.
   b. Topical corticosteroids are commonly prescribed for application directly to the lesions.
   c. Small plaques may be treated with intradermal injections of triamcinolone acetonide aqueous suspension.
   d. Other treatments that may be applied are tars, salicylic acid, Denorex, Anthralin, ultraviolet (UVB) light therapy, psoralens plus ultraviolet A (PUVA), retinoids, and immunosuppressives (e.g., methotrexate; Maurer & Berger, 1998).
   e. Systemic therapy may be used. AZT use may lead to improvement (Merrigan, Bartlett, & Bolognesi, 1999). HAART should be encouraged if appropriate;

efficacy of HAART for psoriasis is unstudied (Maurer & Berger, 1998).

6. Nursing implications
   a. Teach patient not to scratch or rub lesions.
   b. Assist patient to implement self-care measures, such as avoidance of sun exposure and sunburn and maintenance of adequate hydration and nutrition. Patient should avoid bathing more than once daily and avoid use of excessive soap and vigorous scrubbing. Stress and alcohol can trigger exacerbation of psoriasis, so stress management techniques and avoidance or decrease in alcohol consumption should be discussed with patient (Handel, 2001).
   c. Counsel patient about medications, which could exacerbate the condition (i.e., systemic corticosteroids, lithium, chloroquine, beta blockers, and nonsteroidal antiinflammatory agents (NSAIDs).
   d. Instruct patients on proper use of medications.

3.36 Arthritis, Reiter's Syndrome

1. Etiology/Epidemiology
   a. The etiology of arthritis in HIV is unclear; HIV appears to have a cytopathic effect on the joints, and the possibility that HIV is arthrogenic is supported by animal studies of other lentiviruses.
   b. It is not clear whether HIV infection predisposes to arthritis or whether viral or immune mechanisms associated with HIV disease contribute to joint pathology.
   c. Prevalence of inflammatory arthritis in HIV-infected persons in the United States is 15–25% (Keat & Rowe, 1991); prevalence may be underreported due to lack of recognition by clinicians.

2. Pathogenesis
   a. Limited data are available on synovial immunopathology. HIV-related arthritis is characterized by nonspecific, chronic synovial inflammation and high synovial-fluid cell counts. In some cases, signs of inflammatory change are

minimal. Arthritis may be precipitated by other infections.

b. Pathogenesis of HIV-related Reiter's syndrome is complex and may involve decreased CD_4 lymphocytes, increased CD_8 lymphocytes, induction by infectious agents, expression of HLA-B27, and direct and indirect consequences of HIV infection. One third of patients with HIV-associated Reiter's syndrome also have documented enteric infections.

3. Clinical presentation
   a. Arthritis can occur at any stage of HIV disease, but it typically develops when CD_4 lymphocyte counts are low. Arthritis is typically characterized by joint inflammation, pain, and limited range of motion.
   b. Reiter's syndrome is characterized by the classic triad—arthritis, urethritis, and conjunctivitis—and occurs in some HIV-infected patients; all three features may be completely or partially present.
   c. Constitutional features of Reiter's syndrome, including fever, weight loss, malaise, lymphadenopathy, and diarrhea, are common and indistinguishable from symptomatic HIV disease (Lane, 1998).
   d. Most frequent sites of inflammation in Reiters' syndrome are the ankle and foot. Ambulatory patients may demonstrate a broad-based ataxia (sometimes referred to as AIDS foot), shifting their weight to the outer margins of the foot to minimize ankle pain.

4. Diagnosis
   a. Radiologic studies may not reveal features of spondyloarthropathies.
   b. Synovial-fluid biopsy results are variable and may reveal only nonspecific chronic synovitis.
   c. Laboratory results include elevated erythrocyte sedimentation rate (ESR) and C-reactive protein, negative for antinuclear antibody (ANA) and rheumatoid factor; tissue typing reveals strong link between HLA-B27 and Reiter's syndrome.

5. Prevention/Treatment
   a. Pharmacologic agents include nonsteroidal antiinflammatory agents (NSAIDs), phenylbutazone, sulfasalazine, prednisone, depot steroids, Myochrysine, hydroxychloroquine sulfate, etretinate, and cyclosporine. Steroid use may increase risk for invasive candidiasis and cytomegalovirus; cytopenias may limit use of NSAIDs.
   b. Avoid other immunosuppressive agents (e.g., methotrexate, ultraviolet B light therapy for psoriatic disease); their use has been associated with sudden fulminant immunodeficiency and the appearance of Kaposi's sarcoma and severe opportunistic infections.
   c. Physical therapy is an absolute requirement to improve mobility and range of motion of affected joints.

6. Nursing implications
   a. Evaluate response to therapy based on patient self-report and physical findings (e.g., range of motion, ability to carry out activities of daily living).
   b. Observe for possible comorbid conditions (e.g., weight loss), which may result from functional limitations and the inability to obtain food and prepare meals; evaluate the need for home care services.

3.37 Osteopenia, Osteoporosis, Avascular Necrosis

1. Etiology/Epidemiology
   a. Osteopenia: bone thinning; osteoporosis: severe loss of bone mass with disruption of skeletal microarchitecture; avascular necrosis (AVN): bone necrosis secondary to circulatory insufficiency (Powderly, 2001)
   b. Etiology: unknown; may be related to antiretroviral therapy, direct infection of osteogenic cells, cytokine activation, dyslipidemia, hypogonadism, and steroid use (Currier, 2001)
   c. Prevalence: osteopenia: 22% to 50% (Carr, Miller, Eisman, & Cooper, 2001; Tebas et al., 2001); osteoporosis: 10% to 21% (Hoy, Hudson, Law, & Cooper, 2000; Tebas et al., 2001); AVN: 4.4% (Masur et al., 2000)

2. Pathogenesis
   a. Osteopenia and osteoporosis: uncoupling of bone formation and bone resorption (Fairfield, Finkelstein, Klibanski, & Grinspoon, 2001)
   b. AVN: unknown; may involve deposition of lipids in subchondral bone vasculature with subsequent occlusion and ischemia (Currier, 2001)

3. Clinical presentation
   a. Osteopenia and osteoporosis are clinically silent disorders.
   b. AVN most commonly involves the hip. Disabling pain may be insidious or sudden in onset and involves decreased range of motion.

4. Diagnosis
   a. Osteopenia and osteoporosis are diagnosed through bone density evaluations.
   b. AVN is best evaluated by magnetic resonance imaging (MRI).

5. Prevention/Treatment
   a. Osteopenia and osteoporosis: smoking cessation, normalization of lipid profile, weight-bearing exercise, and adequate intake of calcium and vitamin D; biphosphonate therapy for osteoporosis
   b. AVN: activity modification, analgesic therapy, and prosthetic replacement

6. Nursing Implications
   a. Patients who smoke should be advised to quit, as smoking accelerates bone loss.
   b. Evaluate diet for adequate intake of calcium and vitamin D. Consult with nutritionist if indicated.
   c. Teach patient that 30 minutes of weight bearing exercises (walking, jogging, aerobics, dancing, tennis, weight lifting) ≥ 3 times weekly may slow bone loss. This has not been formally evaluated in HIV infected person.
   d. Provide referrals to physical and occupational therapist for design and implementation of a comprehensive exercise and activity program and for fitting of assistive devices if indicated.
   e. Advise short periods of rest (1–2 days) if pain is severe. Teach importance of balancing rest with exercise.

3.38 Nephropathy

1. Etiology/Epidemiology
   a. HIV-associated nephropathy (HIVAN) can be a direct result of HIV infection or a result of secondary infections or adverse effects of medical therapies (Brook & Miller, 2001; Brzosko & Mysliwiec, 2000; Rao, Friedman, & Nicastri, 1987; Wooley et al., 2001).
   b. It is the most common cause of chronic renal disease in HIV-infected patients (Monahan, Tanji, & Klotman, 2001; Sothinathan, Briggs, & Eustace, 2001).
   c. The majority of HIVAN cases in the United States occur in African Americans; it is the leading cause of end-stage renal disease (ESRD) in African Americans (Crowley, Cantwell, Abu-Alfa, & Rigsby, 2001; Monahan et al., 2001; Shahinian et al., 2000).

2. Pathogenesis
   a. The exact mechanism of HIV nephro-pathogenesis remains unclear (Kimmel, 2000).
   b. Pathogenesis likely involves HIV infection of renal tubular and epithelial cells (Betjes, Weening, & Krediet, 2001). HIVAN shares clinical and histopathological features with focal and segmental glomerulosclerosis, suggesting a similar pathophysiological mechanism (Avila-Casado, 1999; Sfakianakis et al., 2000).

3. Clinical presentation
   a. HIVAN is often asymptomatic and undetected until proteinuria is found on a screening urinalysis.
   b. Symptomatic patients present with rapidly progressing azotemia and progressive renal failure (Betjes et al., 2001; Brook & Miller, 2001; Cosgrove, Abu-Alfa, & Perazella, 2002; Kirchner, 2002; Rajvanshi & Gupta, 2001).

4. Diagnosis
   a. Renal biopsy is necessary for a definitive diagnosis of HIVAN (Kimmel, 2000). Histopathological findings include focal segmental glomerulosclerosis with glomerular collapse, acute tubular necrosis, and mild interstitial inflammation.

b. Other components of a diagnostic work-up include ultrasonography, serology, and urinalysis (Betjes et al., 2001; Kimmel, 2000; Kirchner, 2002; Rajvanshi & Gupta, 2001).
  i. Ultrasound will show kidney enlargement.
  ii. Serological studies will reveal rapidly developing azotemia.
  iii. Urinalysis will reveal proteinuria.
5. Prevention/Treatment
  a. HAART has been shown to be effective in managing HIVAN (Betjes et al., 2001; Brook & Miller, 2001; Cosgrove et al., 2002; Kimmel, Bosch, & Vassalotti, 1998; Kirchner, 2002; Rao, 2001; Rajvanshi & Gupta, 2001).
  b. Decreased progression to ESRD can be achieved with cyclosporins, glucocorticoids, and angiotensin-converting enzyme (ACE) inhibitors (Betjes et al., 2001; Cosgrove et al., 2002; Kimmel et al., 1998; Kirchner, 2002; Rajvanshi & Gupta, 2001; Sothinathan et al., 2001).
6. Nursing implications
  a. Educate patient to avoid nephrotoxic agents and to maintain adequate hydration; reinforce self-care strategies to control hypertension (Sothinathan et al., 2001).
  b. Assess nutritional status (i.e., weight, body mass index, serum proteins, usual dietary intake) and risk for developing malnutrition before initiating a low-protein diet to slow renal disease progression.

3.39 Lactic Acidosis

1. Etiology/Epidemiology
  a. Hyperlactatemia is believed to be caused by mitochondrial toxicity induced by nucleoside reverse transcriptase inhibitors (NRTIs; Cote et al., 2002; Glesby, 2002).
  b. Lactic acidosis is a severe form of hyperlactatemia characterized by an arterial pH < 7.35 and venous lactate levels > 2.0 mmol/L (Masur, 2001).
  c. Prevalence of asymptomatic hyperlactatemia in NRTI-treated persons is estimated to range from

8% to 21% (Harris et al., 2000; Vrouenraets et al., 2000).
  d. Incidence of mild symptomatic hyperlactatemia has been reported as 14.5 per 1,000 patient years on NRTIs (Lonergan, Havlir, Barber, & Mathews, 2001).
  e. Lactic acidosis is a rare complication of NRTIs, with incidence estimated to be 0.84 per 1,000 person years (Maulin et al., 1999).
2. Pathogenesis
  a. NRTI-induced mitochondrial dysfunction in the liver leads to inhibition of fatty acid oxidation with subsequent anaerobic metabolism and lactate accumulation (Glesby, 2002).
3. Clinical presentation
  a. Persons with mild or moderate hyperlactatemia may be asymptomatic or have mild GI symptoms (i.e., nausea, abdominal distension, pain). Laboratory findings include increased serum lactate and transaminase levels (McComsey & Lederman, 2002).
  b. Lactic acidosis is characterized by fatigue, dyspnea, nausea and vomiting, abdominal pain, edema, and hepatomegaly. Laboratory findings include elevated serum transaminase levels and liver biopsy shows steatosis, inflammation, and necrosis (Masur, 2001).
4. Prevention/Treatment
  a. Anecdotal data suggest that thiamine and riboflavin may prevent recurrence of hyperlactatemia in persons who must be maintained on NRTI therapy (McComsey & Lederman, 2002).
  b. Monitor lactate levels in NRTI-treated persons who present with suspicious signs or symptoms (i.e., fatigue, nausea and vomiting, increased anion gap, low plasma bicarbonate levels; Masur, 2001).
  c. Discontinue NRTIs in persons with severe lactatemia (5.0–10.0 mmol/L) and symptoms (Masur, 2001).
5. Nursing implications
  a. Educate patient/family/significant other regarding early detection of hyperlactatemia.
  b. Recognize patients who are at higher risk for developing lactic acidosis

(i.e., presence of other mitochondrial toxicity-mediated disorders, such as lipoatrophy and peripheral neuropathy).

3.40 Hepatitis A

1. Etiology/epidemiology
   a. Hepatitis A virus (HAV) is an RNA virus; it is a hepatovirus, a member of the Picornaviridae family (Zuckerman & Zuckerman, 1999).
   b. Seroprevalence of HAV in the United States is approximately 30% and is endemic in third world countries (Centers for Disease Control and Prevention, Advisory Committee on Immunization Practices, 1999).
   c. Predominant route of transmission is oral-fecal (Ida et al., 2002).
      i. Contaminated water, food, and shellfish are vehicles for transmission.
      ii. HAV is sexually transmitted via oral-anal contact.
      iii. Person-to-person contact is through contamination of hands with feces.
   d. Blood-borne outbreaks of hepatitis A have occurred in hemophiliacs through the administration of contaminated blood products.
   e. Mean incubation period is 4 weeks (Zuckerman & Zuckerman, 1999).
   f. The following persons are at risk for hepatitis A (Centers for Disease Control and Prevention, National Center for Infectious Diseases, 2001a):

   • Travelers to areas that have high rates of hepatitis A
   • Men who have sex with men
   • Persons who have chronic liver disease and are anti-HAV negative
   • Persons who have clotting-factor disorders
   • Injection and noninjection drug users
   • Day care workers and attendees
   • Laboratory workers who work with HAV

2. Pathogenesis
   a. HAV is ingested or injected and spreads to the liver (Centers for Disease Control and Prevention, Advisory Committee on Immunization Practices, 1999); histopathologic changes in the liver are most likely the result of immune injury (Ida et al., 2002).
   b. HAV is usually a mild, self-limiting infection and does not progress to chronic liver disease or hepatocellular carcinoma (Zuckerman & Zuckerman, 1999).
   c. HAV load is higher and prolonged in HIV-infected patients compared with HAV mono-infected persons (Ida et al., 2002).

3. Clinical presentation
   a. Signs and symptoms of acute infection can include fatigue, anorexia, fever, jaundice, nausea, vomiting, diarrhea and abdominal pain (Centers for Disease Control and Prevention, National Center for Infectious Diseases, 2001d, 2001e); acute infections can be asymptomatic. (Zuckerman & Zuckerman, 1999).
   b. Severity of symptoms increases with age (Alter & Mast, 1994).

4. Diagnosis
   a. Serologic evidence of IgM anti-HAV is present in the 1st week of symptomatic infection. Anti-HAV IgG peaks 1 month and confers protective immunity to subsequent infections.

5. Prevention/Treatment
   a. HAV vaccine is administered to individuals at high risk for exposure to HAV (e.g., international travelers to regions where sanitation is poor or areas where HAV is endemic).
   b. HIV individuals coinfected with any hepatrophic virus should be vaccinated with the HAV vaccine.
   c. Symptomatic treatment occurs when the patient is ill.

6. Nursing implications
   a. Perform HAV risk assessment for all HIV-positive patients.
   b. Conduct patient, family, and staff teaching regarding meticulous hand washing.
   c. Advise to avoid contact with fecal material.
   d. Teach patient that infectious state in HIV/HAV coinfection may last as long as a year (Ida et al., 2002).

3.41 Hepatitis B

1. Etiology/Epidemiology
   a. Hepatitis B virus (HBV) is a double-stranded DNA virus and is classified as a hepadnavirus (Zuckerman & Zuckerman, 1999).
   b. Seroprevalence of anti-HBV in the United States is approximately 0.5% (John Hopkins University, Division of Infectious Diseases, 2002).
   c. Route of transmission is blood borne and sexual (National Digestive Diseases Information Clearinghouse, 2002).
   d. Incubation period range is 1 to 6 months (Zuckerman & Zuckerman, 1999).
   e. The following persons are at risk for HBV (Centers for Disease Control and Prevention, National Center for Infectious Diseases, 2001f):

   - Men having sex with men
   - Persons with multiple sex partners
   - Persons with an HBV-infected sex partner
   - Injection drug users
   - Hemophiliacs
   - Travelers to areas that have high rates of HBV
   - Infants born to HBV-infected mothers

2. Pathogenesis
   a. Histopathologic changes in the HBV-infected liver are believed to be caused by immune injury (Zuckerman & Zuckerman, 1999).
   b. Chronic liver disease occurs in 2–8% of infected adults; it is more common in children, especially infants, with occurrence as high as 80% (John Hopkins University, Division of Infectious Diseases, 2002).
   c. HBV is a risk factor for development of hepatocellular carcinoma (John Hopkins University, Division of Infectious Diseases, 2002).

3. Clinical presentation (Centers for Disease Control and Prevention, National Center for Infectious Diseases, 2001f)
   a. Signs and symptoms include fatigue, nausea, abdominal pain, diarrhea, loss of appetite, fever, dark urine, and jaundice. Acute infection can also be asymptomatic (Zuckerman & Zuckerman, 1999).
   b. Chronic hepatitis with liver cirrhosis may present with symptoms of jaundice, dark urine, ascites, pruritis, nausea, vomiting, coagulation disorders, and gastrointestinal bleeding.

4. Diagnosis
   a. HBV is diagnosed by serologic evidence of antigens.
   b. Markers of HBV replication are HBV DNA and the surface proteins, hepatitis B surface antigen (HBsAg), and hepatitis e antigen (HBeAg). HBsAg is the earliest indicator of infection and the antigen most routinely measured. HBeAg indicates active infection and a high level of infectivity. HBV DNA is the most certain indicator of HBV infection.
   c. HBV antibodies are produced in response to HBV antigens and are markers for the course of the disease. Anti-HBc (core antibody) is the first antibody to appear and is a lifelong marker of past exposure. The appearance of anti-HBs occurs 1–2 months after HBsAg disappears and is a marker of subsequent immunity (Zuckerman & Zuckerman, 1999).
   d. Liver biopsy may be performed to assess extent of liver injury (National Digestive Diseases Information Clearinghouse, 2002).

5. Prevention/Treatment
   a. Vaccination with the HBV vaccine is the best protection (see Section 2.2). The vaccine should be offered to all HIV-infected persons.
   b. No specific therapy for acute HBV infection is available.
   c. For chronic HBV treatment with a 4-month course of interferon alfa-2b, 5 million units or 10 million units 3 times weekly IM or SC, can achieve hepatitis B e antigen seroconversion, normalization of aminotransferase levels, reduced hepatic inflammation, and possibly reduced progression to cirrhosis and improvement in survival in 20–30% of patients (Lin, 2001).
   d. For chronic infection lamivudine 100 mg PO daily for 12 months achieves a response rate of 20–30%. After 3 years

of therapy response rates increase to 40–65% (Lin, 2001). Lamivudine is now considered first-line therapy.

    i. Cases of fatal reactivation HBV due to lamivudine-associated mutations have been reported in HIV/HBV coinfected persons who have liver cirrhosis (Bonacini, Kurz, Locarnini, & Ayres, 2002).

  e. Tenofovir disoproxil fumarate (tenofovir DF) 300 mg once daily is a nucleotide analogue with demonstrated excellent activity against wild-type and nucleoside-resistant HBV.

6. Nursing implications

  a. Standard precautions should be used on all patients.

  b. Patients with HBV should be screened for hepatitis A (HAV) and hepatitis C (HCV).

  c. Patients with HBV should receive the HAV vaccine, if indicated.

  d. Elicit history of botanical alternative therapy use. Certain botanicals are hepatotoxic (e.g., comfrey, kava; Odom & Finkbine, 2001).

  e. Patients considered for interferon alpha therapy should be screened for mood disorders because this is a relative contraindication to treatment.

  f. Provide patient and family teaching regarding prevention of disease transmission (National Digestive Diseases Information Clearinghouse, 2002).

    i. Condoms should be used to prevent infection with HBV and other sexually transmitted diseases.

    ii. Patient should not share drug needles or injection equipment or share toothbrushes or razors of infected persons.

    iii. Tattoos and body piercings should be performed with sterile equipment by an experienced operator who can practice standard precautions.

    iv. Patient should abstain from alcohol intake.

    v. Review with patient medications and adverse effects.

3.42 Hepatitis C

1. Etiology/Epidemiology

  a. Hepatitis C virus (HCV) is a single-stranded RNA virus and is related to flavivirus (Zuckerman & Zuckerman, 1999). HCV is divided into genotypes 1–6, based on genetic heterogeneity, and these are further subdivided into more than 60 subtypes. The prevalence of HCV genotypes varies in different parts of the world. Genotypes 1–3 predominate in the United States.

  b. Seroprevalence of HCV is variable within the population.

    i. General population: 1.8% (Centers for Disease Control and Prevention, National Center for Infectious Diseases, 2001c)

    ii. HIV-infected persons: between 30% and 40% (Monga et al., 2001)

    iii. HIV-positive injection drug users: between 50% and 90% (Graham et al., 2001)

    iv. Men who have sex with men: 4% (Centers for Disease Control and Prevention, National Center for Infectious Diseases, 2001c)

    v. Infants born to HCV infected mothers: 5% (Centers for Disease Control and Prevention, National Center for Infectious Diseases, 2001b)

    vi. Hemophiliacs treated with products made prior to 1987: 87% (Centers for Disease Control and Prevention, National Center for Infectious Diseases, 2001b)

    vii. Blood recipients receiving blood prior to 1990: 6% (Centers for Disease Control and Prevention, National Center for Infectious Diseases, 2001c)

  c. Route of transmission is blood borne. Sexual transmission is possible but is a less efficient mode of transmission than blood borne. Vertical transmission of HCV is 3.2 times greater in HIV/HCV-coinfected mothers (Poles & Dieterich, 2000).

  d. Mean incubation period is 7 weeks (National Institutes of Health, 1997).

2. Pathogenesis
   a. Histopathologic changes in the HCV-infected liver are believed to be caused by cytopathicity (Poles & Dieterich, 2000).
   b. Chronic infection develops in approximately 80% of persons infected with HCV (Poles & Dieterich, 2000).
   c. HCV is a major risk factor for development of hepatocellular carcinoma (National Institutes of Health, 1997).
   d. Persons with HIV/HCV coinfection have more rapid progression to liver cirrhosis; compliance with HAART in the HIV/HCV-coinfected person has not been shown to decrease HCV RNA levels nor has it changed serum alanine aminotransferase (ALT) levels (Torre et al., 2001).
3. Clinical presentation (National Institutes of Health, 1997)
   a. Approximately 90% of persons who have acute HCV infection are asymptomatic (Centers for Disease Control and Prevention, National Center for Infectious Diseases, 2001c).
   b. Signs and symptoms of chronic HCV infection are usually mild and nonspecific. Fatigue is the most frequent complaint. Anorexia, weight loss, and muscle aches may be present.
   c. If associated with liver cirrhosis, which occurs in 20–30% of patients, symptoms include jaundice, dark urine, ascites, pruritus, nausea, vomiting, coagulation disorders, and gastrointestinal bleeding.
   d. Serum HCV RNA is detectable 1–3 weeks following exposure.
   e. Serum ALT levels become elevated shortly before clinical symptoms appear. HCV viremia is associated with normal ALT levels in 30–40% of persons with chronic HCV (Centers for Disease Control and Prevention, National Center for Infectious Diseases, 2001b).
   f. Morbidity and mortality are increased in HCV/HIV-coinfected people, compared with people who have HCV or HIV mono-infection (Monga et al., 2001).
4. Diagnosis
   a. A third-generation enzyme immunoassay (EIA) HCV antibody test should be used to screen for HCV; early EIA testing may be falsely negative in immunocompromised hosts (Ray, 2002).
   b. A serum HCV RNA qualitative and quantitative test can also be used for hepatitis C detection.
   c. Liver biopsy is performed to evaluate extent of liver injury associated with chronic HCV infection (National Institutes of Health, 1997).
5. Treatment
   a. Current standard treatment is pegylated interferon (IFN) and ribavirin. Typical dosing of IFN for hepatitis is 3 million units by subcutaneous injection, 3 times per week. Pegylated IFN, which results from the attachment of a polyethylene glycol molecule to IFN, has a longer half-life and is typically dosed at 1.5 mg/kg of body weight once per week. Ribavirin is typically dosed at 1,000–1,200 mg per day, given orally.
   b. Hepatitis A and B vaccination is recommended in HCV-infected persons who are not immune; acute HAV and HBV infections can exacerbate HCV infection (Keeffe, 2002).
   c. Antiretroviral-associated hepatotoxicity occurs more frequently in HCV-positive patients (Ray, 2002). Antiretroviral therapy may be required if severe hepatotoxicity occurs.
6. Nursing implications
   a. Standard precautions should be used on all patients.
   b. Screen patients with HCV for HAV and HBV.
   c. Educate patients about adverse effects of medication and monitor patients frequently. Treatment with INF/Ribaviran is associated with many adverse reactions (e.g., injection site reactions, anemia).
   d. Elicit history of botanical alternative therapy use. Certain botanicals are hepatotoxic (Odom & Finkbine, 2001).
   e. Screen patients considered for interferon alpha therapy for mood disorders because this is a relative contraindication to treatment.
   f. Screen for Type 2 diabetes, which has been linked with HCV (Mehta et al., 2000).

g. Provide patient and family teaching regarding prevention of disease and disease transmission including the following:

   i. Alcohol use increases risk for mortality in patients with chronic HCV (National Institutes of Health, 1997).

   ii. Keep open wounds covered (Keeffe, 2002).

   iii. Patient should not share razors or toothbrushes or drug needles or equipment (Keeffe, 2002).

   iv. Tattoos and body piercings should be performed with sterile equipment by an experienced operator who can practice standard precautions.

   v. Condoms should be used to prevent infection with HCV and other sexually transmitted diseases.

   vi. Review with patient medications and adverse effects.

References

Abercrombie, P. (2000). Improving adherence to abnormal Pap smear follow-up. *Journal of Obstetrical, Gynecologic, and Neonatal Nursing, 30*, 80–88.

Aberg, J. A., & Powderly, W. G. (2002). Cryptococcosis and HIV. In *HIV InSite Knowledge Base*. Retrieved February 6, 2003, from http://hivinsite.ucsf.edu/InSite.jsp?doc= kb-05-02-05

Aboulafia, D. M., Bundow, D., Waide, S., Bennet, C., & Kerr, D. (2000). Initial observations on the efficacy of highly active antiretroviral therapy in the treatment of HIV-associated autoimmune thrombocytopenia. *American Journal of Medicine and Science, 320*(2), 117–123.

Abramson, D. I., Steinhart C., & Frascino, R. (2000). Epoetin alfa therapy for anaemia in HIV-infected patients: Impact on quality of life. *International Journal of STD and AIDS, 11*, 659–665.

Abularach, S., & Anderson, J. R. (2001). Gynecological problems. In J. R. Anderson (Ed.), *A guide to the clinical care of women with HIV* (pp. 149–196). Rockville, MD: U.S. Department of Health and Human Services.

Alter, M. J., & Mast, E. E. (1994). The epidemiology of viral hepatitis in the united states. *Gastroenterology Clinics of North America, 23*(3), 437–454.

Andersen, M. D., Smereck, G. A. D., Hockman, E. M., Ross, D. J., & Ground, K. J. (1999). Nurses decrease barriers to health care by "hyperlinking" multiple-diagnosed women living with HIV/AIDS into care. *Journal of the Association of Nurses in AIDS Care, 10*, 55–65.

Augenbraun, M. (1995). Increased genital shedding of herpes simplex virus type 2 in HIV-seropositive women. *Annals of Internal Medicine, 123*(11), 845–847.

Avila-Casado, M. C. (1999). Collapsing glomerulopathy: A new entity associated with nephritic syndrome and end-stage renal failure. *Revista de Investigacion Clinica, 51*(6), 367–373.

Bain, B. J. (1999). Pathogenesis and pathophysiology of anemia in HIV infection. *Current Opinion in Hematology, 6*, 89–93.

Barbaro, G., DiLorenzo, G., Grisorio, B., & Barbarii, G. (1998). Incidence of dilated cardiomyopathy and detection of HIV in myocardial cells of HIV positive patients. *New England Journal of Medicine, 339*, 1093–1099.

Barchiesi, F. (1995). Transmission of fluconazole-resistant *Candida albicans* between patients with AIDS and oropharyngeal candidiasis documented by pulsed-field gel electrophoresis. *Clinical Infectious Diseases, 21*(3), 561–564.

Bartlett, J., & Gallant, J. (2000). *2000–2001 Medical management of HIV infection*. Baltimore: Port City Press.

Bartlett, J. G., & Gallant, J. E. (2001). *Medical management of HIV infection: 2001 edition*. Baltimore: Johns Hopkins University, Department of Infectious Diseases.

Behrens, G., Dejam, A., Schmidt, H., Balks, H. J., Brabrant, G., Korner, T., et al. (1999). Impaired glucose tolerance, beta cell function and lipid metabolism in HIV patients under treatment with protease inhibitors. *AIDS, 13*, 63–70.

Betjes, M. G., Weening, J., & Krediet, R. T. (2001). Diagnosis and treatment of HIV-associated nephropathy. *Netherlands Journal of Medicine, 59*(3), 111–117.

Bick, J. (2001). Prevention of opportunistic infections (OIs) in those with HIV infection. *HIV and Hepatitis Education Prison Project News, 4*(12), 1–7.

Boardman, L., Piepert, J., Hogan, J., & Cooper, A. (1999). Positive cone biopsy specimen margins in women infected with the human immunodeficiency virus. *American Journal of Obstetrics and Gynecology, 181*, 1395–1399.

Bonacini, M. (1990). Prospective evaluation of blind brushing of the esophagus for Candida esophagitis in patients with human immunodeficiency virus infection. *American Journal of Gastroenterology, 85*(4), 385–389.

Bonacini, M., Kurz, A., Locarnini, S., & Ayres, A. (2002). Correspondence-fulminant hepatitis B due to a lamivudine-resistant mutant HBV in a patient coinfected with HIV. *Gastroenterology, 122*, 244–245.

Brew, B. J. (1999). AIDS dementia complex. *Neurologic Clinics, 17*, 861–881.

Brinkman, K. (1999, June). *Mitochondrial toxicity of nucleoside analogue reverse transcriptase inhibitors*. Paper presented at the First International Workshop on Adverse Drug Reactions and Lipodystrophy in HIV, San Diego, CA.

Brinkman, K., Smeitink, J. A., Romijn, J. A., & Reiss, P. (1999). Mitochondrial toxicity induced by nucleoside-analogue reverse-transcriptase inhibitors is a key factor in the pathogenesis of antiretroviral-therapy-related lipodystrophy. *Lancet 354*, 1112–1115.

Brook, M. G., & Miller, R. F. (2001). HIV-associated nephropathy: A treatable condition. *Sexually Transmitted Infections, 77*(2), 97–100.

Brzosko, S., & Mysliwiec, M. (2000). HIV nephropathy and other kidney diseases in patients with human immunodeficiency virus infections. *Przeglad Lekarski, 57*(3), 160–164.

Burbano, X., Miguez, M. J., Lecusay, R., Rodriguez, A., Ruiz, P., Morales, G., et al. (2001). Thrombocytopenia in HIV-infected drug users in the HAART era. *Platelets, 12*(8), 456–461.

Carbonara, S., Fiorentino, G., Serio, G., Maggi, P., Ingravallo, G., Monno, L., et al. (2001). Response of severe HIV-associated thrombocytopenia to highly active antiretroviral therapy including protease inhibitors. *Journal of Infection, 42*(4), 251–256.

Carr, A., Miller, J., Eisman, J. A., & Cooper, D. A. (2001). Osteopenia in HIV-infected men: Association with asymptomatic lactic acidemia and lower weight pre-antiretroviral therapy. *AIDS, 15,* 703–709.

Carr, A., Miller, J., Law, M., & Cooper, D. (2000). A syndrome of lipoatrophy, lactic acidaemia and liver dysfunction associated with HIV nucleoside analogue therapy: Contribution to protease inhibitor-related lipodystrophy syndrome. *AIDS, 14,* 25–32.

Carr, A., Samaras, K., Burton, S., Law, M., Freund, J., Chisholm, D., et al. (1998). A syndrome of peripheral lipodystrophy, hyperlipidemia and insulin resistance in patients receiving HIV protease inhibitors. *AIDS, 12,* 51–58.

Carr, A., Samaras, K., Thorisdottir, A., Kaufmann, G. R., Chisholm, J. J., & Cooper, D. A. (1999). Diagnosis, prediction, and natural course of HIV-1 protease-inhibitor-associated lipodystrophy, hyperlipidaemia, and diabetes mellitus: A cohort study. *Lancet, 353* (9170), 2093–2099.

Cejtin, H., Komaroff, E., Massad, L. S., Korn, A., Schmidt, J. B., Eisenberger-Matityahu, D., et al. (1999). Adherence to colposcopy among women with HIV infection. *Journal of Acquired Immune Deficiency Syndrome, 22,* 247–252.

Centers for Disease Control and Prevention. (1987). Revision of the CDC surveillance case definition for acquired immunodeficiency syndrome. *MMWR, 36,* 3–15.

Centers for Disease Control and Prevention. (1998). 1998 guidelines for the treatment of sexually transmitted diseases. *Morbidity and Mortality Weekly Report, 47*(20).

Centers for Disease Control and Prevention. (1999). USPHS/IDSA guidelines for the prevention of opportunistic infections in persons infected with human immunodeficiency virus: U.S. Public Health Service (USPHS) and Infectious Diseases Society of America (IDSA). *MMWR, 48*(RR 10), 1–59, 61–66.

Centers for Disease Control and Prevention. (2001). Draft of guidelines for the prevention of opportunistic infections (OIs) in persons infected with human immunodeficiency virus. *MMWR, 50*(32), 1.

Centers for Disease Control and Prevention. (2002a). *Cryptococcosis.* Retrieved February 17, 2003, from http://www.cdc.gov/ncidod/dbmd/diseaseinfo/cryptococcosis_t.htm

Centers for Disease Control and Prevention. (2002b). *Epidemiology and prevention of vaccine-preventable diseases* (Pink Book, 6th ed.). Washington, DC: Author.

Centers for Disease Control and Prevention, Advisory Committee on Immunization Practices. (1999). Prevention of hepatitis A through active or passive immunization, *MMWR, 48* (No. RR-12), 1–35.

Centers for Disease Control and Prevention, Division of Bacterial and Mycotic Diseases. (2001). *Listeriosis.* Retrieved November 22, 2002, from http://www.cdc.gov/ncidod/dbmd/diseaseinfo/listeriosis_g.htm

Centers for Disease Control and Prevention, National Center for Infectious Diseases. (2001a). *Hepatitis A virus infection.* Retrieved June 4, 2001, from http://www.cdc.gov/ncidod/diseases/hepatitis/slideset/hep_a/slide_4.htm

Centers for Disease Control, National Center for Infectious Diseases. (2001b). *Hepatitis C clinical features and natural history: Chronic HCV infection.* Retrieved April 23, 2002, from http://www.cdc.gov/ncidod/diseases/hepatitis/c_training/edu/3/clinical-chronic.htm

Centers for Disease Control, National Center for Infectious Diseases. (2001c). *Hepatitis C epidemiology: Prevalence of HCV.* Retrieved December 6, 2002, from http://www.cdc.gov/ncidod/diseases/hepatitis/c_training/edu/1/epidem-demo.htm

Centers for Disease Control and Prevention, National Center for Infectious Diseases. (2001d). *Viral hepatitis: A fact sheet.* Retrieved April 23, 2002, from http://www.cdc.gov/ncidod/diseases/hepatitis/a/fact.htm

Centers for Disease Control and Prevention, National Center for Infectious Diseases. (2001e). *Viral hepatitis A: Frequently asked questions.* Retrieved April 23, 2002, from http://www.cdc.gov/ncidod/diseases/hepatitis/a/faqa.htm#1a

Centers for Disease Control and Prevention, National Center for Infectious Diseases. (2001f). *Viral hepatitis B: Frequently asked questions.* Retrieved April 23, 2002, from http://www.cdc.gov/ncidod/diseases/hepatitis/b/fab.htm

Chapple, I. L. C., & Hamburger, J. (2000). The significance of oral health in HIV disease. *Sexually Transmitted Infections, 76,* 236–243.

Cosgrove, C. J., Abu-Alfa, A. K., & Perazella, M. A. (2002). Observations on HIV-associated renal disease in the era of highly active antiretroviral therapy. *American Journal of the Medical Sciences, 323*(2), 102–106.

Cote, H. C., Brumme, Z. L., Craib, K. J., Alexander, C. S., Wynhoven, B., Ting, L., et al. (2002). Changes in mitochondrial DNA as a marker of nucleoside toxicity in HIV-infected patients. *New England Journal of Medicine, 346,* 811–820.

Coyle, T. E. (1997). Hematologic complications of human immunodeficiency virus infection and the acquired immunodeficiency syndrome. *Medical Clinics of North America, 81,* 449–470.

Crowley S. T., Cantwell, B., Abu-Alfa, A., & Rigsby, M. O. (2001). Prevalence of persistent asymptomatic proteinuria in HIV-infected outpatients and lack of correlation with viral load. *Clinical Nephrology, 55*(1), 1–6.

Currie, P. F., Goldman, J. H., Caforio, A.L., Jacob, A. J., Baig, M. K., Brettle, R. P., et al. (1998). Cardiac autoimmunity in HIV related heart muscle disease, *Heart, 79,* 599–604.

Currier, J. S. (2001). Metabolic complications of antiretroviral therapy and HIV infection. *Medscape HIV/AIDS: Annual Update 2001.* Retrieved, September 2002, from http://www.medscape.com/viewarticle/418630

Deepe, G. S. (2000). Histoplasma capsulatum. In G. L. Mandell, J. E. Bennett, & R. Dolin (Eds.), *Principles and practice of infectious diseases* (pp. 2719–2733). Philadelphia: Churchill Livingstone.

De Luca, A., Giancola, M. L., Ammassari, A., Grisetti, S., Paglia, M. G., Gentile, M., et al. (2000). The effect of potent antiretroviral therapy and JC virus load in cerebrospinal fluid on clinical outcome of patients with AIDS-associated progressive multifocal leukoencephalopathy. *Journal of Infectious Diseases, 182,* 1077–1083.

DeSimone, J. A., Pomerantz, R. J., & Babinchak, T. J. (2000). Inflammatory reactions in HIV-1-infected persons after initiation of highly active antiretroviral therapy. *Annals of Internal Medicine, 133,* 447–454.

Dewsnup, D. H. (1994). Efficacy of oral amphotericin B in AIDS patients with thrush clinically resistant to fluconazole. *Journal of Medical and Veterinary Mycology, 32*(5), 389–393.

Dole, P. (2001). Human papillomavirus management in HIV-infected women. *Nurse Practitioner Forum, 12*(4), 214–222.

Dore, G. J., Correll, P. K., Li, Y., Kaldor, J. M., Cooper, D. A., & Brew, B. J. (1999). Changes to AIDS dementia complex in the era of highly active antiretroviral therapy. *AIDS, 13,* 1249–1253.

Doweiko, J. P. (1999). Hematologic manifestations of HIV infection. In T. C. Merrigan, J. G. Bartlett, & D. Bolognesi (Eds.), *Textbook of AIDS medicine* (2nd ed., pp. 611–627). Baltimore: Lippincott Williams & Wilkins.

Doweiko, J. P., & Groopman, J. E. (1998). Hematologic manifestations of HIV infection. In G. P. Wormser (Ed.), *AIDS and other manifestations of HIV infection* (3rd ed., pp. 541–557). Philadelphia: Lippincott-Raven.

Duerr, A., Kieke B., Warren, D., Shah, K., Burk, R., Peipert, J. F., et al. (2001). Human papillomavirus-associated cervical cytologic abnormalities among women with or at risk of infection with human immunodeficiency virus. *American Journal of Obstetrics and Gynecology, 184,* 584–590.

Duong, M., Petit, J. M., Piroth, L., Grappin, M., Buisson, M., Chavanet, P., et al. (2001). Association between insulin resistance and hepatitis C virus chronic infection in HIV-hepatitis C virus-coinfected patients undergoing antiretroviral therapy. *Journal of Acquired Immune Deficiency Syndromes, 27,* 245–250.

Ellerbrock, T., Chiasson, M. A., Bush, T. J., Sun, X. W., Sawo, D., Brudney, K., et al. (2000). Incidence of cervical squamous intraepithelial lesions in HIV-infected women. *Journal of the American Medical Association. 283,*1031–1037.

Engleson, E. S., Glesby, M., Sheikan, J., Wang, J., & Kotler, D. P. (2000, July). *Body composition changes during and after growth hormone therapy for lipodystrophy and truncal adiposity* [Abstract]. Poster session presented at the XIII International Conference on AIDS, Durbin, South Africa.

Enting, R. H., & Portegies, P. (2000). Cytarabine and highly active antiretroviral therapy in HIV-related progressive multifocal leukoencephalopathy. *Journal of Neurology, 247,* 134–138.

Erlich, K. (1999). Herpes simplex virus. In P. Cohen, M. Sande, & P. Volberding (Eds.), *The AIDS knowledge base* (3rd ed., pp. 699–711). Philadelphia: Lippincott Williams & Wilkins.

Fairfield, W. P., Finkelstein, J. S., Klibanski, A., & Grinspoon, S. K. (2001). Osteopenia in eugonadal men with acquired immune deficiency syndrome. *Journal of Clinical Endocrinology & Metabolism, 86,* 2020–2026.

Ferrando, S., van Gorp, W., McElhiney, M., Goggin, K., Sewell, M., & Rabkin, J. (1998). Highly active antiretroviral treatment in HIV infection: Benefits for neuropsychological function. *AIDS, 12,* 65–70.

Ferri, R., Adinofi, A., Orsi, A., Sterken, D. J., Keruly, J. C., Davis, S., et al. (2002). Treatment of anemia in patients with HIV infection—Part 2: Guidelines for the management of anemia. *Journal of the Association of Nurses in AIDS Care, 1,* 50–59.

Fichtenbaum, C., & Aberg, J. (1999). Candidiasis. In P. Cohen, M. Sande, & P. Volberding (Eds.), *The AIDS knowledge base* (3rd ed., pp. 659–668). Philadelphia, PA: Lippincott Williams & Wilkins.

Flaskerud, J. H., & Ungvarski, P. J. (1999). *HIV/AIDS: A guide to nursing care* (4th ed.). Philadelphia: W. B. Saunders.

Fructher, R., Maiman, M., Sedlis, A., Bartley, L., Camilien, L., & Arrastia, C. D. (1996). Multiple recurrences of cervical intraepithelial neoplasia in women with the human immunodeficiency virus. *Obstetrics and Gynecology, 87,* 338–344.

Galli, M., Ridolfo, A. L., Gervasoni, C. (2001). Cardiovascular disease risk factors in HIV-infected patients in the HAART era. *Annals of the New York Academy of Science, 946,* 200–203.

Germinario, R. J., Colby-Germinario, S. P., Cammalleri, C., & Wainberg M. (2000). The effects of a variety of protease inhibitors on insulin binding insulin-mediated sugar transport and cell toxicity in insulin target and non-target cell cultures. *Antiviral Therapy, 5*(Suppl. 5), 7.

Glesby, M. L. (2002). Overview of mitochondrial toxicity of nucleoside reverse transcriptase inhibitors. *Topics in HIV Medicine, 10,* 42–46.

Goldberg, L. H. (1993). Long-term suppression of recurrent genital herpes with acyclovir. A 5-year benchmark. Acyclovir Study Group. *Archives of Dermatology, 129*(5), 582–587.

Goldie, S. J., Weinstein, M. C., Kuntz, M., & Freedberg, K. A. (1999). The costs, clinical benefits, and cost-effectiveness of screening for cervical cancer in HIV-infected women. *Annals of Internal Medicine, 130,* 97–107.

Goodgame, R. W. (1996). Understanding intestinal spore-forming protozoa: Cryptosporidiosis, microsporidiosis, isospora, and cyclospora. *Annals of Internal Medicine, 124*(4), 429–441.

Gottlieb, S. (1999). Some HIV patients can stop taking prophylaxis against infections. *British Medical Journal, 318*(7193), 1231.

Gowdey, G., Lee, R. K., & Carpenter, W. M. (1995). Treatment of HIV-related hairy leukoplakia with podophyllum resin 25% solution. *Oral Surgery, Oral Medicine, Oral Pathology, 79,* 64–67.

Graham, C. S., Baden, L. R., Yu, E., Mrus, J. M., Carnie, J., Heeren, T., et al. (2001). Influence of human immunodeficiency virus infection on the course of hepatitis C virus infection: A meta-analysis. *Clinical Infectious Diseases, 33,* 562–569.

Greenspan, D., Komaroff, E., Redfore, M., Phelan, J. A., Navzesh, M., Alves, M., et al. (2000). Oral mucosal lesions and HIV viral load in the Women's Interagency HIV Study (WIHS). *Journal of Acquired Immune Deficiency Syndromes, 25*(1), 44–50.

Greenspan, J., & Greenspan, D. (1995). *Oral manifestations of HIV infection.* Carol Stream, IL: Quintessence Publishing.

Hadigan, C., Corcoran, C., Basgoz, N., Davis, B., Sax, P., & Grinspoon, S. (2000). Metformin in the treatment of HIV lipodystrophy syndrome: A randomized controlled trial. *Journal of the American Medical Association, 284,* 472–477.

Handel, J. (2001). Dermatological care of clients with HIV/AIDS. In C. A. Kirton, D. Talotta, & K. Zwolski (Eds.), *Handbook of HIV/AIDS nursing* (pp. 323–325). St. Louis, MO: Mosby.

Harris, M., Tesiorowski, A., Chan, K., Hogg, R., Rosenberg, F., Chan Yan, et al. (2000). Lactic acidosis complicating antiretroviral therapy: Frequency and correlates. *Antiviral Therapy, 15*(Suppl. 2), 31.

Heard, I., Tassie, M., Kazatchkine, M. D., & Orth, G. (2002). Highly active antiretroviral therapy enhances regression of cervical intraepithelial neoplasia in HIV-seropositive women. *AIDS, 16,* 1799–1802.

Hillman, R. S. (1998). Anemia. In A. S. Fauci, J. B. Martin, E. Braunwald, D. L. Kasper, K. J. Isselbacher, S. L. Hauser, et al. (Eds.), *Harrison's principles of internal medicine* (pp. 334–339). New York: McGraw-Hill.

Hitchcock, C. A. (1993). Fluconazole resistance in Candida glabrata. *Antimicrobial Agents and Chemotherapy, 37*(9), 1962–1965.

Holcomb, K., Matthews, R. P., Chapman, J. E., Abulafia, O., Lee, Y., Borges, A., et al. (1999). The efficacy of cervical conization in the treatment of cervical intraepithelial neoplasia in HIV-positive women. *Gynecologic Oncology, 74,* 428–431.

Hou, J., & Major, E. O. (2000). Progressive multifocal leukoencephalopathy: JC virus induced demyelination in the immune compromised host. *Journal of Neurovirology, 6*(Suppl. 2), 98–100.

Hoy, J., Hudson, J., Law, M., & Cooper, D. A. (2000, January–February). *Osteopenia in a randomized,*

multicenter study of protease inhibitor (PI) substitution in patients with the lipodystrophy syndrome and well-controlled HIV viremia [Abstract]. Paper presented at the 7th Conference on Retroviruses and Opportunistic Infections, San Francisco.

Ida, S., Tachikawa, N., Nakajima, A., Daikoku, M., Yano, M., Kikuchi, Y., et al. (2002). Influence of human immunodeficiency virus type 1 infection on acute hepatitis A virus infection. *Clinical Infectious Diseases, 34*(3), 379–385.

Jamieson, D. J., Duerr, A., Burk, R., Klein, R. S., Paramsothy, P., Schuman, P., et al. (2002). Characterization of genital human papillomavirus infection in women who have or who are at risk of having HIV infection. *American Journal of Obstetrics and Gynecology, 186,* 21–27.

John Hopkins University, Division of Infectious Diseases. (2002). *Hepatitis B virus (HBV).* Retrieved August 19, 2002, from http://www.hopkins-id.edu/diseases/hepatitis/hbv_faq.html

Jones, J. L., Hanson, D. L., Dworkin, M. S., Alderton, D. L., Fleming, D. L., Kaplan, J. E., et al. (1999). Surveillance for AIDS-defining opportunistic illnesses, 1992–1997. *MMWR, 48*(SS-2), 1–22.

Jones, J. L., Hanson, D. L., Dworkin, M. S., Ward, J. W., & Jaffe, H. W. (1999). Effect of antiretroviral therapy on recent trends in selected cancers among HIV-infected persons. Adult/adolescent spectrum of HIV disease project group. *Journal of Acquired Immune Deficiency Syndrome Human Retrovirology, 21* (Suppl. 1), 11–17.

Jones, S. P., Doran, D. A., Leatt, P. B., Maher, B., & Pirmohamed, M. (2001). Short-term exercise training improves body composition and hyperlipidaemia in HIV-positive individuals with lipodystrophy. *AIDS, 15,* 2049–2051.

Kahn, J. O., Hecht, F. M., Chesney, M. A., & Walker, B. D. (1999). Early intervention: Acute HIV infection. In R. Dolin, H. Masur, & M. S. Saag (Eds.), *AIDS therapy* (pp. 229–235). New York: Churchill Livingstone.

Keat, A., & Rowe, I. (1991). Reiter's syndrome and associated arthritides. *Rheumatic Disease Clinics of North America, 17,* 25–42.

Keeffe, E. B. (2002). Current treatment of chronic hepatitis C. *Medscape Gastroenterology eJournal.* Retrieved, December 18, 2002, from http: //www.medscape.com/viewarticle/429322_1

Keruly, J. C., Mehta, S., Chaisson, R. E., & Moore, R. D. (1998, September). *Incidence of and factors associated with the development of hypercholesterolemia and hyperglycemia in HIV-infected patients using a protease inhibitor.* Paper presented at the 38th Interscience Conference on Antimicrobial Agents and Chemotherapy, San Diego, CA.

Kimmel, P. L. (2000). The nephropathies of HIV infection: Pathogenesis and treatment. *Current Opinion in Nephrology and Hypertension, 9*(2), 117–122.

Kimmel, P. L., Bosch, J. P., & Vassalotti, J. A. (1998). Treatment of human immunodeficiency virus (HIV)-associated nephropathy. *Seminars in Nephrology, 18*(4), 446–458.

Kirchner, J. T. (2002). Resolution of renal failure after initiation of HAART: Three cases and a discussion of the literature. *AIDS Reader, 12*(3), 103–105.

Klaus, B. D. (1996). Peripheral neuropathy. *Nurse Practitioner, 21*(6), 130–131.

Koehler, J. E. (1999). Bacillary angiomatosis and other unusual infections in HIV-infected individuals. In M. A. Sande & P. A. Volberding (Eds.), *The Medical management of AIDS* (pp. 411–428). Philadelphia: WB Saunders.

Kolson, D. L., & Gonzalez-Scarano, F. (2001). HIV-associated neuropathies: Role of HIV-1, CMV, and other viruses. *Journal of the Peripheral Nervous System, 6*, 2–7.

Kotler, D. P. (1998). *Update on lipid abnormalities and cardiovascular complications in HIV infection.* Retrieved December 28, 2002, from http://www.medscape.com/viewprogram/295

Kotler, D. P. (1999). *Update on metabolic and morphologic abnormalities in HIV.* Retrieved August, 2002, from http://209.67.30.82/Medscape/HIV/TreatmentUpdate/1999/tu11/public/toc-tu11.html

Kovacs, J. A., Gill, V. J., Meshnick, S., & Masur, H. (2001). New insights into transmission, diagnosis, and drug treatment of *Pneumocystic carinii* pneumonia. *Journal of the American Medical Association, 286*(19), 2450–2460.

Kreuzer, K. A., & Rockstroh, J. K. (1997). Pathogenesis and pathophysiology of anemia in HIV infection. *Annals of Hematology, 75*, 179–187.

Krown, S. E. (1998). Clinical overview: Issues in Kaposi's sarcoma therapeutics. *Journal of National Cancer Institute Monograph, 23*, 59–63.

Lane, N. (1998). *Rheumatologic and musculoskeletal manifestations of HIV.* Retrieved December 18, 2002, from http://hivinsite.ucsf.edu/InSite.jsp?page=kb-04&doc=kb-04-01-15

Leenerts, M. H. (1998). Barriers to self-care in a cohort of low-income white women living with HIV/AIDS. *Journal of the Association of Nurses in AIDS Care, 9*, 22–36.

Lenhard, J. M., Croom, D. K., Weiel, J. E., & Winegar, D. A. (2000). HIV protease inhibitors stimulate hepatic triglyceride synthesis. *Arteriosclerosis, Thrombosis, and Vascular Biology, 20*, 2625–2629.

Levine, A. (1998). Oncologic disorders and cytokines. *Clinical Care Options for HIV, 4*(2), 1–19.

Levine, A. (2001). *New developments in AIDS-related hematology and oncology.* Retrieved November 4, 2002, from http://www.medscape.com/viewarticle

Levine, A. M. (1999). *Anemia, neutropenia and thrombocytopenia: Pathogenesis and evolving treatment options in HIV-infected patients.* Retrieved July 8, 2002, from http://hiv.medscape.com/Medscape/HIV/ClinicalMgmt/CM.v10/pnt-CM.v10.html

Lin, O. S. (2001). Current treatment strategies for chronic hepatitis B and C. *Annual Review of Medicine, 52*, 29–49.

Lonergan, J. T., Havlir, D., Barber, E., & Mathews, W. C. (2001). *Incidence and outcome of hyperlactatemia associated with clinical manifestations in HIV-infected adults receiving NRTI-containing regimens* [Abstract 624]. Paper presented at the Eighth Conference on Retroviruses and Opportunistic Infections, Chicago.

Luque, A. E., Demeter, L. M., & Reichman, R. C. (1999). Association of human papillomavirus infection and disease with magnitude of human immunodeficiency virus type 1. *Journal of Infectious Diseases, 179*, 1405–1409.

Mabruk, M. J. E. M. F., Antonio, M., Flint, S. R., Coleman, D. C., Toner, M., Kay, E., et al. (2000). A simple and rapid technique for the detection of Epstein-Barr virus DNA in HIV-associated oral hairy leukoplakia biopsies. *Journal of Oral Pathology Medicine, 29*, 118–122.

Maiman, M., Watts, D. H., Andersen, J., Ciax, P., Merino, M., & Kendall, M. A. (1999). Vaginal 5-fluorouracil for high-grade dysplasia in human immunodeficiency virus infection: A randomized trial. *Obstetrics and Gynecology, 94*, 95–961.

Mandelblatt, J. S., Kanetsky, P., Eggert, L., & Gold, K. (1999). Is HIV infection a cofactor for cervical squamous cell neoplasia? *Cancer Epidemiology Biomarkers and Prevention, 8*, 97–106.

Mannucci, P. M., & Gringeri, A. (2000). HIV-related thrombocytopenia. *Annals of Italian Medicine, 15*(1), 20–27.

Marrazzo, J. M., Koutsky, L. A., Kiviat, N. B., Kiviat, M. D., Kuypers, J. M., & Stine, K. (2001). Papanicolaou test screening and prevalence of genital human papillomavirus among women who have sex with women. *American Journal of Public Health, 91*(6), 947–952.

Martinez, E., & Gatell, J. (1998). Metabolic abnormalities and use of HIV-1 protease inhibitors. *The Lancet, 352*, 821–822.

Massad, L. S., Riester, K. A., Anastos, K. M., Fruchter, R. G., Palefsky, J. M., Burk, R. D., et al. (1999). Prevalence and predictors of squamous cell abnormalities in papanicolaou smears from women infected with HIV-1. *Journal of Acquired Immune Deficiency Syndromes, 21*, 33–41.

Massad, L. S., Schneider, M., Watts, H., Darragh, T., Abulafia, O., Salzer, E., et al. (2001). Correlating Papanicolaou smear, colposcopic impression, and biopsy: Results from the women's interagency HIV study. *Journal of Lower Genital Tract Disease, 5*(4), 212–218.

Masur, H. (2001). Metabolic complications in HIV disease: Lactemia and bone disease. *Topics in HIV Medicine, 9*, 8–11.

Masur, H., Miller, K. D., Jones, E. C., et al. (2000, September). *High prevalence of avascular necrosis of the hip in HIV infection* [Abstract]. Paper presented at the 38th Annual Meeting of the Infectious Diseases Society of America, New Orleans, LA.

Maulin, L., Gerard, Y., de la Tribonniere, X., Amiel, C., Valette, M., Baclet, V., et al. (1999). *Emerging complications of antiretroviral therapy: Symptomatic hyperlactatemia* [Abstract 1285]. Paper presented at the 39th Interscience Conference on Antimicrobial Agents and Chemotherapy, San Diego, CA.

Maurer, T. A., & Berger, T. G. (1998). *Dermatologic manifestations of HIV.* Retrieved December 18, 2002, from http://hivinsite.ucsf.edu/InSite.jsp?page=kb-04-01-01

McCarthy, G. M. (1991). Factors associated with increased frequency of HIV-related oral candidiasis. *Journal of Oral Pathology and Medicine, 20*(7), 332–336.

McComsey, G. A., & Lederman, M. M. (2002). High doses of riboflavin and thiamine may help in secondary prevention of hyperlactatemia. *The AIDS Reader, 12,* 222–224.

McGuire, D., & So, Y. T. (1998). Neurologic manifestations of HIV. In L. Peiperl & P. Volberding (Eds), *HIV InSite knowledge base.* Retrieved February 11, 2002, from http://hivinsite.ucsf.edu/InSite. jsp?page=kb-04&doc=kb-04–01–02

Mehta, S. H., Brancati F. L., Sulkowski, M. S., Strathdee, S. A., Szklo M., & Thomas, D. L. (2000). Prevalence of type 2 diabetes mellitus among persons with hepatitis C virus infection in the United States. *Annals of Internal Medicine,133,* 592–599.

Melton, S., Kirkwood, C., & Ghaemi, S. N. (1997). Pharmacotherapy of HIV dementia. *Annals of Pharmacotherapy, 31*(4), 457–473.

Merrigan, T., Bartlett, J. G., Bolognesi, D. (Eds.). (1999). *Textbook of AIDS medicine.* Philadelphia: Lippincott Williams & Wilkins.

Minkoff, H., Ahdieh, L., Massad, L. S., Anastos, K., Watts, D. H., Melnick, S., et al. (2001). The effect of highly active antiretroviral therapy on cervical cytologic changes associated with oncogenic HPV among HIV-infected women. *AIDS, 15,* 2157–2164.

Minkoff, H., Feldman, J., DeHovitz, J., Landesman, S., & Burk, R. (1998). A longitudinal study of human papillomavirus carriage in human immunodeficiency virus-infected and human immunodeficiency virus-uninfected women. *American Journal of Obstetrics and Gynecology, 178,* 982–986.

Miralles, P., Berenguer, J., Garcia de Viedma, D., Padilla, B., Cosin, J., Lopez-Bernaldo de Quiros, J. C., et al. (1998). Treatment of AIDS-associated progressive multifocal leukoencephalopathy with highly active antiretroviral therapy. *AIDS, 12,* 2467–2472.

Mitsuyasu, R. (1999). Hematologic disease. In R. Dolin, H. Masur, & M. S. Saag (Eds.), *AIDS therapy* (pp. 666–679). New York: Churchill Livingstone.

Monahan, M., Tanji, N., & Klotman, P. E. (2001). HIV-associated nephropathy: An urban epidemic. *Seminars in Nephrology, 21*(4), 394–402.

Monga, H. K., Rodriguez-Barradas, M. C., Breaux, K., Khattak, K., Troisi, C. L., Velez, M., et al. (2001). Hepatitis C virus infection-related morbidity and mortality among patients with human immunodeficiency virus infection. *Clinical Infectious Diseases, 33*(2), 240–247.

Montoya, J. G., & Remington, J. S. (2000). *Toxoplasma gondii.* In G. L. Mandell, J. E. Bennett, & R. Dolin (Eds.), *Principles and practice of infectious diseases* (pp. 2858–2888). Philadelphia: Churchill Livingstone.

Moore, P. S., & Chang, Y. (1995). Detection of herpes virus-like DNA sequences in Kaposi's sarcoma in patients with and those without HIV infection. *New England Journal of Medicine, 332,* 1186–1191.

Moscicki, A. B., Hills, N., Shiboski, S., Powell, K., Jay, N., Hanson, E., et al. (2001). Risks for incident human papillomavirus infection and low-grade squamous intraepithelial lesion development in young females. *Journal of the American Medical Association, 285,* 2995–3002.

Moyle, G. (2000). Clinical manifestations and management of antiretroviral nucleoside analog-related mitochondrial toxicity. *Clinical Therapeutics, 22,* 911–936.

Musher, D. (2000). *Streptococcus pneumoniae.* In G. Mandell, J. Bennett, & R. Dolin (Eds.), *Principles and practice of infectious diseases* (5th ed., pp. 2128–2147). Philadelphia: Churchill-Livingstone.

Mussini, C., Pezzotti, P., Govoni, A., Borghi, V., Antinori, A., d'Arminio Monforte, A., et al. (2000). Discontinuation of primary prophylaxis for *Pneumocystis carinii* pneumonia and toxoplasmic encephalitis in human immunodeficiency virus type 1-infected patients. *The Journal of Infectious Diseases, 181*(5), 1635.

Nakagawa, M., Stites, D., Patel, S., Scott, M., Hills, N., Palefsky, J., et al. (2000). Persistence of human papillomavirus 16 infection is associated with lack of cytotoxic T lymphocyte response to the E6 antigen. *Journal of Infectious Diseases, 182,* 595–598.

Nardi, S. H., Karpatkin, M., Hart, D., Belmont, M., & Karpartkin, S. (1999). Differentiation of autoimmune thrombocytopenia from thrombocytopenia associated with immune complex disease: Systemic lupus erythematous, hepatitis-cirrhosis, and HIV-1 infection by platelet and serum immunological measurements. *British Journal of Hematology, 105*(4), 1086–1091.

National Digestive Diseases Information Clearinghouse. (2002). *What I need to know about Hepatitis B.* Retrieved August 19, 2002, from http://www.niddk.nih.gov/health/digest/pubs/hep/hepb/hepb.htm

National Institutes of Health. (1997). *NIH consensus development conference on management of hepatitis C.* Bethesda, MD: Author.

Nemechek, P. M., Polsky, B., & Gottlieb, M. S. (2000). Treatment guidelines for HIV-associated wasting. *Mayo Clinic Proceedings, 75,* 386–394.

O'Brien, T. R., Kedes, D., Ganem, D., Macrae, D. R., Rosenberg, P. S., Molden, J., et al. (1999). Evidence for concurrent epidemics of human herpes virus 8 and human immunodeficiency virus type 1 in U.S. homosexual men: Rates, risk factors and relationship to Kaposi's sarcoma. *Journal Infectious Diseases, 180,* 1010–1017.

Odom, J., & Finkbine, S. (2001). Overcoming hepatitis. *Alternative Medicine, 42,* 40–48.

O'Farrell, N. (1994). High cumulative incidence of genital herpes amongst HIV-1 seropositive heterosexuals in south London. *International Journal of STD and AIDS, 5*(6), 415–418.

Palefsky, J. (2000). Anal cancer in HIV infection. *International AIDS Society—USA, 8*(7), 14–17.

Palefsky, J. M., Minkoff, H., Kalish, L. A., Levine, A., Sacks, H. S., Garcia, P., et al. (1999). Cervicovaginal human papillomavirus infection in HIV-positive and high-risk HIV-negative women. *Journal of the National Cancer Institute, 91,* 226–236.

Pardo, C. A., McArthur, J. C., & Griffin, J. W. (2001). HIV neuropathy: Insights in the pathology of HIV peripheral nerve disease. *Journal of the Peripheral Nervous System, 6,* 21–27.

Patton, L. L. (1999). Hematologic abnormalities among HIV-infected patients: Associations of significance for dentistry. *Oral Surgery, Oral Medicine, Oral Pathology, Oral Radiology, and Endodontics, 88,* 561–567.

Peel, K. (1995). Premalignant and malignant disease of the cervix. In C. Whitefield (Ed.), *Dewhurst textbook of obstetrics and gynecology for postgraduates* (5th ed., pp. 717–737). London: Blackwell Scientific.

Poles, M. A., & Dieterich, D. T. (2000). Hepatitis C virus/human immunodeficiency virus coinfection: Clinical management issues. *Clinical Infectious Diseases, 31,* 154–161.

Polsky, B., Kotler, D., & Steinhart, C. (2001). HIV-associated wasting in the HAART era: Guidelines for assessment, diagnosis, and treatment. *AIDS Patient Care and STDs, 15*(8), 411–423.

Poncelet, A. N. (1998, February 15). An algorithm for the evaluation of peripheral neuropathy. *American Family Physician.* Retrieved January 31, 2003, from http:// www.aafp.org/afp/980215ap/poncelet.html

Powderly, W. G. (1995). A randomized trial comparing fluconazole with clotrimazole troches for the prevention of fungal infections in patients with advanced human immunodeficiency virus infection. NIAID AIDS Clinical Trials Group. *New England Journal of Medicine, 332*(11), 700–705.

Powderly, W. G. (2001, January/February). Bone disorders in HIV-infected patients. *Medscape HIV/AIDS, 7*(1). Retrieved September, 2002, from http://www. medscape.com/viewarticle/403863

Power, C., Selnes, O. A., Grim, J. A., & McArthur, J. C. (1995). HIV Dementia Scale: A rapid screening test. *Journal of the Acquired Immune Deficiency Syndrome, 8,* 273–278.

Project Inform. (2001). *Mycobacterium avium complex (MAC) fact sheet.* Retrieved March 18, 2002, from http://www. thebody.com/pinf/mac.html

Rabeneck, L. (1994). Esophageal candidiasis in patients infected with the human immunodeficiency virus. A decision analysis to assess cost-effectiveness of alternative management strategies. *Archives of Internal Medicine, 154*(23), 2705–2710.

Rajvanshi, P., & Gupta, B. (2001). Human immunodeficiency virus-associated nephropathy. *Journal of the Association of Physicians of India, 49,* 813–818.

Rao, T. K. (2001). Human immunodeficiency virus infection and renal failure. *Infectious Disease Clinics of North America, 15*(3), 833–850.

Rao, T. K., Friedman, E. A., & Nicastri, A. D. (1987). The types of renal disease in the acquired immunodeficiency syndrome. *New England Journal of Medicine, 316*(17), 1062–1068.

Ray, S. C. (2002). Perspectives: Science and treatment of HIV and hepatitis C virus coinfection. *Topics in HIV Medicine, 9*(6), 11–16.

Richart, R. M., Cox, J. T., Twiggs, L. B., Wilkenson, E. J., & Wright, T. C. (2002). A sea change in diagnosing

and managing HPV and cervical disease—Part 1. *Contemporary OB/GYN, 5,* 42–56.

Roubenoff, R., Weiss, L., McDermott, A., Heflin, T., Cloutier, G. J., Wood, M., et al. (1999). A pilot study of exercise training to reduce trunk fat in adults with HIV-associated fat redistribution. *AIDS, 13*(11), 1373–1375.

Rozenbaum, W., Molina, J. M., Delfraissy, J. F., Bentata, M., DeTruchis, P., & Antoun, Z. (2000, January–February). *Improvements of lipodystrophy in HIV infected subjects switching from 2NRTI/PI to 2NRTI/abacavir* [Abstract]. Poster session presented at the annual Conference on Retroviruses, San Francisco.

Saag, M. S. (2000). Cryptococcosis and other fungal infections (histoplasmosis, coccidioidomycosis). In M. A. Sande & P. Volberding (Eds.), *The medical management of AIDS* (pp. 361–377). Philadelphia: WB Saunders.

Sabella, C., & Goldfarb, J. (1999). *Parvovirus B 19 infections.* Retrieved July 8, 2002, from http://www.aafp. org/afp/991001ap/1455.html

Sacks, S. L. (1996). Patient-initiated, twice-daily oral famciclovir for early recurrent genital herpes. A randomized, double-blind multicenter trial. Canadian Famciclovir Study Group. *Journal of the American Medical Association, 276*(1), 44–49.

Sacktor, N., McDermott, M. P., Marder, K., Schifitto, G., Selnes, O. A., McArthur, J. C., et al. (2002). HIV-associated cognitive impairment before and after the advent of combination therapy. *Journal of Neurovirology, 8,* 136–142.

Safrin, S. (1991a). Clinical and serologic features of herpes simplex virus infection in patients with AIDS. *AIDS, 5*(9), 1107–1110.

Safrin, S. (1991b). A controlled trial comparing foscarnet with vidarabine for acyclovir-resistant mucocutaneous herpes simplex in the acquired immunodeficiency syndrome. The AIDS Clinical Trials Group. *New England Journal of Medicine, 325*(8), 551–555.

Saiag, P., Pavlovic, M., Clerici, T., Feauveau, V., Nicolas, J. C., Emile, D., et al. (1998). Treatment of early AIDS-related Kaposi's sarcoma with oral all-transretinoic acid: Results of a sequential non-randomized phase II trial. Kaposi's sarcoma ANRS study group. Agence Nationale de Recherches sur le SIDS. *AIDS, 12,* 2169–2176.

Saint-Marc, T., & Touraine, J. L. (1999). Effects of metformin on insulin resistance and central adiposity in patients receiving effective protease inhibitor therapy [Letter]. *AIDS, 13*(8), 1000–1002.

Saltzman, R. (1994). Safety of famciclovir in patients with herpes zoster and genital herpes. *Antimicrobial Agents and Chemotherapy, 38*(10), 2454–2457.

Scaradavou, A., Woo, B., Woloski, B. M. R., Cunningham-Rundles, S., Ettinger, L. J., Aledort, L. M., et al. (1997). Intravenous anti-D treatment of immune thrombocytopenic purpura: Experience in 272 patients. *Blood, 89*(8), 2689–2700.

Schacker, T., & Corey, L. (1997). Herpes virus infections in human immunodeficiency virus-infected person. In V. Devita, S. Hellman, & S. Rosenberg (Eds.),

AIDS: Biology, diagnosis, treatment and prevention (4th ed., pp. 267–280). Philadelphia: Lippincott-Raven.

Schambelan, M. (2000). Metabolic and morphologic complications of HIV. *Topics in HIV Medicine, 8*(5), 4–8.

Scherer, P. (1990). How HIV attacks the peripheral nervous system. *American Journal of Nursing, 90,* 67–70.

Schlecht, N. F., Kulaga, S., Robitaille, J., Ferreira, S., Santos, M., Miyamura, R. A., et al. (2001). Persistent human papillomavirus infection as a predictor of cervical intraepithelial neoplasia. *Journal of the American Medical Association, 286,* 3106–3114.

Sfakianakis, G. N., Carmona, A. J., Sharma, A., Strauss, J., Georgiou, M. F., Zilleruelo, G. E., et al. (2000). Diuretic MAG3 scintirenography in children with HIV nephropathy: Diffuse parenchymal dysfunction. *Journal of Nuclear Medicine, 41*(6), 1037–1042.

Shahinian, V., Rajaraman, S., Borucki, M., Grady, J., Hollander, W. M., & Ahuja, T. S. (2000). Prevalence of HIV-associated nephropathy in autopsies of HIV-infected patients. *American Journal of Kidney Diseases, 35*(5), 884–888.

Shepp, D. H. (1985). Oral acyclovir therapy for mucocutaneous herpes simplex virus infections in immunocompromised marrow transplant recipients. *Annals of Internal Medicine, 102*(6), 783–785.

Singer, E. J., & Germaniskis, L. (1995). HIV and peripheral neuropathy. *Journal of the International Association of Physicians in AIDS Care, 1,* 30–33.

Slater, L., & Welch, D. (2000). *Bartonella* species, including cat-scratch disease. In G. L. Mandell, J. E. Bennett, & R. Dolin (Eds.), *Principles and practice of infectious diseases* (pp. 2444–2456). New York: Churchill Livingstone.

Solomon, D., Schiffman, M., & Tarone, R. (2001). Comparison of three management strategies for patients with atypical squamous cells of undetermined significance: Baseline results from a randomized trial. *Journal of the National Cancer Institute, 93*(4), 293–299.

Sothinathan, R., Briggs, W. A., & Eustace, J. A. (2001). Treatment of HIV-associated nephropathy. *AIDS Patient Care and STDs, 15*(7), 363–371.

Spruance, S. L. (1996). A large-scale, placebo-controlled, dose-ranging trial of peroral valaciclovir for episodic treatment of recurrent herpes genitalis. Valaciclovir HSV Study Group. *Archives of Internal Medicine, 156*(15), 1729–1735.

Stewart, J. A. (1995). Herpes virus infections in persons infected with human immunodeficiency virus. *Clinical Infectious Diseases, 21*(Suppl. 1), 114–120.

Subauste, C. S., & Remington, J. S. (2000). AIDS-associated toxoplasmosis. In M. A. Sande & P. Volberding (Eds.), *The medical management of AIDS* (pp. 379–398). Philadelphia: W. B. Saunders.

Sullivan, P. S., Hanson, D. I., Chu, S. Y., Jones, J. L., & Ciesielski, C. A. (1997). Surveillance for thrombocytopenia in persons infected with HIV: Results from the Multistate Adult and Adolescent Spectrum of Disease Project. *Journal of Acquired Immunodeficiency Syndrome and Human Retrovirology, 14*(4), 374–379.

Sullivan, P. S., Hanson, D. L., Chu, S. Y., Jones, J. L., & Ward, J. W. (1998). Epidemiology of anemia in HIV-infected persons: Results from the Multi-state Adult and Adolescent Spectrum of HIV Disease Surveillance Project. *Blood, 91,* 301–308.

Sun, X. W., Kuhn, L., Ellerbrock, T. V., Chiasson, M. A., Bush, T. J., & Wright, T. C. (1997). Human papillomavirus infection in women infected with the human immunodeficiency virus. *New England Journal of Medicine, 337,* 1343–1349.

Swindells, S., Zheng, J., & Gendelman, H. (1999). HIV-associated dementia: New insights into disease pathogenesis and therapeutic interventions. *AIDS Patient Care and STDs, 13*(3), 153–163.

Tate, D. R., & Anderson, R. J. (2001). Recurrence of cervical dysplasia in the human immunodeficiency virus-seropositive patient. *Obstetrics and Gynecology, 97,* 60.

Tavitian, A. (1986). Oral candidiasis as a marker for esophageal candidiasis in the acquired immunodeficiency syndrome. *Annals of Internal Medicine, 104*(1), 54–55.

Tebas, P., Powderly, W. G., Claxton, S., Marin, D., Tantisiriwat, W., Teitelbaum, S. L., et al. (2001). Accelerated bone mineral loss in HIV-infected patients receiving potent antiretroviral therapy. *AIDS, 14,* 63–67.

Thomas, F. P. (2002). HIV encephalopathy and AIDS dementia complex. *eMedicine Journal, 3.* Retrieved, December 19, 2002, from http://www.emedicine.com/NEURO/ topic447.htm

Torre, D., Tambini, R., Cadario, F., Barbarini, G., Moroni, M., & Basilico, C. (2001). Evolution of coinfection with human immunodeficiency virus and hepatitis C virus in patients treated with highly active antiretroviral therapy. *Clinical Infectious Diseases, 33*(9), 1579–1584.

Uberti-Foppa, C., Origoni, M., Maillard, M., Ferrari, D., Ciuffreda, D., Mastrorilli, E., et al. (1998). Evaluation of the detection of human papillomavirus genotypes in cervical specimens by hybrid capture as screening for precancerous lesions in HIV-positive women. *Journal of Medical Virology, 56,* 133–137.

UNAIDS Technical Update. (1998). *HIV-related opportunistic diseases.* Retrieved January 30, 2002, from http://www. unaids.org/publications/documents/impact/opportunistic/opportue.txt

United States Public Health Service, & Infectious Diseases Society of America. (1999). Guidelines for the prevention of opportunistic infections in persons infected with human immunodeficiency virus. *MMWR, 48*(RR-10), 1–59, 61–66.

van der Valk, M. A., Bisschop, P. H., Romijn, J. A., Ackermans, M. T., Lange, Joep, M. A., Endert, E. D., et al. (2001). Lipodystrophy in HIV-1-positive patients is associated with insulin resistance in multiple metabolic pathways. *AIDS, 15,* 2093–2100.

Verma, A. (2001). Epidemiology and clinical features of HIV-1 associated neuropathies. *Journal of the Peripheral Nervous System, 6,* 8–13.

Vrouenraets, S., Treskes, M., Regez, R. M., Troost, N., Weigel, H.M., Frissen, P. H. J., et al. (2000). *The occurrence of hyperlactatemia in HIV-infected patients on*

NRTI treatment [Abstract TuPpB1234]. Paper presented at the XIII International AIDS Conference, Durban, South Africa.

Walli, R., Herfort, O., Michl, G. M., Demant, T., Jager, H., Dieterle, C., et al. (1998). Treatment with protease inhibitors associated with peripheral insulin resistance and impaired oral glucose tolerance in HIV-1 infected patients. *AIDS, 12,* 167–173.

Walli, R., Michl, G. M., Muhlbayer, D., Brinkmann, L., & Goebel, F. D. (2000). Effects of troglitazone on insulin sensitivity in HIV-infected patients with protease-inhibitor-associated diabetes mellitus. *Research in Experimental Medicine, 199*(5), 253–262.

Walling, D. M., Flaitz, C. M., Nichols, C. M., Hudnall, S. D., & Adler-Storthz, K. (2001). Persistent productive Epstein-Barr virus replication in normal epithelial cells in vivo. *Journal of Infectious Diseases, 184*(12), 1499–1507.

Walzer, P. D. (2000). *Pneumocystis carinii.* In G. Mandell, J. Bennett, & R. Dolin (Eds.), *Principles and practice of infectious diseases* (5th ed., pp. 2781–2795). Philadelphia: Churchill-Livingstone.

Wanke, C. E., Silva, M., Knox, T. A., Forrester, J., Speigelman, D., & Gorbach, S. L. (2000). Weight loss and wasting remain common complications in individuals infected with human immunodeficiency virus in the era of highly active antiretroviral therapy. *Clinical Infectious Disease, 31*(3), 803–805.

Wilcox, C. M. (1996). Fluconazole compared with endoscopy for human immunodeficiency virus-infected patients with esophageal symptoms. *Gastroenterology, 110*(6), 1803–1809.

Wooley, I. J., Kalayjian, R., Valdez, H., Hamza, N., Jacobs, G., Lederman, M. M., et al. (2001). HIV nephropathy and the Duffy antigen/receptor for chemokines in African Americans. *Journal of Nephrology, 14*(5), 384–387.

World Health Organization. (1996). *Cancer pain relief, with guide of opioid availability* (2nd ed.). Geneva: World Health Organization.

Wright, T. C., Moscarelli, R. D., Dole, P., Ellerbrock, T. V., Chiasson, M. A., & VanDevanter, N. (1996). Significance of mild cytologic atypia in women infected with human immunodeficiency virus. *Obstetrics and Gynecology, 87,* 515–519.

Wulff, E. A., & Simpson, D. M. (1999). HIV-associated peripheral nervous system complications. *NeuroAids,* 2(3). Retrieved January 31, 2003, from http://aidscience. org/neuroaids/zones/articles/1999/03/Complications/index.asp

Wulff, E. A., Wang, A. K., & Simpson, D. M. (2000). HIV-associated peripheral neuropathy: Epidemiology, pathophysiology and treatment. *Drugs, 59*(6), 1251–1260.

Zuckerman, J., & Zuckerman, A. (1999). Hepatitis viruses. In D. Armstrong & J. Cohen (Eds.), *Infectious diseases* (pp. 4.1–4.3). London: Mosby.

Zwerschke, W., & Jansen-Durr, P. (2000). Cell transformation by the E7 oncoprotein of human papillomavirus type 16: Interactions with nuclear and cytoplasmic target proteins. *Advances in Cancer Research, 78,* 1–29.

Zwolski, K. (2001). Viral infections. In C. Kirton, D. Talotta, & K. Zwolski (Eds.), *Handbook of HIV/AIDS nursing* (pp. 300–316). St. Louis, MO: Mosby.

Zwolski, K., & Talotta, D. (2001). Bacterial infections. In C. Kirton, D. Talotta, & K. Zwolski (Eds.), *Handbook of HIV/AIDS nursing* (pp. 229–253). St. Louis, MO: Mosby.

Section IV

Symptom Management of the HIV-Infected Adolescent and Adult

Symptom management for persons living with HIV/AIDS is recognized as an extremely important component of care management because all patients with HIV experience symptoms throughout the course of their disease. Many of these symptoms are caused by the disorders associated with HIV, whereas others are caused by HIV treatments. Symptoms may impact the health of individuals in many ways: they may affect the patient's ability to adhere to antiretroviral therapy and to seek medical or nursing care, or, most important, they may alter an individual's quality of life. Thus, the prompt recognition and treatment of symptoms cannot be overemphasized.

This section describes common clinical symptoms seen in HIV/AIDS. Nurses, given their history of diagnosing and treating human responses to illness, are well positioned to manage these common responses to HIV. This section is not meant to be an exhaustive list of symptoms but only serves as a guide to the HIV nurse or any nurse in practice to promptly recognize and manage the most common symptoms. The authors, a combination of researchers and clinicians, provide clear descriptions of the symptoms and the nursing assessment and use a nursing diagnosis as the framework for managing symptoms. The importance of pharmacological and nonpharmacological interventions for management of symptoms has been emphasized as well as the acknowledgment that holistic interventions may be an important part of the care plan.

4.1 Anorexia and Weight Loss

1. Etiology
   a. Definitions
      i. Anorexia: loss of appetite resulting in decreased food intake
      ii. Weight loss: involuntary loss of body weight accompanied by loss of body fat and cell mass
   b. Gastrointestinal disorders, medications, psychosocial factors, secondary infections, malabsorption, endocrine disorders, nutrient deficiencies, and proinflammatory cytokines (Keithley, Swanson, & Nerad, 2001; Kotler, 1998)
2. Nursing assessment
   a. Subjective data
      i. Medication review (including alternative therapies)
      ii. Current or previous secondary infections
      iii. Nutrition-related symptoms (e.g., nausea, vomiting, diarrhea, fever, difficulty swallowing, fatigue)
      iv. Dietary patterns (e.g., typical daily intake, food likes and dislikes, food intolerances, special diets, use of dietary/alternative supplements)
   b. Objective data
      i. Measurement of height, weight, body mass index, and fat and muscle mass (Swanson & Keithley, 1998)
      ii. Assessment of functional status, mood, and cognition (Williams, Waters, & Parker, 1999)
      iii. Comprehensive examination of oral cavity for abnormalities affecting nutritional intake
      iv. Assessment of skin, hair, eyes, nails, thyroid, and musculoskeletal system for clinical signs of vitamin and mineral deficiency; assessment for hepatomegaly, splenomegaly, and edema
      v. Laboratory studies: dependent on symptoms—stool cultures, blood cultures, serum testosterone, thyroid profile, serum proteins, and serum micronutrient levels

3. Nursing diagnosis
   a. Altered nutrition: less than body requirements related to inadequate dietary intake, increased energy and nutrient needs, impaired digestion/absorption of nutrients, cognitive changes, and drug interactions as evidenced by nutrition-related symptoms; loss of weight and muscle and fat mass; clinical signs of nutrient deficiency; impaired functional status; and abnormal laboratory studies
   b. Related nursing diagnoses: impaired physical mobility, diarrhea, fatigue, altered mucous membranes, self-feeding deficit, impaired swallowing, and knowledge deficit (Carpenito, 2002)
4. Goals
   a. To maximize nutrient intake
   b. To minimize nutrient losses
   c. To replenish body cell mass
   d. To maintain functional status and quality of life
5. Interventions and health teaching
   a. Nonpharmacological interventions
      i. Assess nutritional status at regular intervals with objective measures.
      ii. Conduct nutrition counseling, including nutritional implications of HIV/AIDS, principles of good nutrition, vitamin/mineral and oral supplements (available as nutrient-dense candy bars, soups, juices, coffees), and nutrition resources.
      iii. Explain food safety measures, including safe handling, storage, and preparation of food; careful cleaning of cooking utensils and cutting boards; avoiding raw or undercooked eggs, meats, or fish; drinking treated water and pasteurized milk.
      iv. Explain nutrition interventions for anorexia/weight loss, such as 1) eat small snacks or meals every 2 to 3 hours; 2) eat high-protein, high-calorie foods and snacks (e.g., peanut butter, cheese, ice cream, nuts); 3) drink high-calorie beverages (e.g., milk shakes, juices, liquid supplements); 4) drink a small glass of wine or

fruit juice before meals to improve appetite; 5) eat cold or lukewarm foods, which have a better flavor than do hot foods; 6) go for a walk or exercise lightly before meals to stimulate appetite; 7) reduce fatigue associated with cooking by using prepared foods, take-out, or home-delivered meals; and 8) eat favorite foods in pleasant, relaxed environment to improve appetite.

   v. Use enteral nutrition when oral intake is adequate accompanied by weight loss. Polymeric formulas (intact/complex nutrients) are used if digestive/absorptive function is normal; elemental formulas indicated if malabsorption is a problem. Enteral formulas fortified with immunostimulatory nutrients (i.e., arginine, omega-3 fatty acids, glutamine, antioxidants) have few or mixed beneficial effects (Keithley & Swanson, 2001).

   vi. Reserve parenteral nutrition for patients with severe gastrointestinal disease or dysfunction (e.g., pancreatitis, intractable vomiting, or diarrhea) because of the high risk for infection and gut atrophy.

   vii. Recommend resistance-type exercise as tolerated to increase lean body mass and improve functional status and energy levels.

   viii. Recommend frequent oral care (after meals and before bedtime) and regular preventive dental care (every 6 months).

   ix. Suggest daily records/checklists of appetite, weight, and symptoms (Holzemer, Hudson, Kirksey, Hamilton, & Bakken, 2001; Lennie, Neidig, Stein, & Smith, 2001)

b. Pharmacological interventions (Corcoran & Grinspoon, 1999; Fairfield et al., 2001)

   i. Appetite stimulants (e.g., megestrol acetate, dronabinol)

   ii. Anabolic agents (e.g., recombinant growth hormone, testosterone, nandrolone, oxandrolone, oxymetholone)

   iii. Other interventions, including thalidomide for aphthous ulcers and wasting syndrome (Wohl et al., 2002)

c. Alternative/complementary therapies used for antianorexia and antiweight loss properties include various dietary supplements (e.g., antioxidants, carotenoids, phytoestrogens, DHEA, flavonoids), herbal therapies, megavitamin/mineral therapy, and juice and enzyme therapy. Presently, little or no evidence exists to support the safety or efficacy of these products.

6. Evaluation

a. Daily caloric intake = 25–35 kcal/kg and daily protein intake = 1.0–1.5 g/kg

b. Weight, body mass index, and fat and muscle mass within 5% of standard

c. Adequate symptom management

d. Improved energy and sense of well-being

4.2 Cognitive Impairment

1. Etiology

a. Cognitive impairment may be secondary to several physical and psychological/emotional problems (Meehan & Brush, 2001; Ungvarski & Trzcianowska, 2000). Possible etiologies include the following:

   i. Systemic infections

     (1) Bacterial infections: bacterial meningitis, sepsis, neurosyphilis

     (2) Fungal infections: cryptococcosis, aspergillosis

     (3) Viral infections: cytomegalovirus, herpes zoster virus, herpes simplex virus, human papovavirus, JC virus

     (4) Mycoplasmic infection: tuberculosis, toxoplasmosis

   ii. Central nervous system cancers: advanced Kaposi's sarcoma, non-Hodgkin's lymphoma, and primary central nervous system lymphoma

   iii. Cerebrovascular disease and accident

iv. Metabolic imbalances: fluid and electrolyte imbalances, nutritional deficits, effects of sleep deprivation

v. Psychological and stress-related illnesses

vi. Medications: histamine blockers, sedatives, anxiolytics, narcotics, steroids, antivirals, anti-TB medications, antidepressants, alcohol, and other recreational drugs

vii. HIV dementia or AIDS dementia complex (ADC)

2. Nursing assessment
   a. Subjective data
      i. Early manifestations
         (1) Cognitive: forgetfulness and loss of concentration, slowed information processing, impaired attention, sequencing problems, and memory loss
         (2) Behavioral: withdrawal, irritability, apathy, and loss of interest in usual activities
         (3) Motor: Slowing, ataxia, tremor, incoordination, weakness, and handwriting change
         (4) Affective: symptoms suggestive of depression and hypomania
      ii. Late manifestations
         (1) Cognitive: severe memory loss, word-finding problems or speech arrest, dysarthria, severe attention and concentration problems, and poor judgment with lack of insight
         (2) Behavioral: increasing severity of behaviors in item (1) plus disinhibition and impetuous actions
         (3) Motor: incontinence, paraplegia, and marked slowing
         (4) Affective: severe depression, organic psychosis, and mania
   b. Objective data
      i. Neuroimaging
         (1) MRI/CT may be normal in the presence of symptoms or may show cortical (sulci may be widened) or ventricular atrophy or diffuse white matter changes or abnormalities.
         (2) Cranial computerized tomography is conducted to look for tumors, lesions, or atrophy.
      ii. Lab work (may be included in the etiologic investigation): CBC with differential, Chemistry panel, Serum B12, folate, albumin, Thyroid function studies, Serum toxoplasmosis IgG titer, Cryptococcal antigen, RPR/VDRL
      iii. Physical examination (especially of nervous system)
      iv. Lumbar puncture to examine the cerebral spinal fluid (CSF) for infectious diseases
      v. Pharmacological history to evaluate for medications that may cause confusion, disorientation, decreased concentration, or memory problems
      vi. Practitioner evaluation of cognition using the Mini-Mental Status Exam and HIV Dementia Scale
      vii. Psychological tests, such as the Beck Depression Scale, Holmes and Rahe Stress Scale, and State/Trait Anxiety Inventory or Depression Anxiety Stress Scale (DASS), to screen for anxiety, stress, and depression
      viii. Patient and family assessment of cognitive, behavioral, motor, and affective symptoms of ADC

3. Nursing diagnosis
   a. Neurocognitive impairment related to systemic and CNS infections, central nervous system cancers, psychological and stress-related illnesses, medications, and ADC

4. Goals
   a. Remove or treat the underlying cause of the cognitive impairment.
   b. Improved cognitive function
   c. Maintenance of self-care activities, including medication adherence
   d. Maintenance of social functioning

e. Maintenance of client safety
f. Prevent disease progression
5. Interventions and health teaching
   a. Nonpharmacological interventions
      i. Refer to psychoeducational groups (Nelson, 1997) that assist the patient in learning ways to overcome cognitive changes, including memory loss.
      ii. Provide memory aids, such as calendars, timers, pill boxes.
      iii. Conduct a safety assessment of home.
      iv. Provide instruction to family/ significant others in monitoring the client for safety issues and use of clear communication.
      v. Assist with advanced directives, wills, trusts, assisted-living referrals and other legal concerns before disease progresses.
      vi. Teach how to prevent HIV-related diseases that cause neurocognitive impairment, such as coccidioidomycosis, cryptococcosis, CMV, histoplamosis, mycobacterial disease, disseminated M. tuberculosis, and progressive multifocal leukoencephalopathy (Ungvarski & Trzcianowska, 2000).
   b. Pharmacological interventions
      i. Antiretrovirals are aimed at decreasing viral replication in the brain; zidovudine best penetrates into the CSF (Portegies & Rosenberg, 1998).
      ii. Psychotropic drugs are used for behavior management.
         (1) Agitation and anxiety: clonazepam, lorazepam, and buspirone; haloperidol, which should be used sparingly at low doses because of a reduction of tolerability to neuroleptics in HIV-positive clients (Mauri, Fabiano, Bravin, Ricci, & Invernizzi, 1997)
         (2) Mood swings and mania: valproic acid and lithium carbonate, which both require monitoring of blood levels

         (3) Depression: fluoxetine, pardetine, sertraline, amitriptyline, and norpranin
         (4) Psychoses: haloperidol, chlorpromazine, molindone (depending on severity of symptoms), and perphenazine
         (5) Psychomotor slowing: methylphenidate and dextroamphetamine (watch for irritability, which can be profound)
   c. Alternative/complementary therapies
      i. Vitamin therapy: Vitamins E, B_6, and B_{12} can be used (Flaskerud & Miller, 1999).
      ii. Chinese herbs: Efficacy and safety of Chinese herbs have not been established, but the herbs are widely used. Clients should consult with a Chinese herbalist because there are no herbs or herbal formulas specific to treating HIV or cognitive impairment. Herbal formulas are individualized to clients' specific symptoms, as diagnosed in traditional Chinese medicine (TCM). Examples include liver Qi stagnation, heart and spleen deficiency, or heat toxins (Ryan & Shattuck, 1994).
      iii. Western herbs: Efficacy and safety of Western herbs also have not been established, but they are still widely used. Gingko biloba is commonly used for memory problems and has little interaction with antiretrovirals but can increase bleeding. Anyone considering using herbs should consult with a licensed herbalist as well as a pharmacist who is knowledgeable about drug–herb interactions.
      iv. Energy work/healing—Anecdotal reports suggest that Reiki, therapeutic touch, and Shen are useful in calming the mind in persons with cognitive impairment. There is no scientific evidence to support this or improvement of cognitive function.

6. Evaluation
   a. Patient will show improved cognitive function.
   b. Patient will be able to perform activities of daily living.
   c. Patient will be able to engage in social interaction, work, and school activities.

4.3 Cough

1. Etiology
   a. Associated with pulmonary conditions, sinusitis, aspiration, esophageal reflux, auditory canal irritation, noxious substances, exercise/activity, and cold air; can occur postbronchoscopy
2. Nursing assessment
   a. Subjective data
      i. When did the cough begin?
      ii. Is the cough productive?
      iii. What is the character of the cough?
      iv. Is there a time of day when the cough is more bothersome?
      v. Is there a relationship to position or posture?
      vi. What makes the cough better? What makes it worse?
      vii. Are there any accompanying signs or symptoms such as, hemoptysis, shortness of breath, wheezing, chest tightness, heartburn, edema or orthopnea, sinus pain, headache, or postnasal drip?
      viii. What are the patient's medical, surgical, and medication histories, including oxygen use and intubation?
   b. Objective data
      i. Pulmonary exam, including rate, amplitude of respiration, rhythm, symmetry of breathing, use of accessory muscles, and breath sounds
3. Nursing diagnosis
   a. Ineffective airway clearance related to smoking or secondhand smoke, airway spasm, mucus/secretions, infection, or allergic airways
   b. Risk for impaired gas exchange
   c. Risk for impaired comfort
4. Goals
   a. Promote optimal respiratory function.
   b. Promote effective cough effort.

c. Eliminate or treat the underlying cause of a chronic cough.
   d. Minimize the discomfort associated with chronic cough.
5. Interventions and health teaching
   a. Nonpharmacological interventions
      i. Prevent stasis of secretions by encouraging deep breathing/incentive spirometry; ambulation/frequent position changes, if on bed rest; and postural drainage/percussion, if necessary.
      ii. Encourage fluid intake of 2.5 to 3L/day to maintain hydration and thin secretions; decrease or eliminate dairy products.
      iii. Use suction to remove secretions if cough is ineffective.
      iv. Promote oral hygiene if cough is productive; instruct on proper disposal of tissues and hand washing.
      v. Position to prevent aspiration and reflux (i.e., elevate head of bed or use wedge-shaped pillow for sleep).
      vi. Teach splinting techniques to minimize pain associated with coughing.
      vii. Offer throat-soothing remedies, such as tea with honey and lemon, cough drops, warm saline gargle, warm mist humidifiers if immunocompetent (follow manufacturer's guidelines for daily cleaning; Althoff, Williams, Molvig, & Schuster, 1997).
      viii. Avoid activities or noxious substances that precipitate cough (e.g., cigarette smoke; Kozier, Erb, Berman, & Burke, 2000).
      ix. Encourage rest periods and energy conservation; plan daily activities with rest periods included.
      x. Evaluate patient's ability to identify effective cough remedies, report changes in frequency and severity of cough, and demonstrate effective cough technique (Kozier et al., 2000).
   b. Pharmacological interventions
      i. Administer cough medications (antitussives, expectorants) on a

scheduled basis rather than prn; schedule expectorants.

c. Alternative/Complementary interventions

    i. Eucalyptus aromatherapy may be useful (Althoff et al., 1997).

6. Evaluation

a. The patient will demonstrate effective coughing and increased air exchange

b. The person will demonstrate an effective respiratory rate and relief of symptoms

c. The individual will describe measures to improve comfort

4.4 Dyspnea

1. Etiology

a. Pulmonary infections include pneumocystis carinii pneumonia (PCP), bacterial pneumonias, mycobacterium avium complex (MAC), *M. tuberculosis,* cytomegalovirus (CMV), *C. albicans,* and *Cryptosporidium.*

b. Pulmonary malignancies include Kaposi's sarcoma (KS) and lymphomas.

c. Autoimmune diseases include lymphocytic interstitial pneumonitis and diffuse infiltrative lymphocytosis syndrome.

d. Anemia

e. Pneumothorax and pleural effusion

f. Exercise intolerance

g. Normal aging process and dying process

2. Nursing assessment

a. Subjective data

    i. Obtain patient's report of breathing difficulty (e.g., presence of orthopnea).

    ii. Ascertain relevant history of the symptoms: onset, duration, frequency of episodes, aggravating or relieving factors, and associated symptoms.

    iii. Two types of patient-rating tools are available.

        (1) Graphic rating scale: Ask patient to quantify the magnitude of dyspnea experienced on a scale of 1 to 5 (1 = *no difficulty breathing,* 5 = *severe difficulty breathing*).

        (2) Visual analog scale is a horizontal or vertical line with

word descriptors or anchors at either end. The patient places a mark on the line indicating the degree of dyspnea experienced.

    iv. Ascertain medical and surgical history, including oxygen use and history of intubation.

    v. Elicit medication, herbal, and nutritional supplement usage.

    vi. Conduct a thorough social assessment: living conditions, support systems, and presence of significant others and pets.

    vii. Obtain patient's report of activities of daily living abilities.

b. Objective data

    i. General appearance and color

    ii. Pulmonary exam: rate, amplitude of respiration, rhythm, symmetry of breathing, use of accessory muscles, nasal flaring, breath sounds, and clubbing

    iii. Cardiovascular exam: blood pressure and pulse

    iv. Lab and diagnostic data: pulse oximetry, chest X-ray, arterial blood gases (ABGs), and sputum studies, if appropriate

3. Nursing diagnosis

a. Activity intolerance related to imbalance between oxygen supply and demand

b. Anxiety related to ineffective breathing pattern

c. Disturbed sleep pattern related to difficulty breathing and positioning required for effective breathing

d. Fear related to threat to state of well-being and potential death

e. Ineffective breathing pattern related to hyperventilation, hypoventilation, pain, anxiety, fatigue, perceptual or cognitive impairment, obesity, body position, and respiratory muscle fatigue

f. Risk for impaired gas exchange

g. Risk for sleep deprivation

h. Risk for impaired comfort

4. Goals

a. Identify and eliminate, or at least control, the causative factors.

b. Promote optimal respiratory functioning.

c. Manage stress and anxiety.

d. Develop strategies to manage dyspnea to provide maximum independence.

5. Interventions and health teaching
   a. Nonpharmacological interventions
      i. Reassess respiratory status at appropriate frequency, including before and after respiratory treatments.
      ii. Eliminate or modify underlying causes of dyspnea.
      iii. Administer oxygen therapy, if indicated; teach patient safety issues, such as flammable hazards.
      iv. Assess need for bronchial hygiene (e.g., aerosol treatments, postural drainage, percussion, suctioning).
      v. Encourage adequate fluid intake to maintain hydration and help thin secretions, unless contraindicated.
      vi. Promote optimal nutrition.
      vii. Position patient to maximize both comfort and ventilation (e.g., sitting upright with pillows under elbows, leaning on overbed table); encourage frequent position changes and ambulation.
      viii. Pace activities and treatments to level of tolerance; encourage energy conservation.
      ix. Assist with activities of daily living, especially those that require use of the upper extremities (e.g., feeding, shaving); keep frequently used items within reach.
      x. Instruct to prolong exhalation phase of breathing using pursed-lip and diaphragmatic breathing techniques and incentive spirometry.
      xi. Counsel to avoid exposure to irritants, such as cigarette smoke, flowers, and perfume.
      xii. Counsel regarding smoking cessation or timing of smoking to occur between activities of daily living and meals to pace with rest periods.
      xiii. Evaluate patient's ability to do the following:

         • Participate in self-care activities, such as energy conservation and pacing activities.

         • Correctly use metered dose inhalers or other medications.
         • Report changes in frequency or severity of dyspnea.
         • Identify contributing factors related to dyspnea.

   b. Pharmacological interventions
      i. Antibiotics, corticosteroids, and bronchodilators, as indicated
      ii. Opioids for palliation
   c. Alternative/complementary therapies: Demonstrate relaxation and panic-control strategies and stress management (e.g., creative visualization, guided imagery, meditation, biofeedback, yoga; Ferrell & Coyle, 2001).

6. Evaluation
   a. The person will identify factors that aggravate activity
   b. The person will identify methods to reduce activity intolerance
   c. The person will progress activity to tolerable level
   d. The person will describe his own anxiety and coping patterns
   e. The person will report an optimal balance of rest and sleep

4.5 Dysphagia and Odynophagia

1. Etiology
   a. Definitions
      i. Dysphagia defined as difficulty swallowing; often described as sensation of food sticking in mouth, pharynx, or esophagus.
      ii. Odynophagia refers to painful swallowing, usually characterized as burning or constricting esophagus.
   b. Dysphagia may be caused by candidiasis; oral, pharyngeal, or esophageal neuromuscular dysfunction; malignancies; decreased saliva production; fatigue
   c. Odynophagia may be caused by opportunisitic infections (candidiasis, HSV, CMV), tumors, and medications (ddC, AZT) associated with mucosal ulceration, inflammation, obstruction, gastroesophageal reflux disease, or all four conditions

2. Nursing assessment
   a. Subjective data
      i. Review of medications (including ASA, NSAIDs, anticholinergics, calcium channel blockers); problematic foods (e.g., peanut butter, spicy foods, citrus, liquids); current and previous opportunistic infections; presence and characteristics of coughing, choking, regurgitation, aspiration, and epigastric pain
   b. Objective data
      i. Inspection of oropharyngeal cavity for infections, lesions, malignancies, saliva production, parotid/ sublingual/submandibular gland enlargement, and adequacy of oral hygiene
      ii. Observation of swallowing of foods and liquids of varying textures and consistencies (Terrado, Russell, & Bowman, 2001)
      iii. Assessment of mental and cognitive status
      iv. Assessment of nutritional status parameters: weight, body mass index, and fat and muscle mass
      v. Laboratory studies: cultures/ biopsies to identify pathogens
3. Nursing diagnosis
   a. Impaired swallowing related to infections, tumors, medications, foods, gastroesophageal reflux disease, fatigue, and dental problems as evidenced by difficult or painful swallowing of food and fluids; coughing, choking, or aspirating when swallowing; and loss of weight and fat and muscle mass.
   b. Related nursing diagnoses include altered mucous membranes, altered nutrition (less than body requirements), risk for aspiration, fatigue, and knowledge deficit (Carpenito, 2002).
4. Goals
   a. Increase knowledge of easy-to-swallow foods and fluids
   b. Improve protein and calorie intake
   c. Reduce swallowing pain and discomfort
   d. Maintain ability to take oral medications
   e. Prevent aspiration
5. Interventions and health teaching
   a. Nonpharmacological interventions

   i. Provide nutrition counseling: 1) eat blenderized or soft foods (e.g., pudding, soups, canned fruits, scrambled eggs); 2) add sauces or gravies to meats and vegetables; 3) dip foods (bagels, cookies) in liquids (tea, coffee); 4) make liquids thicker by adding gravy, mashed potatoes, oatmeal, or Thickit; 5) eat cold or lukewarm foods; 6) avoid sticky foods (e.g., peanut butter, caramels, gummy bears) and milk if problematic; 7) use a straw, tilt head back, or sit upright to facilitate swallowing (Keithley, Swanson, & Nerad, 2001)
   ii. Give oral care counseling: 1) frequent oral care (before and after meals and before bedtime with soft toothbrush and nonirritating, saline or soda-based mouthwash); 2) daily assessment of tongue, pharynx, palate, gingiva, and buccal mucosa for lesions; 3) regular dental checkups and cleanings (every 6 months)
   iii. Refer to swallowing specialist for evaluation and swallowing retraining if indicated
   b. Pharmacological interventions
      i. Topical or systemic pain medications (topical analgesics, oral or subcutaneous morphine)
      ii. Antifungal/antiviral medications based on causative agents
   c. Alternative/complementary therapies
      i. Chamomile, which has antiinflammatory and antispasmodic properties, has been used to treat dysphagia, but its effectiveness is equivocal (Rotblatt & Ziment, 2002).
      ii. Capsaicin is sometimes used to reduce mouth and throat pain, but topical use may increase throat pain and be of limited value (Rotblatt & Ziment, 2002).
6. Evaluation
   a. Daily food/fluid intake meets targeted calorie and protein goals.
   b. Adequate pain relief and comfort occurs when swallowing.

c. Choking, coughing, regurgitation, and aspiration are absent during swallowing.

d. Oral medications are taken without difficulty.

4.6 Oral Lesions

1. Etiology
   a. Infectious causes include Epstein-Barr virus (oral hairy leukoplakia), *Candida albicans* (thrush), bacterial infections (periodontal disease and gingivitis), herpes simplex virus, varicella zoster virus, cytomegalovirus, and human papillomavirus.
   b. Neoplasms include Kaposi's sarcoma and non-Hodgkin's lymphoma.
   c. Possibly autoimmune manifestations include aphthous ulcers.
   d. Treatment-related causes include chemotherapy and radiation-induced stomatitis.
   e. Behavioral factors include smoking and ethanol-induced stomatitis.
   f. Genetic factors include HIV-associated salivary gland disease; may be genetic and has shown associated with HLS-DR5 and HLA-B35 variants (Itescu et al., 1992).
   g. Prevalence of oral lesions has declined since the introduction of protease inhibitors (Patton, McKaig, Strauss, Rogers, & Eron, 2000).

2. Nursing assessment
   a. Subjective data
      i. Current medications (Ketoconazole and zidovudine can induce brown pigmentation of oral mucosa; Greenspan & Greenspan, 1999.)
      ii. Past opportunistic infections and neoplasms
      iii. Unusual oral hygiene practices
      iv. Tobacco, alcohol, and illicit drug use
   b. Objective data
      i. Inspect oropharyngeal cavity for evidence of infection, lesions, or malignancies; note foul breath.
      ii. Inspect teeth and gums for tooth mobility; receding gums with exposure of tooth roots; gingival erythema, which suggests linear gingival erythema, a type of gingivitis (Greenspan, 1998); and necrosis of soft tissue.
      iii. Palpate for parotid/sublingual/submandibular salivary gland enlargement.
      iv. Assess gastrointestinal (GI) system because oral lesions may indicate pathology in other regions of the GI tract (i.e., aphthous ulcers in mouth may be associated with similar lesions in the GI tract; esophageal candidiasis may occur concomitantly with thrush; Greenspan & Greenspan, 1999).
      v. Assess nutritional status: weight, body mass index, muscle mass, and serum albumin.

3. Nursing diagnosis
   a. Impaired oral mucous membrane
   b. Altered nutrition: less than body requirements
   c. Impaired comfort
   d. Impaired swallowing

4. Goals
   a. Maintain adequate protein and calorie intake for metabolic needs.
   b. Reduce pain.
   c. Maintain ability to take oral medications.
   d. Promote knowledge of strategies to manage pain and ensure adequate nutrition.

5. Interventions and health teaching
   a. Nonpharmacologic interventions
      i. See Section 4.5, Dysphagia and Odonophagia
      ii. Provide resources for nonverbal communication if speaking is too painful (e.g., paper and pencil, erasable board and marker).
      iii. Encourage patient to limit or eliminate tobacco and alcohol use.
   b. Pharmacologic interventions
      i. Pharmacological management depends on the etiology (i.e., antibiotic, antiviral, or antifungal medications; thalidomide or steroids for aphthous ulcers).
      ii. Topical or systemic pain medications can be used.
   c. Alternative/complementary therapies

i. Ethanol propolis extract has been shown to have antifungal properties equivalent to nystatin when added to cultured *C. albicans* strains collected from HIV-infected persons (Martins et al., 2002).

ii. Azole-resistant oral candidal lesions in HIV-infected persons have responded to treatments with an oral rinse derived from tea tree oil (Jandourek, Vaishampayan, & Vazquez, 1998) and a commercially available cinnamon preparation (Quale, Landman, Zaman, Burney, & Sathe, 1996).

iii. An oral rinse derived from deglycyrrhizinated licorice has been associated with healing of aphthous ulcers (Das, Das, Gulati, & Singh, 1989).

6. Evaluation
   a. Food and fluid intake adequate for metabolic needs.
   b. Patient describes pain management as satisfactory.
   c. Oral medications are taken without difficulty.

4.7 Fatigue

1. Etiology
   a. Etiology is unknown, but it is likely multifactorial, involving both physiologic and psychological causes.
      i. Physiological causes
         (1) Factors that have been shown to be related to fatigue include nutritional deficiencies, particularly magnesium deficiency (Skurnick et al., 1996); zidovudine-induced myopathy (Cupler et al., 1995; Sinnwell et al., 1995); and low testosterone (Groopman, 1998).
         (2) Fatigue may result from endocrinological dysregulation, including abnormalities in hypothalamic-pituitary-adrenal axis functioning (Clerici et al., 1997; Stolarczyk, Rubio, Smolyar, Young, & Poretsky, 1998) and disruption of circadian variability of thyroid-stimulating hormone (Rondanelli et al., 1997), and liver disease (Bartlett, 1996).
         (3) Fatigue has been associated with the number of current AIDS-related physical symptoms, current treatment for HIV-related medical disorders, antiretroviral medications, and pain (Breitbart, McDonald, Rosenfeld, Monkman, & Passik, 1998).
      ii. Psychological causes
         (1) Depression has been associated with HIV-related fatigue (Barroso, 1999, 2001; Breitbart et al., 1998; Rabkin, Wagner, & Rabkin, 1999); however, explicating the relationship between the two is difficult because fatigue can cause depression, and depression can cause fatigue.
         (2) Anxiety may be related to fatigue as well (Barroso, 2001; Wessely, Hotopf, & Sharpe, 1998).

2. Nursing assessment
   a. Subjective data
      i. The nurse must rely on subjective data because there are no objective clinical indicators.
      ii. There are many fatigue tools available; however, most of them are not appropriate for measuring fatigue in HIV-positive individuals because they simply measure the presence/absence of fatigue or only intensity of fatigue, or they were developed and tested on non-HIV-positive samples (Barroso & Lynn, 2002). The HIV-Related Fatigue Scale was developed specifically for patients with HIV; it contains 56 items, which measure the following:

   - Intensity of fatigue, during that day and over the past week
   - Circumstances surrounding fatigue: factors that make it

better or worse and the individual's patterns of fatigue
- Consequences of the fatigue: how it affects the person with regard to activities of daily living (ADLs) and the ability to think clearly, work, and socialize (Barroso & Lynn, 2002)

   iii. Evaluate the adequacy of the person's sleep pattern

   iv. Inquire about the person's use or abuse of recreational drugs

   v. Conduct an assessment of the person's nutritional intake

b. Objective data

   i. Objective data are of limited usefulness in diagnosing fatigue.

   ii. Laboratory assessment may include hemoglobin, hematocrit, liver function tests, and thyroid function tests. Most studies show no relationship between either CD_4 count or viral load and fatigue (Barroso, 2001; Breitbart et al., 1998; Ferrando et al., 1998, Justice, Rabeneck, Hays, Wu, & Bozzette, 1999).

3. Nursing diagnosis
   a. Impaired physical mobility
   b. Bathing/hygiene self-care deficit
   c. Dressing/grooming self-care deficit
   d. Toileting self-care deficit
   e. Impaired social interaction

4. Goals
   a. Determine the cause of fatigue.
   b. Characterize fatigue: the intensity, the circumstances surrounding the fatigue experience, and the consequences.
   c. Maintain or regain optimal functioning ability.
   d. Assist the patient in locating resources to help him or her cope with fatigue.

5. Interventions and health teaching
   a. Nonpharmacological interventions

   i. Assess for undiagnosed opportunistic infections.

   ii. Assess for and treat underlying depression.

   iii. Control other symptoms that could be causing the fatigue (e.g., diarrhea).

   iv. If fatigue is medication-related, weigh the benefits of the medication against its side effects.

   v. Encourage patients to track their individual patterns of fatigue, keeping a fatigue diary if necessary, so they can best plan their activities each day (e.g., perform most strenuous activities during the times of peak energy, stagger activities to avoid excessive fatigue).

   vi. Napping and reducing strenuous activities have been reported to be helpful (van Servellen, Sarna, & Jablonski, 1998).

   vii. Refer the patient to community-based agencies for assistance with housekeeping and chore support. Evaluate the need for occupational therapy (energy conservation techniques) or physical therapy (reconditioning and strengthening exercises).

b. Pharmacological interventions

   i. One study found that thyroid hormone replacement improved HIV-related fatigue, although participants showed no evidence of thyroid abnormality (Derry, 1996).

   ii. Other successful interventions include dextroamphetamine (Wagner & Rabkin, 2000; Wagner, Rabkin, & Rabkin, 1997), DHEA (Rabkin, Ferrando, Wagner, & Rabkin, 2000), and hyperbaric oxygen (Jordan, 1998; Reillo, 1993).

c. Alternative/complementary therapies

   i. Limited data support the usefulness of hyperbaric oxygen and relaxation training (Fukunishi et al., 1997; Jordan, 1998; Reillo, 1993).

6. Evaluation
   a. The patient will report being able to complete the most pressing tasks through careful planning.
   b. The patient will maintain independence in ADLs.
   c. The patient will access community-based resources, as needed.
   d. The patient will maintain an overall optimal level of functioning.

4.8 Fever

1. Etiology
   a. An abnormally high body temperature. It refers to the entire complex of host defense responses brought about by infectious or noninfectious molecular mediators called pyrogens.
   b. Fever heralds many HIV-related OIs (respiratory and urinary tract, central nervous system, abscesses, gingivitis, gastroenteritis, drug reactions, lymphoma), and noninfectious processes.
   c. Cytokines are believed to be responsible for mediating febrile temperature elevations by increasing synthesis of hypothalamic prostaglandins of the E group (PGE) that readjust the hypothalamic thermostat to a higher set point range (Boulant, 2000; Cooper, 1995).
   d. Several drugs used in treatment of HIV disease are known to induce fever (Lee, 1995): TMP-SMX, atovaquone, amphotericin B (chills or rigors are secondary to fever), ddI, amoxicillin-clavulanic acid, dapsone, ceftazidine, and ganciclovir.

2. Nursing assessment
   a. Subjective data
      i. Review body systems—vomiting, diarrhea, lethargy, rash, cough, congestion, increased irritability, temperature duration
      ii. Review exposure to any animals (cats, dogs, reptiles, farm animals, birds), infectious diseases, or molds. Inquire about whether the patient drinks well or city water at home and whether they live in an older or a newer home. Ask if they have eaten recently at any restaurants, have been exposed to any person from a foreign country, have been incarcerated, or live in a halfway house.
      iii. Inquire about travel history, including any recent travel outside of the state (ascertain which states) or outside of the country.
      iv. Ask about recent immunizations and medications.
      v. Assess all of the above frequently.
   b. Objective data
      i. Select a monitoring schedule consistent with the patient's clinical condition. Routine methods and twice-daily intervals between temperature measurements may not be adequate for detecting febrile episodes in hospitalized patients with evidence of infection, tissue injury, or inflammation (Taliaferro, 1996).
      ii. Increase the frequency of measurements when patients are receiving potentially pyrogenic agents, such as blood or antigenic drugs. Body temperature should be monitored at least every 4 hours.
      iii. Assess whether fever threatens safety. Temperatures approaching 40.5° C impose risk of irreversible central nervous system damage.
      iv. Monitor febrile shivering. During fever, less heat loss is required to elicit shivering and vasoconstriction, making the patient vulnerable to chilling. Low levels of shivering may not be visible but are sufficient to contribute to heat generation and oxygen consumption.
      v. Monitor hydration. Significant amounts of body water are lost by compensatory cooling mechanisms of sweating and hyperventilation during fever.
      vi. Monitor pharmacologic fever therapies. Note responses, side effects, and achievement of therapeutic goals. Body temperature elevations often mark progress when drugs are aimed at controlling underlying infection or pathology.
      vii. Evaluate thermal comfort. Replace clothing with dry, warm clothing after sweating to avoid chilling.

3. Nursing diagnosis
   a. Risk for altered body temperature is related to febrile responses to altered thermoregulatory set point (NANDA, 1996).

b. Altered thermoregulatory set point (an alternative diagnosis) is more precise and calls for attention to the underlying dynamics.

c. Risk for fatigue is related to circulating cytokines and exertion from shivering.

d. Risk for fluid volume deficit is due to fever-related compensatory sweating and insensible loss from respiration.

e. Risk for shivering, hypothermia, and temperature drift occurs during aggressive cooling (Holtzclaw, 1998).

4. Goals

  a. To monitor the patient's response to the febrile symptoms and their treatment

  b. To promote comfort and adequate hydration

  c. To prevent febrile shivering or aggressive chilling

5. Interventions and health teaching

  a. Nonpharmacological interventions

    i. Tepid sponge baths, cooling fans or blankets, ice packs, or alcohol baths are contraindicated because they promote shivering, energy expenditure, and patient discomfort; they may actually raise body temperature.

    ii. Prevent chills and shivering of febrile response at onset of temperature rise by insulating extremities with protective wraps, socks, and absorbent blankets. As chilling subsides, remove heavy covering cautiously to avoid drafts.

    iii. When fever breaks and sweating occurs, remove wet clothing under bed covers to avoid drafts and chilling.

    iv. Avoid giving cold liquids to a febrile patient because rapid ingestion can abruptly cool the body core at a time when the elevated set point is highly sensitive to cooling. The patient can slowly lick or suck frozen juice or flavored Popsicles, which allows gradual ingestion and helps avoid chilling.

  b. Pharmacological interventions

    i. Antipyretic therapy should not be instituted routinely for every febrile episode but should be based on therapeutic goals, relative risk of temperature elevation, and discomfort of fever-related symptoms.

    ii. NSAIDs (e.g., aspirin, acetaminophen, indomethacin) are effective in diminishing fever, but they have significant side effects and may suppress signs of ongoing infection (Styrt & Sugarman, 1990).

    iii. Where not contraindicated, antipyretics can be administered regularly around the clock rather than p.r.n. to people with chronic or frequent fevers to improve patient comfort.

  c. Alternative/complementary therapies

    i. Herbal extracts have long been used to treat fever, but they may interact with prescribed medications.

    ii. White willow bark (*Salix alba*) is similar in origin and action to aspirin.

    iii. Kava kava (*Piper methysticum*) and valerian (*Valeriana officinalis*) can manage fever-induced psychological distress, but they have significant drug interactions.

    iv. Cooling baths or rotary fans to cool the body temperatures can initiate shivering and warming responses that defeat the purpose of cooling.

    v. Warm baths, with temperatures 1 to 2 degrees lower than the body temperature will often sedate the febrile patient and prevent shivering without increasing core temperatures.

6. Evaluation

  a. Evaluate patient's response to the febrile symptoms and their treatment. Surveillance should include threat of neural damage from fever.

  b. During fever, temperature should remain below 40° C.

  c. Evaluate thermal comfort.

  d. Evaluate hydration status.

4.9 Sleep Disturbances

1. Etiology
   a. Sleep disorders contribute to decreased quality of life (Phillips & Skelton, 2001) and can arise from the following:

   - HIV-related symptoms, such as fever, fatigue, and night sweats
   - Side effects from medications, such as efavirenz (Sustiva), which can cause insomnia (Schutz & Wendrow, 2002), and mood-altering drugs
   - Mental health issues, such as depression and anxiety
   - HIV infection of the brain and nervous system
   - Opportunistic infections and neoplasms
   - Social and environmental factors, such as unstable housing, hospitalizations, and limited finances (Nokes, Chidekel, & Kendrew, 1999)

   b. Sleep disorders include the following:

   - Insomnia: poor-quality, insufficient, or nonrestorative sleep
   - Restless legs syndrome: described as a creepy, crawly, unpleasant, burning or itching sensation, usually between the knees and ankles, that sometimes makes it impossible to sit still or lie down for any length of time; can be mistaken for peripheral neuropathy (Rothenberg, 1997)
   - Hypersomnia: sleep-disordered breathing, periodic limb movement disorder, and narcolepsy
   - Parasomnia: a group of sleep disorders, such as nocturnal seizures, REM behavior disorder, and sleepwalking

2. Nursing assessment
   a. Subjective data
      i. Sleep problems may be unreported unless the provider screens for them. Screening questions include the following (based on the responses, a more thorough sleep assessment may be in order; Merritt, 2000):

      - "Does it take you more than 30 minutes to fall asleep?"
      - "When you wake up during the night, do you have trouble going back to sleep?"
      - "Even when you sleep all night, do you feel tired in the morning?"

      ii. With the client's permission, speaking with the bed partner can yield valuable information about the client's sleep pattern.
      iii. Sleep problems are usually aggravated during withdrawal from mood-altering drugs, such as heroin, cocaine, and alcohol. These underlying withdrawal issues should be addressed before arriving at a diagnosis of chronic sleep disturbance.

   b. Objective data
      i. Daily sleep diaries can be used to record naps, sleep latency (i.e., minutes required to fall asleep after going to bed; Allen, 1997), number and duration of awakenings, total sleep, quality of sleep, feelings on awakening, and whether or not the night was typical.
      ii. Self-report instruments, such as the Pittsburgh Sleep Quality Index (Buysse, Reynolds, Monk, Berman, & Kupfer, 1989) are available but may be difficult to administer and score in a clinical setting.
      iii. Actigraphy devices may be used to measure movement over a period of 3 to 5 consecutive days. If there is clear evidence of pathology, a comprehensive assessment in a sleep laboratory using polysomnography is warranted.

3. Nursing diagnosis
   a. Sleep pattern disturbance that may be related to multiple etiologies (Lo & Kim, 1986)

4. Goals
   a. Identify etiology of sleep pattern disturbance
   b. Increase quality and duration of sleep

5. Interventions and health teaching
   a. Nonpharmacological interventions
      i. A number of sleep hygiene strategies have been

identified, including the following:

- Eliminate the bedroom clock.
- Exercise in the late afternoon or early evening for at least 20 minutes, 3–6 hours before bedtime.
- Avoid caffeine, alcohol, nicotine, and other mind-altering drugs. Caffeine reduction has been effective in improving sleep quality in an HIV-infected sample (Dreher, 2000).
- Eat a light snack before going to bed.
- Establish a regular waking time (i.e., get up at the same time, 7 days a week; go to sleep at the same time each night).
- Limit naps to 30 to 50 minutes (Floyd, 1999) and only nap if it does not interfere with nighttime sleep.
- Create enjoyable presleep rituals.
- Schedule thinking time in the early evening.
- Make a list of problems before going to bed (for bedtime worriers).
- Take a hot bath 2 to 4 hours before bedtime.
- If unable to fall asleep within 15 minutes, go to another room and read until drowsy.
- Reserve bed for sleep and sex.
- Create an environment conducive to sleep—clean and dry linens, dark and quiet room, comfortable bed and room temperature (Nokes, Chidekel, & Kendrew, 1999).
- If sleep hygiene strategies are not effective, referral to sleep specialists may be considered.

b. Pharmacological interventions
  i. Benzodiazepines
    (1) The most commonly prescribed hypnotics across all age groups
    (2) Drugs of choice for the treatment of chronic insomnia because of their favorable side-effect profile, wide therapeutic index, and safety in overdose (Buysse & Reynolds, 2000)
    (3) Are metabolized in the liver, which may result in drug–drug interactions
    (4) Contraindicated in patients with a history of abuse of alcohol or other sedatives
    (5) Can be associated with three different types of discontinuance syndromes: a) rebound—an increase in the original symptom beyond the baseline level; b) withdrawal—the appearance of new symptoms, not originally present, upon discontinuance of the drug; and c) recurrence—return of insomnia symptoms when the medication is discontinued
  ii. Antidepressants, which have a wide range of activities on central neurotransmission, are an alternative to benzodiazepines (Buysse & Reynolds, 2000).
  iii. Antihistamines are frequently used as sedatives.
  iv. Many persons with HIV/AIDS have liver disorders that can complicate the biotransformation of hypnotics. Therefore, nonpharmacological interventions should be fully explored before drugs are administered.
c. Alternative/complementary therapies
  i. Melatonin, a pineal gland hormone, has gained widespread use as a sleep-promoting substance.
  ii. Relaxation training such as progressive relaxation or yoga can be helpful.
  iii. Biofeedback, especially EMG (electromyography) feedback, might be beneficial.
  iv. Sleep restriction, which aims to consolidate sleep through the restriction of the amount of time spent in bed (Bootzin & Rider, 1997), can help increase sleep quality.

v. Acupuncture has been shown to be effective in managing insomnia in HIV-infected persons (Phillips & Skelton, 2001).

vi. Noise management using white noises, such as ocean sounds or sounds of a waterfall delivered by sound conditioners (Floyd, 1999), might be helpful.

6. Evaluation

a. Match sleep hygiene strategies to the unique needs of individual clients. To determine which strategies are effective, introduce no more than two different strategies at any one time. Different strategies should be used for at least 1 week before assessing their effectiveness, unless they are exacerbating the problem.

b. Daytime sleepiness can easily be measured by the Epworth Sleepiness Scale (Johns, 1992), which asks clients to rate their chance of falling asleep in eight situations commonly encountered in daily life, such as sleepiness while driving a car.

4.10 Mobility Impairment

1. Etiology

a. Limitation of movement (Carpenito, 2000); inability to move one or more body parts or inability to move freely within one's environment (Bergquist & Neuberger, 2002)

b. May be caused by primary and secondary etiologies and is frequently multifactorial (Holohan-Bell & Brummel-Smith, 1999)

i. Neurological involvement that causes motor impairment or pain (McGuire & So, 1999; Price, 1999)

ii. Metabolic complications that may result in weakness and altered action potential of muscles

iii. Musculoskeletal injury precipitating mild to severe pain (McGuire & So, 1999)

iv. Opportunistic infections and neoplasms

v. AIDS dementia complex (ADC)

vi. Polyneuropathies (primary due to HIV infection; secondary from pharmacologic agents)

vii. Psychological/psychospiritual complications (i.e., depression, bereavement, fear)

2. Nursing assessment

a. Subjective data

i. Impact on quality of life and relationships

ii. Ability to perform activities of daily living (ADL)

iii. Onset, severity, and character of associated signs and symptoms

(1) Weakness (unilateral vs. bilateral; upper vs. lower extremities)

(2) Decreased endurance, increased fatigue

iv. Other associated neurological symptoms (e.g., incontinence, urinary retention, sensory changes)

v. New or different pattern of constitutional signs and symptoms reported by patient (e.g., fever, weight loss)

vi. Recent changes in medication regimen

vii. Nutritional intake

b. Objective data

i. Musculoskeletal assessment: Conduct gait assessment; evaluate upper and lower body for muscle mass, strength, and equality; assess joint and muscle pain.

ii. Neurological assessment: Assess presence of pain or headache, dizziness, tremors, consciousness, and orientation; evaluate sensory testing of upper and lower extremities along with bilateral comparisons.

iii. Environmental assessment (home, institutional, social): Use Home Assessment Profile (Chandler, Duncan, Weiner, & Studenski, 2001; see Engberg & McDowell, 1999, for additional home safety screening information; see Stone & Wyman, 1999, for environmental hazards in institutional setting); Tinetti's Performance Oriented Mobility Test; Karnofsky Performance Status Index; and Katz Index of Activities of Daily Living, Instrumental Activities of

Daily Living (see Sehy & Williams, 1999, for social and functional assessment measures).

iv. Mental status assessment: Use Folstein Mini-Mental Status Exam, Short Portable Mental Status Questionnaire, and Cognitive Capacity Screening Exam (see Williams & Salisbury, 1999).

v. Use the same instrument/ assessment process consistently to track progression throughout the clinical course.

3. Nursing diagnoses
   a. Risk for injury
   b. Risk for impaired skin integrity
   c. Altered role performance
   d. Altered sexuality patterns
   e. Impaired home maintenance
   f. Potential for self-care deficit
   g. Self-esteem disturbance

4. Goals
   a. Maintain or rehabilitate to the maximal mobility level.
   b. Minimize potential for injury.
   c. Enhance well-being.

5. Interventions and health teaching
   a. Nonpharmacological interventions (Bergquist & Neuberger, 2002)
      i. Recommend maintenance of normal physical activity, including activities of daily living, to the extent possible.
      ii. Recommend incorporation of increased physical activity as appropriate, including flexibility training, resistance or strength training, and endurance or aerobic training.
      iii. Recommend consultation with a physical therapist and a primary care provider in the development of an exercise program.
      iv. Assist with adequate nutritional guidelines for age and stage of HIV, considering food–drug interactions and indications.
      v. Instruct in pain control methods (if applicable, see Herr & Mobily, 1999, for more information).
      vi. Recommend use of appropriate assistive devices to correct any sensory deficits and enhance mobility.
      vii. Conduct psychosocial interventions, including use of therapeutic communication with the patient, the family, and significant others. Consider referral to pastoral or psychological counseling, if indicated.
      viii. Assess and recommend environmental adaptations, beginning with safety and functional assessment; be aware of financial or behavioral constraints inhibiting change in this area. Provide appropriate care and community referrals.
   b. Pharmacological interventions
      i. Recommend use of nonpharmacologic interventions as appropriate prior to the use of pharmacologic agents.
      ii. Instruct patient to take pain medications as needed.
   c. Alternative/complementary therapies
      i. There is some evidence to support the efficacy of diet and nutrition therapy, acupuncture, hyperthermia, and oxygen therapy (Goldberg, 1997).
      ii. Herbal therapies, such as *Astragalus*, schisandra, and ginseng may increase stamina and energy. St. John's Wort can be used topically for muscle soreness. Kava and valerian are used to promote skeletal muscle relaxation (LaValle, Krinsky, Hawkins, Pelton, & Willis, 2000).

6. Evaluation
   a. Evaluate physical environment for safety.
   b. Evaluate strength, flexibility, and endurance.
   c. Evaluate for complications of immobility.

4.11 Nausea and Vomiting

1. Etiology
   a. Nausea: an ill-defined and subjective sensation often characterized by an unpleasant feeling in the epigastrium

and the back of the throat; frequently accompanied by autonomic responses, such as salivation, pallor, sweating, and tachycardia (Porth, 1994; Rhodes & McDaniel, 1997).

b. Vomiting: a sudden and forceful expulsion of the gastric contents through the mouth (Fessele, 1996); may be accompanied by dizziness, bradycardia, and a decrease in blood pressure (Porth, 1994).

c. Frequently a side effect of medications

  i. Antiretroviral therapy: nearly all antiretroviral medications can cause nausea and vomiting.

  ii. Medications to treat opportunistic infections may cause nausea and vomiting and include the following:

   • Pneumocystis pneumonia therapy: clindamycin, dapsone, trimethoprim-sulfamethoxazole (TMP-SMX)
   • Mycobacterium avium complex therapy: azithromycin, clarithromycin, ciprofloxacin, rifabutin
   • Antifungal therapy: amphotericin B, fluconazole, flucytosine, itraconazole
   • Antiparasitic therapy: atovaquone, azithromycin, clarithromycin, clindamycin, iodoquinol, metronidazole, paramomycin, pyrimethamine, TMP-SMX
   • Antiviral therapy: acyclovir, foscarnet, ganciclovir
   • Antineoplastic therapy: bleomycin, cyclophosphamide, doxorubicin, etoposide, ifosfamide, methotrexate, vinblastine, vincristine

d. May be due to HIV-related autonomic neuropathy (Konturek, Fischer, Van Der Voort, & Domschke, 1997)

e. OI-induced endocrine dysfunction has been implicated. OIs include cytomegalovirus, cryptococcus, toxoplasma, mycobacteria, and candida (Etzel, Brocavich, & Torre, 1992).

f. May be caused by radiation therapy or food-borne illness

2. Nursing assessment

  a. Subjective data

   i. Pattern of nausea and vomiting: onset, duration, precipitating factors, and associated symptoms

   ii. Remedies used to alleviate symptoms

   iii. Appearance, amount, and odor of vomitus

   iv. Nutritional intake

   v. Impact of nausea and vomiting on lifestyle

  b. Objective data

   i. Intake and output, weight, and blood pressure

   ii. Skin turgor

   iii. Serum electrolytes, renal function, and liver function enzymes

3. Nursing diagnosis

  a. High risk for fluid volume deficit related to loss of fluids from the gastrointestinal tract secondary to vomiting.

  b. Altered nutrition—less than body requirements—is related to the inability to ingest adequate nutrients due to nausea and vomiting.

  c. Nonadherence to a medication regimen may be the side effect of treatment.

4. Goals

  a. Identify and minimize the causative factors.

  b. Control nausea and vomiting with pharmacological and nonpharmacological interventions.

  c. Support nutritional needs while experiencing nausea and vomiting.

5. Interventions and health teaching

  a. Nonpharmacological interventions

   i. Avoid exposing patient to stimuli likely to produce or worsen nausea, which can precipitate vomiting and fluid loss.

   ii. Maintain a calm, quiet environment.

   iii. Avoid moving the patient suddenly.

   iv. Encourage the patient to take deep breaths while nauseated.

   v. Keep room well ventilated and free of strong odors.

   vi. Assist patient in rinsing and cleaning his or her mouth after each episode of vomiting.

vii. When oral intake is resumed, give clear fluids, such as water or ginger ale, in small amounts. If tolerated, gradually add foods such as gelatin, tea, and clear broth.

viii. Teach the patient and caregiver to eat small, frequent meals to avoid early satiety and improve daily caloric intake.

ix. Teach the patient and caregiver to drink beverages between meals, not with meals, to improve daily caloric intake.

x. Teach the patient and caregiver to avoid foods high in fat (e.g., fried, greasy foods).

xi. Refer patient to a nutritionist for meal planning.

b. Pharmacological interventions
   i. Give antiemetics as prescribed.
   ii. Monitor effectiveness of antiemetics.
   iii. Teach the patient and caregiver the name, dose, frequency of use, and side effects of prescribed antiemetics.

c. Alternative/complementary therapies
   i. Deep breathing
   ii. Acupressure
   iii. Progressive muscle relaxation
   iv. Massage

6. Evaluation
   a. Assess patient's symptoms to see if they have resolved or are minimized.
   b. Evaluate patient and caregiver understanding of the appropriate use of antiemetics (e.g., dosing, administration).
   c. Evaluate patient and caregiver understanding of the appropriate use of nonpharmacologic therapies to manage nausea and vomiting.

4.12 Diarrhea

1. Etiology
   a. Side effects of medications, including antiretrovirals and broad-spectrum antibiotics (Anastasi & Capili, 2001)
   b. Diet: ingestion of undercooked food or contaminated food or water
   c. Bacterial infections: salmonella, shigella, campylobacter, *C. difficile* toxin, *E. coli*

d. Parasites: cryptosporidia, microsporidia, isospora, giardia, and amoeba

e. Invasive diseases affecting bowel: *M. avium*, CMV, lymphoma, KS, and colon cancer

f. Other causes: lactose intolerance, low serum albumin levels, zinc deficiency, inadequate digestive enzymes or bile salts, alcohol abuse, idiopathic HIV enteropathy

2. Nursing assessment
   a. Subjective data
      i. Obtain the current history of current and previous medications, GI diseases, stage of illness, weight loss, dietary intake, and travel history.
      ii. Question the patient about the pattern of diarrhea: amount, frequency, appearance, duration, and the associated symptoms. Ask about the precipitating events, cramping, flatus, abdominal distension, tenesmus; impact on lifestyle, quality of life, and ability to care for self.
   b. Objective data
      i. Examine the patient for signs of dehydration, such as a dry skin, dry tongue, decreased skin turgor, decreased urinary output, decreased blood pressure and increased heart rate.
      ii. Perform an abdominal assessment: palpate for masses, observe for distension, auscultate bowel sounds, and conduct rectal examination.
      iii. Obtain laboratory analyses—CBC, chemistry, C reactive protein, erythrocyte sedimentation rate, and stool analyses—O & P (three samples should be sent); culture for enteric pathogens, salmonella, shigella, and campylobacter; assay for *C. difficile* toxin and AFB.

3. Nursing Diagnoses
   a. Diarrhea
   b. Fluid volume deficit
   c. Altered nutrition: less than body requirements

4. Goals
   a. Identify and treat the underlying cause.
   b. Reduce diarrhea with medications and alterations in diet.
   c. Prevent complications of diarrhea.
5. Interventions and health teaching
   a. Nonpharmacological interventions
      i. Maintain hydration by encouraging PO intake and administering IV fluids.
      ii. Replace lost electrolytes with sports drinks (e.g., Gatorade) and saline IV fluids with potassium supplementation, as needed.
      iii. Maintain skin integrity by promoting the use of warm sitz baths, perineal hygiene cleansers, and soft toilet tissue.
      iv. Discuss dietary changes to alleviate diarrhea and meet caloric needs, such as small frequent meals that are calorie dense. Avoid foods that are high in fat. Lactose, caffeine, alcohol, and spicy foods can worsen diarrhea. Encourage intake of foods that bind (i.e., BRAT diet—bananas, rice, applesauce, toast).
      v. Replace lost nutrients (e.g., fat-soluble vitamins, magnesium, potassium, and calcium).
      vi. Refer undernourished patients to dietitian for initiation of oral nutritional supplements.
      vii. Educate patients regarding food safety: wash hands before touching food; discard expired foods; thoroughly cook meat and fish; keep hot foods hot and cold foods cold; thaw frozen foods in the refrigerator, rather than on countertop; clean all kitchen work surfaces with soap and warm water; use plastic rather than wooden cutting boards.
      viii. Encourage patients to use latex barrier condoms for oral and anal sex.
      ix. Teach patients to avoid swimming in lakes or bodies of fresh water because they are likely contaminated with cryptosporidium.
   b. Pharmacological interventions
      i. Antibiotics, if bacterial etiology. If diarrhea is due to C. *difficile*, discontinue antibiotics and treat with oral vancomycin or metronidazole.
      ii. Antidiarrheal agents include opioid preparations (e.g., opium tincture, paregoric) and absorbents (e.g., kaopectate).
      iii. Antispasmodics can be used to treat cramps.
      iv. Pancreatic digestive enzymes are used for malabsorption.
   c. Alternative/complementary therapies
      i. Acupuncture and moxibustion are purported to relieve diarrhea.
      ii. Goldenseal alkaloids (Khin-Maung, Myo-Khin, Nyunt-Nyunt-Wai, Aye-Kyaw, & Tin, 1985) and homeopathic treatments (Jacobs, Jiminez, Gloyd, Gale, & Crothers, 1994) have shown effectiveness.
6. Evaluation
   a. Patient will show a reduction in the frequency and volume of stools.
   b. Patient will show normalization of fluid and electrolyte balance and regain lost weight.
   c. Patient will return to premorbid level of functional status.

4.13 Pain

1. Etiology
   a. Gastrointestinal
      i. Oropharynx/esophageal: fungal infections (e.g., candidiasis, histoplasmosis), aphthous ulcerations, intraoral KS, dental abscesses, necrotizing gingivitis, herpes simplex, CMV ulcers, streptococcal infection, gastric reflux disorders
      ii. Abdominal: CMV colitis/ileitis, intestinal infections (e.g., cryptosporidia, shigella, salmonella, campylobacter, MAC, giardia lamblia, isospora bellis, entameba histolytica, cryptococcus, *Clostridium difficile*), HIV enteropathy/colitis,

lymphoma, KS, pelvic inflammatory disease, cholecystitis related to gallstones, MAC, CMV, cryptosporidium, lymphoma, campylobacter, and KS; pancreatitis related to IV pentamadine, ddI, ddC, CMV, alcohol, and toxoplasmosis; and peritonitis, ectopic pregnancy, appendicitis, perforated ulcer, ileus, and uterine fibroids

   iii. Anorectal: perirectal abscess or fistula; herpes simplex ulcers; anorectal carcinoma; hemorrhoids; foreign object; and proctitis related to herpes, CMV, *C. trachomatus* or *N. gonorrhea*

b. Genito-urinary: herpes simplex virus, epididymitis, cystitis, bartholinitis, and renal calculi

c. Neurological: headaches; CNS toxoplasmosis; meningitis related to *cryptococcus,* syphilis, histoplasmosis, and *M. tuberculosis;* aseptic meningitis; CNS nocardia; herpes encephalopathy; progressive multifocal leukoencephalopathy; sinus infections; migraine; stress/tension; neuropathy; spinal/epidural abscess; spinal MAC; and lymphoma

d. Dermatological: herpes zoster, postherpetic neuralgia, bacterial abscess, and bulky cutaneous KS

e. Musculoskeletal: arthropathy; HIV-related arthralgia, hepatitis C-related arthralgia, or both; psoriatic-related arthritis; avascular necrosis associated with smoking, steroids, trauma, antiretrovirals, dyslipidemia, megace, and pancreatitis; myopathy; and osteopenia/osteoporosis

f. Cardiovascular: pericarditis related to toxoplasmosis, CMV, *mycobacteria,* nocardiosis, Kaposi's sarcoma, lymphoma, herpes simplex, or *cryptococcus;* endocarditis related to *staphylococcus aureus* or nonbacterial thrombosis; angina pectoris related to dyslipidemia; and peripheral vascular disease

g. Pulmonary: infections related to PCP, bacteria, *histoplasmosis, aspergillosis,*

mycobacterium tuberculosis; costal chondritis; and emboli

2. Nursing assessment
   a. Subjective data
      i. Onset and duration, location, character (e.g., burning, sharp, dull), intensity, exacerbating and relieving factors, response to current and past treatments, cultural responses, and meaning of pain to the patient
   b. Objective data
      i. Numerical scale: 0–10 scale (0 = *no pain* 10 = *worst imaginable*)
      ii. Verbal scale (*none, small, mild, moderate, severe*)
      iii. Pediatric faces pain scale (useful when the verbal skills are inadequate)

3. Nursing diagnosis
   a. Alteration in comfort

4. Goals
   a. Achieve optimal level of patient comfort and functioning with the fewest medication-related side effects
   b. Achieve optimal level of patient comfort via the least invasive route
   c. Prevent pain

5. Interventions and health teaching
   a. Nonpharmacological interventions
      i. The nurse should work to individualize each patient's pain regimen.
      ii. Relaxation techniques, imagery, biofeedback, hypnosis, massage, vibration, reflexology, acupressure, and meditation may be helpful as adjunctive therapy.
      iii. Thermal modalities should be used as tolerated.
      iv. Some patients may benefit from prayer.
      v. Rhythmic breathing may be beneficial.
      vi. Ultrasound, physical therapy, and TENS may be helpful.
      vii. Radiation therapy can be used for cancer-related pain (bulky KS, bone metastasis).
   b. Pharmacological interventions (World Health Organization analgesic guidelines; World Health Organization, 1996)
      i. Step 1: Nonopiate

(1) Acetaminophen has no effect on platelet function or renal status and provides no antiinflammatory effect; avoid use with hepatic insufficiency.

(2) Nonsteroidal antiinflammatory agents (NSAIDs): Switch with an NSAID from a different class if sufficient analgesia is not obtained with one NSAID.

    (a) Salsalate and tolmetin produce less inhibition of platelet aggregation than other NSAIDs except for COX-2 inhibitors.

    (b) COX-2 inhibitors should be avoided with ACE inhibitors or diuretics.

    (c) Avoid celecoxib with sulfonamide-derived medications.

    (d) Use for throbbing, aching pain.

(3) Tramadol

    (a) Centrally acting nonopiate

    (b) Can be combined with NSAIDs

    (c) Available alone or with acetaminophen

    (d) Avoid with SSRIs and MAOIs due to serotonin syndrome

    (e) Avoid in persons with seizure history

ii. Step 2: Mild opiates with or without nonopiates

(1) Use caution when using opiates in persons with asthma, increased intracranial pressure (ICP), and hepatic failure.

(2) Maximum dose of combination agents is limited to ceiling dose of the nonopiate (usually acetaminophen or aspirin).

(3) Meperidine and propoxyphene are not recommended due to poor efficacy and accumulation of toxic metabolites.

iii. Step 3: Adjuvants

(1) Add at any step of analgesic ladder.

(2) NSAIDs will provide additive effects to opiates, increasing duration.

(3) Corticosteroids

    (a) Use in treating aphthous ulcers and cerebral edema.

    (b) Use with caution in persons with cavitary infections, bullous lung disease, renal insufficiency, or thrombocytopenia.

(4) Antidepressants (e.g., amitriptyline, doxepin, desipramine) can boost efficacy of opiates.

(5) Provide independent analgesia for neuropathy and postherpetic neuralgia.

(6) Anticonvulsants (e.g., gabapentin, lamotragine) can be helpful in neuropathic pain; avoid carbamazepine due to neutropenia.

(7) Antihistamines (e.g., hydroxyzine) provide additive analgesia, anxiolytic, antiemetic effect.

(8) Caffeine increases opiate effect.

(9) Topicals (e.g., lidocaine patch, lidocaine gel, capsaicin ointment, mentholated creams)

    (a) Remove lidocaine patch every 12 hours.

    (b) Capsaicin ointment must be used QID and can cause initial burning.

iv. Step 4: Strong opiates

(1) Morphine sulfate (MS)

    (a) MS available in short-acting (4 hours) and long-acting (8–12 hours; 24 hours) preparations.

    (b) Do not crush or break the long-acting pill; encourage high fluid intake to activate release of long-acting drug. Long-acting MS may not be released in malabsorptive states: equianalgesic dose: 10 mg/SC = 20–30 mg PO.

(2) Hydromorphone
   (a) Short-acting only (3–4 hours)
   (b) Equianalgesic dose: 2 mg IM/SC = 4 mg PO

(3) Levorphanol
   (a) Length of action: 6–8 hours
   (b) Equianalgesic dose: 2 mg IM/SC = 4 mg PO
   (c) Can accumulate with repetitive dosing

(4) Dolophine
   (a) Length of action: 6–8 hours
   (b) Can accumulate with repetitive dosing
   (c) Phenytoin, efavirenz, rifampin and nevirapine: lower dolophine levels

(5) Meperidine
   (a) Meperidine is not recommended for use > 3 days.
   (b) Length of action is 2–3 hours.
   (c) Oral form is not recommended.
   (d) Toxic metabolites accumulate at doses > 300mg/day, leading to tremors and seizures.
   (e) Meperidine 100 mg IM equals morphine 10 mg IM.
   (f) Avoid use with ritonavir.

(6) Fentanyl
   (a) Long-acting transdermal patch for chronic pain
      (i) Place patch on intact, nonirritated skin.
      (ii) Fever will increase release of patch, so monitor for sedation and decreased duration of analgesia.
      (iii) Avoid use with ritonavir.
   (b) Short-acting submucosal lollipop: Use for breakthrough pain, acute pain, or both; patient should not chew lollipop but rub over buccal mucosa.

(7) Oxycodone
   (a) Available in short-acting and long-acting forms
   (b) Available with and without nonopiate

c. Alternative/complementary therapies
   i. Aromatherapy
   ii. Therapeutic touch/Reiki
   iii. Movement therapy: yoga, stretching, Feldenkreis, Trager, Tai Chi
   iv. Magnets: avoid in pregnancy due to lack of safety data in this population
   v. Acupuncture
   vi. Homeopathy
   vii. Nutritional supplements (Carnitor, alpha lipoic acid) e.g., for neuropathic pain

6. Evaluation
   a. Evaluate the response to the plan continually; change the drug, interval, dose, route, modality; and treat side effects.
   b. Evaluate for sequelae of undermanaged pain.
      i. Physical effects: difficulty sleeping, poor appetite, decreased mobility, shallow breathing, and suppression of immune system
      ii. Psychological effects: anxiety/fear, depression, reduced quality of life, difficulty concentrating, and suicidal ideation
      iii. Social effects: impaired relationships and increased stress on friends/caregivers
      iv. Spiritual effects: human suffering and hopelessness

4.14 Female Sexual Dysfunction

1. Etiology
   a. Organic causes include vascular disease; neurological disease; hormonal/ endocrine disorders; musculogenic,

pelvic, or perineal surgery; trauma to pelvis or spine; pelvic anomalies or disease.

b. Secondary causes of sexual dysfunction may be related to underlying psychiatric disorder such as anxiety disorder, major depression, or a panic disorder.

c. Secondary to medications: antihypertensives, chemotherapeutics, anticholinergics, anticonvulsants, antidepressants, antipsychotics, narcotics, sedatives/anxiolytics, antiandrogens, antiestrogens, birth control pills

2. Nursing assessment
   a. Subjective data
      i. Starting with a general question presented in a nonthreatening manner gives the patient permission to ask further questions. Begin with a question such as "Many women have concerns and questions about sex. What questions do you have?" A more direct approach is "How has this illness affected your sex life?"
   b. Objective data
      i. Evaluation of sexual dysfunction includes a thorough physical examination, including a pelvic examination, psychological and psychosocial assessment, and laboratory or hormonal studies, as indicated. The suggested hormonal profile includes follicle-stimulating hormone, lutenizing hormone, prolactin, total and free testosterone levels, sex hormone-binding globulin, and estradiol levels.
      ii. Tools such as the Female Sexual Function Index (FSFI) can facilitate this discussion (see www.FSFIquestionnaire.com). The FSFI is a brief, valid, and reliable self-report measure of female sexual function. The tool evaluates the following areas of sexual functioning: desire and subjective arousal, lubrication, orgasm, satisfaction, and pain/discomfort (Bayer, Zonagen, Inc., & Target Health, 2000).

3. Nursing diagnosis
   a. Altered sexual pattern
4. Goal
   a. Improved sexual functioning
5. Interventions and health teaching
   a. Nonpharmacological interventions (Phillips, 2000)
      i. Provide education about normal anatomy, sexual function, normal changes of aging, pregnancy, and menopause.
      ii. Enhance stimulation and eliminate routine by encouraging use of erotic materials, masturbation, communication during sexual activity, vibrators, and various positions, times of day, or places. Suggest patient make a date for sexual activity.
      iii. Provide distraction techniques by encouraging erotic or nonerotic fantasy, pelvic muscle contraction and relaxation exercises with intercourse, and use of background music, videos, or television.
      iv. Encourage noncoital behaviors, such as sensual massage, sensate-focus exercises, and oral or noncoital stimulation, with or without orgasm.
      v. Minimize dyspareunia by superficial methods, such as female astride for control of penetration; topical lidocaine; warm baths before intercourse; biofeedback and deep methods, such as position changes so that force is away from pain and deep thrusts are minimized; and use of nonsteroidal antiinflammatory agents before intercourse.
   b. Pharmacological interventions
      i. Aside from hormone replacement therapy, pharmacologic management of female sexual dysfunction is in the early experimental stages. Most of the medications used have been used in the treatment of male erectile dysfunction and are still in experimental stages for use in women.

    ii. Estrogen replacement therapy can be used by menopausal women.

   iii. Methyl testosterone can be used in combination with estrogen in menopausal women for symptoms of inhibited desire, dyspareunia, or lack of vaginal lubrication.

   iv. Sildenafil is a selective type V phosphodiesterase inhibitor that promotes relaxation of clitoral and vaginal smooth muscle.

   v. L-arginine is an amino acid that mediates relaxation of vascular and nonvascular smooth muscle. It has not been used in clinical trials with women, but studies in men look promising.

   vi. Prostaglandin E1 delivered intravaginally is currently under investigation for use in women.

  vii. Phentolamine in oral form causes vascular smooth muscle relaxation. A pilot study in menopausal women showed promise.

  viii. Apomorphine facilitates erectile response in men and is being examined for use in women.

c. Alternative/complementary therapies

   i. Yohimbine bark (Yohimbehe cortex) has been used as an aphrodisiac. It is thought to act as an alpha-adrenergic blocker. Contraindications include existing liver and kidney disease as well as chronic inflammation of the sexual organs (Blumenthal, 1998, 2000).

   ii. Ginkgo biloba leaf extract (Ginkgo folium) has been used to treat patients with antidepressant-induced sexual dysfunction, especially related to the use of selective serotonin reuptake inhibitors (SSRIs). Studies showed women were more responsive to the sexually enhancing effects than men. It has been reported to have a positive effect on all four phases of the sexual response cycle: desire, excitement, orgasm, and resolution. It is thought that Ginkgo biloba leaf extract works by inhibiting platelet activity factor (PAF), which affects prostaglandins and enhances erectile function. Some researchers believe it has some type of norepinephrine repector–induced effects on the brain. Contraindications include a noted hypersensitivity to ginkgo preparations (Blumenthal, 1998, 2000).

   iii. Damiana leaf and herb (*Turnera diffusa*) has been used as an aphrodisiac and for prophylaxis and treatment of sexual disturbances. Little is understood about the mechanism of action as well as any contraindications (Blumenthal, 1998).

   iv. Muira puama (*Ptychopetali lignum*) is used for prevention of sexual disorders as well as an aphrodisiac. The mechanism of action and contraindications are poorly understood (Blumenthal, 1998).

6. Evaluation
   a. Patient will be able to discuss cause of sexual dysfunction.
   b. Patient will discuss alternative, satisfying, and acceptable sexual practices for self and partner.

4.15 Male Sexual Dysfunction

1. Etiology
   a. Premature ejaculation: primarily psychogenic
   b. Erectile dysfunction
      i. Organic causes include vascular disease, neurological disease, endocrine disorders, renal failure, liver disease, malignancies, pelvic or perineal surgeries, trauma to pelvis or spine, penile anomalies or disease, drug abuse, and cigarette smoking.
      ii. Secondary causes of sexual dysfunction may be related to underlying psychiatric disorder such as anxiety disorder, major depression, or a panic disorder
      iii. Secondary to medications: antihypertensives, antidepressants, antiarrhythmics, antihyperlipidemics,

antipsychotics, anticonvulsants, antiandrogens, histamine H$_2$ receptor antagonists, narcotics, nonsteroidal antiinflammatories, antimanics, cytotoxic medications, and ketoconozoles

   iv. Iatrogenic

2. Nursing assessment

  a. Subjective data

    i. Starting with a general question, presented in a nonthreatening manner, gives the patient permission to ask further questions. Begin with a question such as "Many men have concerns and questions about sex. What questions do you have?" A more direct approach is "How has this illness affected your sex life?"

  b. Objective data

    i. Evaluation of sexual dysfunction includes a thorough physical examination, psychological and psychosocial assessment, and laboratory or hormonal studies, as indicated. Diagnostic studies for erectile dysfunction include blood pressure, fasting blood glucose, total low-density and high-density lipoprotein cholesterol and triglycerides, lutenizing hormone and prolactin (looks at bioavailable testosterone), and thyroid studies.

3. Nursing diagnosis

  a. Altered sexual pattern

4. Goal

  a. Improved sexual functioning

5. Interventions and health teaching

  a. Nonpharmacological interventions

    i. Premature ejaculation

      (1) Psychotherapy (Holmes, 2000)

      (2) Couples counseling to improve communication skills

      (3) Behaviorally oriented psychotherapy

    ii. Erectile dysfunction: Advise patient to curtail or eliminate smoking, alcohol, caffeine, and drug abuse.

  b. Pharmacological intervention

    i. Premature ejaculation (Epperly & Moore, 2000; Holmes, 2000): low doses of clomipramine, sertraline, or partoxetine to increase ejaculatory latency

    ii. Erectile dysfunction: A stepped approach to the treatment of erectile dysfunction (Epperly & Moore, 2000) allows the primary caregiver to intervene with patients in Steps 1 and 2, based on a general assessment, before pursuing a urologic referral needed for interventions in Steps 3 and 4.

- Step 1: Oral agents such as Sildenafil, L-arginine (investigational), or testosterone if hypogonadal (Korenman, 1998)
- Step 2: Vacuum or constriction devices
- Step 3: Urethral therapies
  - Intracavernosal injections of prostaglandin E, paperverine, or phentolamine
  - Intraurethral insertion of prostaglandin E
- Step 4: Penile surgery
  - Penile prostheses
  - Penile vascular surgery

  c. Alternative/complementary therapies

    i. Yohimbine bark (Yohimbehe cortex) has been used as an aphrodisiac. It is thought to act as an alpha-adrenergic blocker. Contraindications include existing liver and kidney disease as well as chronic inflammation of the sexual organs (Blumenthal, 1998, 2000).

    ii. Ginkgo biloba leaf extract (Ginkgo folium) has been used as to treat patients with antidepressant–induced sexual dysfunction especially related to the use of SSRIs. Although it is reported that women are more responsive to the sex-enhancing effects than men, it has been used successfully with men. It has been reported to have a positive effect on all four phases of the sexual response cycle: desire, excitement, orgasm, and resolution. It is thought that Ginkgo biloba leaf extract works by inhibiting PAF, which affects prostaglandins and enhances erectile function. Some researchers believe it has some type of norepinephrine repector–induced effects on the brain. Contraindications include a noted hypersensitivity to ginkgo preparations (Blumenthal, 1998, 2000).

   iii. Ginseng root (*Ginseng radix*) has been used to treat erectile dysfunction. The mechanism of action is not understood. Hypertension is a contraindication for the use of ginseng (Blumenthal, 1998).

   iv. Damiana leaf and herb (*Turnera diffusa*) has been used an aphrodisiac and for prophylaxis and treatment of sexual disturbances. Little is understood about the mechanism of action as well as any contraindications (Blumenthal, 1998).

   v. Muira puama (*Ptychopetali lignum*) is used for prevention of sexual disorders as well as an aphrodisiac. The mechanism of action and contraindications are poorly understood (Blumenthal, 1998).

6. Evaluation
   a. Patient will be able to discuss cause of sexual dysfunction.
   b. Patient will discuss alternative, satisfying, and acceptable sexual practices for self and partner.

4.16 Vision Loss

1. Etiology
   a. Vision loss is a state characterized by a change in the amount or patterning of oncoming visual stimuli accompanied by a diminished, exaggerated, distorted, or impaired interpretation (North American Nursing Diagnosis Association, 1996).
   b. Visual impairment from an opportunistic infection may be due to primary or secondary involvement; it

may evolve from the anterior or posterior portion of the eye or the ocular adnexa (Cunningham, 1999).

  c. Anterior involvement (i.e., the cornea, anterior chamber, and iris) originates from tumors and external eye infections (Ahmed, Ai, & Luckie, 1999; Cunningham, 1999).

  d. Posterior involvement (i.e., the retina, choroids, and optic nerve head) originates predominantly from HIV-associated retinopathy and HIV-related opportunistic infections (Ahmed et al., 1999; Cunningham, 1999).

  e. The adnexa (i.e., eyelids, conjunctiva, and lacrimal drainage system) are susceptible to infection with herpes simplex virus (HSV) and Kaposi's sarcoma (KS).

2. Nursing assessment
   a. Subjective data
      i. Impact of visual loss on mood, self-concept, relationships
      ii. Reported symptoms: decreased visual acuity, floaters, light flashes, blurred vision
      iii. Reported date of last ophthalmic/ fundoscopic examination
      iv. Ability to manage activities of daily living
      v. Availability of social support and supportive services
      vi. Emotional responses to changes in visual acuity
   b. Objective data
      i. Unilateral or bilateral field loss; initially, involvement is usually unilateral but becomes bilateral if underlying pathology is left untreated.
      ii. Decreased visual acuity on examination: eye chart test (Snellen, Amsler grid, or Teich Target; Dew & Riley, 1998); ability to read printed materials (determine literacy level before diagnosing a loss of visual acuity)
      iii. Visual field testing: peripheral or central vision loss
      iv. Observed photosensitivity

3. Nursing diagnosis
   a. Altered role performance

b. Impaired home maintenance management

c. Sensory or perceptual alterations (visual)

d. Potential for self-care deficit

4. Goals

a. Prevent visual impairment or loss via early detection and treatment.

b. Promote the patient's safety and autonomy.

c. Support the patient's adaptation to visual impairment or loss.

5. Interventions and health teaching

a. Nonpharmacological interventions

i. Provide symptomatic relief using appropriate pain control techniques (e.g., cool compresses, eye drops, avoidance of bright lights)

ii. Educate the patient, family, and significant other.

(1) Encourage patient to report new or worsening ocular symptoms as soon as they are noticed.

(2) Advise patient to have regular fundoscopic exams from a competent practitioner, especially if CD_4 T lymphocyte count < 50 cells/mm^3.

(3) Refer patient to services for people with visual impairment or blindness for assistance in modifying home environment to maintain safety and promote independence (e.g., magnifying glass, books on tape, individual counseling/support groups; in some instances, occupational therapy may provide additional assistance with adaptive devices and home modifications for visual impairment).

(4) Remind caregivers not to move furniture or rearrange patient's belongings without the patient's consent to avoid disorientation and injury.

(5) Allow for verbalization of feelings (from both HIV-positive person and significant others) regarding visual impairment or vision loss.

(6) Facilitate necessary community referrals to maintain a safe and adequate environment (e.g., Meals on Wheels, home health).

b. Pharmacological interventions

i. Administer or instruct patient or caregiver regarding administration of prescribed eye medications, schedules for medications, and side effects.

ii. When receiving intravenous medications for vision-related problems (e.g., cidofovir), instruct patient or caregiver in correct technique for managing venous access devices (e.g., flushing, site/dressing changes).

iii. For medication side effects impairing vision, clarify with the primary care provider if alternative treatments are possible.

c. Alternative/complementary therapies

i. Stress reduction techniques: Guided imagery and relaxation may reduce fear, enhance feelings of control, and improve immune function.

ii. Herbal therapies include anxiety-reducing herbs, such as valerian, ashwagandha, chamomile, kava, and passion flower (Bascom, 2002). Bilberry and eyebright are used to increase visual acuity. Goldenseal eyewashes are helpful in treating eye infections (Fetrow & Avila, 1999).

6. Evaluation

a. Safety of physical environment

b. Adaptation to visual impairment

c. Progression of visual loss

References

Ahmed, I., Ai, E., & Luckie, A. (1999). Ophthalmic manifestations of HIV infection. In P. T. Cohen, M. A. Sande, & P. A. Volderding (Eds.), *The AIDS knowledge base* (3rd ed., pp. 543–557). Philadelphia: Lippincott Williams & Wilkins.

Allen, R. (1997). The significance and interpretation of the polysomnogram. In M. Pressman & W. Orr (Eds.), *Understanding sleep: The evaluation and treatment of sleep disorders* (pp. 193–208). Washington, DC: American Psychological Association.

Althoff, S., Williams, P. N., Molvig, D., & Schuster, L. (1997). *A guide to alternative medicine.* Lincolnwood, IL: Publications International.

Anastasi, J. K., & Capili, B. (2001). HIV-related diarrhea and outcome measures. *Journal of the Association of Nurses in AIDS Care, 12* (Suppl.), 44–54.

Barroso, J. (1999). A review of fatigue in people with HIV infection. *Journal of the Association of Nurses in AIDS Care, 10*(5), 42–49.

Barroso, J. (2001). "Just worn out": A qualitative study of HIV-related fatigue. In S. G. Funk, E. M. Tornquist, J. Leeman, M. S. Miles, & J. S. Harrell (Eds.), *Key aspects of preventing and managing chronic illness* (pp. 183–194). New York: Springer.

Barroso, J., & Lynn, M. R. (2002). Psychometric properties of the HIV-Related Fatigue Scale. *Journal of the Association of Nurses in AIDS Care, 13*(1), 66–75.

Bartlett, J. G. (1996). *Medical management of HIV infection.* Glenview, IL: Physicians and Scientists Publishing.

Bascom, A. (2002). *Incorporating herbal medicine into clinical practice.* Philadelphia: F.A. Davis.

Bayer, A. G., Zonagen, Inc., & Target Health Inc. (2000). *Female sexual function index (FSFI).* Retrieved December 19, 2002, from www.FSFI questionnaire.com

Bergquist, S., & Neuberger, G. B. (2002). Altered mobility and fatigue. In I. M. Lubkin & P. D. Larsen (Eds.), *Chronic illness: Impact and intervention* (5th ed., pp. 147–177). Boston: Jones and Bartlett.

Blumenthal, M. (Ed.). (1998). *The complete German commission E monographs: Therapeutic guide to herbal medicines.* Boston: American Botanical Council.

Blumental, M. (Ed.). (2000). *Herbal medicine: Expanded commission E monographs.* Newton, MA: Integrative Medicine Communications.

Bootzin, R., & Rider, S. (1997). Behavioral techniques and biofeedback for insomnia. In M. Pressman & W. Orr (Eds.), *Understanding sleep: The evaluation and treatment of sleep disorders* (pp. 315–338). Washington, DC: American Psychological Association.

Boulant, J. (2000). Role of the preoptic-anterior hypothalamus in thermoregulation and fever. *Clinical Infectious Disease, 31*(Suppl. 5), 157–161.

Breitbart, W., McDonald, M. V., Rosenfeld, B., Monkman, N. D., & Passik, S. (1998). Fatigue in ambulatory AIDS patients. *Journal of Pain and Symptom Management, 15,* 159–167.

Buysse, D., & Reynolds, C. (2000). Pharmacologic treatment. In K. Lichstein & C. Morin (Eds.), *Treatment of late-life insomnia* (pp. 231–267). Thousand Oaks, CA: Sage.

Buysse, D., Reynolds, C., Monk, T., Berman, S., & Kupfer, D. (1989). The Pittsburgh Sleep Quality Index: A new instrument for psychiatric practice and research. *Psychiatry Research, 28,* 193–213.

Carpenito, L. J. (2000). *Nursing diagnosis: Application to clinical practice.* (8th ed.). Philadelphia: Lippincott Williams & Wilkins.

Carpenito, L. J. (2002). *Nursing diagnosis: Application to clinical practice* (9th ed.). Philadelphia: Lippincott.

Chandler, J. M., Duncan, P. W., Weiner, D. K., & Studenski, S. A. (2001). Special feature: Assessment profile—A reliable and valid assessment tool. *Topics in Geriatric Rehabilitation, 16*(3), 77–88.

Clerici, M., Trabattoni, D., Piconi, S., Fusi, M. L., Ruzzante, S., Clerici, C., et al. (1997). A possible role for the cortisol/anticortisols imbalance in the progression of human immunodeficiency virus. *Psychoneuroendocrinology, 22*(Suppl. 1), 27–31.

Cooper, K. (1995). Beyond the loci of action of circulating pyrogens: Mediators and mechanisms. In K. Cooper (Ed.), *Fever and antipyresis* (pp. 60–89). New York: Cambridge University Press.

Corcoran, C., & Grinspoon, S. (1999). Treatment for wasting in patients with the acquired immunodeficiency syndrome. *The New England Journal of Medicine, 340*(22), 1740–1750.

Cunningham, E. T., Jr. (1999). Ocular complications of HIV infection. In M. A. Sande & P. A. Volberding (Eds.), *The medical management of AIDS* (6th ed., pp. 171–184). Philadelphia: W. B. Saunders.

Cupler, E. J., Danon, M. J., Jay, C., Hench, K., Ropka, M., & Dalakas, M. C. (1995). Early features of zidovudine-associated myopathy: Histopathological findings and clinical correlations. *Acta Neuropathologica, 90,* 1–6.

Das, S. K., Das, V., Gulati, A. K., & Singh, V. P. (1989). Deglycyrrhizinated liquorice in aphthous ulcers. *Journal of the Association of Physicians of India, 37,* 647.

Derry, D. M. (1996). Thyroid hormone therapy in patients infected with human immunodeficiency virus: A clinical approach to treatment. *Medical Hypotheses, 47,* 227–233.

Dew, T., & Riley, T. A. (1998). Visual changes. In M. E. Ropka & A. B. Williams (Eds.), *HIV: Nursing and symptom management* (pp. 484–492). Boston: Jones and Bartlett.

Dreher, H. (2000). *The effect of caffeine reduction on sleep and well-being in persons with HIV.* (UMI No. 9985695)

Engberg, S. J., & McDowell, J. (1999). Comprehensive geriatric assessment. In J. T. Stone, J. F. Wyman, & S. A. Salisbury (Eds.), *Clinical gerontological nursing: A guide to advanced practice* (2nd ed., pp. 63–80). Philadelphia: W. B. Saunders.

Epperly, T. D., & Moore, K. E. (2000). Health issues in men: Part 1. Common genitourinary disorders. *American Family Physician, 61*(12), 3657–3664.

Etzel, J. V., Brocavich, J. M., & Torre, M. (1992). Endocrine complications associated with human immunodeficiency virus infection. *Clinical Pharmacy, 11,* 705–713.

Fairfield, W. P., Treat, M., Rosenthal, D. I., Frontera, W., Stanley, T., Corcoran, C., et al. (2001). Effects of testosterone and exercise on muscle leanness in eugonadal men with AIDS wasting. *Journal of Applied Physiology, 90,* 2166–2171.

Ferrando, S., Evans, S., Goggin, K., Sewell, M., Fishman, B., & Rabkin, J. (1998). Fatigue in HIV illness: Relationship to depression, physical limitations, and disability. *Psychosomatic Medicine, 60,* 759–764.

Ferrell, B. R., & Coyle, N. (2001). *Textbook of palliative nursing.* New York: Oxford University Press.

Fessele, K. S. (1996). Managing the multiple causes of nausea and vomiting in the patient with cancer. *Oncology Nursing Forum, 23*(9), 1409–1415.

Fetrow, C. W., & Avila, J. R. (1999). *Complementary and alternative medicines.* Philadelphia: Springhouse.

Flaskerud, J. H., & Miller, E. N. (1999). Psychosocial and neuropsychiatric function. In P. J. Ungvarski & J. H. Flaskerud (Eds.), *HIV/AIDS: A guide to primary care management* (4th ed., pp. 255–291). Philadelphia: W. B. Saunders.

Floyd, J. (1999). Sleep promotion in adults. In J. Fitzpatrick (Ed.), *Annual review of nursing research* (pp. 27–56). New York: Springer.

Fukunishi, I., Hosaka, T., Matsumoto, T., Hayashi, M., Negishi, M., & Moriya, H. (1997). Liaison psychiatry and HIV Infection (II): Application of relaxation in HIV-positive patients. *Psychiatry and Clinical Neurosciences, 51,* 5–8.

Goldberg, B. (1997). *Alternative medicine: The definitive guide.* Tiburon, CA: Future Medicine Publishing.

Greenspan, D. (1998). Oral manifestations of HIV. In L. Pieperl & P. Volberding (Eds.), *HIV Insite knowledge base.* Retrieved January 2003, from http://hivinsite. ucsf.edu/InSite.jsp?page=kb-04& doc=kb-04-01-14

Greenspan, J. S., & Greenspan, D. (1999). Oral manifestations of HIV infection and AIDS. In T. C. Merigan, J. G. Bartlett, & D. Bolognesi (Eds.), *Textbook of AIDS medicine* (2nd ed., pp. 521–535). Baltimore: Williams & Wilkins.

Groopman, J. E. (1998). Fatigue in cancer and HIV/AIDS. *Oncology, 12,* 335–341.

Herr, K. A., & Mobily, P. R. (1999). Pain management. In G. M. Bulechek & J. C. McCloskey (Eds.), *Nursing interventions* (3rd ed., pp. 149–171). Philadelphia: W. B. Saunders.

Holmes, S. (2000). Treatment of male sexual dysfunction. *British Medical Bulletin, 56*(3), 798–808.

Holohan-Bell, J. K., & Brummel-Smith, K. (1999). Impaired mobility and deconditioning. In J. T. Stone, J. F. Wyman, & S. A. Salisbury (Eds.), *Clinical gerontological nursing: A guide to advanced practice* (2nd ed., pp. 267–287). Philadelphia: W.B. Saunders.

Holtzclaw, B. J. (1998). Managing fever in HIV disease. *Journal of the Association of Nurses in AIDS Care, 9*(4), 97–101.

Holzemer, W. L., Hudson, A., Kirksey, K. M., Hamilton, M. J., & Bakken, S. (2001). The revised sign and symptom check-list for HIV (SSC-HIVrev). *Journal of the Association of Nurses in AIDS Care, 12*(5), 60–70.

Itescu, S., Mathur-Wagh, U., Skovron, M. L., Brancato, L. J., Marmor, M., Zeleniuch-Jacquotte, A., et al. (1992). HLA-B35 is associated with accelerated progression to AIDS. *Journal of Acquired Immune Deficiency Syndromes, 5,* 37–45.

Jacobs, J., Jiminez, M., Gloyd, S. S., Gale, J. L., & Crothers, D. (1994). Treatment of acute childhood diarrhea with homeopathic medicine: A randomized clinical trial in Nicaragua. *Pediatrics, 93,* 719–725.

Jandourek, A., Vaishampayan, J. K., & Vazquez, J. A. (1998). Efficacy of melaleuca oral solution for the treatment of fluconazole refractory oral candidiasis in AIDS patients. *AIDS, 12,* 1033–1037.

Johns, M. (1992). Reliability and factor analysis of the Epworth Sleepiness Scale. *Sleep, 15,* 376–381.

Jordan, W. C. (1998). The effectiveness of intermittent hyperbaric oxygen in relieving drug-induced HIV-associated neuropathy. *Journal of the National Medical Association, 90,* 355–358.

Justice, A. C., Rabeneck, L., Hays, R. D., Wu, A. W., & Bozzette, S. A. (1999). Sensitivity, specificity, reliability, and clinical validity of provider-reported symptoms: A comparison with self-reported symptoms. *Journal of Acquired Immune Deficiency Syndrome, 21,* 126–133.

Keithley, J. K., & Swanson, B. (2001). Oral nutritional supplements in human immunodeficiency virus disease: A review of the evidence. *Nutrition in Clinical Practice, 16*(2), 98–104.

Keithley, J. K., Swanson, B., & Nerad, J. (2001). HIV/AIDS. In M. Gottschlich (Ed.), *The science and practice of nutrition support: A case-based approach* (pp. 619–641). Dubuque, IA: Kendall/Hunt.

Khin-Maung-U., Myo-Khin., Nyunt-Nyunt-Wai., Aye-Kyaw., & Tin-U. (1985). Clinical trial of berberine in acute watery diarrhea. *British Medical Journal, 291*(6509), 1601–1605.

Konturek, J. W., Fischer, H., Van Der Voort, I. R., & Domschke, W. (1997). Disturbed gastric motor activity in patients with human immunodeficiency virus infection. *Scandinavian Journal Gastroenterology, 32,* 221–225.

Korenman, S. G. (1998). New insights into erectile dysfunction: A practical approach. *The American Journal of Medicine, 105*(2), 135–144.

Kotler, D. P. (1998). Nutritional management of patients with AIDS-related anorexia. *Seminars in Gastrointestinal Disease, 9*(4), 189–199.

Kozier, B., Erb, G., Berman, A. J., & Burke, K. (2000). *Fundamentals of nursing: Concepts, process, and practice* (6th ed.). Upper Saddle River, NJ: Prentice Hall.

LaValle, J. B., Krinsky, D. L., Hawkins, E. B., Pelton, R., & Willis, N. A. (2000). *Natural therapeutics pocket guide.* Hudson, OH: Lexi-Comp.

Lee, B. (1995). Drug interactions and toxicities in patients with AIDS. In P. Cohen, M. Sande, & P. Volberding (Eds.), *The AIDS knowledge base* (4th ed., pp. 161–182). Philadelphia: Saunders.

Lennie, T. A., Neidig, J. L., Stein, K. F., & Smith, B. A. (2001). Assessment of hunger and appetite and their relationship to food intake in person with HIV infection. *Journal of the Association of Nurses in AIDS Care, 12*(3), 66–74.

Lo, C., & Kim, M. (1986). Construct validity of sleep pattern disturbance: A methodological approach. In M. Hurley (Ed.), *Classification of nursing diagnoses: Proceedings of the sixth conference* (pp. 197–206). St. Louis: Mosby.

Martins, R. S., Periera, E. S., Lima, S. M., Senna, M. I., Mesquita, R. A., & Santos, V. R. (2002). Effect of commercial ethanol propolis extract on the in vitro growth of *Candida albicans* collected from HIV-seropositive and HIV-seronegative Brazilian patients with oral candidiasis. *Journal of Oral Science, 44,* 41–48.

Mauri, M. C., Fabiano, L., Bravin, S., Ricci, C., & Invernizzi, G. (1997). Schizophrenic patients before and after HIV infection: A case-control study. *Encephale, 23*(6), 437–441.

McGuire, D., & So, Y. T. (1999). The nervous system in HIV and AIDS. In P. T. Cohen, M. A. Sande, & P. A. Volberding (Eds.), *The AIDS knowledge base* (3rd ed., pp. 445–462). Philadelphia: Lippincott Williams & Wilkins.

Meehan, R. A., & Brush, J. A. (2001). An overview of AIDS dementia complex. *American Journal of Alzheimer's Disease, 16*(4), 225–229.

Merritt, S. (2000). Putting sleep disorders to rest. *RN, 63*(7), 26–31.

Nelson, M. K. (1997). Psychoeducational group work for persons with AIDS dementia complex. In M. B. Winiarski (Ed.), *HIV mental health for the 21st century* (pp. 137–156). New York: New York University Press.

Nokes, K., Chidekel, J., & Kendrew, J. (1999). Exploring the complexity of sleep disturbances in persons with HIV/AIDS. *Journal of the Association of Nurses in AIDS Care, 10*(3), 22–29.

Nokes, K., & Kendrew, J. (2001). Correlates of sleep quality in persons with HIV disease. *Journal of the Association of Nurses in AIDS Care, 12*(1), 17–22.

North American Nursing Diagnosis Association. (1996). *NANDA nursing diagnoses: Definitions and classification 1997–1998.* Philadelphia: Author.

Patton, L. L., McKaig, R., Strauss, R., Rogers, D., & Eron, J. J. (2000). Changing prevalence of oral manifestations of human immunodeficiency virus in the era of protease inhibitor therapy. *Oral Surgery, Oral Medicine, Oral Pathology, Oral Radiology, and Endodontics, 89,* 299–304.

Phillips, K., & Skelton, W. (2001). Effects of individualized acupuncture on sleep quality in HIV disease. *Journal of the Association of Nurses in AIDS Care, 12*(1), 27–39.

Phillips, N. A. (2000). Female sexual dysfunction: Evaluation and treatment. *American Family Physician, 62*(1), 127–136, 141–142.

Portegies, P., & Rosenberg, N. R. (1998). AIDS dementia complex: Diagnosis and drug treatment options. *CNS Drugs, 9*(1), 31–40.

Porth, C. M. (1994). Alterations in gastrointestinal function. In D. Intenzo (Ed.), *Pathophysiology concepts of altered health status* (4th ed., pp. 817–819). Philadelphia: J. B. Lippincott.

Price, R. W. (1999). Management of the neurologic complications of HIV-1 infection. In

M. A. Sande & P. A. Volberding (Eds.), *The medical management of AIDS* (6th ed., pp. 217–240). Philadelphia: W.B. Saunders.

Quale, J. M., Landman, D., Zaman, M. M., Burney, S., & Sathe, S. S. (1996). In vitro activity of *Cinnamomum zeylanicum* against azole resistant and sensitive *Candida* species and a pilot study of cinnamon for oral candidiasis. *American Journal of Chinese Medicine, 24,* 103–109.

Rabkin, J. G., Ferrando, S. J., Wagner, G. J., & Rabkin, R. (2000). DHEA treatment for HIV+ patients: Effects on mood, androgenic and anabolic parameters. *Psychoneuroimmunology, 25,* 53–68.

Rabkin, J. G., Wagner, G. J., & Rabkin, R. (1999). Fluoxetine treatment for depression in patients with HIV/AIDS: A randomized placebo controlled trial. *American Journal of Psychiatry, 156,* 101–107.

Reillo, M. R. (1993). Hyperbaric oxygen therapy for the treatment of debilitating fatigue associated with HIV/AIDS. *Journal of the Association of Nurses in AIDS Care, 4*(3), 33–38.

Rhodes, V. A., & McDaniel, R. W. (1997). Measuring nausea, vomiting and retching. In M. Frank-Stromborg & S. J. Olsen (Eds.), *Instruments for clinical health-care research* (2nd ed., pp. 509–518). Sudbury, MA: Jones & Bartlett.

Rondanelli, M., Solerte, S. B., Fioravanti, M., Scevola, D., Locatelli, M., Minoli, L., et al. (1997). Circadian secretory pattern of growth hormone, insulin-like growth factor type I, cortisol, adrenocorticotropic hormone, thyroid-stimulating hormone, and prolactin during HIV infection. *AIDS Research and Human Retroviruses, 13,* 1243–1249.

Rotblatt, M., & Ziment, I. (2002). *Evidence-based herbal medicine.* Philadelphia: Hanley & Belfus.

Rothenberg, S. (1997). Introduction to sleep disorders. In M. Pressman & W. Orr (Eds.), *Understanding sleep: The evaluation and treatment of sleep disorders* (pp. 57–72). Washington, DC: American Psychological Association.

Ryan, M. K., & Shattuck, A. D. (1994). *Treating AIDS with Chinese medicine.* Berkeley, CA: Pacific View Press.

Schutz, M., & Wendrow, A. (2002). *Quick reference guide to antiretrovirals.* Retrieved September 10, 2002, from http://www.gesidaseimc.com/inforvih/quick.pdf

Sehy, Y. B., & Williams, M. P. (1999). Functional assessment. In J. T. Stone, J. F. Wyman, & S. A. Salisbury (Eds.), *Clinical gerontological nursing: A guide to advanced practice* (2nd ed., pp. 175–199). Philadelphia: W.B. Saunders.

Sinnwell, T. M., Sivakumar, K., Soueidan, S., Jay, C., Frank, J. A., McLaughlin, A. C., et al. (1995). Metabolic abnormalities in skeletal muscle of patients receiving zidovudine therapy observed by ^{31}P in vivo magnetic resonance spectroscopy. *Journal of Clinical Investigation, 96,* 126–131.

Skurnick, J. H., Bogden, J. D., Baker, H., Kemp, F. W., Sheffet, A., Quattrone, G., et al. (1996). Micronutrient profiles in HIV-1-infected heterosexual adults. *Journal of Acquired Immune Deficiency Syndromes and Human Retrovirology, 2,* 75–83.

Stolarczyk, R., Rubio, S. I., Smolyar, D., Young, I. S., & Poretsky, L. (1998). Twenty-four-hour urinary free cortisol in patients with acquired immunodeficiency syndrome. *Metabolism, 47,* 690–694.

Stone, J. T., & Wyman, J. F. (1999). Falls. In J. T. Stone, J. F. Wyman, & S. A. Salisbury (Eds.), *Clinical gerontological nursing: A guide to advanced practice* (2nd ed., pp. 341–367). Philadelphia: W.B. Saunders.

Styrt, B., & Sugarman, B. (1990). Antipyresis and fever. *Archives of Internal Medicine, 150*(8), 1589–1597.

Swanson, B., & Keithley, J. K. (1998). Bioelectrical impedance analysis (BIA) in HIV infection: Principles and clinical application. *Journal of the Association of Nurses in AIDS Care, 9*(1), 49–54.

Taliaferro, D. (1996). *Monitoring fever patterns and hydration in hospitalized persons living with AIDS.* Paper presented at the Southern Nursing Research Society 10th Annual Research Conference, Miami, FL.

Terrado, M., Russell, C., & Bowman, J. B. (2001). Dysphagia: An overview. *MEDSURG Nursing, 10*(5), 233–250.

Ungvarski, P. J., & Trzcianowska, H. (2000). Neurocognitive disorders seen in HIV disease. *Issues in Mental Health Nursing, 21,* 51–70.

van Servellen, G., Sarna, L., & Jablonski, K. J. (1998). Women with HIV: Living with symptoms. *Western Journal of Nursing Research, 20,* 448–464.

Wagner, G. J., & Rabkin, R. (2000). Effects of dextroamphetamine on depression and fatigue in men with HIV: A double-blind, placebo-controlled trial. *Journal of Clinical Psychiatry, 61,* 436–440.

Wagner, G. J., Rabkin, J. G., & Rabkin, R. (1997). Dextroamphetamine as a treatment for depression and low energy in AIDS patients: A pilot study. *Journal of Psychosomatic Research, 42,* 407–411.

Wessely, S., Hotopf, M., & Sharpe, M. (1998). *Chronic fatigue and its syndromes.* Oxford, UK: Oxford University Press.

Williams, B., Waters, D., & Parker, K. (1999). Evaluation and treatment of weight loss in adults with HIV disease. *American Family Physician, 60*(3), 843–854.

Williams, M. P., & Salisbury, S. A. (1999). Cognitive assessment. In J. T. Stone, J. F. Wyman, & S. A. Salisbury (Eds.), *Clinical gerontological nursing: A guide to advanced practice* (2nd ed., pp. 129–154). Philadelphia: W. B. Saunders.

Wohl, D. A., Aweeka, F. T., Schmitz, J., Pomerantz, R., Cherng, D. W., Spritzler, J., et al. (2002). Safety, tolerability, and pharmacokinetic effects of thalidomide in patients infected with human immunodeficiency virus: AIDS clinical trials group 267. *The Journal of Infectious Diseases, 185,* 1359–1363.

World Health Organization. (1996). *Cancer pain relief* (2nd ed.). Geneva: Author.

Section V

Psychosocial Concerns of the HIV-Infected Adolescent and Adult and Their Significant Others

The preceding section focused on the physical responses to the HIV disease, yet we cannot forget that the psychosocial responses are equally important and in fact may be the etiology of many of the physical responses. This section begins with a discussion about how an HIV diagnosis affects individuals and their significant others. The effectiveness of the health care workers' responses might include an assessment of how the person's faith might influence the response; thus, this section is coupled with a beautifully written section on spiritual and religious concerns.

Response to infection can be abnormal or exacerbate baseline psychiatric disorders; thus, this section includes a discussion of common psychiatric complications. Psychiatric disorders may impair quality of life, affect disease progression, and impede treatment. Studies have shown that in patients with psychiatric disease, there is an increase in the likelihood of HIV transmission, either through high-risk behavior or via drug use, which is more prevalent in individuals with psychiatric disorders. This section represents a few of the many disorders that may be seen in the infected individual.

A. Responses to HIV Diagnosis

5.1 Response to an HIV Diagnosis: Infected Person

1. Initial diagnosis
   a. Shock is a common initial reaction. Communication between the patient and primary care provider may be distorted by shock. Encourage the patient to have someone present with the patient during office visits (Nichols, 1983).
   b. Anger can be directed at the diagnosis, the self, or others.
   c. Denial, disbelief, and emotional numbness may be significant enough that the patient will ignore the need for treatment or support. It is important to involve the patient in a supportive group, individual counseling, or in a nonthreatening, structured social activity (Nichols, 1983).
   d. The patient may experience guilt and be concerned with how lifestyle choices impacted his or her HIV status (Nichols, 1983).
   e. Blaming can be directed at self or others.
   f. The nurse must assess the degree of helplessness and hopelessness because these feelings can lead to suicidal ideation.
2. Transitional issues
   a. Relationships must be restructured with loved ones and families that have been altered by the HIV diagnosis (Nichols, 1985). This includes disclosure issues.
   b. The patient must face fear of death and fear of losing the ability to care for him or herself before being able to move into acceptance (Nichols, 1983).
   c. The patient may experience the loss of a job, an income, a home, or all three (Nichols, 1985). Loss of role also occurs (Murphy & Perry, 1988).
3. Acceptance
   a. Focus on living: Patients need to learn to appreciate quality rather than quantity in living and live in the present by celebrating each day (Nichols, 1985).
   b. Active participation in health care: Patients who are actively engaged in their care are more likely to adhere to their treatment plan and medication regimen (Remien & Rabkin, 2001; Roberts, 2002). Stress how health care can assist in living a quality life because antiretroviral therapy has changed the dynamics of the disease, transforming it to a chronic rather than fatal illness.
   c. Reengagement in relationships: It is important for patients to love and be loved throughout the course of the disease (Folkman, Chesney, & Christopher-Richards, 1994).
   d. Sexual functioning and decision making: Dilley, Woods, and McFarland (1997) showed that recent advances in treatment did not reduce the level of concern about infection or perception of risk of infection. Procreation will need to be discussed honestly between partners and negotiated (see Section 6.15, Pregnant Women, for options and concerns)
   e. Evaluation of spiritual beliefs (see Section 5.4)
   f. Rebound of strength and vitality through stability in clinical conditions forces individuals to face the issue of returning to the workforce. This is an effort to master the uncertainty of a chronic illness and restore order in the face of a continued life threat (Rait, 1991).

5.2 Response to HIV Diagnosis: Family and Significant Other

1. Definitions/description
   a. Given the range of family constellations represented by people with HIV infection, a broad definition of family must be used to include both family of origin and family of choice, whether related biologically or legally or not related.
   b. HIV infection presents as a major life transition that is out of sequence with what is expected. Critical points in HIV disease for alterations in family functioning include diagnosis of HIV or AIDS, first hospitalization, first opportunistic infection, new symptoms, recurrences or relapses, and terminal stage of disease.
   c. Alteration in family function occurs when the family is unable to:

- Adapt constructively to crisis or stress
- Communicate openly among family members
- Perform activities associated with family function (e.g., socialization, personal security, acceptance, companionship, and provision of physical necessities, such as food, clothing, shelter, and health care)
- Seek or accept help appropriately

2. Etiology
   a. Similar to risk factors for family/caregiver burden
3. Goals of care
   a. Recognize a family in crisis that needs intervention.
   b. Support the family's adaptation to living with a life-threatening illness of one of its members in a manner that seems appropriate for the particular family.
   c. Identify resources that will support the family and individual members of the family to manage the demands of the loved one's illness.
4. Assessment (Carpentino, 2000)
   a. Family composition
   b. Family strengths
   c. Family rules/discipline
   d. Financial status
   e. Participation in community activities
   f. Family process
   g. Family communication patterns
   h. Family's emotional/supportive pattern (those that are both constructive and destructive)
5. Interventions (Carpentino, 2000)
   a. Acknowledge causative and contributing factors (e.g., sudden illness, hospitalization).
   b. Acknowledge your feelings about the family and their situation.
   c. Provide ongoing information.
   d. Promote cohesiveness.
   e. Discuss the implications for caring for ill family members.

5.3 Caregiver Burden/Strain

1. Definitions/description
   a. There is no consistent, agreed-upon definition of caregiver burden.
   b. The terms *burden* and *strain* have been used interchangeably in the literature to describe the impact of caregiving.
   c. The prevalence is unknown but expected to increase as more people are living with HIV and the trend is moving toward home care.
   d. Signs and symptoms that caregiver burden/strain is present include the following:
      i. Anxiety, fear, and depression: These feelings are common for partners and significant others and are increased in partners who are also HIV infected.
      ii. Disrupted relationships: Person with HIV may have been an important source of support for the partner or spouse, leaving the caregiver feeling unappreciated and discouraged (Turner, Pearlin, & Mullan, 1998).
      iii. Conflicts: Problems can occur with friends and family over caregiving issues as well as with the patient (Turner et al., 1998).
      iv. Grief: Feelings of grief occur throughout the process of illness progression, both for the caregiver and the patient (Folkman, Chesney, & Christopher-Richards, 1994).
2. Etiology
   a. Illness characteristics include severe illness, sudden onset of illness, and manifestations of new symptoms.
   b. Caregiver variables
      i. Gender: Women tend to show higher levels of distress than do men.
      ii. Age: Depending on age, the caregiver may not have had previous caregiving roles (Matheny, Mehr, & Brown, 1997).
      iii. Socioeconomic status and economic burdens: Financial issues can precipitate strain and abuse.
      iv. Other life stressors such as poor health of caregiver or other member of family: Thirty-five percent of families report having several family members (sibling,

Figure 5.3a   Assessment of Social Support

Name, Address, Phone Number	Relationship Relative, Friend, Neighbor, Work Associate	Emotional Closeness High, Medium, Low	Perceived Willingness to Help High, Medium, Low	Types of Support Possible Emotional, Informational, Instrumental	Perceived Ability to Help High, Medium, Low
Jane Doe 123 Friend St. 348-6769	Friend	High	High	Informational	Low

husband, or extended family member) infected with HIV (Fiore et al., 2001).

  v. Other variables: (Ruppert, 1996)

  - Relationship communication style
  - Family developmental stage
  - Social support; see Figure 5.3a for assessment of social support

c. The unrelenting nature of caring for a person with a debilitating condition

d. The vast array and large number of service organizations and providers with whom the caregivers must interact

e. Financial constraints

f. Isolation from friends, family, community

g. Fear of contagion

h. Multiple losses, such as possible death of a loved one, a lifestyle, and a future

i. Pervasive uncertainty about the meaning of the symptoms, the future of caregiving, and strategies to provide the best care

3. Goals of care

a. Enhance the quality of life for both the caregiver and the recipient of care.

b. Prevent illness, disability, and psychiatric and physical morbidity of the caregiver

4. Assessment

a. Risk factors and etiologies

b. Caregivers' subjective perception of tasks they perform

  i. How easy or difficult is each task?

  ii. To what extent does caregiving cause strain with regard to work, finances, social life, and emotional and physical status?

  iii. Are there resultant depression, anxiety, and changes in caregiver's health status? Fatigue is common as demands of caregiving can be relentless.

5. Interventions

a. The nurse works in partnership with the people with AIDS and the caregiver to provide appropriate care (Ramirez, Addington-Hall & Richards, 1998).

  i. Validate the importance of the caregiver's role, their commitment to PWA, and their knowledge base related to caregiving.

ii. Discuss strategies the caregiver can use to interact with health care providers to secure high-quality care for the loved one.

b. Teach universal precautions and basic nursing skills as necessary.

c. Assist caregivers to find meaning in their caregiving experiences by asking, "What does caregiving mean to you?" and "What has caregiving been like for you?"

d. Explore the caregiver's strengths and weaknesses.

e. Discuss the goals of caregiving as perceived by the caregiver.

f. Refer to community services (e.g., caregiver courses, counseling, support groups, respite care services, home care) as needed.

g. Discuss feelings associated with possibility of deciding to institutionalize the ill person or end caregiving role and assist the caregiver in problem solving.

h. Provide information about the disease process, the expected course of illness, diagnostic tests, medical treatments, and symptom management as appropriate with interpretation of new symptoms and manifestations of illness, particularly changes in PWA's mental status.

i. Facilitate problem solving related to treatment decisions.

j. Refer for case management services to assist in coordinating care.

k. Discuss coping options. Encourage caregiver to take each day as it comes, let go of what is not important, put the future on hold, and cherish special moments and time spent with loved ones.

l. Discuss importance of the caregiver taking care of self through health-promotion activities, especially if the caregiver is HIV positive.
  i. Stress-reduction techniques
  ii. Proper nutrition and adequate rest/sleep
  iii. Maintenance of activity and exercise patterns and taking time-out periods
  iv. Avoidance of substance use/abuse

m. Assist in mobilizing resources to help in caregiving activities. Role-play asking for help.

n. Discuss, in conjunction with the PWA, health care durable power of attorney and living will. Refer for legal assistance if necessary.

o. Discuss uncertainty related to caregiving, its sources and manifestations, and ways to manage or accept it.

p. Discuss how the caregiver can promote the PWA's sense of autonomy and independence.

q. Encourage the caregiver to discuss relationship difficulties with PWA.

r. Facilitate caregivers' ability to provide care when PWA is hospitalized.

5.4 Spiritual and Religious Concerns of HIV-Infected Persons

1. Definitions/description
   a. Spirituality: the essence of our being, which shapes our life journey and permeates our living and infuses our unfolding awareness of who and what we are, our purpose in being, and our inner resources (Burkhardt & Nagai Jacobson, 2000, p. 91)
   b. Spiritual wellness: a way of living a lifestyle that views and lives life as purposeful and pleasurable, that seeks out life-sustaining and life-enriching options to be chosen freely at every opportunity and that sinks its roots deeply into spiritual values and/or specific religious beliefs (Pilch, 1998, p. 28)
   c. Spiritual distress: the disruption in the life principle that pervades a person's entire being and that integrates and transcends one's biological and psychosocial nature (North American Nursing Diagnosis Association, 1994). Spiritual distress can manifest itself as guilt, recriminations and self-blame, hyper-religiosity, rejection of significant others, and expressions of despair (Wilson & Kneisl, 1992, p. 600). Although not all individuals identify with a religion or particular belief in a deity, all of humanity is seeking meaning and acceptance.

2. Etiology
   a. Sources of spirituality
      i. Faith tradition of origin or new spiritual journey or practices
      ii. Community, family, and culture

      iii. Love, hope, justice, and forgiveness

      iv. Distant healing/distant prayer (Dossey, 1996; Sicher, Targ, Moore & Smith, 1998)

      v. Peaceful resolve about end of life

  b. Issues affecting spiritual wellness

      i. Anger, shame, guilt, or powerlessness

      ii. Uncertainty and distrust

      iii. Betrayal or forgiveness of self or others

      iv. Loss of perceived future, body image, and relationships

      v. Suffering, anguish, apprehension, and isolation

      vi. Anticipating death or further losses, despair, or hopelessness

      vii. Rejection by family or community (homophobia, intolerance of substance abusers, etc.)

      viii. Chronic illness or mental illness

3. Goal of care

  a. To assist individuals in accessing spiritual resources and maintaining spiritual wellness

      i. All individuals seek meaning to their life and an understanding of devastating predicaments.

      ii. When the self is challenged physically or emotionally, spiritual distress may occur.

      iii. Nurses have the capacity, with nonjudgmental care, to assist patients in drawing on their own spiritual strengths.

4. Assessment

  a. Belief systems, desired spiritual practices, level of connection to a spiritual community

      i. Does the individual belong to a faith tradition or hold particular spiritual beliefs?

      ii. How does the individual draw spiritual strength and with whom? Does patient still experience passion, beauty, or joy?

      iii. How does the individual view God (Allah, Jehovah, Buddha, Great Spirit) or higher power—as a comforter or persecutor? How does the individual feel God sees him or her (Green, Fullilove, & Fullilove, 1998; Williamson, 1998)?

      iv. How does the individual explain life circumstance and illness? Does the individual rely on specific spiritual tenets during times of duress? Is the individual agnostic or atheist?

  b. Indications of spiritual distress (e.g., shame, alienation, unresolved or prolonged anger, inability to consider forgiveness of self/others)

  c. Degree of self-worth/self-esteem

  d. Impact of culture, family, and environment on spiritual beliefs and practices

5. Interventions

  a. Establish a caring, supportive presence.

  b. Include family, significant others, community, and beloved pets in care plans, as appropriate.

  c. Listen with a nonjudgmental ear.

  d. Explore the meaning of illness and how it has affected the individual's self-concept, connections to others, and so on.

  e. Educate self about unfamiliar religions (e.g., Wicca, Santeria), cultural practices, and belief systems (Cantrell, 2001).

  f. Assess degree of hope or despair, anger or alienation.

  g. Refer for psychotherapy if symptoms of depression, anxiety, hopelessness, unremitting anger, guilt, or shame persist.

  h. Encourage self-forgiveness and celebrations of life.

  i. If assisted suicide is requested (assisted suicide is not legal in most states), evaluate patient's reasoning, mental status, and plans. Assess for situations that can impair judgment, including severe depression, compromised mental status, and uncontrolled pain (the major tenet of assisted suicide is patient autonomy; Crock, 1998; Saunders, 2000, 2001).

  j. Reframe self-esteem in light of changes in body image and relationships.

  k. Provide links to pastoral counselors, community programs, vocational training, and volunteerism.

  l. When guilt or shame is present, do the following:

    • Remind individuals that HIV is a medical problem, not a moral issue.

Figure 5.4a   Spirituality: An Integrated Perspective

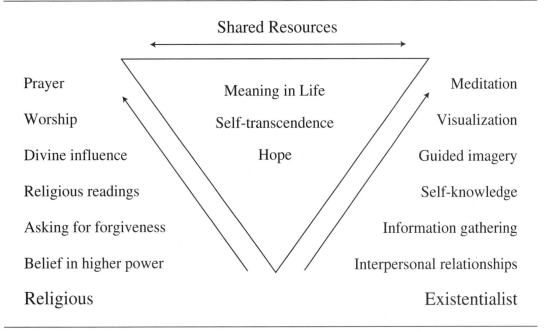

Shared Resources

Prayer

Worship

Divine influence

Religious readings

Asking for forgiveness

Belief in higher power

Religious

Meaning in Life

Self-transcendence

Hope

Meditation

Visualization

Guided imagery

Self-knowledge

Information gathering

Interpersonal relationships

Existentialist

SOURCE: McCormick et al., 2001

- Provide an outlet for verbalizing shame and shameful behaviors.
- Remind individual that sometimes bad things happen to good people (Kushner, 1981) and that HIV is not retribution for falling short of values or ideals.
- Refer to pastoral counselor, confessor, or psychotherapy if guilt is unremitting.

m. Listen for signs of grief, present or unresolved.

n. In cases of impending death, assist patient with good-byes (wills, video legacies, letters, making peace with self and God). Include cultural or personal preferences (e.g., Hindus may prefer dying on the floor close to earth, and Muslims may elect to die facing east toward Mecca; Galanti, 1997; Hall, 1998; Lyon, Townsend-Akpan, & Thompson, 2001).

o. Instill hope and acceptance.
  i. As appropriate, employ touch; even minimal contact implies acceptance.

ii. Discuss what the patient hopes for (e.g., a cure, more time, a reconciliation).

iii. Assess for hopelessness, which is frequently a symptom of depression (see Section 5.5).

iv. Inquire about what brings individual comfort or joy (e.g., music, friends, family, nature, prayer, meditation, yoga or exercise, service to others).

v. Determine which spiritual practices or beliefs provide meaning to life, hope, and transcendence to individual (see Figure 5.4a; Hall; 1998; McCormick, Holder, Wetsel, & Cawthon, 2001).

p. Engage in prayer, meditation, or rituals with patient, as mutual comfort levels and appropriateness dictate.

q. Facilitate patient's involvement in meaningful spiritual practices and outlets, such as worship, meditation, yoga, healing oils, aromatherapy, imagery, and Therapeutic Touch (Buckle, 2002; Foster, 1999).

r. Work for justice, locally and internationally, in accessing appropriate medical care, pain control, medications, and housing.

B. SELECTED PSYCHIATRIC DISORDERS IN HIV DISEASE

5.5 Depression

1. Definitions/description
   a. A mood disorder characterized by symptoms that persist over a minimum of a 2-week period. A person must have at least five of the nine symptoms, one of which must be a depressed mood or loss of interest or pleasure. These symptoms cannot be accounted for by bereavement, a general medical illness, medications, or alcohol/drug use. The presence of these symptoms results in significant impairment in social and occupational function. The other symptoms include feelings of guilt, suicidal thoughts, sleep disturbance, appetite/weight changes, attention/concentration changes, energy level changes or fatigue, and psychomotor disturbance/slowing (American Psychiatric Association, 2000a).
   b. *DSM-IV* includes the following illnesses or disorders of mood or affect: major depressive disorder, either single episode or recurrent; dysthymic disorder (mood disorder lasting more than 2 years); bipolar disorders; cyclothymic disorder; schizoaffective psychosis; mood disorders secondary to medical conditions; substance-induced mood disorder, with depressed mood or with mixed anxiety and depressed mood (American Psychiatric Association, 2000b; Cabaj, 1996).
   c. Bereavement is not considered a major depressive episode, although symptoms are similar unless these symptoms persist more than 2 months. Normal grief generally lasts more than 6 months and is considered a self-limiting condition (Bonanno & Kaltman, 1999).
   d. HIV-infected persons have a two- to fourfold increase in depressive disorders (Morrison et al., 2002). Rates of depressive disorders range between 2–35% in HIV-infected individuals (Bing et al., 2001; Morrison et al., 2002; New York State Department of Health AIDS Institute, 2001). One study of non-substance-abusing participants had depressive disorder rates of 19% for HIV seropositive women versus 5% in a matched HIV seronegative group (Morrison et al., 2002).
   e. Depression increases with disease progression. Rates of major depressive disorder were 2–11% in asymptomatic HIV-infected and 4–18% in symptomatic HIV-infected persons globally (Morrison et al., 2002).
   f. Compared with men with HIV infection, women with HIV infection have higher rates of depressive disorders.

2. Etiology
   a. Genetic: Depression seems to run in some families.
   b. Biological: It is thought to be caused by an imbalance of neurotransmitters, especially norepinephrine, serotonin, and dopamine.
   c. Social and psychological factors: Depression may be triggered by adverse early life events, intrapsychic conflicts, or reactions to life events (i.e., stressors).
   d. Complex psychobiological syndrome is most probable because depression appears to be caused by multiple factors, including some medications.
   e. Medications such as interferon, used for the treatment of hepatitis C or antihypertensives such as clonidine, reserpine and methyldopa (rarely with angiotensin converting enzyme inhibitors)
   f. Chronic illnesses, including disease progression, increase depression.
   g. Substance abuse and alcoholism can cause depression.

3. Goals of care
   a. To reduce symptoms of depression to improve functioning
   b. To help patient learn a more effective coping style

c. Increase hope and optimism, which can lead to more active involvement in care

d. Establish a positive outlook, which research links with improved immune response

e. Increase potential to adhere to medical regimen

4. Assessment
   a. Mental status
      i. Appearance: Lack of self-care may be evident. Patient may exhibit poor eye contact.
      ii. Mood and affect: Patient is depressed or irritable, with sad or blunted affect.
      iii. Cognition: Patient displays poor attention and concentration, which may result in impaired learning ability and short-term memory.
      iv. Thought processes: Themes of guilt, self-deprecation, and worthlessness are common.
      v. Perception: Patient may have distorted perception. The person may perceive everything as bad or their fault. Hallucinations and delusions may present in persons with severe depression.
   b. Tools can be used to differentiate between depression and neurocognitive changes (seen with AIDS, including dementia, prior neurologic assaults, and substance abuse; Herfkens, 2001) and major depression and other mental disorders.
      i. Global Assessment of Functioning (GAF) considers overall psychological, social, and occupational functioning (Hilsenroth et al., 2000).
      ii. PRIME-MD screens for somatoform, depressive, anxiety, eating, and alcohol disorders. The PHQ is the self-administered version of this tool (Spitzer, Kroenke, Williams, & the Patient Health Questionnaire Primary Care Study Group, 1999).
   c. Cognitive assessment tools include the following:
      i. Folstein Mini Mental State Examination (MMSE) is available for a quick cognitive screen for cortical signs. The instrument can be found at www.nemc.org/case1199/index.shtml or www.emedicine.com/splash/etools_xml.pl
      ii. The Johns Hopkins HIV Dementia Scale tests memory-registration, attention, psychomotor speed, memory recall, and constructional abilities in a short, easy to administer format. It is available at www.iapac.org (Power & Selnes, 1996).
   d. Depression assessment tools include the following
      i. Hamilton Depression Rating Scale (HAM-D) is one of the oldest with best-known rating scales (Andreasen & Black, 2001).
      ii. Goldberg Depression Scale is available at www.psychcentral.com/depinv.htm
      iii. PRIME-MD screens for somatoform, depressive, anxiety, eating, and alcohol disorders. The PHQ is the self-administered version of this tool (Spitzer et al., 1999).
      iv. Center for Epidemiologic Studies Depression Scale (CES-D) is a short 20-question Likert-type scale developed by L. Radloff at the National Institutes of Health (NIH) and is commonly used to assess depression in HIV. It is Available at www.hivcorrections.org (Hefkens, 2001).
   e. Suicidality assessment
      i. Assess for presence of ideation, plan, lethality of method, and ability to carry out the plan.
      ii. Degree of depression is significant. Suicide occurs in the middle range of depression, when the patient still feels hopeless but can mobilize energy to act.
      iii. Signs of suicidal thoughts include sadness, downcast facial expression, slumped posture, and slowed movement.
      iv. Symptoms of suicidality include feelings of sadness, reports of feeling empty or hopeless, sleep or

appetite disturbance, inability to experience pleasure in activities that the person found pleasurable, and fatigue or lack of energy.

v. Neuropsychiatric testing can assist in diagnosis.

vi. Suicidality requires immediate psychiatric intervention in the presence of symptoms/etiology. There is a 15% risk of death by suicide in patients who have been previously hospitalized for depression (Andreasen & Black, 2001).

vii. Differentiate from rational suicide when terminally ill. Nurses must examine their own beliefs and philosophies regarding this issue (Fontana, 2002). The American Nurses Association (ANA) and ANAC provide guidelines in this area

5. Interventions

a. Nonpharmacological interventions

i. Depressed individuals experience varied emotions, such as unworthiness. Staff must be able to provide support that can help decrease the patient's sense of loss and promote feelings of being accepted and cared for.

ii. Individual or group support, professional or peer facilitated, can decrease feelings of isolation. Encourage social and community activities to decrease behaviors that create environments that maintain negative self-views.

iii. Determine risk of patient inflicting self-harm.

iv. Provide appropriate coping and social skills training.

v. Provide grief counseling if appropriate.

vi. Monitor and educate the patient regarding purpose and side effects of medications and ways to manage them (see discussion later in this section).

vii. Consider cultural variations in expression of depressed feelings.

(1) Culturally appropriate affects range from open, demonstrative expression to stoicism.

(2) The expression of depression is not a reliable indicator of the degree of feeling.

viii. Provide education and support to significant others.

(1) Understanding by nurturing the patient and encouraging independence can help support the patient.

(2) Patients who have the support of friends and family tend to cope better with their illnesses.

(3) Dealing with illness and concern about mortality of loved one can cause sadness, anger, and ambivalence.

(4) Support groups can decrease feelings of isolation and help in working out feelings and problem solving.

ix. Refer for psychotherapy. Psychotherapy modalities used to treat depression include interpersonal psychotherapy, cognitive-behavioral psychotherapy, and behavioral therapy (Goldman, Wise, & Brody, 1998).

x. Herbal supplements such as St. John's wort (hypericum perforatum) should not be used with protease inhibitors (PIs) or non-nucleoside reverse transcriptase inhibitors (NNRTIs) because it may result in suboptimal antiretroviral drug concentrations (New York State Department of Health AIDS Institute, 2001).

xi. Encourage a balanced diet to offset depletion in essential elements and vitamins. Folate (folic acid) may enhance antidepressants, especially in women (Goodwin, 2001).

xii. Alternative modalities such as body work, therapeutic touch, and acupuncture may be beneficial.

xiii. Encourage exercise for mild depression.
b. Pharmacologic
  i. Selective serotonin reuptake inhibitors (SSRIs)
    (1) SSRIs (fluoxetine, paroyetine, citalopram, escitalopram) are a first-line choice because they are relatively safe and well tolerated, with fewer drug interactions, including having the least effect on hepatic enzymes.
    (2) Most troubling side effect of SSRIs is sexual dysfunction, which can be managed with dose reductions, drug holidays, or switching to another drug in the same class. Other side effects include headache, irritability/agitation, nausea, difficulty sleeping, and dry mouth.
    (3) SSRIs should be used with caution in patients taking PIs and NNRTIs because these drugs inhibit the cytochrome $_p450$ isoenzymes and lead to accumulation of the SSRI. They also interact with hormonal therapies, such as contraceptives (New York State Department of Health AIDS Institute, 2001).
  ii. Atypical antidepressant medications (bupropion, mirtazapine, nefazodone, venlafaxine) are relatively safe and well tolerated, with the exception of buproprion, which has hepatic concerns. Caution should be used in patients taking NNRTIs or PIs because this regimen may lead to an increased level of antidepressant (New York State Department of Health AIDS Institute, 2001).
  iii. Psychostimulants (methyphenidate, dextroamphetamine)
    (1) Psychostimulants are the most effective, rapid-acting antidepressant for HIV-infected patient. They are the first choice for people suffering from AIDS who also have low energy and mild neurocognitive deficits, such as dementia.
    (2) For individuals in recovery from substance abuse, this may not be a good choice because pscyhostimulants have very addictive qualities. It is contraindicated for patients who abuse amphetamines. Other antidepressants are safe to use for individuals with substance abuse issues.
    (3) Side effects include insomnia, paranoia, and psychosis. Use with caution with patients with seizure disorders.
  iv. Tricyclics antidepressants (TCAs)
    (1) TCAs (amitriptyline, desipramine, nortriptyline) are infrequently used due to significant anticholinergic side effects and should not be used in conjunction with other anticholinergic medications.
    (2) TCAs can be lethal in overdose. Assess suicidal ideation regularly.
    (3) Use with PIs or NNRTIs can lead to increased levels of antidepressant (New York State Department of Health AIDS Institute, 2001).
    (4) Side effects include drowsiness, dry mouth, blurred vision, and constipation.
  v. Specific mood stabilizers for the treatment of bipolar disorders
    (1) Valproate (valproic acid)
      (a) Metabolic pathway is not fully known but agent is associated with hepatotoxicity (American Psychiatric Association, 2000a; New York State Department of Health AIDS Institute, 2001).
      (b) Divalproex sodium, another available preparation of valproate,

is better tolerated than valproic acid due to fewer gastrointestinal side effects, and it can be dosed less frequently (American Psychiatric Association, 2000a).

(2) Lithium is used commonly in HIV patients with primary bipolar disorder (American Psychiatric Association, 2000a).

  (a) Clinical experience suggests that lithium use should be avoided in patients with probable AIDS mania or advanced HIV disease due to risk of toxicity (American Psychiatric Association, 2000a).

  (b) Use caution with patients with HIV-related nephropathy because illness can cause decreased lithium clearance and possible lithium toxicity (American Psychiatric Association, 2000a).

(3) Carbamazepine is used less commonly due to potential to cause bone marrow suppression (American Psychiatric Association, 2000a).

5.6 Primary Anxiety-Spectrum Disorders

1. Definitions/description (American Psychiatric Association, 2002)
   a. Generalized anxiety disorder (GAD): A mood disorder characterized by an excessive uncomfortable feeling of dread, apprehension, and worry, which impairs the person's ability to function. This is the most common anxiety disorder.
   b. Panic disorder and agoraphobia are "extreme, overwhelming form[s] of anxiety often experienced when an individual is placed in a real or perceived life-threatening situation" (Boyd, 2002, p. 454). The feeling is so overwhelming that the person fears having another panic attack. It is common in viral syndromes, cocaine abuse, and recreational drug use.
   c. Social phobia and other phobias
   d. Obsessive-compulsive disorder (OCD)
   e. Posttraumatic stress disorder (PTSD) is a response to significant life trauma from a variety of sources, including interpersonal violence, multiple AIDS-related losses, or notification of an HIV test. Symptoms include nightmares, intrusive thoughts and flashbacks, and poor self-care, including HIV management. It occurs twice as often in women.
   f. Acute stress disorder
   g. Anxiety disorder due to medical conditions
      i. Primary psychiatric disorders that have anxiety symptoms include HIV infection, adjustment disorders, depressive disorders, alcohol and other substance abuse, and bereavement.
      ii. Medical disorders that include anxiety symptoms include fever, dehydration, opportunistic central nervous system (CNS) diseases, neurosyphilis, respiratory conditions, endocrinopathies, metabolic complications, cardiovascular disease, and hyperventilation syndrome.
      iii. Neuropsychiatric disorders that contribute to anxiety include neurocognitive disorders (HIV-associated dementia and minor cognitive motor disorder) and delirium.
      iv. Medications that can contribute to anxiety include acyclovir, antiretrovirals (e.g., efavirenz), corticosteroids, isoniazid, interferons, interleukin-2, and pentamidine. Psychotropic medications (e.g., selective serotonin reuptake inhibitors, e.g., venlafaxine, bupropion; psychostimulants, neuroleptics) can have the side effect of anxiety. Polypharmacy can also contribute to anxiety.

v. Many commonly and not so commonly used substances can also contribute to anxiety. These include alcohol, amphetamines, benzodiazepines, caffeine, cocaine, ecstasy, gamma-hydroxybutyrate (GHB), ketamine, opiates, and nicotine.

vi. Normal anxiety from such things as bereavement is not considered a criterion for anxiety disorder.

h. It is estimated that 2% to 40% of HIV-infected persons have an anxiety disorder (American Psychiatric Association, 2002).

i. It is the most common mental health issue encountered in primary care settings.

j. Anxiety disorders are common throughout the spectrum of HIV infection. HIV-related anxiety is common with milestones such as HIV testing; news of HIV-positive status; appearance of first symptoms; declining CD_4 counts; increasing viral loads; onset of AIDS-defining illness; initiation of antiretroviral therapy (ART); onset of functional or cognitive disabilities, including multisystem medical conditions; negotiation of new sexual life; disclosure of HIV status; chronic pain; and end-of-life preparation.

2. Etiology

a. Genetic or familial tendencies

b. Biological factors: Thought that limbic system mediates general anxiety, worry, and vigilance. Gamma-aminobutyric acid (GABA), serotonin, and neuropeptides appear to have a role in the regulation of anxiety.

c. Social and psychological factors: Cognitive-behavioral theory postulates that anxiety stems from an inaccurate assessment of perceived environmental dangers. Psychoanalytic theory proposes that anxiety results from unresolved unconscious conflicts. Many HIV-infected persons have sexual orientation issues, a history of incarceration or interpersonal violence that contributes to high levels of anxiety, chronic and acute, or both. Poor social support and maladaptive coping strategies contribute to anxiety triggers.

d. Effects of medications (see previous discussion)

e. May be seen with drug and alcohol intoxication and withdrawal

3. Goals of care

a. Reduce patient's level of discomfort.

b. Help patient identify source of anxiety.

c. Assist patient in developing alternative ways of coping.

4. Assessment

a. History

i. Tools useful in evaluating anxiety

(1) The Structured Clinical Interview for *DSM-III-R* Non-Patient Version-HIV (SCID-NP-HIV) excludes HIV-related worries but has a module for diagnosing HIV-specific adjustment disorders.

(2) The Modified Hamilton Anxiety Rating Scale (some somatic anxiety symptoms are omitted) can also be useful.

ii. Gather information specific to presenting symptoms.

iii. Obtain a thorough past medical, psychiatric, social history (recent stressful events including homelessness, loss of loved one or job, incarceration, interpersonal violence), and family history.

iv. Assess for underlying medical conditions and substances (prescription, over-the-counter, illicit drugs, herbals) that could cause or exacerbate anxiety.

v. Assess level of stress including suicidality.

vi. Assess past history of interpersonal violence including sexual abuse.

b. Physical signs

i. Autonomic/somatic symptoms can mimic medical conditions: shortness of breath and palpitations, chronic abdominal pain without pathology, gastrointestinal (GI) symptoms, and central and peripheral nervous systems. Sympathetic nervous system response includes increased heart rate, increased blood pressure, and constricted pupils.

ii. Physical symptoms can also indicate anxiety: muscle tension, worried facial expression, tingling hands or feet, hand wringing, tremors or twitching, restlessness, GI disturbance, chest pain, palpitations, headache, shortness of breath, lightheadedness and dizziness, faintness, dry mouth, and increased motor activity.

c. Psychological symptoms: worry, unexplained feeling of discomfort, difficulty with concentration, preoccupation with self, and complaints of chronic fatigue or lack of energy.

5. Interventions
   a. Nonpharmacological
      i. Supportive therapy
         (1) Express empathy.
         (2) Reassure patient about cause of physical symptoms of anxiety.
         (3) Identify patients' strengths and weaknesses.
         (4) Teach patients simple relaxation exercises, such as diaphragmatic breathing, meditation, self-hypnosis, and imagery (American Psychiatric Association, 2002; New York State Department of Health AIDS Institute, 2001).
      ii. Electromyographic biofeedback, acupuncture, Therapeutic Touch
      iii. Aerobic exercise
      iv. Coping strategies, such as goal setting, information seeking, skill mastery, or help seeking
      v. Cognitive-behavioral therapy (Goldman, Wise, & Brody, 1998). Exposure techniques can also be used by experienced therapists for panic disorder.
      vi. Peer support groups that are gender and culturally appropriate can provide basic information to reduce anxiety from knowledge deficit.
      vii. Consider cultural variations in expression of anxiety. Use language and interventions that are culturally appropriate and meaningful to the patient

   b. Pharmacological
      i. Buspirone: used for patients with persistent anxiety. Helpful for patients with anxiety and a history of substance abuse because there is no potential for abuse (American Psychiatric Association, 2002; New York State Department of Health AIDS Institute, 2001). Due to the mechanism of action, the onset of action of buspirone takes 3 to 6 weeks, so benzodiazepine may be used concurrently and then tapered. It is contraindicated with MAO inhibitors and has no anxiolytic effects (American Psychiatric Association, 2002).
      ii. Benzodiazepines: Although most commonly used for anxiety, use with caution due to potential for physical and psychological dependence. Cytochrome $_P450$ inhibition may have drug-to-drug interactions with protease inhibitors (New York State Department of Health AIDS Institute, 2001).
      iii. Selective serotonin reuptake inhibitors (SSRIs) can be used as a first- or second-line treatment for generalized anxiety disorder and are particularly helpful for social phobia, panic disorder, OCD, PTSD, and GAD (American Psychiatric Association, 2002; New York State Department of Health AIDS Institute, 2001). Nefazadone may be helpful for agitated depression and anxiety disorders because of its antianxiety properties; however, it is a potent inhibitor of cytochrome $_P4503A$.
      iv. Antidepressants may be helpful. Venlafaxine for GAD has few drug interactions with HIV medications (American Psychiatric Association, 2002). SSRIs are effective for many anxiety disorders, including social phobias, OCD, and GAD.

5.7 Delirium

1. Definitions/description
   a. Characterized by disturbance of consciousness and a change in cognition that develops over a short period of time and is caused by the direct physiologic consequences of a medical condition
   b. Prevalence: most common neuropsychiatric complication in hospitalized AIDS patients (New York State Department of Health AIDS Institute, 2001)
   c. Patients at high risk for developing delirium: those in advanced stages of immunosuppression; those with a history of opportunistic infections, substance use, or head or brain injury; those with previous episodes of delirium or dementia; or those with infection or malignancies of the central nervous system (CNS; New York State Department of Health AIDS Institute, 2001)
2. Etiology
   a. Single or multiple simultaneous etiologies may be present.
   b. Toxic causes are related to medications, alternative or complementary therapies, or drug or alcohol intoxication/withdrawal. Newly introduced medications should be high on the list of differential diagnoses.
   c. Metabolic causes include electrolyte disturbances, endocrine disorders, hypoxia, fever, and renal or liver insufficiency.
   d. Infectious causes include cryptococcal or toxoplasmosis encephalitis.
   e. Vascular causes include congestive heart failure, cerebrovascular accidents, and anemia.
   f. Neurologic causes include encephalopathy, CNS malignancies and infections, seizures, and postictal state.
   g. Psychiatric causes include severe depression and mania.
3. Goals of care
   a. Swiftly recognize and treat underlying cause(s).
   b. Apply appropriate therapies to reverse or control symptoms.
   c. Prevent injury to patient and others.

4. Assessment
   a. A sudden change in mental status warrants immediate nursing intervention with referral for emergency evaluation.
   b. Level of alertness may vary from agitation to lethargy, stupor, or coma.
   c. Patients are generally drowsy and may require repeated explanations from caregivers and examiners.
   d. Abrupt disturbances in sleep patterns or changes in level of activity should raise suspicions.
   e. Early signs and symptoms of delirium may be inaccurately attributed to anxiety.
   f. Clinical manifestations of delirium in patients with HIV include the following:

   - Impairment of memory, orientation, prefrontal executive functions: difficulty with abstraction, difficulty with sequential thinking, impaired temporal memory, impaired judgment
   - Disturbances in thought and language with decreased verbal frequency
   - Disturbances in perception: visual hallucinations and paranoid delusions
   - Disturbances in psychomotor function: hypoactive, hyperactive, or mixed
   - Disturbances in the sleep-wake cycle with daytime lethargy, nighttime agitation
   - Affective lability: rapidly changes from one emotional state to another
   - Neurologic abnormalities: tremors, myoclonus, asterixis, nystagmus, ataxia, cranial nerve palsies and cerebellar signs (New York State Department of Health AIDS Institute, 2001)

   g. Interview caregiver and observe patient to assess functional status, medications, substance use, other new clinical signs and symptoms, and any history of delirium or precipitating event.
5. Interventions
   a. Nonpharmacological
      i. Correct underlying conditions that have led to delirium, such as metabolic abnormalities, sepsis,

hypoxemia, anemia, CNS infections and malignancies, antiretroviral therapies, opioids, and illicit substance use (New York State Department of Health AIDS Institute, 2001).

ii. Provide safe and consistent environment and increase supervision of patient as indicated.

iii. Institute appropriate treatment for causative condition, monitor patient's response, and report adverse effects of treatment.

iv. Communicate in clear, simple terms to avoid misperceptions.

v. Educate patient, family, and significant other regarding care and diagnostic procedures, medications given and expected effects, and the need to orient the patient to person, time, place, and situation.

vi. Consult with provider if patient is at risk for endangering self or others to determine need for restraints.

vii. Ensure patient's activities of daily living are met.

viii. Attempt to organize care to ensure patient's nighttime sleep is undisturbed.

ix. Evaluate patient/caregiver resources for continuing care when hospitalization is no longer required.

x. If patient does not sleep through the night, nighttime help or temporary placement may be necessary until the patient's sleep and activity needs are reestablished.

b. Pharmacologic
   i. Low doses of neuroleptics, such as haloperidol (Haldol) or risperidone (Risperdal) to treat confusion or agitation

5.8 Mental Illness and Substance Use

1. Definitions/description
   a. Dual diagnosis refers to the cooccurrence of mental health disorders and substance abuse disorders (alcohol or drug dependence or abuse, or both).

b. Dual diagnosis and dual/multiple disorders profiles may include the following:

- Severe/major mental illness and a substance disorder(s)
- Substance disorder(s) and personality disorder(s)
- Substance disorder(s), personality disorder(s), and substance-induced acute symptoms that may require psychiatric care (i.e., hallucinations, depression, and other symptoms resulting from substance abuse or withdrawal)
- Substance abuse, mental illness, and organic syndromes in various combinations. Organic syndromes (e.g., HIV) may be a result of substance abuse, or they may be independent of substance abuse.

c. Acronyms that define various dual disorders
   i. MICAA: mentally ill, chemical abusers, and addicted
   ii. MISA: mentally ill substance abuser

d. Many studies of comorbidity show that people with alcohol and drug use disorders have high rates of personality disorder, depression, and, to a lesser extent, anxiety disorders. Whereas only a small number of substance users suffer from severe psychotic disorders, a sizable portion of people with severe psychotic disorders appear to have comorbid substance abuse disorders (Cournos & McKinnon, 1997).

2. Etiology
   a. The interactions between drug use and high-risk behaviors and mental illness are well known.
      i. Injection-drug users account for an estimated 35.6% of AIDS cases (Health Resources and Services Administration, 2001; Lucas, 2001).
      ii. Bing and colleagues (2001) estimate that noninjection drug users account for 30% to 46% of AIDS cases.
      ii. Sex, especially unprotected sex, may be used as a commodity that can be exchanged for money, drugs, a place to stay, and cigarettes.

iii. Studies of the sexual activity of the mentally ill have demonstrated that a significant portion of the mentally ill are engaging in sexual activity. Moreover, patients who do report recent sexual activity have engaged in multiple risk behaviors (Cournos & McKinnon, 1997).

3. Goals of care
   a. Maintain the safety of the patient regardless of the setting.
   b. Decrease the symptoms associated with the specific mental illness.
   c. Decrease the negative effects of substance use for the patient and others.

4. Assessment
   a. It is difficult to correctly diagnose concurrent problems such as mental illness and substance abuse. Drug use can mimic psychiatric disorders and psychiatric problems may remit once the person has been drug-free.
   b. To correctly assess for diagnose the MICCA patient the nurse must examine the following:

   - Drug and alcohol use patterns
   - Legal history
   - Educational/vocational history
   - Developmental/family history
   - Psychiatric history
   - Medical history
   - Previous treatment history
   - Medical test data: e.g., urine and blood samples, blood alcohol levels
   - Psychological test data

5. Interventions
   a. Nonpharamacologic
      i. Division in treatment philosophy between mental health professionals, addiction specialists, and medical services make treatment for the MICCA difficult.
      ii. Efforts should be made to coordinate and services between psychiatric and chemical dependency treatment programs
      iii. Day treatment programs that include psychiatric, medical, and support groups have been beneficial in stabilizing and increasing medication adherence for MICCA individuals.

   iv. For non-pharmacological treatment of specific psychiatric disorders see the specific mental illness in this section. Non-pharmacological treatments are also discussed in Section 6.17, the substance abuse community.
   b. Pharmacologic
      i. See specific mental illness in this section. Treatments for the substance abuser are discussed in Section 6.17, The Substance Abuse Community.

References

American Psychiatric Association. (2000a). *Diagnostic and statistical manual of mental disorders* (4th ed.). Washington, DC: Author.

American Psychiatric Association. (2000b). *Practice guideline for the treatment of patients with major depressive disorder. American Journal of Psychiatry,* 157(4 Suppl.), 1–45.

American Psychiatric Association. (2002). *HIV and anxiety. Office on HIV Psychiatry-Anxiety.* Retrieved December 23, 2002, from www.psych.org/aids/modules/anxietyon

Andreasen, N. C., & Black, D. W. (2001). *Introductory textbook of psychiatry* (3rd ed.). Washington, DC: American Psychiatric Publishing.

Bing, E. G., Burnnam, M. A., Longshore, D., Fleishman, J. A., Sherbourne, C. D., London, A. S., et al. (2001). Psychiatric disorders and drug use among human immunodeficiency virus-infected adults in the United States. *Archives of General Psychiatry, 58*(8), 721–728.

Bonanno, G., & Kaltman, S. (1999). Toward an integrated perspective on bereavement. *Psychological Bulletin, 125,* 760–776.

Boyd, M. A. (Ed.). (2002). *Psychiatric nursing: Contemporary practice* (2nd ed.). Philadelphia: Lippincott Williams & Wilkins.

Buckle, J. (2002). Clinical aromatherapy. *Journal of the Association of Nurses in AIDS Care, 13,* 81–99.

Burkhardt, M., & Nagai Jacobson, M. G. (2000). Spirituality and health. In B. Dossey, L. Keegan, & C. Guzzetta (Eds.), *Holistic nursing: A handbook for practice* (3rd ed., pp. 91–121). New York: Aspen Publishers.

Cabaj, R. P. (1996). *Management of depression and anxiety in HIV-infected patients.* Retrieved September 1, 2002, from http://www.iapac.org/Text/mandepanxhivinfpat.htm

Cantrell, G. (2001). *Wiccan beliefs and practices: With rituals for solitaries and covens.* St. Paul, MN: Llewellyn.

Carpentino, J. (2000). *Nursing diagnosis: Application to clinical practice* (8th ed.). Philadelphia: Lippincott.

Cournos, F., & McKinnon, K. (1997) *Substance use and HIV risk among people with severe mental illness.* Retrieved

January 5, 2003, from http://www. drugabuse.gov/pdf/monographs/monograph170/ download170.html

Crock, E. A. (1998). Breaking (through) the law—Coming out of the silence: Nursing, HIV/AIDS and euthanasia. *AIDS Care, 10*(Suppl. 2), 137–145.

Dilley, J. W., Woods, W. J., & McFarland, W. (1997). Are advances in treatment changing views about high-risk sex? *The New England Journal of Medicine, 337*(7), 501–502.

Dossey, L. (1996). *Prayer is good medicine: How to reap the healing benefits of prayer.* San Francisco: Harper.

Fiore, T., Flanigan, T., Hogan, T., Cram, R., Schuman, P., Schoenbaum, E., et al. (2001). HIV infections in families of HIV-positive and at-risk HIV-negative women. *AIDS Care, 13*(2), 209–214.

Folkman, S., Chesney, M. A., & Christopher-Richards, A. (1994). Stress and coping in caregiving partners of men with AIDS. *Psychiatric Clinics of North America, 17*(1), 35–53.

Fontana, J. S. (2002). Rational suicide in the terminally ill. *Journal of Nursing Scholarship, 34*(2), 147–151.

Foster, B. (1999, Summer). Yoga for HIV/AIDS: The mind-body connection. *Body Positive, 32*–36.

Galanti, G. A. (1997). *Caring for patients of different cultures: Case studies from different American hospitals* (2nd ed.). Philadelphia: University of Pennsylvania Press.

Goldman, L. S., Wise, T. N., & Brody, D. S. (Eds.). (1998). *Psychiatry for primary care physicians.* Chicago: American Medical Association.

Goodwin, G. M. (2001). The addition of folic acid to fluoxetine for major depression increases response rates especially in women. *Evidenced-based Mental Health, 4,* 41.

Green, L., Fullilove, M. T., & Fullilove, R. (1998). Stories of spiritual awakening: The nature of spirituality in recovery. *Journal of Substance Abuse Treatment, 15*(4), 325–331.

Hall, B. (1998). Patterns of spirituality in persons with advanced HIV disease. *Research in Nursing and Health, 21*(2), 143–153.

Health Resources and Services Administration. (2001). *Substance abuse in the US: An update.* Retrieved January 18, 2003, from http://hab.hrsa.gov/publications/hrsaconv/hrsa501/hrsa501.html

Herfkens, K. M. (2001). Depression, neurocognitive disorders and HIV in prisons. *HEPPNews, 4*(1), 1–9.

Hilsenroth, M., Ackerman, S., Blagys, M., Baumann, B., Baity, M., Smith, S., et al. (2000). Reliability and validity of DSM-IV Axis V. *American Journal of Psychiatry, 157*(11), 1858–1863.

Kushner, H. (1981). *When bad things happen to good people.* New York: Schocken Books.

Lucas, G. M. (2001). *Management of HIV infection in injection-drug users.* Retrieved January 18, 2003, from www.medscape.com/viewarticle/418652_print

Lyon, M., Townsend-Akpan, C., & Thompson, A. (2001). Spirituality and end of life care for an adolescent with AIDS. *AIDS Patient Care and STDs, 15*(11), 555–560.

Matheny, S. C., Mehr, L. M., & Brown, G. (1997). Caregivers and HIV infection: Services and issues. *Primary Care, 24*(3), 677–690.

McCormick, D., Holder, B., Wetsel, M., & Cawthon, T. (2001). Spirituality and HIV disease: An integrated

perspective. *Journal of the Association of Nurses in AIDS Care, 12,* 59–65.

Morrison, M. F., Petitto, J. M., Have, T. T., Gettes, D. R., Chiappini, M. S., Weber, A. L., et al. (2002). Depressive and anxiety disorders in women with HIV infection. *American Journal of Psychiatry, 159*(5), 789–796.

Murphy, P., & Perry, K. (1988). Hidden grievers. *Death Studies, 12,* 451–462.

New York State Department of Health AIDS Institute. (2001). *Mental health care for people with HIV infection: HIV clinical guidelines for the primary care practitioner.* New York: Author.

Nichols, S. E. (1983). Psychiatric aspects of AIDS. *Psychosomatics, 24*(12), 1083–1089.

Nichols, S. E. (1985). Psychosocial reactions of persons with the acquired immunodeficiency syndrome. *Annals of Internal Medicine, 103,* 765–767.

North American Nursing Diagnosis Association. (1994). *Classification of nursing diagnosis. Proceedings of 10th Conference.* St. Louis, MO: Author.

Pilch, J. (1998). Wellness spirituality. *Health Values, 12*(3), 28–31.

Power, C., & Selnes, O. A. (1996). The Johns Hopkins HIV Dementia Scale. *Journal of International Association of Physicians in AIDS Care.* Retrieved February 25, 2003, from www.iapac.org

Rait, D. S. (1991). The family context of AIDS. *Psychiatric Medicine, 9*(3), 423–439.

Ramirez, A., Addington-Hall, J., & Richards, M. (1998). ABC of palliative care: The carers. *British Medical Journal, 316*(7126), 208–211.

Remien, R. H., & Rabkin, J. G. (2001). Psychological aspects of living with HIV disease. *Western Journal of Medicine, 175*(5), 332–335.

Roberts, K. J. (2002). Physician-patient relationships, patient satisfaction, and antiretroviral medication adherence among HIV-infected adults attending a public health clinic. *AIDS Patient Care and STDs, 16*(1), 43–50.

Ruppert, R. A. (1996). Psychological aspects of lay caregiving. *Rehabilitation Nursing, 21*(6), 315–320.

Saunders, J. (2000). AIDS nursing and physician-assisted suicide. Part I. *Journal of the Association of Nurses in AIDS Care, 11*(6), 45–53.

Saunders, J. (2001). AIDS nursing and physician-assisted suicide. Part 2. *Journal of the Association of Nurses in AIDS Care, 12*(1), 71–82.

Sicher, F., Targ, E., Moore, D., & Smith, H. (1998). A randomized double-blind study of the effects of distant healing in a population with advanced AIDS. *Western Journal of Medicine, 169*(6), 356–367.

Spitzer, R. L., Kroenke, K., Williams, J. B. W., & the Patient Health Questionnaire Primary Care Study Group. (1999). Validation and utility of a self-report version of the PRIME-MD. *Journal of the American Medical Association, 282*(18), 1734–1744.

Turner, H. A., Pearlin, L. I., & Mullan, J. T. (1998). Sources and determinants of social support for caregivers of persons with AIDS. *Journal of Health and Social Behavior, 39,* 137–151.

Williamson, R. (1998). Images of God among persons with AIDS. *The Journal of Pastoral Care, 52*(1), 56–61.

Wilson, H. S., & Kneisl, C. R. (1992). *Psychiatric nursing* (4th ed.). Reading, MA: Addison-Wesley.

Section VI

Concerns of Special Populations

Community is derived from the Latin word meaning "fellowship." Fellowship is one kind of relationship an individual can have with other persons. These relationships often define an individual, the collective response to living with HIV/AIDS, or both. To care for a person with AIDS, the nurse needs to have an understanding of the patient's community—not just the patient's age group (e.g., adolescents), gender, or ethnicity but also the groups the client identifies with (e.g., men who have sex with men). This section provides the reader with the understanding of how the disease affects individuals in their communities. Each section comprehensively defines a community and how that community is represented in today's epidemic. Because people are living longer with the disease, it is also important to understand the common health issues of the community and implement health interventions that reflect these specific needs. The challenges to access, treatments, and research initiatives are also discussed, and specific approaches to caring for the individual and the community itself round out the discussion.

6.1 Adolescents

1. Description of the community
   a. Adolescence is a gradual and variable process from onset of puberty until maturity.
   b. For clinical purposes, adolescence extends from ages 12 to 21 years.
   c. Legally, adolescents are minors (under the age of majority) until age 18 in 47 states and age 19 in Alabama, Nebraska, and Wyoming.
   d. A *mature minor,* covered by mature minor doctrine, can understand the benefits and risks of treatment and is able to give informed consent.
   e. An *emancipated minor* is married, serving in the armed forces, or living apart from parents and managing own financial affairs.
   f. A *medically emancipated* minor is, in addition to the previous, above a specified age, a minor parent or runaway, deemed able to provide informed consent and to seek care for a condition that, if left untreated, could jeopardize the health of self or others (e.g., consent for pregnancy-related care, including contraceptive care; diagnosis and treatment of sexually transmitted diseases [STDs], including HIV; treatment for substance abuse).
   g. Demographics
      i. According to a White House report (White House Office of National AIDS Policy, 2000), half of all new HIV infections occur in people under age 25.
      ii. Approximately 16% of all male AIDS cases and 21% of all female AIDS cases are diagnosed in adults ages 20 to 29; given the years of delay from HIV infection to the onset of AIDS, many were infected as teens (Centers for Disease Control and Prevention, 2000a).
      iii. Geographic variation includes higher rates in urban areas, especially the Northeast and South.
      iv. African American and Hispanic adolescents/young adults (male and female) are disproportionately represented in reported AIDS cases (60–65% in 13–24 age group), compared with their representation in the U.S. population (Centers for Disease Control and Prevention, 2000a).
      v. The expanding HIV epidemic in adolescents/young adults is increasingly female, minority, and sexually transmitted.
2. Common health issues
   a. Adolescence is a time of growth and experimentation, a stage of striving for independence/autonomy, and a time of feeling curious and invulnerable. All of these factors may lead to sexual and drug-related risk behaviors that increase exposure to HIV. Social skills and negotiating skills are still evolving.
   b. Adolescents generally are concrete thinkers, especially those under age 18; therefore, they are unlikely to think of the long-term consequences of their actions. Teens process information differently than adults or children do.
   c. Denial is a strong defense mechanism, and peer groups are major directives of behavior.
3. HIV/AIDS in the adolescent community
   a. Transmission, risk behaviors, and prevention issues
      i. Most adolescents are unaware of their HIV status and may unknowingly transmit the virus.
      ii. Primary identifiable mode of HIV transmission among adolescents is sexual activity, mainly heterosexual in females and homosexual in males. Most adolescents do not personalize risk or threat of HIV infection.
      iii. Sexual activity is reported in 37% of 9th graders and 66% of 12th graders; less than 50% of teens use condoms consistently; more than 1 million teen pregnancies occur yearly (about half of homeless youth report pregnancies; U.S. Department of Health and Human Services, Health Resources and Services Administration, HIV/AIDS Bureau, 2001).

iv. Both gender and age power imbalance in a study of African American and Latina adolescent females with older male partners (3 years older or more) were found to increase young women's HIV risk (UCSF Center for AIDS Prevention Studies and AIDS Research Institute, 1999).

v. Twenty-five percent of high school students report being under the influence of alcohol or other drugs the last time they had sex (White House Office of National AIDS Policy, 2000).

vi. Adolescents at highest risk are those out of their homes (e.g., teens in foster care, or incarcerated, runaways, transient/homeless youth), school dropouts, men having sex with men and those exploring same-sex relationships, sexually abused adolescents, teens in a high-prevalence community, and HIV-affected teens or those orphaned by the death of HIV-infected parent.

vii. STDs facilitate transmission of HIV; each year, 1 in 4 sexually experienced teens contracts an STD.

viii. In early puberty, physiologic immaturity of the female cervical transformation zone increases vulnerability for STD acquisition.

ix. Barriers to prevention programs include the following:

- Parents, community organization, school systems often refuse to support HIV/AIDS educational offerings due to their denial, homophobia, and inadequate training.
- A lack of social marketing exists; most teens report not knowing how or where to get tested.
- Many adolescents at highest risk are the most difficult to reach; 10–15% of youth have dropped out of school (U.S. Department of Health and Human Services, Health Resources and Services Administration, HIV/AIDS Bureau, 2001).
- Many adolescents know about transmission, but fewer know to prevent infection or lack the skills to practice safer behaviors.
- Half of teens believe parental permission is needed to get tested, which is often not true. Confidentiality is essential to ensure use of testing and treatment facilities by adolescents. An adolescent has the same right to confidentiality as adults have.

b. Access to care, treatment, and research
  i. Barriers include the following:

- HIV care often is provided to adolescents by people with no training in adolescent health; few providers are trained to serve the specific needs of sexual minority youth.
- The largest gap in health services is the treatment of adolescents with mental health or alcohol and substance-abuse problems.
- Health care is not a top priority for most adolescents; many deny any health threat.
- One in three youths, 18–24 years old, has no public or private health insurance.
- There is a lack of youth-centered services that are accessible, convenient, and confidential.
- There is a lack of a unified support community.
- Adherence barriers related to developmental stage or specific psychosocial issues include chaotic lives, competing interests, fear of disclosure to family or friends, lack of support, conflict between dependency on adults and need

to challenge authority for independence, acceptance of treatment when feeling well, and understanding of complex regimens (U.S. Department of Health and Human Services, Health Resources and Services Administration, HIV/AIDS Bureau, 1999).

- Clinical research is impacted by small numbers of HIV-infected adolescents in care.
- Institutional review boards that examine research proposals to ensure participant safety, confidentiality, and informed consent must weigh potential value of information about youth versus the vulnerability of youth.
- Health care providers of HIV-infected youth are not knowledgeable about opportunities for participation in research

4. Specific care approaches
   a. Individual
      i. Build and maintain trusting relationship based on confidentiality. Assess family disclosure and dysfunction, social relationships, sexual orientation, mental health, parenting/pregnancy, job, school, and shelter.
      ii. Assess risk of STD, alcohol and drug use, and incidents of abuse or violence. Use peer health educators/counselors; teens are more receptive to input from respected peers than from authoritarian adults.
      iii. Provide information to correct common misconceptions (e.g., HIV is transmitted only if sick).
      iv. Promote routine, voluntary, and confidential HIV counseling and testing.
      v. Build communication and negotiation skills.
      vi. Provide risk reduction with condom demonstration and application practice.

   b. Community
      i. HIV-prevention programs are most successful when appropriate adolescents (e.g., appropriate age range and sexual orientation, culturally competent) are involved in the planning and implementation.
      ii. Prevention programs need to be implemented, sustained, and reinforced before practice of risky behavior (before early teen years).
      iii. Include information on sexual practices; most sexual intercourse is spontaneous rather than planned.
      iv. Provide easy access to condoms.
      v. Provide easy access to information on drug use: Alcohol and recreational drugs impair judgment and promote high-risk behaviors.
      vi. Prevention programs should involve various groups, such as media, schools, parents, and community organizations.
      vii. Outreach for those not in home or school include venues such as mobile vans, residential child care facilities, shopping malls, recreation centers, youth shelters, and detention centers; either ORASURE, HIV antibody test by oral swab, or OraQUICK Rapid HIV Antibody Test by finger stick, should be available at these venues.
      viii. Each visit for health care should include STD and pregnancy prevention counseling (Centers for Disease Control and Prevention, 2000b).
      ix. Prevention programs must be linked to HIV counseling and testing, comprehensive health care with support and legal services, and access to research on a continuum.
      x. Use recognized adolescent models as guides for developing teen programs (e.g., U.S. Department of Health and Human Services, Health Resources and Services

Administration, HIV/AIDS Bureau, *Lessons Learned*, 2001a).

6.2 The Blind and Visually Impaired Community

1. Description of the community
   a. Visual impairment: vision not fully corrected by ordinary prescription lenses, medical treatment, or surgery; includes conditions ranging from the presence of good usable vision to low vision to the complete absence of sight
   b. Blindness: lack of usable sight
   c. Legal blindness: defines visual conditions that, when present, connote eligibility for government or other benefits and services. An individual who is legally blind has a visual acuity of 20/200 in the better eye with the best correction or a visual field of no more than 20 degrees and cannot read the big *E* on the Snellen eye chart.
   d. Low vision: not corrected to normal vision with standard eyeglasses or contact lenses, medications, or surgery, after which some good usable vision remains. People with low vision can learn to make the best use of the vision available to them.
   e. Although estimates vary, there are approximately 10 million people who are blind or visually impaired in the United States (American Foundation for the Blind, 2001; National Federation of the Blind, 2000).
   f. Approximately 1.3 million Americans are legally blind (American Foundation for the Blind, 2001; National Federation of the Blind, 2000).
   g. Approximately 109,000 people with visual impairments in the United States use long canes for mobility. Slightly more than 7,000 Americans use guide dogs (American Foundation for the Blind, 2001; National Federation of the Blind, 2000).
   h. Of all Americans who are blind and visually impaired, approximately 80% are White, 18% are Black, 8% are Hispanic, and 2% are other races (American Foundation for the Blind, 2001; National Federation of the Blind, 2000).
   i. Currently 42% of Americans with visual disabilities are married, 33% are widowed, 13% are separated or divorced, and 13% have never been married (American Foundation for the Blind, 2001; National Federation of the Blind, 2000).
   j. Approximately 46% of adult Americans with visual impairments are employed, whereas only 32% of working-age Americans with blindness are employed. People with visual disabilities do not have the same range of opportunities available to them as sighted people (Kestelyn, 2001; Wolffe & Springer, 2002).
   k. Barriers to employment include poverty; discrimination; lack of education, resources, and necessary technology; and employer's lack of awareness.
   l. Forty-five percent of individuals with severe visual impairment or blindness have a high school diploma, compared with 80% of fully sighted individuals. Among high school graduates, those with severe visual impairment or blindness are about as likely to have taken some college courses as those who are sighted, but they are less likely to have graduated.

   Of people with visual impairments, approximately 62% of Whites complete high school or higher education, compared with 41% of Blacks and 44% of Hispanics (American Foundation for the Blind, 2001; National Federation of the Blind, 2000; Wolffe & Springer, 2002).
   m. It is estimated that 50% to 75% of all HIV/AIDS clients will be affected at some point with ocular complications including blindness (Guex-Crosier, 2001; Robinson, 1999; Vrabec, 1996)
2. Common health issues
   a. People with visual impairment suffer from a lack of understanding and research about visual impairment and the idea of sighted people that people with blindness are also deaf and dumb.
   b. Adults over 55 years of age have more psychological and physical problems, such as depression, because of loss,

isolation, and inability to maintain quality of life and activities of daily living.

c. Only 1% of the elderly with visual impairment who need assistance and education are able to get help due to lack of funding.

3. HIV/AIDS in the visually impaired community (Kapperman et al., 1993; Jamie et al., 2001)

a. Transmission, risk behaviors, and prevention issues

i. Gaps in sexuality education, including HIV/AIDS and STDs

ii. Lack of educational material for visually impaired

b. Access to care, treatments or research

i. Access to health care is difficult to assess. Most studies look at either children younger than 21 years of age or adults over 55 years when discussing psychosocial effects of blindness.

ii. Lack of employment leads to lack of private insurance coverage.

iii. Lack of having own transportation must rely on public transportation, family, or friends, which leads to a lack of independence.

iv. Children have fewer mobility difficulties and adapt more quickly to their surroundings. More are being mainstreamed in public schools to prevent social isolation.

c. Specific care approaches

i. Individual

(1) Points of etiquette when interacting with a person who is blind or visually impaired include the following:

- Introduce yourself using your name and position, especially if you are wearing a name badge containing this information.

- Speak directly to people who are blind or visually impaired, not through a companion, guide, or other individual.

- Speak using a natural conversational tone and speed. Do not speak loudly or slowly, unless the person also has a hearing impairment.

- Address the person by name when possible. This is especially important in crowded areas.

- Immediately greet the person when he or she enters a room or a service area. This allows you to let the person know you are present and ready to assist, and it eliminates uncomfortable silences.

- Indicate the end of a conversation to avoid the embarrassment of leaving a person speaking when no one is actually there (especially those totally blind).

- Feel free to use words that refer to vision, such as *look*, *see*, and *watch*; they are part of everyday verbal communication. The words *blind* and *visually impaired* are also acceptable in conversation.

- Be precise and thorough when you describe people, places, or things to people who are totally blind. Don't leave things out or change a description because you think it is unimportant or unpleasant.

- Feel free to use visually descriptive language. Making reference to colors, patterns, designs, and shapes is perfectly acceptable.

- Offer to guide people who are blind or visually impaired by asking if they would like assistance. Offer them your arm. It is not always necessary to provide guided assistance; in some instances it can be disorienting and disruptive. Respect the desires of the person.

- Guide people who request assistance by allowing them to take your arm just above the elbow with your arm bent. Walk ahead of the person you are guiding. Never grab a person who is blind or visually impaired by the arm and push him or her forward.
- Do not leave a person who is blind or visually impaired standing in free space when you serve as a guide. Always be sure that the person has a firm grasp on your arm or is leaning against a chair or a wall if you have to be separated momentarily.
- Guide dogs are working mobility tools. Do not pet them, feed them, or distract them while they are working.
- Be calm and clear about what to do if you see a person who is blind or visually impaired about to encounter a dangerous situation. For example, if a person is about to bump into a stanchion in a hotel lobby, calmly and firmly call out, "Wait there for a moment; there is a pole in front of you."

ii. Community
(1) Sexuality education is generally acquired from conferences.
(2) Programs should assist individuals with visual impairments to be able to access conferences and conference material.
(3) Outreach efforts need to include people with visual

impairments and other disabled groups.

6.3 Commercial Sex Workers

1. Description of the community
   a. Sex industry workers are men, women, or transgendered individuals who exchange sexual services for money, gifts, drugs, a place to sleep, and so on. General work locations include the street, massage parlors, escort services, and brothels.
   b. Economic need is the driving force behind the entry into the industry. Individuals remain in this job until their economic situation changes, substance abuse issues are resolved, or individuals are able to leave coercive relationships or domination by other persons (e.g., pimp, madame). As in other professions, the more autonomy the worker has, the less vulnerable he or she is to stressors. For example, a number of peer organizations have been formed around the world that function to keep sex workers informed about health and other issues.
2. Common health issues
   a. Sex industry workers are often from oppressed groups (e.g., youth; women; ethnic or racial minorities; gay, lesbian, bisexual, transgendered people; homeless people with mental illness; or people living with addiction).
   b. Psychosocial issues include low educational or vocational skills, poor social support or connectedness with caring adults, complex social entanglements, and likelihood of criminalized lifestyle.
   c. Psychological issues include low self-esteem and low self-efficacy, decreased assertiveness, depression, posttraumatic stress, hopelessness, stigma, and multiple losses of support persons with HIV, which often place individuals at risk for increased risk-taking behaviors.
   d. There is often a history of living with violence and sexual and physical abuse during childhood. Sex industry workers continue to be victims of violent crimes

by patrons, employers, partners, police, and vigilantes.

3. HIV/AIDS in the sex industry worker community
   a. Transmission, risk behaviors, and prevention issues
      i. Sex workers who use IV drugs, heroin or crack cocaine are at very high risk for infection, transmission, and risk-taking behavior.
      ii. Risk for workers is often higher than it is for patrons because workers have multiple contacts and are more likely to perform higher risk-receptive acts (e.g., patrons will often pay 2 to 3 times normal rates for unprotected sex).
      iii. There is an increased risk of partner being an IV drug user.
      iv. Sex industry workers are at increased risk for developing and transmitting multidrug resistance to antiretrovirals from sexual partners, both prior to and after HIV infection.
      v. Sex industry workers are at increased risk of transmitting HIV secondary to high HIV viral loads if not on antirtrovirals.
      vi. There is an increased risk of contracting and transmitting multiple HIV subtypes, opportunistic infections (OIs), and sexually transmitted diseases (STDs).
   b. Access to care, treatment, and research
      i. Barriers to care include financial issues, such as lack of health insurance, and a knowledge deficit concerning how to access the health care system. If the worker does not work, there is no income to pay for care.
      ii. Addiction and mental illness may be barriers to health care access.
      iii. There is often a decreased self-care efficacy.
      iv. Sex workers' fear and avoidance by health care workers and health systems related to stigma of sex work.
      v. There is a societal and health care provider indifference to women, substance users, and marginalized groups.
      vi. There is poor access to experimental and complementary therapies that may improve quality of life.
      vii. Poor treatment outcomes are affected by numerous factors, including barriers to health care, late diagnosis and treatment of HIV disease and OIs, and chaotic interaction with health care system (e.g., lack of consistent care, incomplete treatment regimens, poor baseline health/nutritional status).

4. Specific care approaches
   a. Individual
      i. Establish trust through open, nonjudgmental exploration of lifestyle, issues related to substance use, and health history. Obtain an in-depth sexual history, which many sex industry workers do not want to disclose to health care providers.
      ii. Allow time for relationship to develop, be patient, and ask direct questions.
      iii. Foster hope and independence while recognizing functional and social limitations.
      iv. Assess legal history and current legal problems and be aware of current laws related to sex work and HIV. Provide referrals when necessary.
      v. Assess knowledge of and provide education about healthy lifestyles, safer sex practices, and harm-reduction modalities (if pertinent). Provide written educational resources at fifth-grade reading level.
      vi. Assess connection to financial support systems, such as Social Security.
      vii. Social assistance and other forms of financial assistance may allow sex workers to stop working. HIV diagnosis can increase eligibility for financial assistance.

viii. Refer for educational and career counseling where appropriate.

ix. Discuss available support services with the client to reduce isolation and hopelessness and to begin the healing process.

x. Refer to a peer group for support if one is available or if the patient has access to Internet resources.

xi. Refer to family, psychiatric, or addiction services and drug treatment if appropriate, preferably with a primary care provider who is able to provide sensitive, consistent care. Knowledge of working hours and substance abuse habits can assist in making appointments that can be kept.

b. Community

i. Use outreach teams to provide education about safer sex and safer substance use and provide a connection to health care, legal services, and drug treatment.

ii. Use outreach workers recruited from the community of former sex industry workers because they are familiar with the community and culture.

iii. Organize a multidisciplinary team of health care providers educated about the needs of this population and implement consciousness raising regarding possible bias.

iv. Services and supplies (e.g., condoms, female and male) should be accessible, affordable, accompanied with negotiation skills, and modeled by peers (Witte, Takeshi, El-Bassel, Gilbert, & Wallace, 2000).

v. The goal is to reduce risky behavior through the provision of needed health care services that include, but are not limited to, counseling to reduce drug abuse and sexual and physical abuse and to support those seeking alternative employment opportunities.

vi. Work with law enforcement to provide useful interventions when sex workers are incarcerated.

vii. Direct education and outreach to sex industry consumers about risks related to HIV infection and transmission.

viii. Focus on using a holistic approach to care by providing integrated programs that include substance abuse treatment (e.g., needle exchanges, drug treatment, methadone maintenance programs), abuse counseling, and the provision of basic primary care from a single care facility.

ix. Expand use of community-based clinics, mobile units, and home care nursing to provide services in the areas where sex workers live and work.

6.4 Gay and Bisexual Men

1. Description of the community

a. While the label men who have sex with men (MSM) continues to be used as a risk category in statistical reporting of HIV/AIDS, many men consider it offensive and reductionistic, connoting mere physicality between men. Gay identity development involves a holistic appreciation of intimacy, emotional attachment, and relationships between men in addition to sexual responses and behaviors. In a discussion of HIV and AIDS, the gay male community includes sexually active males who a) identify as gay (i.e., mainly having sex with men and socializing with gay community), b) bisexual men (i.e., having sex with both men and women; these men may or may not socialize in the gay community), and c) who have sex with men but do not self-identify as gay or socialize in the gay community (i.e., these men may or may not have sex with women).

b. Sexual identity is influenced by emotional, affectionate, and spiritual aspects of relationships with men; varying levels of affiliation with the gay culture and community; and the presence of familial, social, and political pressures (e.g., stigma, antigay prejudice, legal discrimination).

c. Gay and bisexual men are not a homogeneous group. They may be White (65%), Black (20%), Hispanic (13%), or Asian/Pacific Islander (1%); impoverished, blue collar, middle- or upper class; adolescent or elderly; or Baptist, Jewish, or Catholic. They may use injection drugs or have hemophilia. They may be single, partnered, married, or divorced and may have children (Centers for Disease Control and Prevention, 1997).

2. Common health issues

a. Health care providers maintain social stereotypes, prejudices, and disdain of gay men. Programs to educate and adjust provider attitudes are limited. Health care professionals need to be comfortable with sensitively discussing gay and bisexual sexuality and become familiar with the complex emotional, interpersonal, and sociopolitical issues affecting prevention behaviors.

b. Mental health care professionals are often uneducated and insensitive to gay issues and physiologic/sociologic needs, especially related to the coming-out process. Few mental health providers are equipped to counsel about multiple losses and grief and bereavement overload for gay men experiencing unprecedented losses of partners, friends, and acquaintances to AIDS.

c. Increased rates of sexually transmitted diseases facilitate the transmission of HIV to uninfected partners.

   i. Syphilis rates are on the rise among MSM.

   ii. Rectal gonorrhea and chlamydia rates continue to increase among young MSM.

   iii. Trichomonas is highest among Black and Caribbean Americans and is asymptomatic in men.

   iv. Stigma associated with same-sex behaviors may be a barrier to the prevention and treatment of sexually transmitted diseases.

   v. Rates of alcoholism and tobacco use are high among gay men; the use of illicit and recreational drugs is a concern, especially among young gay men who then participate in increased risky behavior.

3. HIV/AIDS and the gay and bisexual male community

a. Transmission, risk behaviors, and prevention issues

   i. MSM continue to be disproportionately affected with the highest incidence of annual AIDS cases. It remains the leading cause of death for men ages 25–44.

   ii. Approximately 54% of all persons in the United States diagnosed with AIDS have been gay males; more than 60% of all AIDS deaths have been in the gay male community.

   iii. HIV seroprevalence estimates in urban U.S. gay communities range from 10% to 30%, and HIV seroconversion rates for gay men remain highest of all risk categories.

   iv. In 2000, gay males accounted for 62% of new male HIV infections among adolescents ages 13–19 years old and 53% of new infections in the 20–24 age group.

   v. Men of color—particularly Black and Hispanic men—are disproportionately represented in the numbers of new HIV infections and AIDS cases.

   vi. Social stigma associated with homosexuality encourages internalized homophobia and may promote unhealthy dissociation of sexual behaviors and sense of self.

   vii. Public disdain, harassment, even violence is directed to gays (gay bashing).

   viii. Sexual behavior between men is illegal in many U.S. states.

   ix. Some MSM feel the need to hide sexual orientation to preserve treasured aspects of life (e.g., employment, family and social relationships, religious affiliations).

   x. Entrance and orientation to gay culture is often clandestine, guilt laden, or even dangerous; sensitive and accurate information about the gay community, culture, or sexual practices is often difficult to locate, especially for adolescents.

xi. Bisexual men may remain peripheral to the gay culture, feeling a lack of support and isolation. This may be especially true for MSM who do not identify as gay and who may be in otherwise heterosexual relationships.

xii. Gay men developed successful, short-term behavior-change programs early in the epidemic; new programs should focus on strategies for lifelong, sustained sexual behavior change. Teens must be targeted as well.

b. Access to care, treatment, and research

i. Gay men—particularly White men—have historically been eager and willing participants in clinical trials; as a group, they have exhibited high levels of compliance to research protocols, contributed to the knowledge base, and provided researchers with important feedback with which to guide their science.

ii. Marginalized populations in the gay community (e.g., ethnic minority gay men, bisexual men) have faced financial and social barriers in accessing equitable HIV care and may carry an understandable distrust of research protocols because of historical exploitation by unethical research practices (e.g., Black men in the Tuskegee syphilis experiment).

iii. Access to care and research protocols has been enhanced by skills in assertiveness, negotiation, and empowerment that have been developed by gay men throughout the HIV epidemic.

iv. Treatment outcomes vary by socioeconomic status, psychosocial characteristics, and availability of personal support systems. Gay men fare better than many

persons with AIDS in overall health-related quality of life, adherence to HAART medications, and longevity.

4. Specific care approaches

a. Individual

i. In addition to printed brochures, advertisements, and posters, HIV prevention approaches may include one-on-one counseling, personal skill-building activities, and group discussions.

ii. The unique issues for HIV-negative gay men (e.g., survivor guilt, social isolation, contradictory desires to become HIV infected for the secondary gains) have been ridiculed and undervalued; prevention programs must address these issues openly and assist uninfected gay men to manage the complexities of their emotional and sexual lives.

iii. Targeted, and culturally appropriate, prevention services for men in minority populations and other marginalized subpopulations of the gay community (e.g., gay men with visual or hearing impairments, teens, bisexual men) need to be developed.

iv. Developing targeted prevention services for men who have sex with men—but do not identify as gay or bisexual—must be a priority.

v. Gay men have experienced unprecedented levels of death, grief, and bereavement. The traumatic outcomes may affect HIV prevention behaviors and erode the individual's resolve to remain uninfected; HIV prevention programs can facilitate grief, acknowledge the traumas, and explore the effects on the health and well-being of HIV-negative gay men.

vi. Peer education and social and community networks should be used.

(1) Employ gay and bisexual men as outreach workers, clinicians, and counselors.

    (2) Use HIV-positive gay and bisexual men to educate and motivate HIV-positive men, and use HIV-negative gay and bisexual men to educate and motivate HIV-negative men.

  vii. Provide education, networking, counseling, and support for gay men coming out of the closet to reduce internalized homophobia, increase self-esteem, and build skills in negotiating safer sex.

b. Community

  i. Homophobia must be identified, exposed, and publicly denounced; provide education and training for researchers, clinicians, and staff.

  ii. Reevaluate safer-sex messages for subtle sexual or moral judgments or messages that are culturally insensitive or inappropriate.

  iii. Prevention messages must acknowledge gay and bisexual men, not just as individuals but as social beings with complex family, group, and community roles and relationships.

  iv. Many community events center around supporting HIV-positive gay and bisexual men and foster a sense of gay community, not just HIV community in high seroprevalence areas, by involving uninfected gay and bisexual men with an equal voice.

  v. In research studies, rather than simply having HIV-negative gay men serving as controls, provide needed services and treatments.

  vi. Mandatory name reporting following HIV testing (required by law in a majority of states) is incongruent with the need to hide one's sexual behavior from others to avoid stigma, ostracism, and discrimination; the real and perceived threats must be minimized to encourage HIV testing.

  vii. Provide separate discussion and bereavement groups for both HIV-positive and HIV-negative men to reduce grief and bereavement overload.

  viii. Use the gay and bisexual media (e.g., newspapers) regularly to educate the gay and bisexual male community and build trust and familiarity with health care providers.

  ix. Collaborate with gay and bisexual community-based organizations on the development, implementation, and evaluation of prevention programs.

6.5 HIV-Infected Health Care Workers

1. Description of the community (Centers for Disease Control and Prevention, 2001d)

  a. Through June, 2001, 461,495 AIDS cases were reported for whom occupational information is available and reported in the United States. Of these cases, 23,473 (5.1%) were employed in health care, and 5,106 were nurses.

  b. Most of these health care workers were infected from non-occupational exposure to HIV. There are 57 occupationally acquired HIV infections in health care workers (26 have developed AIDS); 24 of these cases involved nurses, 19 involved laboratory workers, 6 involved physicians, 2 involved surgical technicians, 1 involved a dialysis technician, 1 involved a respiratory therapist, 1 involved a health aide, 1 involved an embalmer/morgue technician, and 2 involved housekeepers/maintenance workers.

2. Common health issues

  a. Physical concerns

  i. Dealing with HIV-related fatigue while at work (evaluate sleep patterns, anemia, medications, and inadequate nutrition; Association of Nurses in AIDS Care, 2001)

  ii. Pushing too hard to prove one is healthy and can perform job responsibilities

  iii. Limiting exposure to opportunistic infections in the workplace (see Work Issues section later)

iv. Remembering to take care of self (e.g., getting an annual flu vaccine, eating a balanced diet, exercising, getting plenty of sleep; Association of Nurses in AIDS Care, 2001)

b. Psychosocial concerns

   i. Overidentifying with own HIV patients' physical and psychosocial issues

   ii. Need to be attentive to issues of grief overload, including loss of roles and changes in body image

   iii. Balancing the amount of HIV/AIDS work and volunteering

   iv. Allowing self to be the patient, not the nurse, with health care providers involved in own care

   v. Adjusting to having friends and colleagues who are now one's caregivers

   vi. Allowing self to be a receiver rather than solely a giver of care

   vii. Working with own state nurses' association and ANAC chapter

   viii. Learning to know how and what to ask for regarding own needs

c. Financial/Legal concerns

   i. Deciding when to go on disability (earlier vs. later in course of illness); changing from full- to part-time employment, which may affect insurance eligibility or cost of premiums for health, life, and disability insurance

   ii. Confidentiality issues if employed at the same place where one received health care

   iii. Insurance issues

      (1) Preexisting condition clauses on new policies

      (2) How to pay premiums when no longer working

   iv. Requirements to report HIV status to regulatory/licensing authorities

      (1) Become familiar with laws

      (2) Bring a support person to any formal meetings regarding reporting HIV status or proposed restrictions on practice

d. Work issues

   i. Deciding whom to tell (e.g., supervisor/manager, employee health department, coworkers, infection control practitioner)

      (1) It may be helpful to practice first, talking it through with someone not outside of place of employment.

      (2) Pros of telling include scheduling flexibility and avoidance of exposure to opportunistic and other infections.

      (3) Evaluate whom one can trust with this sensitive information.

   ii. Working to develop practice guidelines to protect nurses from infections in patients and vice versa. Using Centers for Disease Control and Prevention (CDC) and Occupational Safety and Health Administration (OSHA) guidelines such as *Universal (Blood and Body Fluid) Precautions*, and *Isolation Techniques for Use in Hospitals*

   iii. Dealing with coworker issues: potential nonacceptance of HIV status, helplessness, knowing how to help, and overprotectiveness

   iv. Becoming familiar with the American's with Disabilities Act (ADA) and employer compliance (World Health Organization, 1999)

   v. Determining continued ability to work (e.g., fatigue, mental slowing)

3. HIV in the infected health care worker community

   a. Transmission, risk behaviors, and prevention issues

      i. Health care personnel living with HIV infection have a right to continue working as health care providers and to be assured of confidentiality about their HIV status in all cases. Health care workers with HIV infection should not be required to disclose their HIV status to their patients (Association of Nurses in AIDS Care, 1999).

      ii. The Centers for Disease Control and Prevention did not document a single case of HIV transmission from 63 HIV-infected health care workers to any of their more then 22,000 patients (Gostin, 2000).

   iii. Based on the lack of any confirmed cases, the risk of transmission of HIV from provider to patient is judged to be so small that practice restrictions do not appear warranted.

   iv. All health care workers should be informed about mechanisms of transmission and preventative strategies for blood-borne pathogens, and these should be universally applied.

b. Access to care, treatment, and research (World Health Organization, 1999)

   i. Seek care where confidentiality can be maintained.

   ii. Maintain medical appointments.

   iii. Seek counseling when necessary to maintain health and well-being.

4. Specific care approaches

a. Individual

   i. Nurses caring for or working with an HIV-positive colleague

     (1) Be aware of your own feelings of discomfort.

       (a) If you feel any awkwardness, and it seems appropriate to talk about this, acknowledge this with your colleagues.

       (b) Failure to recognize your own feelings may lead to isolation of or withdrawal from your colleagues.

       (c) Sometimes saying, "I don't know what to say or do; how can I help?" may be very supportive or helpful.

     (2) Respect the right of your colleague not to talk about her or his health status or not to want support; your colleague needs to be the one to decide when and from whom to get support.

     (3) If your colleague is also your patient, be particularly cautious about protecting confidentiality (e.g., access to medical records, disclosure of medical information, informal conversations in the elevators or other public areas).

     (4) Be supportive without being overprotective.

     (5) Make reasonable accommodations when making work assignments.

   ii. Nursing manager supervising an HIV-positive nurse

     (1) Be aware of the implications of the ADA and the need for reasonable accommodations.

     (2) Refer HIV-positive or other staff members to employee assistance if appropriate and available.

     (3) Know that job expectations and performance need to be fair and equitable for all employees; difficulties may arise if other coworkers feel they are not treated in the same manner as their HIV-positive colleague.

b. Community

   i. Encourage involvement with HIV-positive health care workers for support and information.

   ii. Refer to resources, if appropriate, such as *HIV+ NURSE,* the newsletter of the HIV+ Nurses Committee of the Association of Nurses in AIDS care, retrievable at http://www.anacnet.org/products/publications.htm

6.6 The Deaf and Hearing-Impaired Community

1. Description of the community

a. Approximately 28 million persons in the United States have a significant hearing loss in one or both ears. However, persons who identify socially as Deaf—usually associated with using sign language as their main mode of communication—number nearly two million. Other modes of communication include lip-reading and drawing. The

Deaf community is characterized by a unique culture with common language, beliefs, customs, and social norms. The use of American Sign Language (ASL) bonds the community.

b. The Deaf culture is often misunderstood by outsiders who fail to appreciate the richness of ASL. ASL is used by 75% of the Deaf community, whereas others in the Deaf community use Pidgin Signed English (PSE) or Signed Exact English (SEE) to communicate.

c. Deaf persons often reject the label of disabled (deficit model), preferring to have pride in the richness and diversity of the Deaf culture.

d. Definitions used to describe the community include the following:

- Deafness usually means that the hearing loss precludes the learning of language through hearing.
- Hard of hearing is less severe than Deafness and permits the learning of language with the use of hearing aids or related technological devices.
- Hearing impairment includes all degrees of hearing loss from minor to profound.
- Social affiliation often correlates with self-identification (Gaskins, 1999). Persons with significant hearing loss who don't self-identify or socialize with the Deaf community are often referred to as deaf, whereas persons who mainly communicate in sign language and identify as culturally Deaf are called Deaf (capital *D*). Both deaf and Deaf persons have a high risk for acquiring HIV infection.

e. Substance abuse is higher (1 in 7) among Deaf persons than among hearing persons (1 in 10), and Deaf persons have limited access to support groups or drug programs.

f. Many Deaf persons have experienced discrimination, marginalization, or abuse in the health care setting that has resulted in a distrust of health care providers.

g. Health care providers rarely know or use sign language interpreters with Deaf clients; many of the health-related educational materials are written at a level above the average fifth-grade reading level of Deaf adults; many Deaf persons are unfamiliar with basic facts about sexually transmitted diseases, safer sex strategies, or medication adherence principles. One study among Deaf persons in a substance abuse treatment program reported only 15% of participants had HIV transmission facts (Health Resources and Services Administration, HIV/AIDS Bureau, 2001).

h. Many Deaf persons have only minimal anatomy and physiology knowledge necessary to comprehend the complexities of HIV/AIDS.

2. Common health issues

a. Stigma, discrimination, and denial within the Deaf community are barriers.

   i. There are small, tightly knit communities in which confidentiality is often lost, leading to denial and secrecy.

   ii. Deaf people may be unempowered, have poor self-esteem, lack adequate skills in written and spoken English, and lack negotiation skills; behaviors common in Deaf culture are often misinterpreted by non-Deaf persons (e.g., direct communications that are misunderstood as aggressive or rude).

b. Marginalization and isolation of Deaf persons are due to real and perceived barriers in health care communications.

c. Deaf persons have limited or nonexistent access to HIV prevention, family planning, mental health, sexually transmitted diseases information, and substance abuse resources; one study revealed that 94% of AIDS service organizations surveyed provided no services for Deaf persons.

d. Published research on the Deaf experience in health care is virtually nonexistent.

e. Erroneous beliefs and stereotypes about Deaf and hearing impaired people are a barrier to effective care. Health care workers may believe the following:

- Hearing impairment equals intellectual impairment.
- The Deaf cannot learn like hearing people.
- Writing back and forth is effective communication and fosters comprehension.
- Anyone who knows even a little sign language can act as an interpreter.

    f. Ninety percent of Deaf people were born to hearing parents; parents may not accept their child's deafness, respect the Deaf culture, or learn their child's sign language and are likely to hide or deny the child's deafness by forbidding the use of sign language. Deaf persons often develop a family of choice with other Deaf persons; conflicts with the family of origin may surface in the health care setting.

3. HIV/AIDS and the Deaf community
    a. Transmission, risk behaviors, and prevention issues
        i. Precise numbers of Deaf persons with HIV/AIDS are unknown (Gaskins, 1999); the Centers for Disease Control and Prevention does not collect data on numbers of Deaf persons with AIDS, and a sampling frame is unavailable.
        ii. The HIV seroprevalence rates of Deaf persons is higher than that of the general population; infection rates for Deaf gay men are as high as—or higher than—that of hearing gay men.
        iii. Deaf persons are often diagnosed late in HIV/AIDS disease, when they present with symptoms.
            (1) Transmission modes are similar to that of hearing persons.
            (2) Deaf gay men are isolated from Deaf community and marginalized from the gay community, resulting in few skills to negotiate safer sex and manage risk behaviors.
            (3) Children with disabilities are at an increased risk for sexual abuse and subsequent increased risk for substance abuse as adults.
    b. Access to care, treatment, and research
        i. Deaf persons with HIV infection are a minority within a minority community and lack necessary support structures to successfully manage their treatment.
        ii. Communication barriers limit access to care and treatment or research protocols. Few medical facilities own a TTY machine, reducing most communication with the Deaf, including directions to the clinic.
        iii. Low employment rates for Deaf persons translates to less private insurance coverage, poorer health status, and fewer options for personal transportation to attend appointments. Deaf persons may be diagnosed with HIV late in the disease (when symptomatic) and die sooner than their hearing peers due to a decreased comprehension of HIV disease, limited assistance with medication adherence, and inadequate social support systems.
        iv. Deaf persons may not understand the concept of taking medicines before getting sick (prophylaxis), the specificity of medications (e.g., mistakenly assuming all antibiotics can be used interchangeably), or the importance of HAART adherence.

4. Specific care approaches
    a. Individual
        i. Assure accurate and consistent interpreting services; interpreters vary in fluency with specific levels of sign language (e.g., minimal language skills vs. signed English).
        ii. Use telecommunication devices for the Deaf (TDD or TTY) or telephone relay systems so that Deaf clients have access to providers via the telephone.
        iii. Use Deaf counselors or peer educators whenever possible.
        iv. Use visual aids for comprehension and encourage peer discussion for skill building.

v. Encourage emotional expression and facilitate grieving.

vi. Offer guidance and support in navigating the health care system.

vii. Empower individuals to take responsibility for actions and understand consequences of personal decision making. Role play safer sex negotiation.

viii. Do not assume understanding of crucial vocabulary; explain all terminology and validate by encouraging the Deaf person to explain concepts back to the counselor.

b. Community

i. Increase communication with the Deaf and hard of hearing community.

(1) Provide interpreting services at community forums and prevention/care sites.

(2) Provide training to nurses and health care providers in TTY machine use and ASL.

(3) Decrease stereotypes and lack of understanding about the Deaf community.

ii. Involve high-risk Deaf persons in all levels of prevention planning.

iii. Develop an appreciation for the richness of Deaf culture and identify beliefs, values, and needs; develop a culturally appropriate approach to providing HIV-prevention and clinical care services.

iv. Recruit, educate, and hire Deaf peer counselors to provide services, perform outreach activities, and build capacity in the Deaf community. Provide outreach efforts to all levels of the Deaf community, including schools, rehabilitation centers, organizations, social groups, and mobile vans for difficult to reach individuals.

v. Develop targeted services (e.g., Deaf gay men, Deaf women, Deaf drug users, Deaf African Americans).

vi. Provide HIV case managers and health care providers with specialized training to serve disadvantaged Deaf persons who lack skills in American Sign Language.

vii. Install TTY machines in clinics.

6.7 People With Hemophilia

1. Description of the community

a. Hemophilia is a sex-linked genetic disorder characterized by an absence or deficiency of a plasma-clotting protein; because of inheritance patterns, most people with hemophilia are male. Additionally, there are numerous other inherited bleeding disorders, such as von Willebrand disease, which are generally less severe in nature.

b. Types of hemophilia

i. Hemophilia A (classic hemophilia) is caused by deficiency of clotting protein factor VIII; it is 4 times more prevalent than hemophilia B.

ii. Hemophilia B (Christmas disease) is caused by a deficiency of clotting protein factor IX.

c. Hemophilia A and B are characterized by the severity of the clotting disorder (normal factor level is approximately 100%)

i. Severe hemophilia: < 1% baseline clotting factor level

ii. Moderate hemophilia: 1% to 5% baseline clotting factor level

iii. Mild hemophilia: 5% to 50% baseline clotting factor level

d. U.S. incidence: 1 in 7,500 live male births; there are approximately 20,000 people with hemophilia in the United States (National Hemophilia Foundation, 2002a).

e. Many people with hemophilia have been instructed in self-infusion with factor concentrates to immediately treat bleeding episodes. Thus, they are very knowledgeable about recognition of bleeding episodes and infusion techniques.

f. Between 1978 and 1985, people with hemophilia were exposed to HIV through infusions of plasma-derived factor concentrates used to treat hemorrhages. It is estimated that approximately 8,000 people with hemophilia or other bleeding disorders became HIV seropositive through plasma factor products (National Hemophilia Foundation, 2002b).

g. In 1982, the Centers for Disease Control and Prevention (CDC) reported the first case of AIDS in a person with hemophilia (Centers for Disease Control and Prevention, 1982).

h. As of June 2001, 5,471 people with inherited bleeding disorders have been diagnosed with AIDS in the United States (Centers for Disease Control and Prevention, 2001a). Of these, 237 were < 13 years old when diagnosed.

i. It is estimated that 50% of those infused with clotting factors between 1978 and 1985 became HIV seropositive and that 70% of those with severe hemophilia (baseline factor level < 1%) became HIV seropositive (Augustyniak et al., 1990) because of the amount of infected infusion products used.

j. Some HIV-infected people with hemophilia subsequently transmitted the virus to their sexual partners.
   i. Between 15% and 30% of the sexual partners of people with hemophilia became HIV seropositive.
   ii. Vertical transmission has also occurred.

k. CDC reported two cases of HIV transmission occurring from one HIV-infected person with hemophilia to another person residing in the same household. One case occurred through IV or percutaneous exposure from home infusion (Centers for Disease Control and Prevention, 1992). In the second case, the mechanism of exposure was from an unrecognized or unreported incident of blood contact (Centers for Disease Control and Prevention, 1993).

l. Viral inactivation of all factor concentrates began in 1984; since 1987, through surveillance methods, no new infections have been identified from factor infusions that have been virally inactivated and donor screened (Frick et al., 1992).

m. As with other people who have a chronic illness, people with hemophilia do not want to be identified by a disease (i.e., "hemophiliacs") but rather as people with a disease.

2. Common health issues
   a. Hemarthrosis, a complication of hemophilia, may affect treatment for HIV (e.g., painful arthropathy is commonly treated with ibuprofen; however, the combination of antiretrovirals and ibuprofen may cause bleeding; Ragni et al., 1988).
   b. HIV therapies that may cause thrombocytopenia may be contraindicated or need to be monitored more cautiously.
   c. It is extremely important to consider the underlying bleeding disorder if procedures are planned that may induce bleeding, such as biopsies, arterial punctures, and bronchoscopy. Hemophilia treatment center staff should be consulted prior to any planned procedures.
   d. People with hemophilia are more likely to experience significant bleeding if they develop idiopathic thrombocytopenia purpura (ITP) because of their underlying bleeding disorder.
   e. Septic arthritis may develop in joints previously damaged by hemarthrosis and in joints with arthroplasties.
   f. Lymphomas may present as pseudohematomas.

3. HIV/AIDS in the hemophilia community
   a. Transmission, risk behaviors, and prevention issues
      i. Sexual partners of HIV-seropositive people with hemophilia are at risk for HIV infection and need to cope with changing their sexual practices to incorporate safer sex practices.
   b. Access to care, treatment, and research
      i. During the early 1980s, people with hemophilia lived in constant fear of their HIV infection becoming known and of being

associated with a high-risk group; stigma presented a significant barrier to care.

ii. In the 1980s, people with hemophilia frequently lacked access to clinical trials because of the geographic location of research sites or exclusion from particular trials because of elevated liver function tests associated with complications of hemophilia, particularly hepatitis C.

iii. Historically, the National Hemophilia Foundation coordinated the AIDS Clinical Trial Unit (ACTU) Without Walls to coordinate and monitor NIAID research protocols at hemophilia treatment centers nationwide (Kramer et al., 1990). Today, HIV-infected people with hemophilia are referred to local resources for research opportunities.

iv. The National Hemophilia Foundation continues to advocate for research protocol inclusion criteria considerations so as not to exclude people with hemophilia.

v. Most people with hemophilia are already connected to a hemophilia treatment center for coordination of their bleeding disorder; thus, many also have access to HIV care coordination through their established nurse coordinator.

4. Specific care approaches
   a. Individual
      i. Counsel about standard precautions to prevent viral transmission, including the handling and disposal of infusion products and equipment.
      ii. Refer patient to local hemophilia support groups and services.
      iii. Teach and reinforce safer sex practices.
   b. Community
      i. Promote hemophilia support services and programs, including peer programs.
      ii. Participate in public policy discussions about access to hemophilia and HIV care, treatment, and advocacy in schools and other public institutions or in community-based organizations that provide services to people with HIV infection.

6.8 Homeless Persons

1. Description of the community
   a. The Stuart B. McKinney Homeless Assistance Act (1988) defines the homeless as an individual or family who meet the following criteria:

   - Lacks a fixed, regular, and adequate nighttime residence
   - Have a primary nighttime residence that is supervised, such as a publicly or privately operated shelter
   - Use a public or private place not designed for or ordinarily used as a regular sleeping accommodation for human beings
   - Use a place for shelter that is designed to provide temporary living, such as welfare hotels, congregate shelters, or transitional housing for the mentally ill
   - Have limited shelter resources or are living temporarily with friends or relatives

   b. HIV/AIDS is three times higher in homeless compared with nonhomeless populations, and HIV/AIDS is even higher among the mentally ill. One third to one half of AIDS cases are among the homeless or those at risk of being homeless (Song & HRSA, 2000).
   c. Diverse factors that contribute to homelessness include the following:

   - Unemployment/underemployment, lack of affordable housing, failure of the social safety net, and poverty
   - Indigence following overwhelming medical cost for care of physical disabilities or chronic illness
   - Abusive/neglectful home environments that force women, children, and adolescents onto the streets without shelter or social support

- Problems related to drug and alcohol use
- Problems related to mental illness (an estimated 30% to 49% of homeless people suffer some degree of mental illness; they are easily victimized and unlikely to receive appropriate treatment; Song & HRSA, 2000)
- Dual or multiple diagnoses of addiction, mental health, HIV, tuberculosis, and hepatitis C
- Stigmatization related to any of the previous conditions
- Discriminatory treatment by health care and service providers
- Illegal immigrant status

2. Common health issues
   a. Common comorbidities (e.g., respiratory, foot, skin, parasitic intestinal infections; dental and periodontal disease; infestations; tuberculosis, hepatitis C)
   b. No or limited access to hygiene facilities (toilets, bathrooms, shower, laundry); inadequate clothing in inclement weather
   c. Poor diet (inadequate caloric and nutrient intake reduces resistance to illness and ability to regain health)
   d. Few opportunities for purposeful activity, leading to boredom, low self-esteem, and an exacerbation of existing mental problems
   e. Special concerns of homeless families include the following:

   - Fifty percent of teens report pregnancies while homeless.
   - Homeless people lack support structures for child rearing.
   - Homeless people are more likely to drop out of school or miss school due to a chaotic lifestyle.
   - Homeless people engage in minimal health maintenance (e.g., immunizations, especially for hepatitis; early detection of HIV; recognition of early developmental problems).
   - Homeless people receive little or no teaching concerning safer sexual practices and problems arising from drug use, for parents or children.

   f. Social issues of homeless individuals include the following:

   - There is a high incidence of trauma-related injuries.
   - Medications are often stolen or lost.
   - There is a high incidence of physical (60%) and sexual abuse to individuals and children (75% women, 30% men, and 35% to 50% out of home youth).
   - Client-centered services are frequently unavailable.
   - Low-cost housing is unavailable in areas adjacent to available services.
   - Programs that deal with addiction (e.g., needle exchange, methadone, detoxification) are inadequate.
   - Few service resources are available to assist with child rearing and education.
   - Fewer shelters are available in rural areas.

3. HIV/AIDS in the homeless community
   a. Transmission, risk behaviors, and prevention issues
      i. The longer a person is homeless, the greater the likelihood he or she will fall into one or more high-risk behaviors, such as sharing needles and using unsafe sexual practices (e.g., sex with multiple partners, exchanging sex for money).
      ii. Homeless teens' intention to use condoms is based on present needs, social connectedness, self-efficacy, and lack of resources for condoms. (Rew, Fouladi, & Yockey, 2002). Homeless teens do not receive social support of caring adults to guide decision making. They often use sex to acquire the bare necessities (e.g., food, shelter, drugs, companionship). They have decreased self-care because of despair, hopelessness, and untreated mental illness, and they lack social and assertive skills that might help reduce their risk for HIV.
      iii. Sexual and physical abuse rates are disproportionately high, contributing to poor self-care.
      iv. All activities of daily living, including consensual and

nonconsensual sex, take place in unsafe and unclean conditions.

  v. Lack of housing leads to affronts to the immune system due to extremes in temperatures.

  vi. Food and shelter become first priority, leaving few economic resources for condoms.

  vii. Infrequent access to health care may delay diagnosis of multiple health problems, including HIV, tuberculosis, hepatitis C, and sexually transmitted diseases, which in turn may increase rates of HIV transmission, including vertical transmission.

b. Access to care, treatment, and research

  i. Barriers include lack of health insurance and inability to pay for care, primarily due to having no fixed address and inability to receive social and medical entitlements.

  ii. Fifty-six percent of homeless people have no regular source of health care, which contributes to poor continuity (Song & HRSA, 2000).

  iii. Homeless people are not able to navigate the difficult and confusing health care system without assistance.

  iv. Homeless people are not able to tolerate long waits for care due to substance use, mental illness, and risk of losing belongings or place in food or shelter lines.

  v. Homeless people lack knowledge of where to go for care and lack transportation (or the means to pay for it).

  vi. Homeless people do not trust in the system because of previous negative experiences of discriminatory treatment by care providers.

  vii. Homeless people have a limited ability to adhere to research protocols because of a chaotic lifestyle.

  viii. Treatment outcomes are affected by lack of continuity of care because homeless people may use the emergency room instead of a doctor's office when seeking care. Homeless people may have poor adherence to medication schedules due to a chaotic lifestyle (e.g., can not pay, unable to wait to have prescriptions filled, might have prescriptions stolen), mental illness, substance abuse and treatment failure due to developing resistance to medications, interactions with street drugs, or failure to take medications consistently. Homeless peoples' lack of refrigeration restricts choices of antiretroviral medications that require special diets or cooling.

4. Specific care approaches

a. Individual

  i. Establish trust through open, direct, nonjudgmental exploration of individual's beliefs, risk factors, and perceived needs and barriers to care.

  ii. Use client-centered approach to care and treatment.

  iii. Relationship may take time to develop; complete history may not emerge for weeks or months due to mistrust; be patient.

  iv. Listen carefully to what clients are trying to say; ask direct questions to clarify.

  v. Assess cultural, legal, social service, and daily living needs; be aware that shelter, food, money, and drug and alcohol needs often take priority over health care; be prepared to assist with meeting basic needs first.

  vi. Assess financial support and eligibility for financial benefits: e.g., general assistance, Social Security income, AIDS Drug Assistance Program, and Aid to Families with Dependent Children (AFDC) can help get homeless people off the street, but there may be little left over for food or other essentials. Stable housing improves appointment keeping.

  vii. Base interventions on realistic picture of individual's lifestyle, daily needs, and functional capabilities. Homeless people often do not keep calendars or wear watches; drop-in hours are more appropriate than strictly scheduled appointments.

viii. Use multidisciplinary team approach to ensure all needs are being addressed.
  (1) HIV education
  (2) Immunizations to protect from hepatitis and other infections
  (3) Dental care
  (4) Nutrition: food pantries, emergency meal, or voucher programs
  (5) Harm reduction
  (6) Confidentiality
  (7) Consistency of services through nursing case management
  (8) Plan of care development
  (9) Referrals for education, skills building, and so on as individual is ready

b. Community
  i. Explore the perceptions and reported needs of homeless people in the community (individuals and families) to identify geographic location, social and community support, and available resources.
  ii. Use culturally representative outreach workers to gain entrance and trust in the community and to provide consistent presence, care, and messages within the community.
  iii. Expand use of community-based clinics, mobile units, and home care or public health nursing to increase accessibility to health care.
  iv. Incorporate services that meet the housing, legal, financial, and health care (including mental health) needs into existing community clinic structures to provide one-stop health care or housing facilities.
  v. Provide appropriate, comprehensive mental health services and treatment centers to expand care options.

vi. In areas where the need for services for the homeless is not being met, consider the possibility of providing mobile services to meet the need (i.e., take the service to the client).

vii. Use models that have worked to develop new programs (US Department of Health and Human Services, Health Resources and Services Administration, HIV/AIDS Bureau, 2001).
  (1) Interdisciplinary teams composed of a registered nurse, an addiction counselor, and a peer leader
  (2) Health advocate to liaison within clinic with health care provider and client
  (3) Flexibility to modify organizational structure and goals when needed
  (4) Engaged and challenged client, using stages of change (transtheoretical model)
  (5) Links with community agencies and learning to coexist with different services
  (6) Collaboration with public officials for fair housing issues; provision of stability, which will have a positive impact on behaviors that may put the person at risk for HIV infection/transmission
  (7) Collaboration with community to identify and develop plans to fill in needed service gaps for HIV-infected individuals who are homeless
  (8) Support for continued needle-exchange and free or affordable methadone maintenance programs
  (9) Support for day programs to provide stimulus to relieve boredom and build skills around activities of daily living
  (10) Support for programs to help integrate persons who have been homeless back into the workforce

6.9 Incarcerated Persons

1. Description of the community
   a. The term *incarcerated* refers to inmates in federal prisons, state prisons, and county or city jail systems; prisoners within jail systems are either being detained prior to trial or serving sentences.
   b. By end of 1999, nearly 6.3 million adults were incarcerated or on parole compared with 1 million in 1994 (AIDS Action, 2001; HRSA, 2000).
   c. Eighty-five percent of state inmates and 58% of federal offenders have a history of substance abuse, a reflection of the tighter 1994 drug enforcement laws (Beck & Harrison, 2001).
   d. Incarcerated people have a long history of violence exposure, with 75% of women and 30% of men reporting a history of sexual abuse, which places them at increased risk for HIV infection, if they are not already infected (Browne, Miller, & Maguin, 1999; Cohen et al., 2000; Dilorio, Hartwell, & Hansen, 2002; HRSA, 2000).
   e. Gender characteristics of incarcerated people
      i. Incarcerated women
         (1) Women have higher HIV rates; in the Northeast 21% are HIV infected (DeGroot, 2000). The majority are minority individuals with similar risk factors as other women.
         (2) HIV-infected female inmates are often serving sentences for drug-related crimes, including exchanging sex for money.
         (3) HIV-infected female inmates often have dependent children, and many had their children taken away because of substance abuse.
         (4) Most learned they were HIV infected while incarcerated.
      ii. Incarcerated men
         (1) Men have multiple incarcerations and represent 88% of overall population (Maruschak & Beck, 2001).
         (2) Among incarcerated men, 25% to 33% have previous convictions for violent crimes and therefore are serving long sentences.
         (3) HIV-infected incarcerated men who were symptomatic when entering the correctional system often become sicker while incarcerated.
         (4) HIV-infected incarcerated men often deny having sex with other men; they are more willing to report injecting drug use (IDU).

2. Common health issues
   a. Inmates have increased rates and outbreaks of tuberculosis, hepatitis, sexually transmitted diseases (STDs). These health risks are a part of being in overcrowded settings that present enormous public health hazards and challenges.
   b. Predetention behaviors that compromise health status include IDU, homelessness, poverty, poor self-care skills, poor social skills, concrete thinking, decreased motivation to seek care, and nonadherence to treatment if care has been received. Inmates also have mental health issues. The prevalence of anxiety disorders is as high as 90% (Keaveny & Zauszniewski, 1999), depression is often seen, and inmates within maximum security prison systems are often found to have severe personality and thought disorders. Higher numbers of individuals with mental illness are incarcerated in jails, not prisons, for lesser crimes (Cox, Banks, & Stone, 2000).
   c. Literacy levels are low and are generally masked by the individual. This places offenders at risk for low-paying jobs, poor social adjustment, and poor comprehension abilities that may affect adherence to medical regimens. Sixty-five percent have not finished high school (Hayes, 1994; HRSA, 2000;

National Center for Education Statistics, 1994).

3. HIV/AIDS in the incarcerated community
   a. Transmission, and risk behaviors, and prevention issues
      i. The incidence of HIV/AIDS continues to increase behind bars, reflecting the community rates. Within state prisons, rates are 1% in Midwest prisons, 29% in Northeast, and 5% in federal penitentiaries (Maruschack & Beck, 2001). These trends contribute to the widely held perception that inmates living with HIV/AIDS are the epidemic's most underserved and disadvantaged group, often coming from communities of poverty (Flaskerud & Winslow, 1998). African Americans and Latinos are disproportionately represented among the incarcerated.
      ii. HIV seroprevalence rates among female inmates are actually higher than those among males.
      iii. Reports of inmates transmitting HIV infection to correctional officers (and vice versa) are poorly documented because these sexual acts are considered nonconsensual (inability of offenders to consent) and fall under federal felonies (Human Rights Watch Women's Rights Project, 1996; Amnesty International, 1999; Gollub, 1999). In June 2002, the U.S. Congress convened a task force to investigate ongoing allegations of sexual abuse within prisons.
         (1) State laws vary regarding sexual assault behind bars, with approximately half having no laws. Exchanging sex for money or necessities is common.
         (2) The Centers for Disease Control and Prevention (CDC) reported that sexual abuse is 8 to 10 times higher in prison, compared with the general population, with rates as high as 27% among incarcerated women (Centers for Disease Control and Prevention, 2002a). Stop Prison Rape reported 20% of incarcerated men suffer a sexual assault and 10% suffer a rape (Centers for Disease Control and Prevention, 2002a).
         (3) *Not Part of My Sentence: Violations of the Human Rights of Women in Custody* (Amnesty International, 1999) is part of a human rights violations campaign for female offenders in custody. Numerous examples of misuse of power, humiliation, sexual assault, and inappropriate conduct of male guards with female prisoners during pat downs and body searches were reported.
      iv. Of the inmate population, 3.2% acquire HIV infection during incarceration from having sex, sharing needles for IDU, body piercings, or tattooing; or exchanging blood from altercations (HRSA, 2000; HRSA 2001a; Lichenstein, 2000). This is not well documented because of obvious legal implications.
      v. Few correctional systems allow distribution of condoms and dental dams to inmates, considering them contraband. Some U. S. jails have allowed condoms only if individuals proclaim themselves as gay.
      vi. No correctional facility allows drug paraphernalia for injecting or bleach for cleaning needles, although injecting drug use is known to occur.
      vii. The major strategies for controlling communicable disease within correctional systems are screening, control, and security.
      viii. HIV and STD preventive educational information is

available within most correctional systems.

ix. HIV testing of inmates

(1) There are no clear CDC recommendations for testing.

(2) Sixteen states perform mandatory testing of inmates on entry to the system.

(3) Within some jail systems, anonymous testing is available through local health department representatives.

(4) All federal and many states test inmates on release.

(5) Some counties and states permit mandatory inmate testing in cases of possible exposure to correctional staff.

(6) Some inmates are tested by court order or are automatically tested following commission of certain crimes.

(7) Within all correctional systems, voluntary testing under the order of a qualified health care provider is available.

(8) Centerforce leads a peer-led HIV educational program with partners to reduce HIV transmission during visits with male offenders (Grinstead, Zack, & Faigles, 1999).

(9) Pre- and posttest counseling

(a) For medical testing, HIV counseling is available throughout all correctional systems.

(b) With mass or mandatory testing of inmates, it is often difficult to provide both pre- and posttest counseling.

(c) Counseling is sometimes provided by health assistants rather than professional health care workers.

(10) Confidentiality/Disclosure

(a) Infected inmates whose serostatus is known to others are often subjected to physical and emotional harm and intense discrimination because of homophobia, racism, and misinformation.

(b) Because of the efficiency of the rumor mill, it is often difficult to maintain confidentiality.

(c) HIV disease is often treated during specialty clinic sessions that can inadvertently disclose HIV serostatus by association.

(d) Some states require disclosure of inmates' HIV serostatus to correctional administrators.

(11) Medical care to infected inmates is limited by state taxpayer funding.

(12) Some state prison systems segregate infected inmates from the general prison population, which has been upheld as constitutional (Vicini, 2000).

b. Access to care, treatment, and research

i. AIDS is the second cause of death (29%) for inmates, although the rate is decreasing in the post-HAART era (Centers for Disease Control and Prevention, 1999a).

ii. The incarcerated are not eligible for Medicaid or Medicare benefits, relying on state and local budgetary allocations.

iii. Budgetary constraints, limited staffing, and few HIV/AIDS specialists within correctional systems can present barriers to adequate HIV care.

iv. The quality of HIV care in correctional systems differs widely; localities with higher community HIV seroprevalence are more likely to have HIV experienced health care providers.

v. Eighth amendment rights ensure medical care for offenders (Sylla & Thomas, 2000).

vi. Standards of care are set by the National Commission on Correctional Health Care (National Commission on Correctional Health Care, 1997).

(1) Access to antiretroviral therapies and prophylactic regimens is generally available to inmates when indicated; however, access to mental health and drug rehabilitation services is often quite restricted.

vii. Since the federal regulations were enacted in 1983 to protect inmates against research abuse, strict requirements have resulted in inmates often being excluded from clinical trials. Currently, this is under review again as inmates push for participation in HIV clinical trials (DeGroot, Bick, Thomas, & Stubblefied, 2001).

viii. Obtaining informed consent and ensuring confidentiality for research studies are believed to be extremely difficult in most correctional systems, with questions arising from ability of offender to give consent freely.

ix. Inmates of color may be distrustful of researchers, given past practices of abuse (e.g., the Tuskegee experiment and other coercive prison studies).

x. A recent landmark study conducted behind bars contrasting antiretroviral therapy that was directly observed (DOT) versus keep on person (KOP) showed that the DOT group reached an 85% viral suppression compared with 50% in the KOP group (Fischl et al., 2000).

xi. Many areas of prison life can interfere with ART adherence and continuity. Examples include lockdowns for security reasons, security transfers to other facilities, out of facility medical appointments, court appearances, Bible study and other groups, visiting hours, and work release (Miller & Rundio, 1999).

xii. Treatment outcomes

(1) For inmates who come from unstable environments, incarceration with its limited access to drugs and alcohol may actually result in better treatment outcomes (Eichold, 1995).

(2) Increasing consistent relationships with health care providers has been reported as a primary factor in increasing adherence to medical regimens including antiretroviral treatment (Altice & Buitrago, 1998; Holzemer, 1999; Roberts, 2002).

4. Specific care approaches
   a. Individual
      i. Counsel inmates individually about ways to reduce the risk of HIV transmission (see Preventing the Transmission of HIV Infection, Section 1.3) and allow time for questions.

      ii. Encourage participation in peer education classes when available or use of educational videos shown by health care staff (Fink, Walker, Dole, & Lang, 2001). Videos are available from a number of pharmaceutical companies and from Albany Medical Center HIV Project.

      iii. Provide individual coaching with a matter-of-fact and future-oriented approach, which may be more effective than a group approach.

      iv. Assess literacy levels and design education strategies appropriately. Low-literacy educational materials, such as comic books, that target incarcerated populations are available from pharmaceutical companies in both English and Spanish. Some resources include *Cell War* and *Sister Story* by Bristol-Meyers Squibb and *My Gramma Has HIV* and *Women First* by Agouron. The HIV Invading T-cell Model by Merck provides a visual model because Web access is prohibited.

   v. Educate inmates about preventive health behaviors and provide information that enhances decision making and self-care abilities. (Leenerts, 1999; Nicodemus & Paris, 2001). Offenders have the right to refuse care.

   vi. Provide treatment for psychiatric illness and substance abuse before addressing other issues.

   vii. Avoid labeling and stigmatizing HIV-infected inmates.

   viii. Assess eating habits, prison food versus cubicle/cell, and availability of food when there are medication or food restrictions or needs.

   ix. For inmates who are parents, involve other family members in planning for dependent children (Thompson & Harm, 2000).

   x. Prerelease planning is critical to decrease recidivism and ensure continuity of HIV care, including adherence to antiretroviral therapy. Offenders require referrals and linkages with medical, housing, and social services (HRSA, 2001b). Whenever possible, results from tuberculosis screening and immunization records, summaries of medical records, and an adequate supply of medications should be provided. Application for Medicaid may be required. Unfortunately, unplanned releases from court appearances jeopardize the best plans.

b. Community

   i. Increase offenders participation in peer-led programs such as the AIDS Counseling and Education (ACE) program, currently available at approximately 66% of facilities (Boudin et al., 1999).

   ii. Provide HIV education at all levels

     (1) Correctional officers also lack HIV knowledge (Frank 1999).

     (2) Health care providers, including nurses, who comprise 20% of the correctional staff, may be isolated and lack HIV knowledge.

       (a) An HIV nurse at each facility would be beneficial at all levels.

       (b) Use free educational venues specific to HIV and correctional health care issues that can be facilitated by use of video simulcasts and newsletters such as *HEPPNews* (www.hivcorrections.org) and *HIV Inside.* AIDS Education and Training Centers (AETC) can also provide assistance in HIV education.

       (c) Provide Web sites that can provide guidance to HIV care such as ANAC (www.anacnet.org), Medscape (www.medscape.com), or HIV Medication Guide (http://www.jag.on.ca).

     (3) Prison administration also require HIV education.

   iii. Develop policies that reduce barriers to medication administration to provide for the highest quality of care. This includes policies regarding DOT and KOP, HIV clinical trials, food restrictions, and activities that interfere with administering medications (Babudieri, Aceti, D'Offizi, Carbonara, & Starnini, 2000). Linkages with the community are imperative. Models that have been successful include ex-offender–run, public-health run, and university affiliated programs that organize multifaceted programs that include making medical appointments, meeting housing needs, and assisting with social services (AIDSAction, 2001; HRSA, 2001b; Freudenberg, Wilets, Greene, & Richie, 1998). Telemedicine is a helpful bridge to the community providing medical consultation.

    iv. Apply public health practices to reduce transmission of HIV, tuberculosis, and STDs, including harm reduction (Gaiter, Jurgen, Mayer, & Hollibaugh, 2000).

    v. Amnesty International (1999) suggests increasing same-sex correctional officers (CO) in living and bathing areas of prisons as one method of reducing sexual assault by opposite-sex COs.

    vi. Advocate at all levels for harm reduction and accessible preventive devices (condoms and bleach) behind bars (Gaiter et al., 2000; Leh, 1999).

    vii. Advocate regarding alternatives to incarceration for substance abusers and increased funding for rehabilitation behind bars. This would include detoxification, education and counseling, and self-help groups such as Alcoholics Anonymous and Narcotics Anonymous during incarceration. On release, inmates need to be referred to halfway houses or day treatment programs.

6.10 Lesbians and Bisexual Women

1. Description of the community
   a. Lesbian: female who is primarily attracted emotionally and physically to other females
   b. Bisexual woman: woman who identifies self as emotionally and physically attracted to males and females
      i. Women who have sex with women (WSW) may self-identify as heterosexual or may not identify at all as lesbians for various reasons related to culture,

ethnicity, occupation, or peer support.
      ii. Women, especially women of color or of non-White cultural backgrounds, may not identify themselves for fear of rejection by their family and cultural supports.

2. Common health issues
   a. Sexual orientation identity does not predict sexual behaviors.
   b. WSW are visible to society as women with the same gender biases, and women who fear social retaliation may not identify themselves as lesbian.
   c. Access to health care and quality of care is a major concern of WSW.
      i. Many use complementary health care providers to seek care that is more holistic and less discriminatory.
      ii. Health care practices emerge from heterosexual assumptions with perspectives that neglect to address lesbian concerns, which establish alienating practices.
      iii. Providers should use unbiased language and questions.
      iv. Lack of sexual history that includes sexual orientation fails to assess risk behaviors (e.g., toys, sexual play during menses, other specific sexual risks).
   d. A social history is important in making appropriate recommendations about preventive health screenings, preventive behaviors, and treatment options. Social history should include the following:

   - Substance use and abuse history
   - Physical or emotional abuse
   - Social systems and employment
   - A complete history that assesses behavior placing women at risk for HIV transmission

   e. Clinicians should take a careful sexual history.
      i. It is important to include history of sexual activity with men because past and current sexual partners may not be limited to women. Of WSW, 53% to 99% report having had sex with men, and 20% to 30% continue to have

sex with men as well as women (Marrazzo, Koutsky, & Handsfield, 2001). Unprotected sexual activity with men increases the likelihood of risk for past acquisition of chronic viral STD, such as HIV, HSV, and HPV.

ii. Sexual history should also include the following:

- Use of words about sexual behaviors that are understandable to the client
- Prior sex with gay, bisexual, or IV drug using men and women
- Number of lifetime male sex partners
- Exchange of sex for drugs or money
- Age at first vaginal or anal intercourse
- Unprotected anal intercourse
- Use of condoms
- How sex toys are cleaned and whether they are shared
- Is there sex during menses
- Evaluate other sex behavior placing women at risk for HIV transmission

3. HIV/AIDS in the lesbian and bisexual community of women
   a. Transmission, risk behaviors, and prevention issues
      i. Through December 1998, 2,220 of the 109,311 women reported with AIDS are reported to have had sex with women; however, most had other risk factors.
      ii. Of the 2,220 women, 347 reported having had sex only with women, and 98% of them had another risk factor, mainly IV drug use (Centers for Disease Control and Prevention, n.d.).
      iii. Information regarding WSW is missing in half of the 109,311 reports, which is possibly due to lack of solicitation of information by the provider (Centers for Disease Control and Prevention, n.d.).
      iv. Female-to-female transmission is uncommon; however, the

possibility exists, though other behaviors can mask it. Further research is needed in this area.

v. Evidence exists that herpes simplex virus, *Trichomonas vaginalis, Gardnerella vaginalis,* and possibly human papillomavirus may be transmitted from woman to woman. However, transmission of HIV is less clear (Diamant, Schuster, McGuigan, & Lever, 1999).

vi. There are several case reports of HIV-infected women whose only known potential route of transmission was woman to woman.

vii. One prospective study found no woman-to-woman transmission of HIV after 6 months among 18 HIV-discordant couples. The researchers suggest transmission is biologically and reasonably possible; however, the following factors were noted to hinder transmission:

- Lack of traumatic sex (for many WSW)
- Lowered rate of sex in lesbian couples
- Lower risk in lesbian sexual practices
- Lower level of HIV in cervicovaginal secretions
- Efficacy of defensive biological mechanisms
- Higher attention to risk practices (Raiteri, Baussano, Giobbia, Fora, & Sinicco, 1998)

viii. Modes of HIV transmission among WSW include the following:

- IV drug use (most common mode of transmission)
- Donor insemination for pregnancy through fresh and frozen semen
- Sexual risk behaviors for WSW

(1) WSW, like heterosexual women, engage in a wide variety of sexual behaviors and practices.

(2) Some factors can increase the chance of transmission. These factors include concurrent STDs, especially ulcerative conditions; sores on the lips and mouth; cuts on the hands; and transfer of fluid by hand, glove, toy, or insertion device.

(3) Sex toys or other insertion devices may play a role in transmission. These objects can cause trauma, which may become a portal of entry for HIV during activities; cause exchange of infected fluids if they are shared without disinfection; draw blood or cause abrasion if used in traumatic or sadomasochistic activities; transfer virus through contact with urine, feces, or menstrual blood on partner's broken skin or mucous membranes.

ix. Spermicides added or found on condoms can kill HIV and STDs; however, they can increase inflammation that can increase transmission.

x. Douches and enemas may irritate vaginal and rectal linings and cause microscopic tears or abrasions, which increase risk for HIV transmission.

4. Specific care approaches
   a. Individual
      i. Use of universal precautions and latex barriers during traumatic or sadomasochistic activities.
      ii. Avoid use of semen from HIV-infected men and avoid using fresh semen unless donor has been properly screened for HIV.
      iii. Precautions should be used to avoid sexual transmission.
         (1) Use protective barriers during cunnilingus or anilingus.
         (2) Use dental dams.
         (3) Condoms may be cut at the tip and the side to lie flat as a barrier.
         (4) Plastic wrap, such as Glad Wrap or Saran Wrap, are unofficially advocated as body fluid barriers. Effectiveness of these methods has not been researched.
      iv. Wear protective gloves (latex or polyurethane) on hands during mutual masturbation to avoid sharing of body fluids, especially during menstruation.
      v. Use female condom with sex toys in the vagina or for anal sex. Do not use female condoms for cunnilingus because they do not cover the entire vaginal opening.
      vi. Use precautions with toys and devices. Each partner should have their own toy or device, and condoms should be applied on dildos or other toys at each use. Disinfect toys and devices (depending on the toy's material), using one of the following methods:
      (Note: Electric and battery-operated devices, such as vibrators, cannot be immersed in water.)
         (1) Wash with soap and water, then rinse.
         (2) Boil the toy for 20 minutes.
         (3) Soak in isopropyl alcohol for 30 minutes and rinse with water.
         (4) Rinse three times with full-strength bleach, then rinse with water.
   b. Community (see also Section 6.4)
      i. Screening programs targeted toward women of all sexual orientations and socioeconomic levels for early identification and management of HIV disease
      ii. Assistance accessing health care
      iii. Increasing awareness among all nurses and health care providers regarding HIV risks among lesbian and bisexual women
      iv. Increasing awareness among lesbian and bisexual women

regarding risk factors for HIV transmission

6.11 Migrant and Seasonal Farm Workers

1. Description of the community
   a. Migrant and seasonal farm workers (MSFM) are agricultural laborers who cultivate and harvest crops during growing seasons and who migrate with the change of season.
   b. There are major streams of MSFWs in the United States.
      i. The East Coast stream consists of native African Americans, Latinos, and Mexican Americans.
      ii. The Central stream is made up of Mexicans and Mexican Americans.
      iii. The West Coast stream is made up primarily of Mexicans.
   c. The majority of MSFWs are Mexican.
   d. The largest number of MSFWs are employed in California, Texas, Florida, North Carolina, and Washington.
   e. The total number of MSFWs is difficult to determine but is estimated to be more than four million (Go & Baker, 1995; Organista & Organista, 1997).
   f. The majority of MSFWs are young (average age is 25) and male and often live and work in rural areas.
2. Common health issues
   a. Most live in poverty.
   b. Education is limited.
   c. Environmental stressors include the following:

   - Poor housing
   - Inadequate diet and difficulty taking medication with specific dietary needs
   - Limited sanitation facilities
   - Isolation (often due to illegal immigrant status)
   - Long, harsh working hours

   d. Cultural and language barriers to care are present.
   e. There is a lack of knowledge about or ability to qualify for care in the communities.
   f. Health beliefs about HIV/AIDS may delay HIV testing.

3. HIV/AIDS in the MSFW community
   a. Transmission, risk behaviors, and prevention issues
      i. HIV/AIDS is 10 times higher in the MSFW community than in the general population.
      ii. Unprotected sex is the major mode of HIV transmission.
      iii. Latino culture may contribute to high-risk sexual behaviors (i.e., gender-role beliefs related to extramarital sex and submissiveness of women and intolerance of homosexual behavior).
      iv. Condom use practices are inconsistent, and knowledge of condoms is lacking.
      v. Exchanging sex for money is common at many migrant camps.
      vi. Lay injections of vitamins, antibiotics, hormones, pain killers, and steroids is common among MSFWs from Mexico.
   b. Access to care, treatment, and research
      i. MSFWs often are not privy to or eligible for mainstream HIV/AIDS prevention and education programs.
      ii. Continuity of care and adherence to complex treatment regimens is extremely challenging.
      iii. Community-based agencies have been found to provide more effective prevention services than federal state or private agencies (Organista, & Organista, 1997).
      iv. MSFWs often delay seeking HIV testing and care after diagnosis.
      v. Medication side effects and dietary requirements impact ability to work. Some individuals stop migrating, which affects earning ability.
4. Specific care approaches
   a. Individual
      i. Care should be culturally sensitive and gender specific.
      ii. Acknowledge existing care-seeking practices.
      iii. Assist with skills building if patient is no longer migrating.

iv. Treatment regimens need to be coordinated between health care sites or agencies.

b. Community

i. Programs need to consider the level of acculturation and the mobility of the population.

ii. Brief interventions need to be developed that include HIV testing and counseling.

iii. Generational differences in the camps (*colonia*) need to be considered (Ford, King, Nerenberg, & Rojo, 2001).

iv. Farmworker Health Services, Inc. provides outreach and education to MSFWs by creating and maintaining linkages between the MSFWs and existing local health care providers, including lay health workers.

v. User-friendly and language-appropriate services, such as mobile units and extended hours, would increase accessibility to care.

vi. Existing models should be used to develop new programs (U.S. Department of Health and Human Services, Health Resources and Services Administration, HIV/AIDS Bureau, 2001).

6.12 Older Persons

1. Description of the community

a. For years, the Centers for Disease Control and Prevention (CDC) grouped all cases of middle-aged and older adults AIDS cases into one category of age 50 or older. In some states, this practice continues. As of December 2000, 774,463 AIDS cases have been reported, 11% in men ages 50 and older ($n = 71,428$) and 9% in women ages 50 and older ($n = 12,616$). Despite a prevalence rate of approximately 10% since the beginning of the epidemic, middle-aged and older people living with HIV/AIDS are invisible (Centers for Disease Control and Prevention, 2002a).

2. Common health issues

a. The incidence of chronic illnesses increases with aging. The interaction of chronic illnesses (such as diabetes and hypertension) with HIV results in complex health management plans. Antiretrovirals can further complicate treatment plans already consisting of numerous medications.

b. With increased age, there is decreased organ functioning.

c. Older injecting drug users often have acquired injection-related chronic illnesses, such as kidney problems, cardiac changes, and blood-borne infections, such as hepatitis and HIV.

d. Hyperlipidemia and insulin resistance associated with some antiretrovirals are particularly problematic in middle-aged and older persons already at increased risk for heart disease and stroke. African Americans are at even higher risk for these health problems (see Section 6.14 for more information on African Americans).

e. Early work indicated that mortality rates after an AIDS diagnosis were twice as high for persons ages 50 and older, compared with younger persons, but this may be due to delayed diagnosis of HIV disease resulting in missed opportunities for treatment.

3. HIV/AIDS in the middle-aged and older community

a. Transmission, risk behaviors, prevention issues

i. Prevention messages do not target the community, sending the message that HIV is a problem that only affects younger people.

ii. In the United States, the life expectancy for women exceeds that of men. Heterosexual women are at particular disadvantage if they are interested in being sexually active because there are many fewer male partners in their age cohort available to them. Middle-aged and older women may have lost a steady partner to death or divorce and are reentering the dating scene with few skills in condom negotiation and facing fierce competition for an attractive, sexually competent male partner (Nokes, 1996).

iii. Older adults disclose their HIV status to fewer persons.
   (1) Heightened fear of stigmatization and rejection after disclosure
   (2) Fewer persons in the middle-aged and older person's social network

iv. Middle-aged and older persons report difficulty in learning their HIV status, even when they request an HIV screening test.

v. Before the spring of 1985, receipt of infected blood products was the major route of infection, especially for older White women. Since the advent of widespread testing of blood and body products, that route of infection has been virtually eliminated. There are currently no differences based on age in routes of HIV infection.

vi. Prevention messages do not target middle-aged and older adults. To illustrate, using the search engine on the CDC HIV surveillance Web page, the key word "older adult" yielded 1 citation, "middle-aged" yielded 4 citations, and "adolescents" yielded 543 citations.

vii. Middle and older age is a period in which people have ideally acquired wisdom based on life experiences and education. There is an assumption that, unlike younger people, older people should know better and control their urges to prevent exposure to HIV.

viii. Older adults may perceive that fear of infection is outweighed by the desire for intimate sexual contact and deny possible risk associated with sexual behaviors.

ix. The two major risk behaviors for HIV infection are unprotected male-male sex and injection drug use, presenting unique challenges for middle-aged and older persons in the gay male and injection drug use communities.

x. Physical changes associated with aging require tailored HIV prevention messages for middle-aged and older adults (Klein et al., 2001). The gay male community values youth and physical fitness, and body changes associated with aging are often not perceived as desirable. Many middle-aged and older gay men have lost their extensive social network to HIV/AIDS and find themselves relatively isolated.

xi. Substance abuse presents several issues.
   (1) Substance abusers often have a history of incarceration that limits their employment opportunities, and they may have strained relationships with their non-drug-using social support network.
   (2) Persons with a family history of drug use are more likely to have a drug use issue; older adolescent and younger adult children may be repeating the mistakes of their parents, which causes much pain, guilt, and regret.

xii. Middle-aged and older men may experience erectile dysfunction, which results in difficulty in applying condoms because the penis may not sustain an erection. Medications to treat erectile dysfunction, such as Viagra, have resolved the problem of condom application. Men who believed that they had lost the ability to be sexually active are now enjoying their increased skills, but there has been little effort to link prevention messages to prescriptions for medications to treat erectile dysfunction (Sadeghi-Nejad et al., 2000).

xiii. Middle-aged and older women are experiencing the symptoms of menopause, which usually includes decreased vaginal secretions. The lack of lubrication may increase microabrasions that would increase the possibility of HIV infection during unprotected sex. Although there are a variety of strategies that women can use to increase vaginal lubrication, they are not tied to an HIV prevention message.

xiv. Health care providers may be reluctant to screen middle-aged and older adults for risky sexual and drug use behaviors because they fear offending the older person and may feel embarrassed to ask personal questions of clients who may remind them of their parents.

b. Access to care, treatment, and research

i. There are very few health care providers who have expertise both in HIV treatment and biological changes associated with aging. Using many providers results in fragmented health care. When middle-aged and older persons fail to disclose their HIV status to providers who are treating their aging problems, unexpected and possibly dangerous outcomes of treatment can result.

ii. Medications are metabolized differently as people age, yet there are no guidelines for HIV medication protocols for middle-aged and older persons. Because the numbers of participants in clinical trials are low (less than 50), it is not clear how these findings can be used in this age group.

iii. Research trials conducted to explore the interrelationship of menopause treatment and HIV disease in these aging women have been small and lack the rigor of a clinical trial such as PACTG 076 B, the study of AZT during pregnancy.

iv. Research is needed to determine if there are differences in treatment outcomes between middle-aged and older adults and younger persons. The problem of comorbidities, often present in this population, complicates treatment plans and may result in increased morbidity and mortality (Nokes et al., 2000). On the other hand, these people are survivors and have learned skills that younger populations may not have learned. Although it is acknowledged that, in general, older people die more frequently than younger people do, the key issue is excess mortality. How many older people in the United States with HIV are dying years before their average life expectancy?

4. Specific care approaches

a. Individual

i. Health care providers need to anticipate that these individuals may need more activity of daily living supports to maintain themselves at home. Functional impairments related to activities such as walking up steps and carrying groceries occur more often in this community than in persons ages 49 and younger.

ii. Middle-aged and older adults reported that they want to be respected for their age and sometimes find it difficult to be lectured by health care providers who are the age of their children. A fine balance needs to be achieved because the younger provider has knowledge and skills needed by the older person, but these contributions must be conveyed in a manner that promotes acceptance.

b. Community

i. Middle-aged and older adults with HIV/AIDS may have a pivotal role in an extended family network. They may be the grandmother, mother, wife, and friend who comforts, cooks, and nurtures. Illness of this significant hub in the social network will affect many people and destabilize the social equilibrium of many.

ii. The gay and lesbian communities have created social supports that provide vital services that cannot be accessed from the broader, heterosexual community because of real or perceived stigma. These services are often provided free of charge, and the more widespread use of the Internet has facilitated access to resources for gay and lesbian persons who live in more remote areas.

iii. Further work is needed to determine the extent of the excess mortality that an HIV diagnosis causes in different racial, gender, and age groups.

6.13 Rural Communities

1. Description of the community
   a. Rural versus nonmetropolitan (U.S. Department of Agriculture, 2001)
      i. Rural or nonmetropolitan residents represent approximately 25% of the U.S. population.
      ii. Rural area is a population density of fewer than 2,500 residents.
      iii. Frontier area is fewer than six people per square mile.
      iv. Nonmetropolitan refers to a county without a core area that has more than 50,000 residents (a standard metropolitan statistical area [SMSA])
   b. Characteristics of a rural community (Bushy, 2000; Ricketts, 1999)
      i. The South has largest proportion of rural residents and the Northeast has smallest.
      ii. People in rural communities often have better access to extended family than urban residents.
      iii. Rural residents are self-reliant and independent.
      iv. People in rural communities have strong, informal support resources.
      v. Insiders are long-time residents, and outsiders are newcomers.
      vi. Rural communities are characterized by a lack of anonymity (lack of privacy).
      vii. A large proportion of other special populations are in some areas (e.g., Native Americans, Hispanics, seasonal migrant farm workers).
      viii. Employment rates in agriculture, forestry, and fishing are higher in rural than in urban areas and is declining. Most employment is in manufacturing and services.

2. Common health issues
   a. Residents are generally poorer, older, less insured, have higher rates of unemployment, and are less educated than residents in urban areas.
   b. Residents experience isolation due to geographical remoteness.
   c. There is often difficulty receiving health care due to lack of a nearby public transportation system.
   d. Rural residents often delay seeking health care until gravely ill.
   e. Fewer health care providers, including HIV specialists, are in rural areas.
   f. There is a reluctance of nurses in rural areas to care for HIV/AIDS clients (Preston, Forti, Kassab, & Koch, 2000).
   g. Higher rates of chronic disease and infant mortality occur in rural than in urban areas.

3. HIV/AIDS in the rural community
   a. Transmission, risk behaviors, and prevention issues
      i. The Centers for Disease Control and Prevention began reporting nonmetropolitan cases of AIDS in 1991.
      ii. New cases of rural HIV/AIDS are increasing at a higher rate than they are in urban areas (Voelker, 1998; Whetten–Goldstein, Nguyen, & Heald, 2001).
      iii. Higher incidence of HIV/AIDS in minorities and women than in urban areas. Some states report a 170-fold increase in AIDS among rural African American women in past decade (Crosby, Yarber, DiClemente, Wingood, & Meyerson, 2002).
      iv. The South is experiencing the most rapid growth of rural cases of HIV/AIDS.

v. According to Bushy (2000) the following conditions contribute to the continued spread of HIV in rural communities:

- Rural residents are less likely to seek testing, and health care providers are less likely to test for HIV.
- Rural pregnant women are less likely to receive HIV counseling.
- Confidentiality is an issue in all areas of care (local residents know each other).
- Stigma prevents seeking care and increases social isolation (coming home if HIV infected vs. leaving for urban area).
- HIV/AIDS education not well accepted, particularly in the schools.
- Transmission is more likely to be heterosexual than in urban areas.

vi. People perceive they are at low risk for HIV transmission. Rural women are more likely than their nonrural counterparts to accept partner statements regarding risk or testing.

vii. Prevention programs may not be targeted to those with the least amount of knowledge about HIV.

viii. In states with high agriculture/farms, individuals may have easier access to clean needles because of veterinary supplies.

b. Access to care, treatment, and research

i. There is an overall shortage of health care providers for local care, and local health care providers often have less experience with HIV diagnoses and treatment protocols.

ii. Limited HIV/AIDS resources and services in rural communities is coupled with fewer integrated case management systems and professional networks to assist patients and families.

iii. Treatment outcomes are negatively affected by lack of access to care (transportation, medical insurance), limited services and resources, and difficulty understanding complex medical regimens.

4. Specific care approaches

a. Individual

i. Adopt culturally sensitive care because rural communities often contain people of different cultures.

ii. Acknowledge social isolation and that there are fewer helpers (family, neighbors, professionals) to draw on. Assess and intervene to solve problems where nurses can offer real help (e.g., HIV education to willing caregivers).

iii. Increase frequency of contact through outreach from experts who use telephone callbacks and telephone education and support systems through the use of telehealth/telemedicine technology, if available, and visiting nurses.

b. Community

i. Identify appropriate HIV educational Web sites that the community can use.

ii. According to St. Lawrence (1999), the following activities can be used at the community level:

- Build professional-community partnerships for prevention activities.
- Assess HIV needs of the community.
- Involve community members in discussing and planning prevention activities among both uninfected and infected.
- Conduct targeted community outreach intervention campaigns.
- Form cooperative networks with schools and work sites.
- Align with state health department prevention plans: school health programs; Women, Infants, and Children (WIC) program; sexually

transmitted disease clinics; and public health workers.

- Educate young adults about prevention strategies and conduct media campaigns geared to rural facts and situations.

iii. Build professional-community partnerships for services to diagnosed population and families.

iv. Educate community groups about the needs of local HIV/AIDS populations (e.g., the faith-based organizations).

v. Use county fairs to disseminate HIV information.

vi. Identify local social gathering spots (e.g., elders, diners, grange, 4H, church) and then target for prevention efforts.

vii. Educate and consult with urban and state task forces about local needs.

viii. Identify resources and obtain funding for services and support with the help of local business leaders and professionals.

ix. Ease interactions with local authority systems, such as police.

x. Build alliances with other rural HIV/AIDS workers and organizations and increase HIV education to nurses and other health care providers via continuing education (CEU) or continuing medical education (CME) and nursing/medical curriculums that integrate HIV.

6.14 The African American Community

1. Description of the community
   a. The majority of African Americans are descendants of West Africans living in the Western Hemisphere. This definition includes African descendants in the West Indies, Canada, Cuba, Central and South America, and Mexico. The terms *African American* and *Black* are used interchangeably to include those individuals who self-identify as either. Generally speaking, for people of the older generation, the word *Black* is more widely acceptable, whereas the younger generation might prefer the term *African American*.
   b. According to Census 2000, 36.4 million people, or 12.9% of the total population, reported being Black or African American. About 60% live in 10 states that contain almost half of the total U.S. population (U.S. Census Bureau, 2001).

2. Common health issues
   a. Disparities in health and illness experienced by African Americans, compared with the U.S. population as a whole, is varied, and despite efforts to improve the health of African Americans, disparities persist (U.S. Department of Health and Human Service, 2001).
      i. Diabetes is the sixth leading cause of death for this population. The African American death rate due to diabetes is more than twice that for Whites.
      ii. Heart disease is the leading cause of death for all racial and ethnic groups. African Americans are 30% more likely to die of heart disease than are Whites.
      iii. African Americans are 30% more likely to die of cancer than are Whites.
      iv. Data from 1999 held that African Americans were 40% more likely to die of stroke than were Whites, when differences in age distributions were taken into account.
      v. African American women are less likely to receive care, and when they do receive it, they are more likely to have received it late.
      vi. According to the 2001 Surgeon General's report (U.S. Department of Health and Human Services, 2001) on mental health, the prevalence of mental disorders is believed to be higher among African Americans than among Whites, and African Americans are more likely than Whites to use the

emergency room for mental health problems.

3. HIV/AIDS in the African American community
   a. Transmission, risk behaviors, and prevention issues
      i. Approximately 1 in 50 African American men and 1 in 160 African American women are believed to be infected with HIV. By comparison, 1 in 250 White men and 1 in 3,000 White women are believed to be infected (Kaiser Family Foundation, n.d.).
      ii. Each year, more than 50% of the new HIV infections occur in African Americans.
      iii. Of all ethnic populations, the African American community has the largest number of people living with AIDS.
      iv. African Americans view AIDS as the number one health problem facing the nation and the world (Kaiser Family Foundation, n.d.).
      v. Subgroups in the African American community are overrepresented in the epidemic.
         (1) African American women comprise 13% of the U.S. population and in the year 2000 represented 63% of the reported AIDS cases in women.
         (2) African American teens (13–19 years old) comprise 15% of the U.S. population and account for 64% of the reported AIDS cases in teenagers.
         (3) African American children represent 58% of all pediatric AIDS cases.
         (4) For African American men ages 25–44 years, HIV infection is the leading cause of death and the third most common cause of death for African American women.
      vi. Anemia is a frequent complication of HIV disease and is an independent predictive marker for disease progression and death in HIV-infected patients. Blacks are almost twice as likely as Whites to have non-drug-related anemia (Sullivan, Hanson, Chu, Jones, & Ward, 1998). The factors associated with this finding have not been elucidated.
      vii. The highest mortality from HIV-related illness occurs in African American men and women.
      viii. According to the 2001 National Health Interview Health Survey, the vast majority of African Americans are aware of the basics of HIV and how the virus is transmitted. There does continue to be some misconception about the transmission of HIV through casual contact, such as kissing and sharing a drink with an HIV-infected person (Kaiser Family Foundation, n.d.).
      ix. A national survey showed that the median age at first vaginal intercourse for African American men is lower than that of Whites (15 years vs. 17 years). In the same study, coital frequency did not differ significantly by race (Billy, Tanfer, Grady, & Klepinger, 1993).
      x. Sexually transmitted diseases are reported more often in African Americans than in Whites and remain an important biological risk factor for the transmission of HIV.
      xi. African Americans are much more likely to be tested late in the course of HIV disease (Wortley et al., 1995).
   b. Access to care, treatment, and research
      i. Being African American or of any race is not a risk factor for AIDS, but social determinants such as poverty, discrimination, social segregation and lower quality of HIV care have contributed to the continued spread of the disease.
      ii. Multiple barriers to care exist in the African American community:
         (1) Studies have found that African Americans continue

to be discriminated against in a variety of areas, ranging from face-to-face interactions, housing, employment, and health and social services (Klonoff & Landrine, 1999).

(2) African Americans are less likely than other groups to have health insurance and correspondingly are less likely to benefit from early intervention and preventive treatment.

(3) A national study found that inferior patterns of HIV care were seen for many of the measures studied in Blacks and Latinos compared with Whites and in the uninsured and Medicaid-insured compared with the privately insured. Even with multivariate adjustment, many differences remained statistically significant. Even by early 1998, fewer Blacks, women, and uninsured and Medicaid-insured persons had started taking antiretroviral medication (Shapiro et al., 1999).

(4) One study of patients in the Baltimore area found that Blacks were less likely than Whites to receive HARRT (Keruly, Conviser, & Moore, 2002).

(5) African Americans are underrepresented in AIDS research. Researchers have difficulty recruiting African Americans into clinical trials.

   (a) One study of Blacks of unknown HIV status confirmed that many African Americans still believe that HIV is an artificially created virus designed by the federal government to exterminate the Black population. Interestingly, this belief was most associated with those of higher levels of education. Men rather than women are likely to hold this view (Klonoff & Landrine, 1999).

   (b) In a separate study, also of Blacks of unknown HIV status, more than half disagreed with the U.S. government's involvement in AIDS research as being beneficial to the African American community. Two thirds of the respondents ($n = 301$) had heard of the Tuskegee Study (where Black men were knowingly not treated for syphilis) and often cited this as the reason why Blacks do not participate in clinical trials. Of those, 50% reported that today's AIDS scientists are more honest and respectful of Blacks than their Tuskegee counterparts (Sengupta et al., 2000).

   iii. Researchers have established that the stigma associated with AIDS is more negative among minorities than among Whites (Herek & Capitanio, 1993).

4. Specific care approaches
   a. Individual
      i. Appreciate the role racism has played and continues to play in the lives of the African American patient. Nurses of all ethnic origins must understand and accept their own values to effectively work with others from different cultures.
      ii. Do a client cultural assessment that includes beliefs, values, biases, taboos, customs, traditions, language, and relationships with family and community.
      iii. Recent evidence has demonstrated that about one third of men with a

sexually transmitted disease are never tested for HIV. The nurse must ensure that individuals at high risk for HIV are appropriately tested (Ciesielski & Boghani, 2002).

    iv. Studies demonstrate that culture-sensitive risk education and interventions are effective in promoting greater use of condoms and reducing risky behaviors (Jemmott, Jemmott, Fong, & McCaffree, 1999). Long-term studies are needed to see if the effects of the interventions are sustained.

b. Community

    i. Belief in AIDS-conspiracy theories among Blacks must be acknowledged and addressed in culturally tailored AIDS prevention and education programs.

    ii. The continued spread of HIV in the African American community is multifactorial. One social theory suggests that when residential, educational, and social segregation exists, African Americans are more likely to engage in sexual and drug-use behaviors that may lead to HIV transmission with other African Americans than with members of other racial groups (Smith et al., 2000).

    iii. Systematic social support has been demonstrated to be influential in controlling the epidemic in certain groups (e.g., the gay community). Adequate and effective support mechanisms are essential if epidemic control is to occur in this and other communities (e.g., injection drug users).

    iv. The Black church has throughout the 20th century promoted education, business, and political activism with the Black community. The church is an ideal setting in which to offer health promotion activities for African Americans (Markens, Fox, Taub, & Gilbert, 2002).

6.15 Pregnant Women

1. Description of the community

    a. The majority of women infected with HIV are of childbearing age.

    b. Vertical or perinatal transmission refers to pregnant women with HIV transferring HIV to their unborn children.

        i. Vertical transmission rates are 15–25% in industrialized countries, such as the United States and Western Europe.

        ii. In developing countries, vertical transmission rates are 25–45%.

    c. HIV can be transmitted antepartally, intrapartally (during delivery), and postpartally through breast-feeding; the majority of all infections are thought to occur late in pregnancy (20–33%) or during delivery (45–80%), with breast-feeding adding an additional 15–35% globally (Newell, 1998; Rouzioux et al., 1995).

2. Common heath issues

    a. Reproductive decisions of HIV-infected women are similar to uninfected women and are influenced by profound meaning of childbearing across cultures and class (Mitchell, Brown, Loftman, & Williams, 1990; Sunderland, Minkoff, Handle, Moroso, & Landesman, 1992).

    b. Pregnancies are often unplanned in both HIV-infected and uninfected women. In the Women's Interagency Health Study (WIHS) study, 3.5% of HIV-infected women versus 9% of uninfected women had unplanned pregnancies (Wilson et al., 1999).

    c. Women are often economically dependent on men and unable to leave abusive relationships. Children often represent bonding in intimate or coercive relationships between a man and woman. Abuse increases during pregnancy, especially in women in relationships with a history of domestic violence. It is important to assess the client's safety and ability to access care, which is often decreased in this population.

3. HIV/AIDS in pregnant women

    a. Transmission, risk behaviors, and prevention issues

i. For serodiscordant couples (one HIV seronegative and one HIV seropositive partner), conception counseling is often omitted by health care professionals for fear of medical legal repercussion should the HIV-uninfected partner seroconvert.

ii. Failure to discuss risks associated with unsafe sex or to provide guidance as to how to reduce or minimize HIV transmission risks actually places discordant couples at an increased risk for unsafe behavior. HIV transmission risks should be discussed often with both individuals present, and the discussion needs to be documented. It is important to know your institution's policy on this topic before doing counseling.

iii. Explore options such as adoption, in vitro fertilization (IVF), intracytoplasmic sperm injection (ICSI), or intrauterine insemination. These methods have low to no HIV transmission reported. Economics and insurance will dictate most options.

iv. If the woman is HIV infected, reduce the partner's risk of contracting HIV by considering intrauterine insemination or self-insemination. Self-insemination methods include fertility timing and turkey basting (Macaulay, Kitzinger, Green, & Wight, 1995). Turkey basting is an unconventional self-insemination, where sperm from the HIV negative partner is self-inserted using a 20 cc syringe or turkey baster. This is an affordable option, decreasing risk for the HIV negative partner. Fertility time can reduce unsafe sexual practices from 30 days/month to 1–2 days/ month reduces overall risks significantly. Menstrual calendars for at least 3 months with basal body temperatures can assist in identifying ovulation and should be kept prior to attempting

conception. Safer sex must be encouraged during this time and at nonfertile times. It is essential that the HIV viral load is undetectable.

v. If the man is HIV infected, consider sperm donation. Recent studies with sperm washing or the previously mentioned alternatives have been encouraging (Ball, 2000; Gilling-Smith, 2000; Mandelbrot, Heard, Henrion-Geant, & Henrion, 1997).

vi. Preconception counseling for men should include education regarding the impact of antiretroviral therapy (ART) on HIV concentrations in semen. HIV in semen is twice as high as serum blood levels. Most men believe that an undetectable HIV serum blood level means that semen is also undetectable and as a result may abandon safer sex practices (Kalichman et al., 2002). After 6 months of ART therapy, 15–34% of men had detectable HIV viral load in the semen. After 18 months of ART, most men have undetectable HIV semen viral loads; however, one study found several men to still have detectable HIV after 2 years of ART treatment (Leruez-Ville et al., 2001; Zhang et al., 1998).

vii. Infertility issues related to HIV can complicate a woman's desire for pregnancy.
   (1) HIV increases spontaneous abortions and stillborns and preterm delivery, if not on antiretroviral therapy (Olaitan et al., 1996; Shapiro et al., 2000).
   (2) There is an increased incidence and severity of pelvic inflammatory disease with HIV (6.7–22%), which causes blocked fallopian tubes.
   (3) Substance use (marijuana, cocaine, heroine, methodone, alcohol, and central nervous

system agents, such as barbiturates and PCP) can disrupt the hypothalamic-pituitary-ovarian (HPO) axis, altering fertility at various levels (Goeders, 1998). Chemical toxins, such as those found in plastics manufacturing, farming, and lead smelters, can also alter the HPO, altering fertility (Silbergeld & Flaws, 1999).

(4) HIV-infected partners may have decreased sperm count or impaired sperm motility, especially if CD_4 cell count is less than 200 (Muller, Coombs, & Krieger, 1998; Umapathy, Simbini, Chipata, & Mbizvo, 2001).

viii. Some states have mandatory (e.g., New York and Connecticut) prenatal testing for all women.

(1) The Centers for Disease Control and Prevention (CDC; 1994) has expressed concern regarding mandatory testing, stating testing may interfere with a woman's rights to participate in reproductive decisions and fearing that pregnant women would avoid prenatal care.

(2) CDC guidelines recommend universal counseling and voluntary HIV testing for pregnant women (Centers for Disease Control and Prevention, 2001e).

(3) Many women learn their seropositivity during pregnancy.

b. Access to care, treatment, and research

i. Early prenatal care has significantly reduced morbidity and mortality associated with pregnancy. Early detection of maternal HIV infection along with intervention and prenatal care can significantly reduce vertical transmission.

ii. Prenatal care includes the following:

- Assessing knowledge about perinatal transmission, partner's HIV status, and patient's HIV status. Is partner notification necessary (refer to state laws regarding this issue)? Pregnancy does not lower CD_4 cell counts (vanBenthem, Vernazza, Coutinho, & Prins, 2002).
- Stabilizing all chronic illnesses, including HIV, anemia, and so on to maximize maternal and fetal outcomes. This includes assessing HIV disease, CD_4 cell counts, and viral load. Screen and treat sexually transmitted diseases and obtain a Pap smear. Immunize for hepatitis, rubella, influenza, tetanus and diphtheria, and pneumonia as appropriate prior to conception.
- Screening for rubella titers, blood type, and hemoglobin levels
- Placing patient on folate 0.4 mg PO prior to conception and 1 mg during pregnancy
- Initiating and managing ART, which does not differ between HIV-pregnant and HIV-nonpregnant women, with the exception of contraindicated medications. Women who have not initiated ART and do not have an impending need to begin therapy may wish to delay therapy until the 2nd semester, when organogenesis is complete.
- Assessing readiness for ART or evaluating current ART regimen, modifying ART as necessary (Anderson, 2001)
- Suggesting initiation of ART by 2nd semester. Although monotherapy is not recommended, adding zidovudine (ZDV) to current regimens is the current recommendation of the CDC (Centers for Disease Control and Prevention, 2000b; see

Table 6.15a *Perinatal transmission prophylaxis regimen*

Antepartum	Initiated at 14–34 weeks gestation and continued throughout pregnancy A. PACTG 076 regimen: ZDV 100 mg 5 times daily B. Acceptable alternative regimen: • ZDV 200 mg 3 times daily Or • ZDV 300 mg 2 times daily
Intrapartum	During labor, ZDV 2 mg/kg IV over 1 hr, followed by a continuous infusion of 1 mg/kg IV until delivery
Postpartum	Oral administration of ZDV to the newborn (ZDV syrup, 2 mg/kg every 6 hr) for the first 6 weeks of life, beginning at 8-12 hours after birth

SOURCE: Centers for Disease Control and Prevention, 2000b

Table 6.15a). Single dose nevirapine is currently being studied in HIVNET 012 or PACTG 250/316 as an alternate to ZDV. Although nevirapine (Viramune) is not accepted as standard therapy at this time. The U.S. Public Health Service does list ZDV, with 3TC (Epivir) or nevirapine as alternative therapies (Guay et al., 1999; U.S. Public Health Service, 2002). Nelfinavir is being studied under ACTG 353 (Beckerman, 2000; for newborn ART recommendations, see Section VII, Clinical Management of Pediatric HIV Patients). Report all suspected adverse ART events to the Antiretroviral Pregnancy Registry (phone: 800–258–4263; address: 1410 Commonwealth Drive, Wilmington, NC 28403).

• ARTs that are contraindicated during pregnancy: Efavirez (Sustiva) and Hydroxyurea.
• Use the following medications with caution and careful monitoring: Indinivir (Crixivan), d4T (Zerit), ddi (Videx), Agenerase (Amprenavir).
• Beginning ART prior to conception allows for adjustment and treatment of side effects so that pregnancy-related nausea does not occur concurrently.

iii. Mental illness (including substance abuse) presents challenging problems in that many psychiatric medications are contraindicated during pregnancy, which can then compromise adherence to ART and prenatal appointments. These are factors contributing to perinatal (vertical) transmission

iv. Maternal risk factors with strong evidence-based support include individuals with advanced HIV disease as evidenced by decreased CD_4 cell count or CD_4-CD_8 ratio, or HIV viral load greater than 1,000. Individuals not on ART are at highest risk for transmitting HIV to their unborn child.

v. Maternal risk factors with limited evidence include individuals with vitamin A deficiency, sexually transmitted diseases, active genital herpes simplex virus lesion if in labor, anemia, genetic factors, illicit drug use, smoking, and seroconversion.

vi. Obstetrical risk factors for transmitting HIV to the unborn child include prolonged rupture of membranes (> 4 hrs), with a 2% increased risk for each hour until delivery (Read et al., 2001), vaginal delivery, and lack of ART during labor and delivery. Additionally, chorioamnionitis, invasive fetal procedures, and episiotomies may also contribute to increased rates of HIV transmission.

vii. Characteristics of those who were least likely to complete zidovudine therapy included older maternal age, CD_4 counts greater than 500, preterm birth, smoking or alcohol use, and cocaine or heroin use during pregnancy, especially at birth (Orloff et al., 2001).

viii. See Section VII for additional risk factors to children postpartum.

4. Specific care approaches
   a. Individual
      i. Hold frank discussions about the pros and cons of pregnancy, being HIV infected and pregnancy, risk of HIV transmission to the unborn child, and to discordant partners. All discussions should be documented.
      ii. Provide basic education about fertility and ovulation, including how to time conception.
      iii. Keep menstrual calendar for 3–6 months.
      iv. Discuss guardianship issues and support of partner, family, and friends.
      v. Discuss safer sex and contraception postpartum.
      vi. Educate regarding stages of pregnancy, intrapartum and postpartum.
      vii. Assess obstetrical history, outcomes, and any children born HIV seropositive. Are children living with patient or have they been lost to protective services or adoption?
      viii. Assess need for parenting classes.
      ix. Assess nutritional intake, economic ability to buy food, history of eating disorders, obesity or underweight issues, and housing (ability to prepare food and bottles for and bathe an infant).

      x. Assess stability of housing and whether or not housing is needed.
      xi. Provide social work and nutrition referrals.
      xii. Provide mental health and substance abuse referrals as needed with appropriate harm reduction when needed.
      xiii. Assess smoking history and encourage cessation program prior to conception.
      xiv. Refer to primary care provider for routine HIV care and to obstetrics/gynecology provider for Pap smear, sexually transmitted disease screening, and prenatal care. If patient has cervical dysplasia, refer for colposcopy and biopsy in preconception because biopsies cannot be done during pregnancy.
      xv. Assess partner's HIV status and involvement in the pregnancy or desire for pregnancy, including discussions about discordant couples and disclosure issues.
      xvi. Council regarding cesarean section at delivery with all women. Current studies have shown no difference in perinatal transmission rates between women on ART who had vaginal (5.5%) versus cesarean section (4.5%) deliveries (Patel et al., 2002). There is no evidence of cesarean section benefit if the woman is in labor or has ruptured membranes, so the cesarean section must be scheduled prior to 38–39 weeks of gestation. Cesarean section is only beneficial if viral load is ≥ 1,000 copies/ml near term, even if on ART, or with women who are not on ART (Watts, 2002). The risk of morbidity is increased with cesarean versus vaginal deliveries, especially with low CD_4 cell counts.
   b. Community
      i. Continue to educate health care providers and policymakers about the importance of voluntary HIV testing for pregnant women.

ii. Encourage and support outreach to all women in a variety of community places for the purposes of early HIV identification and HIV education.

iii. Educate community-based organizations and peer advocates about the importance of early prenatal care to reduce vertical transmission.

iv. Educate health care providers and related ancillary professionals regarding management of HIV in pregnancy.

6.16 Recent Immigrants

1. Definition of the community
   a. By definition, an immigrant is a person who is foreign born, who is not a U.S. citizen, and who has resettled in the United States with or without legal authorization.
   b. In 2000, 28.4 million foreign-born residents were in the United States. They comprised 10.4% of the total population (Lollock, 2000).
   c. Percentage of immigrants in United States
      i. Latin American (includes Central American, Caribbean, and South American): 51% (Lollock, 2000)
      ii. Asian (includes Chinese [Cantonese, Mandarin, Fukinese], Vietnamese, Korean, Cambodian, Filipino, Thai, Japanese, and Laotian): 25.5% (Lollock, 2000; United States Embassy, 1997)
      iii. European: 15.3%
   d. There were 8.7 million illegal immigrants in the United States in 2000 (Lollock, 2000).
      i. Illegal residents comprise 1.9 % of the U.S. population (Immigration and Naturalization Service, 2002).
      ii. Mexico is the leading country of origin, with 3.9 million (44%) illegal immigrants (Immigration and Naturalization Service, 2002).
      iii. Other countries of origin for illegal immigrants include El Salvador, Guatemala, Canada, Haiti, Philippines, the Dominican Republic, and China (Immigration and Naturalization Service, 2002).
   e. More than 16% of immigrants live below poverty level (Lollock, 2000).
   f. Seventy-nine percent of immigrants are between ages 18 and 64 years, the age at most risk for HIV infection (Lollock, 2000).

2. Common health issues
   a. Immigrants face many multicultural, economic, and political barriers to health care access in the United States.
      i. More than 32% of immigrants lack health insurance; illegal immigrants make up 26.8% of those without insurance. It is estimated that 14 million immigrants will be without insurance in the next decade (Camarota, 2001).
      ii. Many immigrants hold jobs that do not offer health insurance. Low incomes make it difficult to purchase health insurance.
      iii. Many immigrants are unfamiliar with health care system.
      iv. Among immigrants there is a mistrust of Western health care services. Immigrants may seek care from traditional healers and may fall victim to scams that take advantage of immigrants' ignorance of health care.
      v. Many immigrants fear HIV disclosure and being reported to the Immigration and Naturalization Service (INS), with subsequent deportation.
   b. Immigration and the law
      i. In 1987, the Immigration and Nationality Act (INA) banned HIV-infected immigrants from entering the United States (Goldberg, 2002).
      ii. In October of 1990, the Immigration Act of 1990 (IMMACT90) amended the INA and provided waivers for short-term visits, such as conferences and athletic events (Goldberg, 2002).
      iii. Since 1996, the INS has allowed HIV-infected immigrants to apply for individual asylum based on past or future persecution if they

return to the country of origin. Inadequate medical care and social ostracism are not considered persecution (Goldberg, 2002).

iv. An HIV-infected immigrant already living in United States cannot be deported if he or she maintains legal status.

v. All immigrants applying for legal permanent status must take an HIV test. HIV counseling is often unavailable, if not provided. The immigrant may be denied residency if found HIV positive. A waiver may be granted if the immigrant has close family ties in the United States or has applied for asylum.

vi. Medical facilities have no legal right or obligation to report undocumented HIV-infected immigrants to the INS.

3. HIV/AIDS in the immigrant community
   a. Transmission, risk behaviors, and prevention issues
      i. Racial and ethnic minorities are disproportionately affected by HIV. From 1981–2000, Blacks and Hispanics accounted for 56% of all HIV cases, although they only represented 25% of U.S. population (Centers for Disease Control and Prevention, 2001b).
      ii. Transmission modes vary among immigrant populations.
         (1) MSM (men who have sex with men) transmission is common among Latin Americans and Asian/Pacific Islanders.
         (2) Mother-to-child transmission is common in sub-Saharan Africa.
         (3) Heterosexual transmission is a common mode of transmission among Latin Americans, Asian/Pacific Islanders, and in sub-Saharan Africa.
      iii. Unique cultural risk behaviors include the following:
         - Lack of condom use and multiple sexual partners are common among Latin Americans, Africans, and Asian/Pacific Islanders.
         - Needles are commonly shared for medications and vitamins taken in the homes of Latin Americans.
         - Breastfeeding is common among Africans due to lack of potable water.
         - Blood products may not be screened for HIV and other sexually transmitted diseases (STDs), and selling of blood by commercial sex workers is common among Asian/Pacific Islanders.
   b. Access to care, treatment, and research
      i. Immigrants often arrive in poor health and only receive medical care when ill.
      ii. Immigrants often arrive with infectious diseases and are at increased risk for tuberculosis, hepatitis, and parasitic diseases (including giardia lamblia; Roberts & Kemp, 2001).
      iii. Many immigrants mistakenly believe that HIV is a gay White male disease and do not see themselves at risk. HIV-testing rates among Asians and women are low due to cultural stereotypes about risks (Maldonado, 1999).
      iv. Among some immigrants, HIV is often considered taboo, generating shame and guilt. Isolation and nondisclosure about HIV status is common.
      v. Underreporting and misclassification of Asian Pacific Islander cases occurs because many states collect or report data as "other ethnicity."

4. Specific approaches
   a. Individual
      i. Awareness of cultural characteristics and health beliefs is important in developing a plan of care (Marin, Rissmiller, & Beal, 1995; Mercer, 2002).
         (1) Illness may be perceived as disharmony/imbalance or act

of God. Hot/cold, yin-yang themes exist in many cultures.

(2) Immigrants may seek traditional healers and herbal (botanical) remedies before seeking care from Western practitioners.

(3) Incorporate cultural beliefs in treatment plans, so they do not interfere with prescribed treatment. For example, encourage the client to think of their life as a gift from God that should be protected if that is the belief system.

(4) Provide clinic office hours accessible to clients who work long hours, such as evening clinics or weekend hours.

(5) Clinics and other health care facilities should have available primary care providers who speak the same language and dialect as the client or have competent translators who understand medical terminology (Mercer, 2002).

ii. Immigrants may view sex as private and personal and not something discussed with outsiders.

iii. Nutritional assessment should be done to assess unique cultural food. Incorporate medication schedule with meals.

iv. Respect the client's culture and incorporate medical treatments as needed.

v. Where appropriate, include family or the head of the household in discussions of health care.

vi. Provide culturally appropriate information and referral sources.

b. Community

i. Form interagency linkages and referrals with immigrant community-based organizations.

ii. Use peer advocates for outreach programs, which can build trust and bridge cultural barriers (Chin, Kang, Martinez, Kim, & Schluter, 2001).

iii. Include immigrant representation in prevention planning and community groups (Maldonado, 1999).

iv. Prevention programs should include minorities, immigrants, women, intravenous drug users, commercial sex workers, and incarcerated populations.

v. Develop prevention materials that are culturally appropriate or in the native language.

6.17 Substance Users

1. Description of the community

   a. People who use legal or illegal substances with the intent to alter consciousness; addiction, substance abuse, and substance misuse are terms generally applied when use becomes harmful or uncontrolled.

   b. Substance use can interfere with a person's ability to access the health care system and manage his or her HIV disease to maximize health and quality of life.

   c. Substance use exists on a continuum from minimal to maximal impact and within a social context that is value laden and tends to marginalize and criminalize users.

   d. Types of substance users and their relation to HIV disease

      i. Injecting drug users (IDUs)

         (1) IDUs currently make up more than 32% of total AIDS cases and 37% of HIV cases; many pediatric HIV cases are related to mothers who are IDUs (Nwanyanwu, Chu, Green, Buehler, & Berkelman, 1999).

         (2) Active IDU negatively affects disease progression, transmission, and access to care.

         (3) Previous use also has implications for care (e.g., possibilities for relapse, pain control, stress management).

         (4) Heroin, amphetamines, and cocaine are the most commonly injected drugs.

Each substance has specific psychological, social, and physical effects on the user and requires providers to tailor patient care plans specific to the patient's drug use. How the provider addresses care depends on the drugs used.

(5) IDUs, though often poor and marginalized, exist at all socioeconomic levels of society.

ii. Non-IDUs

(1) Crack cocaine is highly addictive and is associated with many infections. Smoking increases the risk of infections related to the lungs, such as asthma and many different pneumonias (e.g., aspergillus pneumonia, asthma).

(2) Individuals who inhale, smoke, or ingest substances such as alcohol, prescription drugs, heroin, LSD, marijuana, and ecstasy are at greater risk for other infections related to the method of administration.

(3) Non-IDUs may have been injectors in the past and are at risk for becoming injectors again.

e. Substance use is complex and multifaceted; users often use more than one substance or route of administration depending on availability, desired high, or ability to procure.

2. Common health issues

a. Mental illness, childhood sexual or physical abuse, and history of familial addiction and dysfunction are highly correlated with substance use.

b. Race, ethnicity, gender, sexual preference, and class affect drug use, health, and access to health care.

c. Criminalization of lifestyle leads to marginalization and a distrust of authority and institutions; access to housing, food, and health care is often compromised by restrictions on serving active users. The Americans with Disabilities Act prohibits withholding of health services to people who are addicts.

d. Adverse health effects of substance use

i. Infections (e.g., abscesses; sepsis; endocarditis; central nervous system [CNS], hepatic, and renal infections) related to unclean injection equipment, unsafe techniques, and impurities in substances injected

ii. Organic syndromes related to direct effect of substances/impurities on tissues; affects skin, muscular, CNS, hepatic, renal, and vascular systems

iii. Causation or exacerbation of depression, psychosis, suicidal tendencies, isolation from social support systems, stigmatization, and poor self-esteem

iv. Self-medication for pain or mental illness with illicit substances often results in underlying problems becoming masked and undiagnosable.

v. Associated risks of substance abuse include malnutrition, homelessness, and poor coping mechanisms. These added risks increase the challenges health care providers face in delivering care to these clients.

vi. Poor health related to lifestyle and substance abuse add to the challenges in providing care. Adherence issues become a problem when the treatment plan is believed to be incompatible with street and prescribed drugs.

vii. Substance abuse places individuals at increased risk for infectious diseases, such as tuberculosis, sexually transmitted diseases (STDs), hepatitis, and HIV.

viii. Substance use, particularly rational or moderate, may provide positive coping strategies for some and improve quality of life; some substance use (e.g., marijuana, opiates) may provide symptom relief as well as have positive effects on mental status or sense of well-being.

3. HIV/AIDS in the substance abuse community
   a. Transmission, risk behaviors, and prevention issues
      i. Substance use may increase a person's risk of contracting HIV and transmitting it to others.
      ii. The risk increases because the person engages in risk behaviors (e.g., shared equipment, unsafe sex) while high or in exchange for substances.
      iii. Drug cravings may lead to risky practices, such as unsafe sexual practices, unsafe injection practices, and interpersonal violence.
   b. Access to care, treatment, and research
      i. Structural barriers such as insurance, finances, and knowledge deficit may create a confusing health care system.
      ii. Substance users are often labeled as immoral, noncompliant, manipulative, and drug seeking. This puts an undue burden on the client to access appropriate care.
      iii. Users are often disorganized due to lifestyle and altered mental status; appointments, records, and medication refills may be lost, not kept, or stolen.
      iv. Conflicts over pain medication often undermine relationships with provider. Pain management is often undertreated.
      v. Restrictions, rules, and requirements for persons to be clean and sober deter users from accessing care while using substances.
      vi. Users of illicit substances may fear arrest and thus may have distrust of authority including medical institutions.
      vii. Providers often refuse to treat active users who are mentally ill.
      viii. Active users are usually denied access to clinical trials for experimental treatments.
      ix. Addiction (craving) must be addressed by user before other needs, especially those involving stress (stress triggers craving), are met.
      x. Barriers to care often prevent diagnosis of HIV disease and related problems until too late for treatment.
      xi. Interactions between street drugs and prescribed medications are poorly understood. However, some amounts of alcohol in nelfinavir may be a contraindication for recovering addicts and alcoholics. Sustiva can give the sensation of being high for some individuals and is often abused by active addicts.
      xii. Methadone does interact with some HIV medications and may require dose adjustments (Barlett & Gallant, 2001; Rainey et al., 2000):
         (1) Increases delavirdine and fluconazole
         (2) Decreases the effect of abacavir, amprenavir, efavirenz, lopinavir, nelfinavir, ritonavir, phenytoin, rifabutin, and rifampin
         (3) No effect on didanosine (ddi), stavudine (d4t), and zidovudine (AZT)

4. Specific care approaches
   a. Individual
      i. Provider needs to have working knowledge of substance-use culture; ask questions if you do not know.
      ii. Establish trust through open, nonjudgmental exploration of substance use.
      iii. Users will often cover or minimize use until trust is established; allow time for relationship to develop (can be months to years).
      iv. User may not perceive substance use as primary problem; assess immediate needs and offer assistance.

v. Understand the user's relationship with substances and work to provide safer alternative.

    (1) Harm reduction: a model that attempts to reduce or eliminate risk of HIV infection/transmission by changing high-risk sex and substance-use behaviors (e.g., teaching safe injection use/techniques, initiating needle/syringe exchange programs; Patten, Vollman, & Thurston, 2000)

    (2) Abstinence: one option in a multifaceted approach

    (3) Peer programs such as Alcoholics Anonymous (AA) and Narcotics Anonymous (NA) are free, with high a success rate

vi. Provide information on demand drug treatment programs that are accessible, flexible, and noncoercive.

vii. Acknowledge difficulty accessing health care; express willingness to work to overcome barriers.

viii. Discuss benefits of substance use for person as well as costs; substance use is often related to primary coping mechanisms; do not attempt to remove this coping mechanism without providing a substitute.

ix. Comprehensive substance use history may take time to complete; be patient.

x. Substance users are capable of making decisions concerning treatment and quality-of-life issues; respect their ability to do so.

xi. Differentiate between the person and the effects of the drug to identify with a person and his or her life.

xii. Construct interventions with substance users' culture in mind: Be aware that users often do not keep appointments (drop-in schedules and rescheduling several times may be necessary) and do not schedule appointments that coincide with peak use times (beginning and midmonth when person gets paid) because appointments will usually not be kept.

xiii. Offer drug treatment/detoxification regularly after trust is established; avoid making recovery a requirement for continued care.

xiv. Manipulation and scamming are survival tools for many users; expect and acknowledge this. Do not take it personally if you are scammed. Respect, trust, and negotiation are the best tools to minimize manipulation.

xv. Assess support networks and family relationships; remember that dysfunctional relationships are sometimes better than none.

xvi. Interventions in the acute setting

    (1) Assess substance use and most recent use.

    (2) Anticipate and treat withdrawal symptoms; know that opiate and alcohol withdrawal are better understood and treated than amphetamine and cocaine withdrawal.

    (3) Users expect to be judged and treated punitively; anticipate this and reassure them that this will not happen.

    (4) Stress, fear, and poor coping mechanisms without drugs potentiate cravings.

    (5) Despite best attempts, users may leave against medical advice (AMA); begin discharge planning early. Provide medications and referrals if possible.

    (6) Attempt referral to home care agencies to complete IV therapy and provide follow-up.

    (7) Primary care/ community-based agency referrals are important to break the cycle of using the

ER and hospital as only source of health care.

xvii. Clear, reasonable, firm limits help patient understand expectations.

xviii. Patient advocacy remains central to the nurse's role in caring for the substance user with HIV disease.

xix. A team approach with excellent communication reduces impact of attempts to split and manipulate.

xx. Assess and treat pain adequately (often the precipitating factor in users leaving AMA).

b. Community

i. Expanded services for substance users

(1) Day treatments where the client can still work in the evening or return to home provide advantages to the drug user.

(2) Outreach clinics and services in areas populated by users are more easily accessed.

(3) Drug treatment centers need child care services for single parents.

(4) Develop alternatives to prison for nonviolent drug-related offenses, especially for women and individuals from lower socioeconomic levels (Freudenberg, 2002).

(5) Create needle exchange centers that are legal and provide free access to clean injection equipment (Burris, Lurie, Abrahamson, & Rich, 2000).

(6) Expand access to drug treatment and detox, including methadone (an estimated 2.8 million users of illicit drugs reside in the United States, with only 600,000 treatment slots available; Schoener, Hopper, & Pierre, 2002).

(7) Develop housing options for active users. Active users are often restricted from subsidized AIDS housing.

(8) Expand use of community-based clinics, walk-in clinics, mobile vans, and public health and home care nursing to provide as much health care as possible in the areas users live (Thompson et al., 1998).

(9) Expand harm-reduction services to meet people where they are; for example, IDUs often require wound care services, so nurses could provide harm reduction at the same time (Grau, Arevalo, Catchpool, & Heimer, 2002).

ii. Design outreach and case management programs targeting substance users in a multidisciplinary approach to connect them with housing, food, health care, and financial support.

iii. Rework the traditional model of hospice and palliative care to accommodate the needs of substance users with HIV disease; this would include adequate pain control.

iv. Expand research into treatment of withdrawal and detoxification from cocaine and amphetamines.

v. Educate professionals and patients about available resources such as the following:

- National Harm Reduction Coalition, Oakland, CA 94610; phone (510) 444–6969
- Alcoholics Anonymous, www.alcoholics-anonymous.org
- Al-Anon/Alateen, www.al-anon.org
- Narcotics Anonymous, http://www.na.org/index.html
- National Clearinghouse for Alcohol and Drug Information, www.health.org
- National Institute on Drug Abuse, www.nida.nih.gov
- Substance Abuse and Mental Health Services, www.samhsa.gov

- Web of Addictions, www.well.com/user/woa
- World Health Organization, www.who.org

6.18 Transgender/Transsexual Persons

1. Description of the community
   a. Transgender is an umbrella term that includes intersex, transsexual, transvestite, transgender, and other gender-deviant presentations.
      i. Lexicon for transgender community is growing; *trans* is often used as most inclusive term.
      ii. It is not necessary to have genital surgery to define oneself as trans, and many people have no intention to do so.
      iii. Many people who have had sexual reassignment surgery (SRS) obtain all legal documentation in the new gender and no longer consider themselves trans.
      iv. Statistical reporting of HIV exposure does not include trans identity as a category; the supposition is most data are subsumed into men having sex with men (MSM) data.
      v. Two broad categorizations exist within trans-community:

         - Female-to-male (FTM): transman: born phenotypically female, seeking masculine identity/presentation
         - Male-to-female (MTF): transwoman: born phenotypically male, seeking feminization of identity/presentation

      vi. Trans community reflects society at large; majority identify as heterosexual, from perspective of gender identity not birth gender
      vii. Most HIV-positive trans identified people are MTF, legally male and having sex with men.
   b. Trans community has been affected from the beginning of the HIV outbreak in the United States.

   c. People of trans experience are not a homogeneous group. They may be White, African American, or Hispanic; impoverished, blue collar, middle or upper class; adolescent or elderly; or Baptist, Jewish, or Catholic. They may be injection drug users (IDUs), hemophiliacs, or have received blood transfusions.
   d. Without accurate statistics, the impact of AIDS on the trans community is difficult to quantify; it may be possible to extrapolate from the MSM data in this section.

2. Common health issues
   a. Social stigma associated with trans identity
   b. Public disdain, harassment, even violence directed to trans community (i.e., transphobia)
   c. Lack of acceptance by other marginalized communities (i.e gay populations, non-White cultures)
   d. Protective impulse to hide gender identity and affectional (sexual) orientation
   e. Need to hide gender identity to preserve employment, family, social relationships, and religious affiliations
   f. Entrance and orientation to trans culture often clandestine, guilt laden, and occasionally dangerous
   g. Lack of access to medical supervision of hormone use often leads to procurement from illicit sources.
      i. Eighty-two percent of hormone injectors obtained hormones from medical source (Clements-Nolle, Marx, Guzman, & Katz, 2001).
      ii. Potentially harmful doses of estrogen and testosterone, including Serostim (human growth hormone), are taken.
      iii. Injecting oils and other substances to achieve altered body image are potential sources of abscesses and other health problems (Lombardi & vanServellen, 2000).
   h. Reliable information about trans community and culture is usually difficult to locate.
   i. Health care workers maintain social stereotypes, prejudices, and disdain

of people of trans experience; programs to educate and adjust attitudes are limited.

j. Mental health care professionals are often uneducated and insensitive to trans issues and their psychological/sociologic needs; few mental health providers are equipped to counsel about routine mental health concerns as separate from experience of living with trans identity.

k. Rate of alcoholism, illegal drug use, and sex work is understood to be disproportionately high in trans community.

l. Commercial sex work is used to pay for medications and procedures often not covered by medical insurance (Lombardi & vanServellen, 2000).

3. HIV/AIDS in the trans community
   a. Transmission, risk behaviors, and prevention issues
      i. There are no behavior-change programs specifically targeting the trans communities, MTF or FTM, except for what is learned from MSM programs.
      ii. Health care professionals remain uncomfortable with trans sexuality and are largely unaware of the complex sexual, emotional, and personal issues affecting prevention.
      iii. Prevention efforts must account for myriad gender presentations (emotional as well as physical) and sexual practices that complicate message diffusion.
      iv. Mandatory name reporting for HIV testing (required by law in most states) is incongruent with need to hide gender/sexuality from society.
      v. It is difficult to target prevention messages for trans people if they are not self-identified, or, if self-identified, they may not be connected to larger community.
      vi. Word choice and vocabulary limitations make direct, sensitive, and inclusive materials difficult to create.

   b. Access to care, treatment, and research
      i. Pursuit of hormones (over HIV) is the major reason transgender persons seek health care (Clements-Nolle et al., 2001).
      ii. There are no known treatment or research protocols targeting the trans community.
      iii. Public assistance to the uninsured is often awarded under person's legal name and gender; this may no longer reflect the person's reality and prevent the person from accessing benefits.
      iv. Historically, the medical professions have not respected the trans experience, engendering distrust in the trans community.

4. Specific care approaches
   a. Individual
      i. Medical management (The Harry Benjamin International Gender Dysphoria Association Inc., 2001; Israel & Tarver, 1997; Tom Waddell Health Center, 1998)
      ii. HIV-positive people of trans experience may not initially reveal trans identity to health care providers, appearing for appointments in clothing, hairstyle, and so on of the legal gender until trust is established.
      iii. Although some data exist, cross-gender hormone therapy (CGHT) does not have a medically recognized standard of care.
         (1) Feminizing and masculinizing hormone treatments both impact interpretation of standard lab data (i.e., hemoglobin, hematocrit, lipid profile).
         (2) Estrogen therapy will lower both hemoglobin and hematocrit into the normal female range; conversely, increased hemoglobin and hematocrit values in trans men has led to unnecessary work-up for polycythemia, secondary erythrocytosis due to cardiopulmonary disease, or malignant neoplasm, and

so on, especially if client has not disclosed testosterone use to medical provider or if provider is not knowledgeable about trans care.

 (3) Dyslipidemia can be a result of non-nucleoside reverse transcriptase inhibitor (NNRTI), protease inhibitor (PI), nucleoside reverse transcriptase inhibitor (NRTI), or testosterone therapy.

 (4) Clients with hepatitis or liver damage may need increased hormone doses or use injectable or transdermal delivery systems, which bypass the liver.

iv. Minimal data related to effects of antiretroviral medications on hormones, and vice versa, are available. It is known that protease inhibitors decrease the metabolism of estrogens, whereas some NNRTIs, such as Sustiva, increase the metabolism of estrogen. (See 6.19 Women)

v. Cosmetic surgeries (e.g., breast reduction or enlargement, body sculpting) may be pursued separate from SRS and performed by surgeons not in communication with client's primary health center.

 (1) The reasons to seek unconnected surgical care may be due to stigma, refusal of U.S. surgeons to perform the surgery, or the cost of procedures in the United States, among others.

 (2) Failure of client to disclose HIV status

 (3) Healing may be compromised by a high viral load (especially if this is unknown to surgeon) and travel or recuperation in a country with decreased access to standard hygiene measures.

 (4) Patient education related to possible outcomes of surgeries and importance of postop self-care is of high priority.

vi. Health care workers must validate individual's experience with gender as personally and socially important.

vii. Reassure the trans client of the provider's intention to be sensitive, despite own lack of training or experience with people of trans experience.

viii. Offer to use client's preferred name and gender expression to fullest extent allowed by charting system and medical-legal restrictions.

ix. Many people of trans experience also belong to other disenfranchised groups (e.g., the unemployed, the homeless, sex workers, racial/ethnic minorities, youth), which creates additional hurdles to optimizing care.

x. Provide education, networking, counseling, and support for trans men and trans women to reduce internalized transphobia and increase self-esteem.

xi. Establish connections to trans-sensitive specialists for routine referrals.

xii. Offer to monitor/prescribe CGHT for client, especially as harm-reduction measure for those clients accessing hormones from illicit/illegal sources. (*Note:* Client will often engage in medical care for hormone therapy when still precontemplative of initiating antiretroviral therapy.)

xiii. Provide additional counseling and education regarding long-term effects on CGHT (Leon, 2002).

 (1) Explore options for sperm/egg banking as result of possible/probable infertility.

 (2) Educate that estrogen therapy will cause erectile dysfunction.

 (3) Educate MTF clients on estrogen therapy about increased risk of a deep vein

thrombosis or pulmonary embolus and increased risk with smoking.

xiv. Offer mental health and substance abuse counseling/treatment and needle exchange resources (Gomez, Bates, & Taylor, 2002; Nemoto et al., 2002).

xv. Reinforce safer sex practices.

xvi. Offer life skills counseling as needed to reduce sex industry work and related risks (Gomez et al., 2002; Nemoto et al., 2002).

xvii. Offer legal counseling as needed.

b. Community

i. Transphobia must be identified, exposed, and publicly denounced; provide education and training for clinicians and staff.

ii. Reevaluate safer sex messages for messages and language that are culturally insensitive or inappropriate or contain moral judgments.

iii. Prevention messages must acknowledge people of trans experience, not only as individuals but also as social beings with complex family, group, and community roles and relationships.

iv. Explore medical-legal issues related to feminization/virilization within practice setting.

v. Employ people of trans experience as outreach workers, clinicians, and counselors, especially to sex worker community, which has a disproportionate number of trans women.

vi. Use existing trans media (e.g., magazines, Web sites) regularly to educate and reach the community to build trust and familiarity.

vii. Work with trans-identified community-based organizations, if available.

viii. Identify trans-friendly health care providers for client referral.

ix. Develop outreach projects that access trans community, such as mobile vans.

6.19 Women

1. Description of the community

   a. Since the first female case of AIDS was reported in 1981, the number has quadrupled, now accounting for 32% of all AIDS cases in the United States and 55% globally (Centers for Disease Control and Prevention, 2001).

   b. As of 1998, AIDS became the fifth leading cause of death among U.S. women ages 25 to 44 years (decreasing from the third leading cause of death, reflecting the HAART era) and the third leading cause of death among African American women (Centers for Disease Control and Prevention, 1999, 2000).

   c. Female rates have risen each year of the epidemic. Since 1998, 76% of new AIDS cases are women, demonstrating the lack of prevention efforts targeted toward women (Centers for Disease Control and Prevention, 1999, 2000, 2001).

   d. In 1993, the Centers for Disease Control and Prevention (CDC) expanded its AIDS surveillance case definition for adolescents and adults. The expanded definition included invasive cervical carcinoma. The impact of the expanded definition has been more sensitive in identifying HIV disease manifestations in women.

   e. Poor women of color disproportionately account for 79% of AIDS cases, and Hispanic women account for 21% (AIDSAction, 2002).

   f. There is significant geographic variability in the prevalence of AIDS in women. Most of the women who have CDC identified as having AIDS live in large cities on the U.S. coasts, principally in the Northeast. The number of women with AIDS in rural areas and smaller communities continues to grow, particularly in the Southeast.

2. Common health issues

   a. Most opportunistic infections (OIs) are seen equally in men and women, with the exception of Kaposi's sarcoma, which rarely occurs in women (2%).

   b. There is a greater incidence of candida esophagitis.

c. Vaginal candidiasis is more persistent, especially as the CD_4 cell counts drop.

d. Cervical dysplasia is the most prominent and problematic OI.

e. Sexually transmitted diseases (STDs) and pelvic inflammatory disease (PID) are more severe and difficult to treat.

f. Women not on antiretroviral therapy (ART) have twice as much anemia as women on ART (Levine et al., 2001).

g. Impact of HIV on hormonal levels (Cu-Uvin et al., 2000; Greenblatt, Ameli, Grant, Bacchetti, & Taylor, 2000)

   i. In HIV, levels of progesterone and estradiol are not affected.

   ii. Luteinizing hormone (LH) surges may increase CD_4 cells.

   iii. Follicle stimulating hormone (FSH) surges may decrease CD_4 cells while increasing CD_8 cells.

   iv. Interruption of the hypothalamic-pituitary-ovarian axis (HPO) can be altered or suppressed by OIs, HIV medications, and opiates (prescription and illicit drugs), including methadone. In HIV there is a threefold increased risk for amenorrhea, especially with lower CD_4 counts, serum albumin less than 3, or current use of amphetamine or heroine (Levine et al., 2001). Lower CD_4 counts appear to contribute to anovulation in 48% of HIV-infected women (Clark et al., 2001).

   v. Generally intermenstrual bleeding occurs more commonly in AIDS than in HIV disease, except with conditions such as hepatitis C and cervical dysplasia, where it occurs in both stages of the disease (Cohen et al., 1996; Ellerbrock et al., 1996; Levine et al., 2001).

   vi. HIV infected women on average enter menopause at age 47, whereas uninfected women have an average age of 51 (Clark et al., 2001). Hot flashes occurred twice as frequently in women with CD_4 counts greater than 500 (54%) than in women with CD_4 counts less than 200 (Clark et al., 2000).

3. HIV/AIDS and women

a. Transmission, risk behaviors, and prevention issues

   i. The incidence of woman-to-woman transmission of HIV is low (less than 0.04% contact from oral-vaginal, oral-anal, and digital penetration); larger studies of lesbians with HIV have found that other risk factors (e.g., injecting drug use, sex with men, transfusions) could not be ruled out as the mode of disease acquisition (Anderson, 2001).

   ii. By 1995, heterosexual acquisition surpassed injecting drug use (IDU) transmission as the leading mode of HIV acquisition in women diagnosed with AIDS in the United States and is now the predominant mode of transmission worldwide. Women who have IDU partners (17%) are at increased risk for HIV transmission.

   iii. Power imbalances (economic, gender, cultural) make it difficult for women to negotiate safe sexual relationships (Gollub, 1999; Wyatt et al., 2002).

   iv. Drug dependence may increase women's exposure to unsafe situations (e.g., needle use, sex, multiple partners, exchanging sex for money) and decrease the ability to negotiate safe ones.

   v. Domestic violence rates among HIV-infected women are approximately 67%, and women are less likely than men to disclose HIV status in these relationships (Browne, Miller, & Maguin, 1999; Cohen et al., 2000; El-Bassel, Witte, Wada, Gilbert, & Wallace, 2001; Zierler et al., 2000).

   vi. Heterosexual women (who may believe that monogamy means they are not at risk) may have partners with past or current hidden risks. There is a lack of a sense of vulnerability or risk for

HIV, particularly for women unaware of their partner's current or past risk behaviors. Women who are re-entering the sexual arena after a long hiatus may lack knowledge about the risks of acquiring HIV (Rich, 2001).

vii. Acquiring and transmitting HIV is enhanced by the following circumstances:

- Both circulating and prescription hormones contribute to HIV transmission. This includes the presence of progesterone and combination hormonal therapy found in hormonal contraceptives and megestrol acetate (Megace) (Crowley-Nowick, Douglas, & Moscicki, 2002; Sager et al., 2002). HIV-1 RNA shedding is lowest just prior to the LH surge, and a rapid increase occurs from the LH surge until menses (Hawes, Critchlow, Redman, Sow, & Kiviat, 2002).
- Transmission risk increased during the menses, postpartum, and postabortion and following cervical biopsies.
- Douching disturbs the vaginal ecosystem, making transmission of HIV and also other sexually transmitted infections easier.
- Non-oxynol 9 (N-9) use tends to create vaginal abrasions (deZoysa, 2000).
- Presence of STDs facilitates HIV transmission fourfold.

viii. No single prevention strategy will work with this heterogeneous group because different subgroups require discrete prevention efforts; women are at risk through IDU or sexual contact. Age, gender, and cultural considerations must be applied.

b. Access to care, treatment, and research

i. Access to treatments may be impaired by socioeconomic/lifestyle barriers, lack of transportation or child care, employment that grants no sick leave or health care benefits, or active drug use. Disorganized lifestyles may reduce drug users' ability to follow through with care needs; health care may be a low priority.

ii. Women with stigmatized lifestyles or who are illegal immigrants may shy away from contact with mainstream providers or may not fully disclose relevant information.

iii. Some women are dependent on unsupportive or abusive partners.

iv. Psychosocial/cultural barriers may impair access: Women may have a tendency to take care of themselves last. Caregiving responsibilities as a mother for other HIV family members may consume all available time and energy. As many as 35% of HIV-infected women report another family member (sibling, husband, or child) as also HIV infected (Fiore et al., 2001). Women may not understand the language or medical vocabulary of educators and providers, health care environments may not be sensitive to women, and some primary care provider(s) are untrained in HIV/AIDS and related issues.

v. Women are underrepresented in experimental HIV/AIDS protocols. They may be barred from participation in protocols by virtue of gender, presence of a uterus, and lack of surgical sterilization.

(1) Female AIDS Clinical Trials Group (ACTG) participants between 1987 and 1990 represented 6.7% of all participants. Nearly half were White, with different socioeconomic and demographic profiles than most HIV women. Only 22.6% had a history of IDU (Levine, 1999).

(2) Women participating in clinical trials today are approximately 17%, and the small numbers may jeopardize identifying specific gender differences in ART.

4. Specific care approaches
   a. Individual
      i. Response to ARV
         (1) ARV has extended survival time—twice as long in men as in women—and may reflect initiating therapy later in their disease with poor access to care.
         (2) Protease inhibitors can impact the menstrual cycle (Barlett & Gallant, 2001): Viracept (nelfinavir) and Norvir (ritonavir) may cause menorrhagia (i.e., prolonged and heavy menses). About 23% of women taking Crixivan (indinavir) or Invirase (saquinavir) report menstrual changes.
         (3) ARV can impact hormonal contraceptives. Other contraceptive methods or medication adjustments may be necessary (Barlett & Gallant, 2001).
         (4) The following reduce estrogen in hormonal contraceptives or hormone replacement therapy: Viracept (nelfinivir; by 47%, and progesterone, 18%); Norvir (ritonavir; by 40%); Viramune (nevirapine; by 20%); Kaletra (LPV/RTV; by 42%). The following increase estrogen: Crixivan (indinavir; by 24%, and progesterone, 26%) and Sustiva (efavirenz; by 37%).
         (5) Proportionately, fewer women than men receive ARV. This was reflected in 1997, when there was a 3% increase in deaths among women while morbidities declined in all other categories (Centers for Disease Control and Prevention, 1999b).
         (6) Gender differences in ARV metabolism may explain increased side effects, increased risk of lactic acidosis and hyperglycemia, and a twofold trough level with delavirdine and higher blood levels of ritonavir as compared to men (Currier, Yetzer, Potthoff, Glassman, & Heath-Chiozzi, 1997; Currier et al., 2000; Hader, Smith, Moore, & Holmberg, 2001; "Women and Pharmacology," 2001).
         (7) Fat maldistribution occurring in women both on and off ARV generally results in increased breasts and abdominal girth differing from patterns in men.
      ii. Survival rates of women with HIV
         (1) Early studies found shorter survival rates in women than in men, with HIV diagnosis at decreased CD_4 counts, socioeconomic status, lack of access to treatment, and later initiation of ART being major contributors (Hader et al., 2001).
         (2) CD_4 counts are generally higher in healthy women than they are in men. CD_4 counts often drop faster in women but then level off similar to men; however, women were diagnosed with AIDS with 146 CD_4 cells versus 49 in men, and they have higher CD_4 counts at death, 44 versus 22 in men (Anastos et al., 1999; Junghans, Ledergerber, Chan, Weber, & Egger, 1999). Higher CD_4 may be more predictive of survival in women than low HIV RNA (viral load). Women generally have lower HIV RNA than do men, with similar CD_4 counts, especially in early infection

(Anastos et al., 2000; Farzadegan et al., 1998; Rompalo et al., 1999). Hormonal variance may be a contributing factor. No changes in prophylaxis or initiation of ART are indicated at this time because studies continue to contradict one another.

iii. Don't assume heterosexuality; ask directly about relationships and sex with both men and women to develop an appropriate plan of care (Morrow & Allsworth, 2000).

iv. Facilitate empowerment of women to assist them in making healthy and safe choices. Assist in developing positive life skills that can alter negative appraisal related to HIV illness (Bova, 2001). This includes education about sexuality, anatomy and physiology, as well as STDs and HIV disease. Reframing negative appraisals of illness, which are often linked to cultural health beliefs, can assist in managing symptoms and adjusting to chronic illness (Bova, 2001). Provide assistance to heal from interpersonal violence to increase self-care practices (Leenerts, 1999).

v. The client's relationship with his or her provider is the most significant factor in predicting adherence to medical regimes, including ART (Carr, 2001; Roberts, 2002).

vi. Discuss long-term planning for minor children.

b. Community

i. Coordinate clinical care and services where possible to facilitate one-stop shopping for HIV care, gynecologic services, and HIV care for children. Arrange clinic times to allow for visits by women with school-age children. Make provisions for child care in clinic.

ii. Have other resources that women use frequently (e.g., drug treatment, colposcopy, support groups, family planning, case management, legal services) available for immediate referral.

iii. Discuss clinical drug trials with all women and need for contraception if of reproductive age.

iv. Educate health care providers regarding the special needs of women with HIV, including research.

References

AIDSAction. (2001). *What works in HIV prevention for incarcerated populations.* Retrieved February 28, 2003, from www.aidsaction.org

AIDSAction. (2002). *Communities of color and HIV/AIDS.* Retrieved January 11, 2002, from www.aidsaction.org

Altice, F. L., & Buitrago, M. I. (1998). Adherence to antiretroviral therapy in correctional settings. *Journal of Correctional Health Care, 5,* 179–200.

Amnesty International. (1999). Rights for all. In *Not part of my sentence: Violations of the human rights of women in custody.* New York: Author.

Anastos, K., Gange, S. J., Lau, B., Weiser, B., Detels, R., Giorgi, J. V., et al. (2000). Association of race and gender with HIV-1 RNA. *Journal of Acquired Immune Deficiency Syndrome, 24*(3), 218–226.

Anastos, K., Kalish, L. A., Hessol, N., et al. (1999). The relative value of CD_4 cell count and qualitative HIV-1 RNA in predicting survival in HIV-1-infected women: Results of the women's interagency HIV study. *AIDS, 13,* 1717–1726.

Anderson, J. R. (Ed). (2001). *A guide to the clinical care of women with HIV.* Rockville, MD: U. S. Department of Health and Human Services, Health Resources and Services Administration.

Association of Nurses in AIDS Care. (1999). *Position paper: Discrimination protections for people with HIV infection: Reviewed and revised by the ANAC board August 14, 1999.* Retrieved March 1, 2003, from http://www.anacnet.org/about/policy.htm

Association of Nurses in AIDS Care. (2001). Work issues for the HIV+ nurse. *+ Nurse, 2,* 1–4.

Augustyniak, L., Kramer, A.S., Frick, W., Brownstein, A.P., Evatt, B. (1990, June). *Regional seropositivity rates for HIV infection in patients with hemophilia.* Paper presented at the Sixth International Conference on AIDS, San Francisco.

Babudieri, S., Aceti, A., D'Offizi, G. P., Carbonara, S., & Starnini, G. (2000). Directly observed therapy to treat HIV infection in prisoners. *Journal of the American Medical Association, 284,* 179–180.

Ball, S. C. (2000). Addressing the issue of childbearing in heterosexual couples discordant for HIV. *The AIDS Reader, 10,* 144–145.

Barlett, J. G., & Gallant, J. E. (2001). *2001–2002 medical management of HIV infection.* Baltimore: Johns Hopkins University Press.

Beck, A. J., & Harrison, P. M. (2001). *Prisoners in 2000.* Washington, DC: U.S. Department of Justice, Bureau of Justice Statistics.

Beckerman, K. P. (2000). Principles of management of HIV disease during pregnancy. *Journal of the International AIDS Society, 8*(7), 18–25.

Billy, J. O. G., Tanfer, K., Grady, W. R., & Klepinger, D. H. (1993). The sexual behaviors of men in the United States. *Family Planning Perspective, 25,* 52–60.

Blindness Statistics. (2000). National Federation of the Blind. Retrieved March 2003, from www.nfb.org

Boudin, K., Carrero, I., Clark, J., Flournoy, V., Loftin, K., Martindale, S., et al. (1999). ACE: Peer education and counseling program meets the needs of incarcerated women with HIV/AIDS issues. *Journal of the Association of Nurses in AIDS Care, 10*(6), 90–98.

Bova, C. (2001). Adjustment to chronic illness among HIV-infected women. *Journal of Nursing Scholarship, 33,* 217–224.

Browne, A., Miller, B., & Maguin, E. (1999). Prevalence and severity of lifetime physical and sexual victimization among incarcerated women. *International Journal of Law and Psychiatry, 22*(3–4), 301–322.

Burris, S., Lurie, P., Abrahamson, D., & Rich, J. D. (2000). Physician prescribing of sterile injection equipment to prevent infection: Time for action. *Annals of Internal Medicine, 133*(3), 218–228.

Bushy, A. (2000). HIV/AIDS: The silent enemy within rural communities. In A. Bushy (Ed), *Orientation to nursing in the rural community.* Thousand Oaks, CA: Sage.

Camarota, S. A. (January 2001). *Immigrants in the United States: A snapshot of America's foreign born. Publication of the Center for Immigration Studies.* Washington, DC: Author.

Carr, G. S. (2001). Negotiating trust: A grounded theory study of interpersonal relationships between persons living with HIV/AIDS and their primary health care providers. *Journal of the Association of Nurses in AIDS Care, 12,* 35–43.

Centers for Disease Control and Prevention. (1982). Update on acquired immunodeficiency syndrome (AIDS) among patients with hemophilia. *MMWR, 31,* 48.

Centers for Disease Control and Prevention. (1992). HIV infection in two brothers receiving intravenous therapy for hemophilia. *MMWR, 41,* RR-14.

Centers for Disease Control and Prevention. (1993). HIV transmission between two adolescent brothers with hemophilia. *MMWR, 42,* RR-49.

Centers for Disease Control and Prevention. (1994). Zidovudine for the prevention of HIV transmission from mother to infant. *Morbidity and Mortality Weekly Report, 43,* 285–287.

Centers for Disease Control and Prevention. (1997). *HIV/AIDS trends among U.S. men who have sex with men (MSM).* Retrieved September, 2002, from http://www.thebody.com/cdc/msm.html

Centers for Disease Control and Prevention. (1999a). Decrease in AIDS-related mortality in a state correctional system—New York, 1995–1998. *MMWR, 47*(51), 1115–1117.

Centers for Disease Control and Prevention. (1999b). *HIV/AIDS surveillance report* (Vol. 11). Atlanta, GA: U.S. Deptartment of Health and Human Services, Public Health Service.

Centers for Disease Control and Prevention. (2000a). *HIV/AIDS surveillance report.* Atlanta, GA: U.S. Department of Health and Human Services, Public Health Service.

Centers for Disease Control and Prevention. (2000b). *Most teens not provided STD or pregnancy prevention counseling during check-ups.* Retrieved, December 6, 2000, from http://www.thebody.com/cdc/std/teen_checkup.html

Centers for Disease Control and Prevention. (2001a). *HIV/AIDS surveillance report, 12*(2). Retrieved, August, 2001, from http://www.cdc.gov/hiv/stats/hasr1202/table7.htm

Centers for Disease Control and Prevention. (2001b). HIV testing among racial/ethnic minorities—United States, 1999. *MMWR, 50*(47), 1054–1058.

Centers for Disease Control and Prevention. (2001c). HIV/AIDS—United States, 1981–2000. *MMWR, 50,* 430–434.

Centers for Disease Control and Prevention. (2001d). *Preventing occupational HIV transmission to healthcare personnel.* Retrieved February 27, 2003, from http://www.cdc.gov/hiv/pubs/facts/hcwsurv.htm

Centers for Disease Control and Prevention. (2001e). Revised recommendations for HIV screening of pregnant women. *Morbidity and Mortality Weekly Report, 50,* RR-19.

Centers for Disease Control and Prevention. (2002a). Deaths among persons with AIDS through December 2000. *HIV/AIDS Surveillance Supplemental Report, 8*(1). Retrieved January 5, 2003, from http://www.cdc.gov/hiv/stats/hasrsupp81.pdf

Centers for Disease Control and Prevention. (2002b). Prison rapes spreading deadly diseases. *HIV/AIDS, sexually transmitted diseases, and tuberculosis prevention news update.* Retrieved August 28, 2002, from www.cdc.gov

Centers for Disease Control and Prevention. (n.d.). *HIV/AIDS and U.S. women who have sex with women (WSW).* Retrieved February 12, 2002, from http://www.cdc.gov/hiv/pubs/facts/wsw.htm

Chin, J. J., Kang, E., Martinez, J. M., Kim, J. H., & Schluter, D. P. (2001). Training providers to improve service delivery to Asians and Pacific Islanders. In R. E. Sember (Ed.), *Lessons learned.* Rockville, MD: Department of Health and Human Services, HIV/AIDS Bureau.

Ciesielski, C., & Boghani, S. (2002, March). *HIV infection among men with infectious syphilis in Chicago 1998–2000.* Paper presented at the Ninth Annual Retrovirus Conference, Seattle, Washington.

Clark, R. A., Cohn, S. E., Jarek, C., Craven, K. S., Lyons, C., Jacobson, M., et al. (2000). Perimenopausal symptomatology among HIV-infected women at least 40 years of age. *Journal of Acquired Immune Deficiency Syndrome, 23,* 99–100.

Clark, R. A., Mulligan, K., Stamenovic, E., Chang, B., Watts, J. A., Squires, K., et al. (2001). Frequency of anovulation and early menopause among women enrolled in selected adult AIDS clinical trials group studies. *Journal of Infectious Diseases, 184,* 1325–1327.

Clements-Nolle, K., Marx, R., Guzman, R., & Katz, M. (2001). HIV prevalence, risk behaviors, health care use, and mental health status of transgender persons: Implications for public health intervention. *American Journal of Public Health, 91,* 915–921.

Cohen, M., Deamant, C., Barkan, S., Richardson, M., Young, M., Holman, S., et al. (2000). Domestic violence and childhood sexual abuse in HIV-infected women and women at risk for HIV. *American Journal of Public Health, 90,* 560–565.

Cohen, M. H., Greenblatt, R., Minkoff, H., Barkan, S. E., Burns, D., Denenberg, R., et al. (1996, July). *Menstrual abnormalities in women with HIV infection.* Paper presented at the XI International Conference on AIDS, Vancouver, BC.

Cox, J. F., Banks, S., & Stone, J. L. (2000). Counting the mentally ill in jails and prisons. *Psychiatric Service, 51*(4), 533–534.

Crosby R. A., Yarber, W. L., DiClemente, R. J., Wingood, G. M., & Meyerson, B. (2002). HIV-associated histories, perceptions, and practices among low-income African American women: Does rural residence matter? *American Journal of Public Health, 92,* 655–659.

Crowley-Nowick, P., Douglas, D., & Moscicki, A. B. (2002, July). *Hormonal contraceptive use and IL-12 concentration in cervical secretions are associated risks for high grade squamous intra-epithelial lesion.* Paper presented at the XIV International AIDS Conference, Barcelona, Spain.

Currier, J. S., Spino, C., Grimes, J., Wofsky, C. B., et al. (2000). Differences between women and men in adverse events and CD_4+ responses to nucleoside analogue therapy for HIV infection. *Journal of Acquired Immune Deficiency Syndromes, 24,* 316–324.

Currier, J. S., Yetzer, E., Potthoff, A., Glassman, H., & Heath-Chiozzi, M. (1997, May). *Gender differences in adverse events on ritonivir: An analysis from the Abbott 247 study.* Paper presented at the First National Conference on Women and HIV, Pasadena, CA.

Cu-Uvin, S., Wright, D. J., Anderson, D., et al. (2000). Hormonal levels among HIV-1 seropositive women compared with high-risk HIV-seronegative women during the menstrual cycle. *Journal of Women's Health and Gender Based Medicine, 9,* 857–863.

DeGroot, A. S. (2000). HIV infection among incarcerated women: Epidemic behind bars. *The AIDS Reader, 10*(5), 287–295.

DeGroot, A. S., Bick, J., Thomas, D., & Stubblefied, E. (2001). HIV clinical trials in correctional settings: Right or regression? *AIDS Reader, 11,* 34–40.

DeZoysa, I. (2000, July). *Non-oxynol 9 (M-9) significantly increases heterosexual transmission to women.* Paper presented at the XIII International AIDS Conference, Durban, South Africa.

Diamant, A. L., Schuster, M. A., McGuigan, K., & Lever, J. (1999). Lesbians' sexual history with men: Implications for taking a sexual history. *Archives of Internal Medicine, 159,* 2730–2736.

Dilorio, C., Hartwell, T., & Hansen, N. (2002). Childhood sexual abuse and risk behaviors among men at high risk for HIV infection. *American Journal of Public Health, 92,* 214–219.

Eichold, S. (1995). HIV care in correctional facilities. *Journal of Correctional Health Care, 2,* 111–112.

El-Bassel, N., Witte, S. S., Wada, T., Gilbert, L., & Wallace, J., et al. (2001). Correlates of partner violence among female street-based sex workers: Substance abuse, history of child abuse, and HIV risks. *AIDS Patient Care and STDs, 15,* 41–51.

Ellerbrock, T. V., Wright, T. C., Bush, T. J., Dole, P., Brudney, K., & Chiasson, M. A. (1996). Characteristics of menstruation in women infected with human immunodeficiency virus. *Obstetrics and Gynecology, 87*(8), 1030–1034.

Farzadegan, H., Hoover, D. R., Astemborski, J., et al. (1998). Sex differences in HIV-1 viral load and progression to AIDS. *Lancet, 352,* 1510–1514.

Fink, M. J., Walker, S., Dole, P., & Lang, A. (2001, November). *Educational videotapes for incarcerated women: Using focus groups to learn and teach.* Paper presented at the 25th National Conference on Correctional Health Care, the National Commission on Correctional Health Care, and the Academy of Correctional Health Professionals, Albuquerque, NM.

Fiore, T., Flanigan, T., Hogan, J., Cram, R., Schuman, P., Schoenbaum, E., et al. (2001). HIV infection in families of HIV-positive and at-risk HIV-negative women. *AIDS Care, 13,* 209–215.

Fischl, M., Rodriguez, A., Scerpella, E., Monroig, R., Thompson, L., & Richtine, D. (2000, January). *Impact of directly observed therapy on outcomes in HIV clinical trials.* Paper presented at the Seventh Conference on Retroviruses and Opportunistic Infections, San Francisco.

Flaskerud, J. H., & Winslow, B. J. (1998). Conceptualizing vulnerable populations health-related research. *Nursing Research, 47*(2), 69–78.

Ford, K., King, G., Nerenberg, L., & Rojo, C. (2001). AIDS knowledge and risk behaviors among Midwest migrant farm workers. *AIDS Education and Prevention, 13*(6), 551–560.

Frank, L. (1999). Prisons and public health: Emerging issues in HIV treatment adherence. *Journal of the Association of Nurses in AIDS Care, 10*(6), 25–31.

Freundenberg, N. (2002). Adverse effects of U.S. jail and prison policies on the health and well-being of women of color. *American Journal of Public Health, 92,* 1895–1899.

Freudenberg, N., Wilets, I., Greene, M. B., & Richie, B. E. (1998). Linking women in jail to community services: Factors associated with rearrest and retention of drug-using women following release from jail. *Journal of American Women's Association, 53*(2), 89–93.

Frick, W., Augustyniak, L., Laurence, D., Brownstein, A., Kramer, A., & Evatt, B. L. (1992). Human immunodeficiency virus infection due to clotting factor concentrates: Results of the Seroconversion Surveillance Project. *Transfusion, 32,* 8.

Gaiter, J., Jurgen, R., Mayer, K., & Hollibaugh, A. (2000). Harm reduction inside and out: Controlling HIV in and out of correctional facilities. *AIDS Reader, 10,* 45–52.

Gaskins, S. (1999). Special populations: HIV/AIDS among the Deaf and hard of hearing. *Journal of the Association of Nurses in AIDS Care, 10,* 75–78.

Gilling-Smith, C. (2000). Assisted reproduction in HIV-discordant couples. *The AIDS Reader, 10,* 581–587.

Go, V., & Baker, T. (1995). Health problems of Maryland migrant farm laborers. *Maryland Medical Journal, 4*(1), 606–608.

Goeders, N. E. (1998). Stress, the hypothalamic-pituitary-adnexal axis, and vulnerability to drug use. *NIDA Research Monograph, 169,* 83–104.

Goldberg, S. B. (2002). Immigration issues and travel restrictions. The body. *Encyclopedia of AIDS.* Retrieved January 9, 2003, from http://www.thebody.com/encyclo/immigration.html

Gollub, E. B. (1999). Human rights is a US problem, too: The case of women and HIV. *American Journal of Public Health, 89*(10), 1476–1485.

Gomez, M., Bates, C., & Taylor, M. (2002, July). *Transgendered persons and the HIV/AIDS in communities of color.* Paper presented at the XIV International AIDS Conference, Barcelona, Spain.

Gostin, L. (2000). National policy on HIV-infected healthcare workers questioned. *Journal of the American Medical Association, 284,* 1965–1970.

Grau, L. E., Arevalo, S., Catchpool, C., & Heimer, R. (2002). Expanding harm reduction services through a wound and abscess clinic. *American Journal of Public Health, 92,* 1915–1917.

Greenblatt, R, M., Ameli, N., Grant, R. M., Bacchetti, P., & Taylor, R. N. (2000). Impact of the ovulatory cycle on virologic and immunologic markers in HIV-infected women. *The Journal of Infectious Diseases, 181,* 82–90.

Grinstead, O. A., Zack, B., & Faigles, B. (1999). Collaborative research to prevent HIV among male prison inmates and their female partners. *Health Education and Behavior, 26*(2), 225–238.

Guay, L. A., Musoke, P., Fleming, T., Bagenda, D., Allen, M., Nakabiito, C., et al. (1999). Intrapartum and neonatal single-dose nevirapine compared with zidovudine for prevention of mother-to-child transmission of HIV-1 in Kampala, Uganda: HIVNET 012 randomised trial. *Lancet, 354,* 795–802.

Guex-Cosier, Y. & Telenti, A. (2001). An epidemic of blindness: A consequence of improved HIV care? *Bulletin of the World Health Organization, 79*(3), 180–181.

Hader, S. L., Smith, D. K., Moore, J. S., & Holmberg, S. D. (2001). HIV infection in women in the United States. *Journal of the American Medical Association, 285,* 1186–1192.

The Harry Benjamin International Gender Dysphoria Association Inc. (2001). *The HBIGDA standards of care for gender identity disorders.* Retrieved February 1, 2002, from http://www.hbidgda.org/soc.html

Hawes, S., Critchlow, C. W., Redman, M., Sow, P., & Kiviat, N. (2002, February). *A longitudinal study of the detection of human immunodeficiency virus (HIV) type-1 and type-2 RNA in vaginal secretions among Senegalese women.* Paper presented at the Ninth Conference on Retroviruses and Opportunistic Infections. Seattle, Washington.

Hayes M. (1994). *Social skills: The bottom line for adult LD success.* Retrieved February 28, 2003, from www.ldonline.org/ld_indepth/social_skills/social-1.html

Health Resources and Services Administration, HIV/AIDS Bureau. (2001). *HRSA care to action: HIV/AIDS in the Deaf and hard of hearing.* Retrieved, December 6, 2002, from http://hab.hrsa.gov/programs/factsheets/deaffact.htm

Herek, G. M., & Capitanio, J. P. (1993). Public reactions to AIDS in the United States: A second decade of stigma. *American Journal of Public Health, 83,* 574–577.

Holzemer, W.L. (1999). Predictors of self-reported adherence in persons living with HIV disease. *AIDS Patient Care and STDs, 13,* 185–97.

HRSA. (2000). *Incarcerated people and HIV/AIDS.* Washington, DC: U.S. Department of Health and Human Services.

HRSA. (2001a). Incarcerated populations and HIV/AIDS. *AIDSAction.* Retrieved March 3, 2003, from http://www.aidsaction.org/legislation/pdf/pol_facts_prison.pdf

HRSA. (2001b). *Lessons learned.* Rockville, MD: Author.

Human Rights Watch Women's Rights Project. (1996). *All too familiar: Sexual abuse of women in U.S. state prisons.* New York: Author.

Immigration and Naturalization Service. (2002). *Statistics.* Retrieved January 9, 2002, from http://www.ins.usdoj.gov/graphics/aboutins/statistics/Est2000.pdf

Israel, G. E., & Tarver, D. E. (1997). *Transgender care: Recommended guidelines, practical information and personal accounts.* Philadelphia: Temple University Press.

Jaimie, P. L., Ortiz, M.D.C.S., Torres, R.D., Torres, L., & Diaz, M. A. (2001). Conocimiento en sexualidad y practicas sexuales en estudiantes universitarios con impedimentos visuales: Necesidad de materiales educativos (Knowledge about sexuality and sex behavior in university students with visual impairment: Need of educational materials). *Puerto Rican Health Science Journal, 20*(3), 269–275.

Jemmott, J. B., Jemmott, L. S., Fong, G. T., & McCaffree, K. (1999). Reducing HIV risk-associated sexual behavior among African American adolescents: Testing the generality of intervention effects. *American Journal of Community Psychology, 27,* 161–187.

Junghans, C., Ledergerber, B., Chan, P., Weber, R., & Egger, M. (1999). Sex differences in HIV-1 viral load and progression to AIDS. *Lancet, 353,* 589–591.

Kaiser Family Foundation. (n.d.) *African Americans view of the HIV/AIDS epidemic at 20 years: Findings from a national survey.* Retrieved, January 6, 2002, from http://www.kff.org/docs/AIDSat20/

Kalichman, S. C., Rompa, D., Cage, M., Austin, J., Luke, W., Barnett, T., et al. (2002). Sexual transmission risk perceptions and behavioural correlates of HIV concentrations in semen. *AIDS Care, 14,* 343–349.

Kapperman, G., Matsuoka, J., & Pawelski, C. (1993). *HIV/AIDS prevention: A guide for working with people who are blind or visually impaired* (First ed.) New York: AFB Press.

Keaveny, M. E., & Zauszniewski, J. A. (1999). Life events and psychological well-being in women sentenced to prison. *Issues in Mental Health Nursing, 20,* 73–89.

Keruly, J. C., Conviser, R., & Moore, R. D. (2002). Association of medical insurance and other factors with receipt of antiretroviral therapy. *American Journal of Public Health, 92,* 852–857.

Kestelyn, P. G., & Cunningham, E. T. (2001). HIV/AIDS and blindness. *Bulletin of the World Health Organization, 79*(3), 208–211.

Klein, S., Nokes, K., Devore, B., Holmes, J., Wheeler, D., & St. Hilaire, M. (2001). Age-appropriate HIV prevention messages for older adults: Findings from focus groups in New York State. *Journal of Public Health Management Practice, 7*(3), 11–18.

Klonoff, E., & Landrine, H. (1999). Do blacks believe that HIV/AIDS is a government conspiracy against them? *Preventive Medicine, 28,* 451–457.

Kramer, A., & Brownstein, A.P. (1990, June). *ACTU without walls.* Paper presented at the Sixth International Conference on AIDS, San Francisco.

Leenerts, M. H. (1999). The disconnected self: consequences of abuse in a cohort of low-income white women living with HIV/AIDS. *Health Care for Women International, 20,* 381–400.

Leh, S. K. (1999). HIV infection in U.S. correctional systems: Its effect on the community. *Journal of Community Health Nursing, 16,* 53–63.

Leon, W. (2002, March). *HIV and transgendered persons.* Lecture presented at Hunter College School of Nursing, New York.

Leruez-Ville, M., Dulioust, E., Costabliola, D., Salmon, D., Tachet, A., Finkielsztein, L., et al. (2001). Decrease in HIV-1 seminal shedding in men receiving highly active antiretroviral therapy: An 18-month longitudinal study (ANS EP012). *AIDS, 16,* 486–488.

Levine, A. (1999). HIV disease in women. *HIV Clinical Management, 9,* 8–11.

Levine, A. M., Berhane, K., Masri-Lavine, L., et al. (2001). Prevalence and correlates of anemia in a large cohort study of HIV-infected women: Interagency study. *HIV Treatment Bulletin, 26,* 28–35.

Lichenstein, B. (2000). Secret encounters: Black men, bisexuality, and AIDS in Alabama. *Medical Anthropology Quarterly, 14*(3), 374–393.

Lollock, L. (2000). *Profile of the foreign born population in the United States: 2000. Current population reports.* Washington, DC: U.S. Census Bureau.

Lombardi, E. L., & vanServellen, G. (2000). Correcting deficiencies in HIV/AIDS care for transgendered individuals. *Journal of the Association of Nurses in AIDS Care, 11,* 61–69.

Macaulay, L., Kitzinger, J., Green, G., & Wight, D. (1995). Unconventional conceptions and HIV. *AIDS Care, 7,* 261–276.

Maldonado, M. (1999). *HIV/AIDS: Asian and Pacific Islanders.* Retrieved January 9, 2003, from http://www.NMAC.org

Mandelbrot, L., Heard, I., Henrion-Geant, E., & Henrion, R. (1997). Natural conception in HIV-negative women with HIV-infected partners. *Lancet, 349,* 850–851.

Marin, M. A., Rissmiller, P., & Beal, J. A. (1995). Health-illness beliefs and practices of Haitians with HIV disease living in Boston. *Journal of the Association of Nurses in AIDS Care, 6,* 45–53.

Markens, S., Fox, S. A., Taub, B., & Gilbert, M. L. (2002). Role of Black churches in health promotion programs: Lessons from the Los Angeles Mammography Promotion in Churches Program. *American Journal of Public Health, 92,* 805–810.

Marrazzo, J. M., Koutsky, L. A., & Handsfield, H. H. (2001). Characteristics of female sexually transmitted disease clinic clients who report same-sex behaviour. *International Journal of STD and AIDS, 12,* 41–46.

Maruschak, L. M., & Beck, A. J. (2001). *Medical problems of inmates, 1997.* Retrieved February 28, 2003, from www.ojp.usdoj.gov/bjs/

Mercer, T. A. (2002). New frontier of care. *Advance for Nurses, 2*(14), 14–17.

Miller, S. K., & Rundio, A. (1999). Identifying barriers to the administration of HIV medications to county correctional facility inmates. *Clinical Excellence for Nurse Practitioners,* 286–290.

Mitchell, J., Brown, G., Loftman, P., & Williams, S. (1990). HIV infection in pregnancy: Detection, counseling, and care. *Pediatric AIDS and HIV Infection: Fetus to Adolescent, 1,* 78–82.

Morrow, K. M. & Allsworth, J. E. (2000). Sexual risk in lesbians and bisexual women. *Journal of the Gay and Lesbian Medical Association, 4*(4), 159–165.

Muller, C. H., Coombs, R. W., & Krieger, J. N. (1998). Effects of clinical stage and immunological status on semen analysis results in human immunodeficiency virus type 1-seropositive men. *Andrologia, 30*(Suppl. 1), 15–22.

National Center for Education Statistics. (1994). *Literacy behind prison walls.* Washington, DC: Author.

National Commission on Correctional Health Care. (1997). *Standards for health services in prison.* Chicago: Author.

National Hemophilia Foundation. (2002a). *Hemophilia A: What is it?* Retrieved February 20, 2003, from http://www.hemophilia.org/bdi/bdi_types1.htm

National Hemophilia Foundation. (2002b). *Nurses' guide to bleeding disorders.* New York: Author.

Nemoto, T., Keatley, J., Operario, D., Soma, T., Eleneke, M., Arista, P., et al. (2002, July). *Implementing HIV prevention, drug abuse treatment, and mental health services in transgender community in San Francisco.* Paper presented at the XIV International AIDS Conference, Barcelona, Spain.

Newell, M. L. (1998). Mechanism and timing of mother-to-child transmission of HIV-1 infection. *AIDS, 12,* 831–837.

Nicodemus, M., & Paris, J. (2001). Bridging the communicable disease gap: Identifying, treating and counseling high-risk inmates. *HEPPNews, 4*(8–9). Retrieved March 3, 2003, from www.hivcorrections. org

Nokes, K. (Ed). (1996). *HIV/AIDS and the older adult.* Washington DC: Taylor & Francis.

Nokes, K., Holzemer, W., Corless, I., Bakken, S., Brown, M. A., Powell-Cope, G., et al. (2000). Health-related quality of life in persons younger and older than 50 who are living with HIV/AIDS. *Research on Aging, 22*(3), 290–310.

Nwanyanwu, O., Chu, S., Green, T., Buehler, J., & Berkelman, R. (1999). Acquired immunodeficiency syndrome in the United States associated with injecting drug use. *American Journal of Drug and Alcohol Use, 19*(4), 399–408.

Olaitan, A., Reid, W., Mocroft, A., McCarthy, K., Madge, S., & Johnson, M. (1996). Infertility among human immunodeficiency virus-positive women: Incidence and treatment. *Journal European Society of Human Reproduction and Embryology, 243,* 2793–2796.

Organistra, K. C., & Organistra, P. B. (1997). Migrant laborers and AIDS in the United States: A review of the literature. *AIDS Education and Prevention, 9*(1), 83–93.

Orloff, S. L., Bulterys, M., Vink, P., Nesheim, S., Abrams, E. J., Schoenbaum, E., et al. (2001). Maternal characteristics associated with antenatal, intrapartum, and neonatal zidovudine use in four cities, 1994–1998. *Journal of Acquired Immune Deficiency Syndromes, 28,* 65–72.

Patel, J., Melville, S., Heath, C., Sukalac, K. Dominguez, M. G. Fowler, I., et al. (2002, February). *Role of combination antiretroviral therapy and mode delivery in perinatal HIV transmission (PHT). Pediatric Spectrum of Disease Project (PSD) United States, 1995–2000.* Paper presented at the Ninth Conference on Retroviruses and Opportunistic Infections, Seattle, WA.

Patten, S., Vollman A., & Thurston, W. (2000). The utility of the transtheoretical model of behavior change for HIV risk reduction in injection drug users. *Journal of the Association of Nurses in AIDS Care, 11*(1), 57–66.

Preston, D. B., Forti, E. M., Kassab, C., & Koch, A. (2000). Personal and social determinants of rural nurses' willingness to care for persons with AIDS. *Research in Nursing and Health, 23,* 67–78.

Quick facts and figures on blindness and low vision. (2001). American Foundation of the Blind. Retrieved March 2003 from www.afb.org

Ragni, M. V., Tama, G., Lewis, J. H., & Ho, M. (1988). Increased frequency of haemarthroses in haemophilic patient treated with zidovudine. *Lancet, 8600,* 1454–1455.

Rainey, P. M., Friedland, G., McCance-Katz, E. F., Andrews, L., et al. (2000). Interaction of methadone with didansine and stavudine. *Journal of Acquired Deficiency Syndromes, 24*(3), 241–248.

Raiteri, R., Baussano, I., Giobbia, M., Fora, R., & Sinicco, A. (1998). Lesbian sex and risk of HIV transmission. *AIDS, 12,* 450–451.

Read, J. S., Tuomala, R., Kpamegan, E., et al. (2001). Mode of delivery and postpartum morbidity among HIV-infected women: The Women and Infants Transmission Study. *Journal of Acquired Immune Deficiency Syndrome, 26,* 236–245.

Rew, L., Fouladi, R. T., & Yockey, R. D. (2002). Sexual practices of homeless youth. *Journal of Nursing Scholarship, 34,* 139–145.

Rich, R. R. (2001). Negotiation of HIV preventive behaviors in divorced and separated women reentering the sexual arena. *Journal of the Association of Nurses in AIDS Care, 12,* 25–35.

Ricketts, T. C. (Ed.). (1999). *Rural health in the United States.* New York: Oxford University Press.

Roberts, A., & Kemp, C. (2001). Infectious diseases of refugees and immigrants: Giardiasis (giardia lamblia). *Journal of the American Academy of Nurse Practitioners, 13,* 532–533.

Roberts, K. J. (2002). Physician-patient relationships, patient satisfaction, and antiretroviral medication adherence among HIV-infected adults attending a public health clinic. *AIDS Patient Care and STDs, 16*(1), 43–50.

Robinson, M. R., Ross, M. L., & Whitcup, S. M. (1999). Ocular manifestations of HIV infection. *Current Opinion in Ophthalmology, 10*(6), 431–437.

Rompalo, A. M., Astemborski, J., Schoenbaum, E., Schuman, P., Carpenter, C., Holmberg, S. D., et.al. (1999). Comparison of clinical manifestations of HIV infection among women by risk group, CD_4+ cell count, and HIV-1 plasma viral load. *Journal of Acquired Immune Deficiency Syndrome and Human Retrovirology, 20,* 448–454.

Rouzioux, C., Costalgliola, D., Burgand, M., et al. (1995). Estimating timing of mother-to-child human immunodeficiency virus type 1 (HIV-1) transmission by use of a Markov model. *American Journal of Epidemiology, 142,* 1330–1337.

Sadeghi-Nejad, H., Watson, R., Irwin, R., Nokes, K., Gern, A., & Price, D. (2000). Lecture 5: Erectile dysfunction in the HIV-positive male: A review of medical, legal, and ethical considerations in the age of oral pharmacotherapy. *International Journal of Impotence Research, 12*(Suppl. 3), 49–53.

Sager, R., Lavreys, L., Baeten, J., Richardson, B., Mandaliya, K., Kreiss, J., et al. (2002, February). *Correlates of viral diversity in primary HIV-1 infection in women.* Paper presented at the Ninth Conference on Retroviruses and Opportunistic Infections, Seattle, WA.

St. Lawrence, J. S. (1999). Emerging behavioral strategies for the prevention of HIV in rural area. *The Journal of Rural Health, 15*(3), 335–339.

Schoener, E., Hopper, J., & Pierre, J. (2002). Injecting drug use in North America. *Infectious Disease Clinics of North America, 16*(3), 1–14.

Sengupta, S., Strauss, R. P., DeVellis, R., Quinn, S. C., DeVellis, B., & Ware, W. B. (2000). Factors affecting African-American participation in AIDS research. *Journal of Acquired Immune Deficiency Syndromes & Human Retrovirology, 24*(3), 275–284.

Shapiro, D., Tuomala, R., Samelson, R., et al. (2000, January). *Antepartum antiretroviral therapy and pregnancy outcome in 462 HIV-infected women in 1998–1999 (PACTG 367).* Paper presented at the

Seventh Conference on Retroviruses and Opportunistic Infections, San Francisco.

Shapiro, M. F., Morton, S. C., McCaffrey, D. F., Senterfitt, J. W., Fleishman, J. A., Perlman, J. F., et al. (1999). Variations in the care of HIV-infected adults in the United States: Results from the HIV Cost and Services Utilization Study. *Journal of the American Medical Association, 281,* 2305–2315.

Silbergeld, E. K., & Flaws, J. A. (1999). Chemicals and menopause: Effects on age at menopause and on health status in the postmenopausal period. *Journal of Women's Health, 8,* 227–234.

Smith, D. K., Gwinn, M., Selik, R. M., Miller, K. S., Dean-Gaitor, H., Ma'at, P. I., et al. (2000). HIV/AIDS among African Americans: Progress or progression? *AIDS, 14,* 1237–1248.

Song, J., & HRSA. (2000). *HIV/AIDS and homelessness: Recommendations for clinical practice and public policy.* Washington, DC: Bureau of Primary Health Care and HIV/AIDS Bureau, Health Resources and Services Administration.

Sullivan, P. S., Hanson, D. L., Chu, S. Y., Jones, J. L., & Ward, J. W. (1998). Epidemiology of anemia in human immunodeficiency virus (HIV)-infected persons: Results from the multistate adult and adolescent spectrum of HIV disease surveillance project. *Blood, 91*(1), 301–308.

Sunderland, A., Minkoff, H., Handle, J., Moroso, G., & Landesman, S. (1992). The impact of serostatus in women's reproductive decisions. *Obstetrics and Gynecology, 79,* 1027–1031.

Sylla, M., & Thomas, D. (2000, November). The rules: Law and AIDS in corrections. *HEPPNews.* Retrieved February 28, 2003, from www.hivcorrections.org

Thompson, A. S., Blankenship, K. M., Selwyn, P. A., Khoshnood, K., et al. (1998). Evaluation of an innovative program to address the health and social service needs of drug-using women with or at risk for HIV infection. *Journal of Community Health, 23*(6), 419–440.

Thompson, P. J., & Harm, N. J. (2000). Parenting from prison: Helping mothers and children. *Issues in Comprehensive Pediatric Nursing, 23,* 61–81.

Tom Waddell Health Center. (1998). *Protocols for hormonal reassignment of gender.* Retrieved January 11, 2003, from http://hivinsite.ucsf.edu/InSite.jsp?page=kbr-07–04–16&doc=2098.3d5a

UCSF Center for AIDS Prevention Studies and AIDS Research Institute. (1999). *What are adolescents' HIV prevention needs?* San Francisco: Author.

Umapathy, E., Simbini, T., Chipata, T., & Mbizvo, M. (2001). Sperm characteristics and accessory sex gland functions in HIV-infected men. *Archives of Andrology, 46,* 153–158.

United States Embassy. (1997). *Flying blind on a growing epidemic: AIDS in China.* Retrieved April 26, 2002, from http://www.usembassy-china.org.cn/english/sandt/webaids1.htm

U.S. Census Bureau. (2001). *Profiles of general demographic characteristics: 2000 census of population and housing, United States, 2000.* Retrieved January 15, 2003, from http://www.census.gov/prod/cen2000/dp1/2khus.pdf

U.S. Department of Agriculture. (2001). *Measuring rurality.* Retrieved, January 15, 2003, from http://www.ers.usda.gov/briefing/rurality/

U.S. Department of Health and Human Services. (2001). *Mental health: Culture, race, and ethnicity supplement.* Rockville, MD: Author.

U.S. Department of Health and Human Services, Health Resources and Services Administration, HIV/AIDS Bureau. (1999). *Helping adolescents with HIV adhere to HAART, 1999.* Washington, DC: Author.

U.S. Department of Health and Human Services, Health Resources and Services Administration, HIV/AIDS Bureau. (2001a). *Lessons learned.* Washington, DC: Author.

U.S. Department of Health and Human Services, Health Resources and Services Administration, HIV/AIDS Bureau. (2001b). *Youth and HIV/AIDS.* Washington, DC: Author.

U.S. Public Health Service. (2002.). U.S. Public Health Service task force recommendations for the use of antiretroviral drugs in pregnant HIV-1 infected women for maternal health and interventions to reduce perinatal HIV-1 transmission in the United States. *MMWR, 51*(RR18), 1–38.

vanBenthem, B. H. B., Vernazza, P., Coutinho, R. A., & Prins, M. (2002). The impact of pregnancy and menopause on CD_4 lymphocyte counts in HIV-infected women. *AIDS, 16,* 919–924.

Vicini, J. (2000, January 18). Supreme court upholds segregation of HIV-infected inmates. *Reuters Medical News on Medscape.* Retrieved February 28, 2003, from www.hiv.medscape.com

Voelker, R. (1998). Rural communities struggle with AIDS. *Journal of the American Medical Association, 279,* 5–6.

Watts, G. H. (2002). Management of human immunodeficiency virus infection in pregnancy. *New England Journal of Medicine, 346,* 1879–1891.

Whetten-Goldstein, K., Nguyen, T. Q., Heald, A. E. (2001). Characteristics of individuals infected with the human immunodeficiency virus and provider interaction in the predominantly rural southeast. *Southern Medical Journal, 94*(2), 212–222.

White House Office of National AIDS Policy. (2000). *Youth and HIV/AIDS 2000: A new American agenda.* Washington, DC: Author.

Wilson, T. E., Massad, L. S., Riester, K. A., Barkan, S., Richardson, J., Young, M., et al. (1999). Sexual, contraceptive, and drug behaviors of women with HIV and those at high risk for infection: results from the Women's Interagency HIV Study. *AIDS, 13,* 591–598.

Witte, S. S., Takeshi, W., El-Bassel, N., Gilbert, L., & Wallace, J. (2000). Predictors of female condom use among women exchanging street sex in New York City. *Sexually Transmitted Diseases, 27,* 93–100.

Wolffe, K.E., & Spungin, S.J. (2002). A glance at worldwide employment of people with visual impairments. *Journal of Visual Impairment and Blindness, 96*(4), 245–354.

Women and pharmacology. (2001, March). *PI Perspective, 32,* 11.

World Health Organization. (1999). Managing work and HIV. *HIVFrontline, 38,* 1–8.

Wortley, P. M., Chu, S. Y., Diaz, T., Ward, J. W., Doyle, B., Davidson, A. J., et al. (1995). HIV testing patterns: Where, why, and when were persons with AIDS tested for HIV? *AIDS, 9*(5), 487–492.

Wyatt, G. E., Myers, H. F., Williams, J. K., Kitchen, C. R., Loeb, T., Carmona, J. V., et al. (2002). Does a history of trauma contribute to HIV risk for women of color? Implications for prevention and policy. *American Journal of Public Health, 92,* 660–665.

Zhang, H., Domadula, G., Beaumont, M., et al. (1998). Human immunodeficiency virus type 1 in the semen of men receiving highly active antiretroviral therapy. *New England Journal of Medicine, 339,* 1803–1809.

Zierler, S., Cunningham, W. E., Andersen, R., Shapiro, M. F., Nakazono, T., Morton, S., et al. (2000). Violence victimization after HIV infection in U.S. sample of adult patients in primary care. *American Journal of Public Health, 90,* 208–215.

Section VII

Clinical Management of the HIV-Infected Infant and Child

N ew to this edition is an expanded focus on the care of infected children. Much has been learned about perinatal transmission and the treatment of HIV infection in children, and, because of the successful implementation of the U.S. Public Health Service's (PHS) recommendation for testing of women and for treatment during pregnancy, the incidence of HIV infection in children in the United States has declined dramatically. This is not the case abroad in some of the hard-hit areas, such as in Botswana, where almost 10,000 HIV-infected infants are born annually. Statistics such as this provide the strongest rationale for expanding this section. This curriculum is for nursing everywhere, not just in the United States. Moreover, as our infected children live longer with the disease, often into adulthood, nurses require a knowledge base to provide care across the life span.

This section describes the prevention, classification, diagnosis, staging, and management of HIV disease in infants and children. Special issues related to the initiation of antiretroviral therapy in children are discussed, including a section about the unique pediatric and family issues related to the adherence to antiretroviral therapy.

7.1 Perinatal Transmission of HIV Infection

1. Prevention of perinatal transmission
   a. Treatment with antiretroviral (ARV) medications during pregnancy, labor, and delivery, and treatment of the newborn, reduces the risk of mother-to-child or perinatal transmission of HIV from 25% to as low as 2% (U.S. Public Health Service Task Force, 2002).
   b. Results of PACTG 076, a study of 477 pregnant women randomly assigned to receive a placebo or zidovudine (ZDV) during pregnancy and intravenously (IV) during labor and delivery (the newborns received treatment for 6 weeks) showed that treatment reduced transmission from 22.6% to 7.6% (Connor et al., 1994).
   c. Subsequent research found shorter course ZDV regimens and other ARVs also can reduce perinatal transmission significantly. A study in Thailand found that a short course of ZDV—oral ZDV given to a pregnant woman from 36 weeks gestation and during labor in a non-breast-feeding population—reduced transmission from 50% to 9.4% (Shaffer et al., 1999). The PETRA study in four African countries compared a regimen of oral ZDV/3TC given from 36 weeks through labor and delivery and given to the mother and newborn for a week postpartum or given intrapartum and postpartum to a placebo and to an intrapartum-only regimen. In this breast-feeding population, the study found that intrapartum-only treatment was no more effective than placebo treatment but that the ZDV/3TC regimens reduced transmission to 9% and 11%, thus supporting the need for a postexposure component (Saba, 1999). The HIVNet 012 study, also in a breast-feeding population, found that a single dose of nevirapine to the mother at the onset of labor and to the newborn in the first 72 hours of life could reduce transmission to 12% compared with 21% for a short course ZDV regimen (Guay et al., 1999). The simplicity and low cost of the HIVNet 012 regimen makes it particularly applicable to low resource settings. A retrospective study in New York State found that intervening with ZDV treatment even during labor and delivery or only with the newborn still would significantly reduce the risk of transmission. Transmission rates were 10% with only intrapartum ZDV and 9.8% if only the newborn was treated for 6 weeks, compared with a 26.6% transmission rate if no treatment was initiated (Wade et al., 1998).
   d. The U.S. Public Health Service Perinatal HIV Guidelines Working Group on the use of antiretroviral drugs in pregnant HIV-infected women issues and routinely updates guidelines for maternal health and for reducing perinatal transmission. Current guidelines are available at http://www.aidsinfo.nih.gov/guidelines. The recommendations are shown in Table 7.1a.
2. Breast-feeding
   a. Breast-feeding increases the risk of HIV transmission to newborns by 12% to 16% (Fowler, Simonds, & Roongpisuthipong, 2000; Mbori-Ngacha et al., 2001).
   b. Studies suggest that most transmission occurs in the first few weeks and months of life (Miotti et al., 1999; Nduati et al., 2000).
   c. Mechanism of transmission is thought to be frequent and prolonged exposure of the infant's oral and gastrointestinal (GI) tract to breast milk that is infected with HIV.
   d. Women with HIV infection in the United States and other countries where safe substitute feeding is available are urged not to breast-feed.
   e. Breast-feeding is the norm among many cultural groups in the United States, particularly among recent immigrants from developing countries. Decisions not to breast-feed may raise issues regarding confidentiality of a mother's HIV diagnosis and require sensitivity and supportive interventions (National Pediatric and Family HIV Resource Center, 2002).

Table 7.1a Clinical Scenarios and Recommendations for the Use of Antiretroviral Drugs to Reduce Perinatal HIV Transmission

Clinical Scenario	Recommendations
Scenario 1 HIV-infected women who have not received prior antiretroviral therapy	Pregnant women with HIV infection must receive standard clinical, immunologic, and virologic evaluation. Recommendations for initiation and choice of antiretroviral therapy should be based on the same parameters used for persons who are not pregnant, although the known and unknown risks and benefits of such therapy during pregnancy must be considered and discussed. The three-part ZDV chemoprophylaxis regimen, initiated after the first trimester, should be recommended for all pregnant women with HIV infection regardless of antenatal HIV RNA copy number to reduce the risk for perinatal transmission. The combination ZDV chemoprophylaxis with additional antiretroviral drugs for treatment of HIV infection is recommended for infected women whose clinical, immunologic, or virologic status requires treatment or who have HIV RNA over 1,000 copies/mL regardless of clinical or immunologic status. Women who are in the 1st trimester of pregnancy may consider delaying initiation of therapy until after 10–12 weeks' gestation.
Scenario 2 HIV-infected women receiving antiretroviral therapy during the current pregnancy	HIV-1 infected women receiving antiretroviral therapy and in whom pregnancy is identified after the 1st trimester should continue therapy. ZDV should be a component of the antenatal antiretroviral treatment regimen after the 1st trimester whenever possible, although this may not always be feasible. Women receiving antiretroviral therapy and in whom pregnancy is recognized during the 1st trimester should be counseled regarding the benefits and potential risks of antiretroviral administration during this period, and continuation of therapy should be considered. If therapy is discontinued during the 1st trimester, all drugs should be stopped and reintroduced simultaneously to avoid the development of drug resistance. Regardless of the antepartum antiretroviral regimen, ZDV administration is recommended during the intrapartum period and for the newborn.
Scenario 3 HIV-infected women in labor who have had no prior therapy	Several effective regimens are available; these include (1) single dose nevirapine at the onset of labor, followed by a single dose of nevirapine for the newborn at age 48 hours; (2) oral ZDV and 3TC during labor, followed by 1 week of oral ZDV/3TC for the newborn; (3) intrapartum intravenous ZDV followed by 6 weeks of ZDV for the newborn; and (4) the two-dose nevirapine regimen combined with intrapartum intravenous ZDV and 6 weeks of ZDV for the newborn. In the immediate postpartum period, the woman should have appropriate assessments (e.g., CD₄ count and HIV-1 RNA copy number) to determine whether antiretroviral therapy is recommended for her own health.
Scenario 4 Infants born to mothers who have received no antiretroviral therapy during pregnancy or intrapartum	The 6-week neonatal ZDV component of the ZDV chemoprophylactic regimen should be discussed with the mother and offered for the newborn. ZDV should be initiated as soon as possible after delivery—preferably within 6–12 hours of birth. Some clinicians may choose to use ZDV in combination with other antiretroviral drugs, particularly if the mother is known or suspected to have ZDV-resistant virus. However, the efficacy of this approach for prevention of transmission is unknown, and appropriate dosing regimens for neonates are incompletely defined. In the immediate postpartum period, the woman should undergo appropriate assessments (e.g., CD₄ count and HIV-1 RNA copy number) to determine if antiretroviral therapy is required for her own health. The infant should undergo early diagnostic testing so that if HIV infected, treatment can be initiated as soon as possible.

NOTE: Discussion of treatment options and recommendations should be noncoercive, and the final decision regarding the use of antiretroviral drugs is the responsibility of the woman. A decision to not accept treatment with ZDV or other drugs should not result in punitive action or denial of care. Use of ZDV should not be denied to a woman who wishes to minimize exposure of the fetus to other antiretroviral drugs and who therefore chooses to receive only ZDV during pregnancy to reduce the risk for perinatal transmission.

SOURCE: U. S. Public Health Service Task Force, 2002

3. Diagnosis and evaluation of the HIV-exposed infant
   a. All infants born to mothers with HIV infection will have transplacentally acquired HIV antibody (Nielsen & Bryson, 2000; Working Group on Antiretroviral Therapy and Medical Management of HIV-Infected Children, 2001).
   b. Maternally acquired antibody can be present for up to 18 months of age (Working Group on Antiretroviral Therapy and Medical Management of HIV-Infected Children, 2001).
   c. Diagnosis of HIV in infants should be made using virologic assays that identify the presence of the HIV antigen (Nielsen & Bryson, 2000).
   d. HIV polymerase chain reaction (PCR) has a sensitivity of 90% at 3 months and nearly 100% at 6 months of age (Nielsen & Bryson, 2000).
      i. Presumptive diagnosis of HIV infection can be made on one positive HIV PCR and definitive diagnosis with a confirmatory test on a different blood sample (Working Group on Antiretroviral Therapy and Management of Children with HIV Infection, 1998)
      ii. HIV can be reasonably excluded with two negative HIV PCR results on different samples if both are obtained after 1 month of age and the second is after 4 months of age; some clinicians also use a confirmatory negative ELISA at > 18 months of age (Working Group on Antiretroviral Therapy and Management of Children with HIV Infection, 1998).
   e. Children > 18 months of age can be diagnosed with a positive HIV ELISA and confirmatory Western blot (Working Group on Antiretroviral Therapy and Management of Children with HIV Infection, 1998).
   f. AIDS can be diagnosed based on clinical symptoms in conjunction with laboratory evidence of dysfunction of humoral and cellular immunity using the 1994 Centers for Disease Control and Prevention (CDC) Pediatric HIV Classification System (Centers for Disease Control and Prevention, 1994).

4. Classification system for human immunodeficiency virus in children less than 13 years of age (Centers for Disease Control and Prevention, 1994)
   a. The system is based on three parameters: infection, clinical, and immunologic status with mutually exclusive categories.
   b. Infection status
      i. Infants whose infection status has not been definitively established are categorized with the prefix "E" for "perinatally exposed."
      ii. "E" is rarely used now due to the availability of more rapid diagnosis.
   c. Immunologic categories (see Table 7.1b)
      i. Immunologic categories are based on CD_4 lymphocyte count or a percentage that has been adjusted for age using the more severe of the two if the absolute count and percentage are different.
      ii. Classification may not be changed even if the CD_4 count or percentage improves.
   d. Clinical categories (see Table 7.1c): The four mutually exclusive clinical categories are based on signs, symptoms, or diagnoses related to HIV infection.
      i. Category N (not symptomatic)
      ii. Category A (mildly symptomatic)
      iii. Category B (moderately symptomatic)
      iv. Category C (severely symptomatic): AIDS-defining conditions in the 1987 case definition, except lymphoid interstitial pneumonia (LIP), which is in Category B
   e. Classification is less useful because treatment for children has improved.
      i. Once categorized, a child's category cannot be changed, although a child's clinical condition may improve.
      ii. The CDC category may not accurately reflect a child's current clinical condition when his or her immunologic or clinical condition improves with ARV treatment.

Table 7.1b   1994 Revised Pediatric HIV Classification System: Immunologic Categories Based on Age-Specific CD_4+ Lymphocyte Count and Percentage

Immune Category	Age of Child					
	< 12 months No./mm3 (%)		1–5 years No./mm3 (%)		6–12 years No./mm3 (%)	
Category 1: No Suppression	> 1,500	(> 25%)	> 1,000	(> 25%)	> 500	(< 25%)
Category 2: Moderate Suppression	750–1,499	(15–24%)	500–999	(15–24%)	200–499	(15–24%)
Category 3: Severe Suppression	< 750	(< 15%)	< 500	(< 15%)	< 200	(< 15%)

SOURCE: Centers for Disease Control and Prevention (1994)

5. Natural history of HIV disease in children
   a. Perinatal HIV has two patterns of presentation
      i. Fifteen to 20% of infants present early in life, with rapid onset of severe symptoms, rapid progression, and poor prognosis (Grubman & Oleske, 1995; Lindegren, Steinberg, & Byers, 2000).
         (1) Rapid progression may represent infants infected in utero. Infants are considered to have been infected in utero if viral diagnostic assays (HIV DNA PCR) are positive within 48 hours of birth and are positive on subsequent tests (Nielsen & Bryson, 2000).
         (2) If left untreated, these infants present with severe opportunistic infections (OIs) (e.g., PCP), encephalopathy, failure to thrive, and moderate to severe immune suppression within the 1st year of life.
      ii. Eighty percent of perinatally infected infants become symptomatic after 1 year of age with slower progression of disease with or without immune suppression (European Collaborative Study, 2001; Grubman & Oleske, 1995; Lindegren et al., 2000).
         (1) Infants may be considered to be infected intrapartally if virologic assays within the first 48 hours of life are negative but testing after 1 week of age is positive in the absence of breastfeeding (Nielsen & Bryson, 2000).
         (2) Lymphoproliferative symptoms, including generalized lymphadenopathy and LIP, are common in untreated children.
         (3) HIV-infected children often present with general clinical manifestations of HIV, including recurrent or chronic symptoms of normal childhood illness (e.g., otitis media, reactive airway disease).

6. Prognosis and survival
   a. Progression of HIV disease is frequently rapid in untreated children.
      i. Children usually have evidence of severe immune compromise.
      ii. They frequently have evidence of end organ failure, such as primary HIV encephalopathy and HIV cardiomyopathy.

Table 7.1c   1994 Revised HIV Pediatric Classification System: Clinical Categories

Category N: Not Symptomatic

Children who have no signs or symptoms considered to be the result of HIV infection or who have only ONE of the conditions listed in Category A.

Category A: Mildly Symptomatic

Children with TWO or more of the conditions listed below but none of the conditions listed in Categories B and C.

- Lymphadenopathy (> 0.5 cm at more than two sites; bilateral = one site)
- Hepatomegaly
- Splenomegaly
- Dermatitis
- Parotitis
- Recurrent or persistent upper respiratory infection, sinusitis or otitis media

Category B: Moderately Symptomatic

Children who have symptomatic conditions other than those listed for Category A or C that are attributed to HIV infection. Examples of conditions in clinical Category B include but are not limited to:

- Anemia (< 8 gm/dL), neutropenia (< 1,000/mm^3), or thrombocytopenia (< 100,000/mm^3) persisting > 30 days
- Bacterial meningitis, pneumonia, or sepsis (single episode)
- Candidiasis, oropharyngeal (thrush) persisting (> 2 months) in children > 6 months of age
- Cardiomyopathy
- Cytomegalovirus infection, with onset before 1 month of age
- Diarrhea, recurrent or chronic
- Hepatitis
- Herpes simplex virus (HSV) stomatitis, recurrent (more than two episodes within 1 year)
- HSV bronchitis, pneumonitis, or esophagitis with onset before one month of age
- Herpes zoster (shingles) involving at least two distinct episodes or more than one dermatome
- Leiomyosarcoma
- Lymphoid interstitial pneumonia (LIP) or pulmonary lymphoid hyperplasia complex
- Nephropathy
- Nocardiosis
- Persistent fever (lasting > 1 month)
- Toxoplasmosis, onset before 1 month of age
- Varicella, disseminated (complicated chickenpox)

Category C: Severely Symptomatic

Children who have any condition listed in the 1987 surveillance case definition for acquired immunodeficiency syndrome, with the exception of LIP (which is a Category B condition)

- Serious bacterial infections, multiple or recurrent (i.e., any combination of at least two culture-confirmed infections within a 2-year period), of the following types: septicemia, pneumonia, meningitis, bone or joint infection, or abscess of an internal organ or body cavity (excluding otitis media, superficial skin or mucosal abscesses, and indwelling catheter-related infections)
- Candidiasis, esophageal or pulmonary (bronchi, trachea, lungs)
- Coccidioidomycosis, disseminated (at site other than or in addition to lungs or cervical or hilar lymph nodes)
- Cryptococcosis, extrapulmonary
- Cryptosporidiosis or isosporiasis with diarrhea persisting > 1 month
- Cytomegalovirus disease with onset of symptoms at age > 1 month (at a site other than liver, spleen, or lymph nodes)
- Encephalopathy (at least one of the following progressive findings present for at least 2 months in the absence of a concurrent illness other than HIV infection that could explain the findings): a) failure to attain or loss of developmental milestones or loss of intellectual ability, verified by standard developmental scale or neuropsychological tests; b) impaired brain growth or acquired microcephaly demonstrated by head circumference measurements or brain atrophy demonstrated by computerized tomography or magnetic resonance imaging (serial imaging is required for children < 2 years of age); c) acquired symmetric motor deficit manifested by two or more of the following: paresis, pathologic reflexes, ataxia, or gait disturbance

(Continued)

Table 7.1c Continued

- Herpes simplex virus infection causing a mucocutaneous ulcer that persists for >1 month; or bronchitis, pneumonitis, or esophagitis for any duration affecting a child > 1month of age
- Histoplasmosis, disseminated (at a site other than or in addition to lungs or cervical or hilar lymph nodes)
- Kaposi's sarcoma
- Lymphoma, primary, in brain
- Lymphoma, small, noncleaved cell (Burkitt's), or immunoblastic or large cell lymphoma of B-cell or unknown immunologic phenotype
- *Mycobacterium tuberculosis*, disseminated or extrapulmonary
- *Mycobacterium*, other species or unidentified species, disseminated (at a site other than or in addition to lungs, skin, or cervical or hilar lymph nodes)
- *Mycobacterium avium* complex or *Mycobacterium kansasii*, disseminated (at site other than or in addition to lungs, skin, or cervical or hilar lymph nodes)
- *Pneumocystis carinii* pneumonia
- Progressive multifocal leukoencephalopathy
- Salmonella (nontyphoid) septicemia, recurrent
- Toxoplasmosis of the brain with onset at >1month of age
- Wasting syndrome in the absence of a concurrent illness other than HIV infection that could explain the following findings: a) persistent weight loss >10% of baseline OR b) downward crossing of at least two of the following percentile lines on the weight-for-age chart (e.g., 95th, 75th, 50th, 25th, 5th) in a child ≥1 year of age OR) < 5th percentile on weight-for-height chart on two consecutive measurements, ≥30 days apart PLUS a) chronic diarrhea (i.e., at least two loose stools per day for ≥30 days) OR b) documented fever (for ≥30 days, intermittent or constant)

SOURCE: Centers for Disease Control and Prevention (1994)

iii. In children who are not symptomatic by age 1 year, disease progression is less rapid between ages 1 and 5 years and slow between ages 5 and 10 years (European Collaborative Study, 2001).

iv. Less than 10% of children will remain asymptomatic up to age 5 years (European Collaborative Study, 2001).

b. Availability of ARV therapy has led to a slower progression of disease and improved quality of life in children receiving ARV treatment (European Collaborative Study, 2001; Laufer & Scott, 2000).

c. Children receiving treatment may have a history of recurrent normal childhood infections (e.g., otitis media, sinusitis, reactive airway disease) but no apparent symptoms of HIV infection for years.

d. They often have moderate immune suppression evidenced by decreased CD$_4$ lymphocyte counts and percentage but may have nonfunctional antibody responses (B-cell function).

i. Mortality from HIV disease in one cohort of 1,028 children indicated a decline from 5.3% in 1996 to 0.7% in 1999 (Gortmaker et al., 2001).

ii. Initiation of combination ARV therapy, including a protease inhibitor, was independently associated in this cohort with reduced mortality (Gortmaker et al., 2001).

7.2 Clinical Manifestations and Management of the HIV-Infected Infant and Child

1. Initial visit and baseline assessment: The initial visit and baseline assessment provide an opportunity to obtain a comprehensive history and physical examination. The quantity and quality of the historical information obtained may be dependent on the age of the child as well as the relationship of the child to the guardian. Every effort should be made to obtain as complete a profile as possible.

   a. Health history

i.   Birth history: Information contained in the birth history includes the maternal history, including the mother's antiretroviral history, CD_4 count and viral load at the time of delivery, and any significant maternal illnesses that occurred during the pregnancy or any preexisting chronic conditions. Intrauterine drug exposure to other prescription and nonprescription medications as well as alcohol, tobacco, and illicit drugs should also be included. If available, the infant's gestational age at birth; birth parameters, such as weight, length, and head circumference; and the route of delivery should be documented. Results of any neonatal screenings are also useful historical information.

ii. Medical history: Because of their potential to result in ongoing health concerns for the child, all illnesses, including respiratory, infectious, metabolic, neurologic, and cardiac problems, should be included in the medical history. For chronic illnesses, the date of onset should be recorded, and for episodic illnesses onset and resolution dates are useful if available. Additionally, dates of and reasons for hospitalizations are also significant components of the health history.

iii. Surgical history: All surgical procedures, whether extensive or minor, and their outcomes should be recorded during the initial health history and intake.

iv. Medication history: A detailed medication history, including the initiation and discontinuation of all medications, is essential. Chronic and episodic medications, including those used for infections, HIV prophylaxis, nutritional supplementation, or chronic conditions such as asthma or dermatitis along with medication allergies, are included in a thorough pediatric medication history.

v.   Childhood illnesses and immunizations: During the initial history, it is essential to obtain accurate information on diseases of childhood, such as varicella, including dates of illness and a description of the disease course. The most up-to-date record of immunizations should also be obtained to determine any need for implementation of a catch-up immunization schedule.

vi. Family history: If possible, a detailed family medical history should be obtained to determine the child's risk of certain inherited physical and mental conditions.

vii. Social history: Any history of substance abuse and housing or financial issues should be elicited for further intervention during the initial intake. A clear determination of the family constellation, members of the household, and key involved members of the extended family or community must also be identified.

viii. Nutrition history: If available, serial measurements of weight, height, should be documented to serve as a basis for comparison of future growth. Additionally, a detailed diet history and food preferences as well as food allergy information may also be useful information that can serve as the basis for future dietary and adherence-related interventions.

b. Review of systems

i.   General review: A thorough review of systems should be completed at each visit with a notation of the onset and course of the problem so far. Particular attention should be paid to new problems, problems associated with fever, and those that have not responded as expected to prescribed therapies.

ii. Skin: Make note of all dermatological complaints, including rashes, skin discoloration, ulceration, itching, or bruising.

iii. Head: Problems of the scalp, including areas of hair loss, scaling, flaking, oozing, and any swellings, should be noted.

iv. Eyes: Any history of visual disturbances, eye pain, discharge, or trauma is a significant part of the review of systems.

v. Ears: Hearing disturbances, including diminished hearing or tinnitus as well as ear pain or discharge, should be noted.

vi. Nose and sinuses: Information about the quantity and quality of any nasal discharge as well as sinus pain or tenderness assists in the diagnosis of infectious upper airway processes and should be noted in the review of systems.

vii. Mouth and throat: A history significant for oral problems, such as bleeding, pain, ulceration, lesions, discharge, drooling, difficult or painful swallowing, and problems with dentition and decreased oral intake seemingly related to any of these factors, may indicate serious HIV-related disease processes in infants and children.

viii. Respiratory: Characteristics and duration of respiratory symptoms, including wheezing, cough, sputum production, shortness of breath, chest pain, and exposure to others with similar symptoms, are frequently reported among infants and children with HIV infection and may be representative of common childhood illnesses or more serious underlying HIV-related illnesses.

ix. Cardiovascular: A history of pallor, cyanosis, shortness of breath, edema, or irregular heartbeat, if identified, should be documented and in some cases followed with a detailed cardiology work-up.

x. Gastrointestinal: Of note in this section of the review of systems is any report of abdominal pain, bloating, or cramping. Nausea, vomiting, diarrhea, and the history that preceded the onset of these symptoms should also be noted. Frequency of symptoms, exacerbating and mitigating factors, as well as quality and quantity of stool should also be noted. Exposure to family members or other children with similar complaints is also of significance.

xi. Genitourinary: Notable symptoms and complaints often consistent with genitourinary infections or renal problems include any history of urgency, frequency, pain on urination, lower back pain, or strong smelling or discolored urine, including urine containing blood.

xii. Gynecologic: When age appropriate, menstrual history and onset and norms (duration, pain, clotting) should be ascertained. Pregnancy history including live births, miscarriages, and abortions may also be pertinent for adolescent females. Any history of discharge, pain, or lesions should also be documented.

xiii. Musculoskeletal: Muscle aches, pains and cramps, joint pain, stiffness, or swellings, history of trauma, events and activities preceding onset, and exacerbating and mitigating factors are significant components of this portion of the history.

xiv. Neurologic: Neurologic changes, including alterations in level of consciousness and loss of neurological function, are often hallmark signs of HIV disease progression or an infectious process. Onset and specific symptoms identified in the review of systems assists with further diagnostic work-up of these complaints.

xv. Nutrition assessment: Any history of significant nutritional deficiencies, eating disorders, lead toxicity, other dietary problems including problems with food intake, and a dietary recall are contained in this component of the review.

xvi. Psychiatric and emotional: Significant problems uncovered in this portion of the review of systems may include symptoms of depression, acting-out behavior at home or at school, interpersonal relationships with family members and peers, school performance, and knowledge of HIV diagnosis.

c. Physical examination: In general, unless there is an extremely specific reason for the health care visit, infants and children with HIV infection should have a complete physical examination at each health care encounter. This approach assists with the monitoring of ongoing problems and allows for the early diagnosis of new health issues as they are emerging.

   i. General: Growth parameters and vital signs are essential components of every examination because they are often the first indicator of significant underlying HIV and non-HIV-related problems.

   ii. Growth and development: An initial screening of growth and development is indicated for every infant and child entering HIV services. This assessment may be performed by a developmental specialist or by providers trained in the administration of tests, such as the Denver Developmental Screening Test, to establish a developmental baseline against which future assessments can be compared.

   iii. Neurological examination: Because HIV is a disease that can especially affect the neurological functioning of infants and children, a comprehensive neurological exam is warranted at the initial visit. Particular attention should be paid to cranial nerve, reflex, and developmental status to determine the extent of any current neurological problems and to provide comparison for future determinations, which may be able to show static or progressive changes.

   iv. Mouth and throat examination: Oral problems and oral health can have a significant impact on the growth and well-being of infants and children with HIV infection. Notable findings include lesions such as aphthous ulcers and oral candida, dental caries, and herpetic lesions.

   v. Cardiovascular examination: HIV-related cardiomyopathy may present in infants and children with HIV infection; therefore, findings including cardiac murmurs and abnormalities of heart rate, rhythm, or blood pressure warrant further evaluation by a trained cardiology practitioner.

   vi. Respiratory examination: Viral and bacterial pneumonias as well as asthma, bronchiectasis, and LIP can be causes of diminished respiratory function in infants and children with HIV. Findings of cough, wheezing, shortness of breath, poor aeration, and crackles may be indicative of diseases of childhood that will respond well to treatment of underlying progressive HIV-related processes.

   vii. Abdominal examination: Significant findings in infants and children with HIV infection include abdominal pain, masses, and organomegaly.

   viii. Musculoskeletal examination: Muscle tone and bulk as well as range of motion and tenderness or swelling of joints should be evaluated at each visit.

   ix. Skin examination: Infants and children with HIV infection are prone to various types of dermatological problems, including tinea, herpes zoster, eczema, staphylococcal skin infections, rashes resulting from adverse drug reactions, and various viral exanthems.

d. Laboratory and diagnostic evaluation: The initial visit provides the opportunity to obtain a comprehensive baseline laboratory profile as well as determine immunologic and virologic status and history of exposure to infectious agents.

   i. Immunologic profile: CD_4 T-lymphocyte counts and percentages should be obtained at baseline and compared with age-specific norms to stage the child's degree of immunocompromise and risk for opportunistic infection. Baseline measurements also allow for assessment of the effectiveness of therapeutic regimen changes.

   ii. HIV RNA PCR (viral load): Initial determinations serve as a useful comparison to subsequent counts in determining the need for and the effectiveness of therapeutic regimens and may serve as an indicator of adherence problems as well.

   iii. Complete blood count (CBC) with differential: The CBC with differential is performed at the initial visit to screen for anemia, neutropenia, thrombocytopenia, and other hematologic abnormalities that may be HIV related.

   iv. Multichannel chemistry panel: Blood chemistries are useful in identifying pancreatic, liver, cardiac, and electrolyte abnormalities in infants and children with HIV infection.

   v. Urinalysis (UA): A screening UA is recommended at baseline to identify asymptomatic infection and other abnormalities, such as proteinuria or glucosuria, which may be indicative of other HIV and non-HIV-related disease

processes. Subsequently, annual UAs are recommended (Laufer & Scott, 2000).

   vi. Tuberculin skin test (TST): TST is recommended for children age 6 months and older. Due to the increased risk of the development of tuberculosis (TB) in TB- and HIV-coinfected persons, this is an essential baseline screening test that should be repeated annually or more often if a question of exposure arises.

   vii. Chest X-ray: Chest X-rays are often performed for baseline evaluation purposes and then performed annually to determine current disease processes and to serve as a reference for later episodes of respiratory problems.

   viii. Toxoplasmosis serologic test: Initial toxoplasmosis titers provide information about intrauterine exposure and possible risk of the development of toxoplasmosis if immunocompromise becomes an issue. The test is performed at baseline, and, if negative, should be repeated annually.

   ix. Cytomegalovirus (CMV) serology: This blood test is recommended for initial screening and, if negative, should be repeated on an annual basis due to the risk of the development of CMV disease in severely immunocompromised children.

   x. Varicella serologic test: Varicella titers are useful in establishing a child's potential immunity to this common childhood illness. Because varicella can have especially severe sequelae in HIV-infected children, knowledge of immune status is essential in identifying children most at risk for complications and in need of aggressive treatment.

   xi. Syphilis screening–rapid plasma reagin test (RPR): This test is recommended at baseline to determine the presence of congenital syphilis infection.

xii. Baseline triglycerides: The high incidence of triglyceride elevation in children on certain types of ARV therapy warrants a baseline determination at the initial visit, which can be used for future comparison.

xiii. Hepatitis profile (A, B, C): Determination of a child's hepatitis exposure status, infection status, and immunity are a component of the initial diagnostic evaluation and staging of HIV infection and should be repeated on an annual basis.

2. Immunizations: modifications to the childhood immunization schedule are presented in Table 7.2a. General immunization principles that apply to children with HIV infection are listed in this section.

   a. Inactivated polio vaccine is recommended for routine childhood polio vaccination in the United States (U.S. Public Health Service and Infectious Diseases Society of America & USPHS/ISDA Prevention of Opportunistic Infections Working Group, 2001). Live attenuated viruses, such as oral polio, should not be given to persons with HIV infection or their household contacts.

   b. Measles/mumps/rubella immunization should be given only in children in CDC immunologic classification categories 1 and 2 and should be given as soon after the first birthday as possible. Providers may consider administering the second dose as early as 1 month after the initial vaccine. Cases of immunization-related disease have been reported in the severely immunocompromised patient.

   c. Haemophilus influenza B immunization is routinely recommended for HIV-infected infants and children due to the common and potentially severe nature of these infections.

   d. Influenza vaccine (split-virus for children younger than 13 years old) is recommended for all HIV-infected children older than 6 months of age on an annual basis as well as for their household contacts.

   e. Pneumococcal vaccination is recommended for all children 2 years of age and older due to the increasing incidence of antibiotic resistant *S. pneumoniae* in HIV-infected children. Revaccination should be offered in 3 to 5 years if a child was younger than 10 years at the time of initial immunization or in 5 years for children who were older than age 10 years.

   f. Hepatitis B vaccine is routinely recommended for all HIV-infected infants and children.

   g. Varicella vaccine is not recommended in persons with cellular immune deficiencies. Because children with HIV infection are at increased risk for morbidity from varicella and herpes zoster, the USPHS/ISDA committee recommends that the vaccine be given only to asymptomatic, nonimmunocompromised children with HIV infection (U.S. Public Health Service and Infectious Diseases Society of America & USPHS/ISDA Prevention of Opportunistic Infections Working Group, 2001).

   h. Immune globulin preparations may be indicated for HIV-infected children with specific problems, including intractable thrombocytopenia, recurrent bacterial infections, or evidence of inadequate humoral immunity.

3. Prophylaxis for opportunistic infections

   a. Prophylaxis against *Pneumocystis carinii* pneumonia (PCP) is critical for HIV-exposed infants.

      i. PCP remains the most common AIDS-defining illness in children (Abrams, 2000).

      ii. Most infants present with PCP at 4 to 6 months of age. Risk for PCP in the 1st year of life for a perinatally infected infant not receiving prophylaxis is estimated at 12% (Abrams, 2000).

      iii. All HIV-exposed infants from age 4 weeks to 12 months should receive PCP prophylaxis regardless of CD_4 count (Centers for Disease Control and Prevention, 1995).

Table 7.2a   Recommended Immunization Schedule for HIV-Infected Children

Vaccine	Age											
	Birth	1 mo	2 mos	4 mos	6 mos	12 mos	15 mos	18 mos	24 mos	4-6 yrs	11-12 yrs	14-16 yrs
⬇ Recommendations for these vaccines are the same as those for immunocompetent children. ⬇												
Hepatitis B[1]		Hep B #1									Hep B	
			Hep B #2			Hep B #3						
Diphtheria and Tetanus toxoids, Pertussis[2]			DTaP	DTaP	DTaP		DTaP			DTaP	Td	
Haemophilus influenzae type b[3]			Hib	Hib	Hib	Hib						
Inactivated Polio[4]			IPV	IPV		IPV				IPV		
Hepatitis A[5]										Hep A in selected areas		
⬇ Recommendations for these vaccines differ from those for immunocompetent children. ⬇												
Pneumococcus[6]			PCV	PCV	PCV	PCV			PPV23	PPV23 (age 5-7 yrs)		
Measles, Mumps, Rubella[7]	Do not give to severly immuno-suppressed (Category 3) children.					MMR				MMR	MMR	
Varicella[8]	Give only to asymptomatic non-immunosuppressed (category 1) children. Contraindicated in all other HIV infected children.					Var	Var				Var	
Influenza[9]						A dose is recommended every year						

- ☐ Range of recommended ages for vaccination.
- ⬭ Vaccines to be given if previously recommended doses were missed or were given earlier than the recommended minimum age.
- ▨ Recommended in selected states and/or regions.

This schedule indicates the recommended ages for routine administration of currently licensed childhood vaccines as of November 1, 2000, for children through age 18 years. Additional vaccines may be licensed and recommended during the year. Licensed combination vaccines may be used whenever any components of the combination are indicated and the vaccine's other components are not contraindicated. Providers should consult the manufacturer's package inserts for detailed recommendations.

1. *Infants born to hepatitis B surface antigen (HBsAg)-negative mothers* should receive the first dose of hepatitis B vaccine (Hep B) *at birth and no later than* age 2 months. The second dose should be administered at least 1 month after the first dose. The third dose should be administered at least 4 months after the first dose and at least 2 months after the second dose but not before age 6 months. *Infants born to HBsAg-positive mothers* should receive Hep B and 0.5 mL hepatitis B immune globulin (HBIG) within 12 hours of birth at separate sites. The second dose is recommended at age 1 to 2 months and the third dose at age 6 months. *Infants born to mothers whose HBsAg status is unknown* should receive Hep B within 12 hours of birth. Maternal blood should be drawn at delivery to determine the mother's HBsAg status; if the HBsAg test is positive, the infant should receive HBIG as soon as possible (no later than age 1 week). *All children and adolescents (through age 18 years)* who have not been immunized against hepatitis B should begin the series during any visit. Providers should make special

(Continued)

Table 7.2a   Continued

efforts to immunize children who were born in or whose parents were born in areas of the world where hepatitis B virus infection is moderately or highly endemic.

2. The fourth dose of diphtheria and tetanus toxoids and acellular pertussis vaccine (DTaP) may be administered as early as age 12 months, provided 6 months have elapsed since the third dose and the child is unlikely to return at age 15 to 18 months. Tetanus and diphtheria toxoids (Td) is recommended at age 11 to 12 years if at least 5 years have elapsed since the last dose of diphtheria and tetanus toxoids and pertussis vaccine (DTP), DTaP, or diphtheria and tetanus toxoids (DT). Subsequent routine Td boosters are recommended every 10 years.

3. Three Haemophilus influenzae type b (Hib) conjugate vaccines are licensed for infant use. If Hib conjugate vaccine (PRP-OMP) (PedvaxHIB or ComVax [Merck]) is administered at ages 2 and 4 months, a dose at age 6 months is not required. Because clinical studies in infants have demonstrated that using some combination products may induce a lower immune response to the Hib vaccine component, DTaP/ Hib combination products should not be used for primary immunization in infants at ages 2, 4, or 6 months unless approved by the Food and Drug Administration for these ages.

4. An all-inactivated poliovirus vaccine (IPV) schedule is recommended for routine childhood polio vaccination in the United States. All children should receive four doses of IPV at age 2 months, age 4 months, between ages 6 and 18 months, and between ages 4 and 6 years. Oral poliovirus vaccine should not be administered to HIV-infected persons or their household contacts.

5. Hepatitis A vaccine (Hep A) is recommended for use in selected states or regions and for certain high-risk groups such as those with Hepatitis B or Hepatitis C infection. Information is available from local public health authorities.

6. The heptavalent pneumococcal conjugate vaccine (PCV) is recommended for all HIV-infected children ages 2 to 59 months. Children 2 years and older should also receive the 23 valent pneumococcal polysaccharide vaccine; a single revaccination with the 23 valent vaccine should be offered to children after 3 to 5 years. Refer to the Advisory Committee on Immunization Practices recommendations (80) on dosing intervals for children starting the vaccination schedule after 2 months of age.

7. MMR should not be administered to severely immunocompromised (*Category 3*) children. HIV-infected children without severe immunosuppression would routinely receive their first dose of MMR as soon as possible after reaching their first birthday. Consideration should be given to administering the second dose of MMR as soon as 1 month (i.e., a minimum of 28 days) after the first dose rather, then waiting until school entry.

8. Varicella zoster virus vaccine should be given only to asymptomatic, nonimmunosuppressed children. Eligible children should receive two doses of vaccine with at least a 3-month interval between doses. The first dose may be given as early as 12 months of age.

9. Inactivated split influenza virus vaccine should be administered to all HIV-infected children 6 months of age each year. For children ages 6 months to < 9 years who are receiving influenza vaccine for the first time, two doses given 1 month apart are recommended. For specific recommendations, see Centers for Disease Control and Prevention (2001).

SOURCE: U.S. Public Health Service (USPHS) and Infectious Diseases Society of America (ISDA) & USPHS/ISDA Prevention of Opportunistic Infections Working Group (2001)

    iv. Prophylaxis can be stopped after 4 months of age if HIV infection has been excluded (Centers for Disease Control and Prevention, 1995; Working Group on Antiretroviral Therapy and Medical Management of HIV–Infected Children, 2001).

    v. PCP prophylaxis for children older than age 1 year is based on adjusted CD$_4$ count (Centers for Disease Control and Prevention, 1995).

    (1) Ages 1 to 5 years: CD$_4$ count < 500/μL or CD$_4$ percentage less that 15%

    (2) Age 6 to 12 years: CD$_4$ count < 200/μL or CD$_4$ percentage less that 15%

    vi. All children treated for PCP should receive prophylaxis.

Table 7.2b   Recommendations for PCP Prophylaxis and CD_4 Monitoring for HIV-Exposed Infants and HIV-Infected Children, by Age and HIV-Infection Status

Age/HIV Infection Status	PCP Prophylaxis	CD_4 Monitoring
Birth to 4–6 weeks, HIV exposed	No prophylaxis	1 month
4–6 weeks to 4 months, HIV exposed	Prophylaxis	3 months
4–12 months HIV infected or indeterminate HIV infection reasonably excluded*	Prophylaxis No prophylaxis	6, 9, and 12 months None
1–5 years, HIV infected	Prophylaxis if: CD_4 count is < 500 cells/μL or CD_4 percentage is < 15%[§‡]	Every 3–4 months[†]
6–12 years, HIV infected	Prophylaxis if: CD_4 count is < 200 cells/μl or CD_4 percentage is < 5%[‡]	Every 3–4 months[†]

* HIV infection can be reasonably excluded among children who have had two or more negative HIV diagnostic tests (i.e., HIV culture or PCR), both of which are performed at = 1 month of age and one of which is performed at = 4 months of age, or two or more negative HIV IgG antibody tests performed at > 6 months of age among children who have no clinical evidence of HIV disease.

† More frequent monitoring (e.g., monthly) is recommended for children whose CD_4 counts or percentages are approaching the threshold at which prophylaxis is recommended.

§ Children 1–2 years of age who were receiving PCP prophylaxis and who had a CD_4 count of < 750 cells/μl or percentage of < 15% at < 12 months of age should continue prophylaxis.

‡ Prophylaxis should be considered on a case-by-case basis for children who might otherwise be at risk for PCP, such as children with rapidly declining CD_4 counts or percentages or children with Category C conditions (16). Children who have had PCP should receive lifelong prophylaxis.

SOURCE: Centers for Disease Control and Prevention (1995)

vii. Tables 7.2b and 7.2c present PCP prophylaxis recommendations and regimens for infants and children.

4. Counseling and educating the family and child
   a. Every health care encounter represents an opportunity for ongoing disease counseling and education. The often overwhelming and complex nature of the information requires frequent assessment of the patient and family's understanding. The clinician may need to reinforce previously discussed information on an ongoing or episodic basis.
   b. Comprehensive HIV education, including relaying information about modes of transmission, the effect of HIV on the immune system and other body systems, and issues of confidentiality and disclosure, is a process that continues over the course of the disease. Information should be tailored to the readiness and developmental level of the learners as well as their emotional and psychosocial support needs.
   c. Families and children, as appropriate, should be educated regarding the guidelines for ARV treatment in children with HIV infection as well as available clinical trial opportunities.
   d. The frequency and complexity of HIV care visits often result in difficulty or reluctance on the part of families to continue seeing a primary care provider. The need for a primary care provider and discussions about how the primary care provider and the HIV specialist will

Table 7.2c   Drug Regimens for PCP Prophylaxis for Children = 4 Weeks of Age

---

Recommended Regimen

Trimethoprim/sulfamethoxazole (TMP-SMX) 150 mg TMP/m^2/day with 750 mg SMX/m^2/day administered orally in divided doses twice a day 3 times per week on consecutive days (e.g., Monday-Tuesday-Wednesday).

Acceptable Alternative TMP-SMX Dosage Schedules

* 150 mg TMP/m^2 day with 750 mg SMX/m^2/day administered orally as a single daily dose 3 times per week on consecutive days (e.g., Monday-Tuesday-Wednesday)
* 150 mg TMP/m^2/day with 750 mg SMX/m^2/day orally divided BID and administered 7 days per week
* 150 mg TMP/m^2/day with 750 mg SMX/m^2/day administered orally divided BID and administered 3 times per week on alternate days (e.g., Monday-Wednesday-Friday)

Alternative Regimens If TMP-SMX Is Not Tolerated

* Dapsone[§] 2 mg/kg (not to exceed 100 mg) administered orally once daily
* Aerosolized pentamidine[§] (children = 5 years of age) 300 mg administered via Respigard II inhaler monthly

---

[§] If neither dapsone nor aerosolized pentamidine is tolerated, some clinicians use intravenous pentamidine (4 mg/kg) administered every 2 or 4 weeks.

SOURCE: Centers for Disease Control and Prevention (1995)

collaborate are essential components of patient education. Families should be told which provider they should call for various types of problems that may arise.

e. The role of a balanced diet and adequate nutrient intake should be reiterated with patients and families at each visit.

5. First and subsequent health care follow-up visits: Follow-up visits, though comprehensive, are generally symptom or issue driven. The main goals include assessing the infant, child, and family for new or potential issues related to HIV infection, its symptoms or treatment, and new or ongoing educational needs.

a. Review of previous visit and available diagnostic results: The follow-up visit affords an opportunity to revisit issues raised at the previous encounter and to reinforce issues or information of importance, such as prophylactic and nutritional needs, care of the child with HIV infection, immunization recommendations, and so on.

b. Review of systems: A comprehensive review of systems is an essential component of every visit. Particular attention should be paid to systems where previous or ongoing problems have been reported.

c. Physical examination: A comprehensive physical examination is essential to identify emerging health issues and provide reassurance to patients and families when normal findings are identified.

d. Nutrition assessment: Dietary habits, height, weight, and growth percentiles are evaluated at each visit to allow for early identification of potential nutritional or growth problems.

e. Laboratory and diagnostic evaluation: Subsequent to the initial HIV health care visit, laboratory and diagnostic testing may be driven by accepted monitoring guidelines, symptomatology, history of exposure to certain infectious processes, or for the purposes of monitoring for toxicities of anti-HIV medications and prophylactic regimens.

f. Immunologic profiles: CD$_4$ cell counts and percentages are routinely monitored every 3 months or more frequently if significant changes in values are noted.

g. HIV RNA PCR testing (viral load): Viral load monitoring is routinely performed every 3 months. More frequent testing is indicated when initiating therapy to identify a response to treatment, when viral load values are noted to be increasing, or if adherence problems are suspected.

h. CBC with differential is performed every 3 months or more often as indicated.

i. Multichannel chemistry panel should be performed every 3 months or more often as indicated.

j. Other diagnostics may be performed as indicated based on the need for follow-up of prior visit findings or for newly identified problems.

6. Interventions
   a. Follow-up of initiation of antiretroviral therapy: If antiretroviral therapy has been initiated, assessment of adherence, administration issues, and dosing is a key component of each follow-up visit.
   b. Nutrition intervention: Nutrition education, recommendation of dietary changes or nutritional supplementation, and follow-up may be necessary components of each follow-up visit depending on the growth parameters and nutritional well-being of the infant or child.
   c. Counseling and education: Each health care visit should be seen as an opportunity to enhance the patient or family's knowledge of HIV infection, the patient's disease status, HIV treatment, and issues related to living with HIV infection.

7.3 Managing Antiretroviral Therapy in HIV-Infected Infants and Children

1. Antiretroviral (ARV) therapy
   a. Only some of the ARVs approved for adults are available to children.
      i. Some do not have FDA approval because of lack of clinical trials in children.
      ii. Some pose a particular risk of adverse effects in children.
      iii. Other ARVs are not available in a formulation appropriate for young children (e.g., liquid or tablet that can be crushed).
      iv. Table 7.3a presents antiretroviral medications and their associated drug classification currently approved for children and infants.

2. Prescribing guidelines
   a. Goals of therapy
      i. Principals of general infectious disease treatment should be applied to pediatric HIV disease.
         (1) Early diagnosis and treatment optimizes outcome.
         (2) Changes in the quantity of the infectious agent measures the effectiveness of antimicrobial therapy.
         (3) The goal of therapy is to eradicate the infectious agent or achieve a sustained decrease in replication.
         (4) Combination antimicrobial therapy should be used because single-drug therapy leads to drug resistance.
         (5) Combination antimicrobial therapy should use drugs with different sites or mechanisms of action and nonoverlapping toxicities.
         (6) If eradication of the infectious agent is not possible, therapy should be changed if the patient shows clinical or laboratory progression.
         (7) For a fatal infection, aggressive treatment and greater tolerance for adverse drug side effects are acceptable risks.
         (8) The goal of ARV therapy is to reduce viral load to undetectable levels with therapeutic regimens that support adherence to medications.
         (9) ARV therapy is most likely to be effective in children naive to treatment who are less likely to have resistant strains of the virus.

Table 7.3a   Antiretroviral Drugs in Children

Nucleoside Reverse Transcriptase Inhibitor (NRTI)

Drug	Pediatric Labeling	Liquid Formulation	Neonate/Infant Dose
Zidovudine (ZDV)	Yes	Yes	Yes
Didanosine (ddI)	Yes	Yes	Yes
Zalcitabine (ddC)	No	No	No
Stavudine (d4T)	Yes	Yes	In trial
Lamivudine (3TC)	Yes	Yes	Yes
Abacavir (ABC)	Yes	Yes	Over 3 months, Yes
Tenofovir	No	No	No

Nonnucleoside Reverse Transcriptase Inhibitor (NNRTI)

Drug	Pediatric Labeling	Liquid Formulation	Neonate/Infant Dose
Nevirapine (NVP)	Yes	Yes	In trial
Delavirdine (DLV)	No	No	No
Efavirenz (EFV)	Yes	No	No

Protease Inhibitor (PI)

Drug[+]	Pediatric Labeling	Liquid Formulation	Neonate/Infant Dose
Saquinavir (SQV)	No	No	No
Ritonavir (RTV)	Yes*	Yes	In trial
Indinavir (IDV)	No	No	No
Nelfinavir (NFV)	Yes*	Yes	In trial
Amprenavir (APV)	Yes**	Yes	Age >4 years**
Lopinavir (LPV/RTV)	No	No	No

+ Data on combination PI in pediatrics not available at this time

* Although used in younger children, not labeled for < 2-year-olds

** Approved for children > 4 years of age

SOURCE: Working Group on Antiretroviral Therapy and Medical Management of HIV-Infected Children (2001)

(10) Parents and children must be active participants in the decision making (Working Group on Antiretroviral Therapy and Medical Management of HIV-Infected Children, 2001).

b. Risks and benefits of therapy
   i. Lack of adherence and subtherapeutic levels of ARV may enhance the development of resistance.
   ii. Growth failure and central nervous system (CNS) disease may need specific ARV targeting.
   iii. Children who receive combination therapy have decreased mortality (Gortmaker et al., 2001).
   iv. Children who are treated before they reach Category C have slower disease progression (European Collaborative Study, 2001).
   v. Early aggressive treatment allows for preservation of immune function and minimizes the risk of ARV resistance (Palumbo, 2000).
   vi. Failure of a drug regimen, however, may limit the ARV options available for treatment because of cross-resistance within classes of drugs.

c. Readiness to start treatment
   i. A careful assessment of family readiness to start treatment in an infant or child with HIV infection is essential.

ii. A range of considerations from palatability to scheduling to family understanding of illness must be weighed before treatment is begun.

iii. The clinician and the family must work together as a team to ensure that the regimen chosen is appropriate for the child and the family.

3. Initiating therapy in infants and children: A working group of clinicians, researchers, and family representatives developed guidelines for antiretroviral management of children with HIV infection (Working Group on Antiretroviral Therapy and Management of Children with HIV Infection, 1998). Those guidelines are updated regularly by the group and are available online at the HIV/AIDS Treatment Information Service Web site (http://www.aidsinfo.nih.gov/guidelines).

a. ARV therapy is recommended for all children with HIV infection who show the following:

- Clinical symptoms of HIV infection (Clinical Category A, B, or C) or
- Evidence of immune suppression (Immune Category 2 or 3) or
- HIV RNA levels of > 100,000 copies/ml regardless of clinical or immune status because of high risk for mortality

b. Most pediatric HIV experts would start ARV in all HIV-infected infants < 12 months of age as soon as the diagnosis is confirmed, regardless of clinical or immune status or viral load.

c. Many pediatric HIV experts would start ARV as early as possible in all HIV-infected children regardless of age, symptoms, or immunologic or virologic status before the child experiences immune deterioration.

d. When considering initiating ARV therapy in asymptomatic children > 1 year of age, some pediatric HIV experts would start therapy in children who have the following:

- Normal immune status but rapidly falling CD_4 counts or percentage

- High or increasing viral loads
- Developing clinical symptoms

4. Recommendations for initial therapy: Four categories of recommendations for a particular antiretroviral drug or drug combination are outlined in Table 7.3b.

5. Changing antiretroviral therapy

a. Failure of ARV therapy may be based on the following:

- Clinical, immunologic, or virologic parameters
- Toxicity or intolerance of the current therapy
- New data demonstrating that another regimen is superior to the current regimen

b. Clinical failure is demonstrated by evidence of one of the following:

- Progressive neurodevelopment deterioration should be a strong consideration in evaluating clinical ARV failure.
- Growth failure despite adequate nutritional support and with no other explanation may be evidence of ARV failure.
- Disease progression as evidenced by symptoms or conditions that leads to the advancement to another clinical category

6. Immunologic failure is present when the following occurs:

- Laboratory findings lead to a change in immune classification.
- For children with CD_4 cell percentage of < 15%, the percentage shows a persistent decline of 5 percentiles or more (e.g., 15% to 10%).
- The child has evidence of a rapid and extensive decrease in absolute CD_4 cell count.

7. Virologic failure is suspected when the following occurs:

- Less than a minimally acceptable HIV RNA response after 8 to 12 weeks

  – With a triple combination of ARV < 10 fold (1.0 log) decrease from baseline

Table 7.3b   Recommended Antiretroviral Regimens for Initial Therapy for HIV Infection in Children

Strongly Recommended

Clinical trial evidence of clinical benefit and/or sustained suppression of HIV replication in adults and/or children.

- One highly active protease inhibitor (nelfinavir or ritonavir) plus two nucleoside analogue reverse transcriptase inhibitors.
  - Recommended dual NRTI combinations: The most data on use in children are available for the combinations of ZDV and ddI, ZDV and 3TC, and d4T and ddI. More limited data are available for the combinations of d4T and 3TC and ZDV and ddC.*
- For children who can swallow capsules: the nonnucleoside reverse transcriptase inhibitor (NNRTI) efavirenz** plus two NRTIs , or efavirenz plus nelfinavir and one NRTI

Recommended As an Alternative

Clinical trial evidence of suppression of HIV replication, but (1) durability may be less in adults and/or children than with strongly recommended regimens or may not yet be defined; or (2) evidence of efficacy may not outweigh potential adverse consequences (i.e., toxicity, drug interactions, cost); (3) experience in infants and children is limited.

- NVP and two NRTIs
- ABC in combination with ZDV and 3TC
- Lopinavir/ritonavir with two NRTIs or one NRTI and NNRTI[†]
- IDV or SQV soft-gel capsule with two NRTIs for children who can swallow capsules

Offered Only in Special Circumstances

Clinical trial evidence of either (1) virologic suppression that is less durable than for the Strongly Recommended or Alternative regimes; or (2) data are preliminary or inconclusive for use as initial therapy but may be reasonably offered in special circumstances.

- Two NRTIs
- APV in combination with two NRTIs or ABC

Not Recommended

Evidence against use because (1) overlapping toxicity may occur and/or (2) use may be virologically undesirable

- Any monotherapy[‡]
- d4T and ZDV
- ddC* and ddI
- ddC* and d4T
- ddC* and 3TC

---

* ddC is not available commercially in a liquid preparation, although a liquid formulation is available through a compassionate use program of the manufacturer (Hoffman-La Roche Inc., Nutley, New Jersey, http://www.rocheusa.com). ZDV and ddC is a less-preferred choice for use in combination with a PI.

** EFV is currently available only in capsule form, although a liquid formulation is available through an expanded access program of the manufacturer (Bristol-Myers Squibb Company, http://www.bms.com). There are currently no data on appropriate dosage of EFV in children under age 3 years.

† The data presented to the Food and Drug Administration for review during the drug approval process provided significant data on the pharmacokinetics and safety in children receiving lopinavir/ritonavir (Kaletra) for 24 weeks. The combination of lopinavir/ritonavir with either two NRTIs or one NRTI and an NNRTI may be moved up to the *Strongly Recommended* category as experience with this drug is gained by U. S. investigators.

‡ Except for ZDV chemoprophylaxis administered to HIV-exposed infants during the first 6 weeks of life to prevent perinatal HIV transmission; if an infant is confirmed as HIV infected while receiving ZDV prophylaxis, therapy should be changed to a combination antiretroviral drug regimen.

SOURCE: Working Group on Antiretroviral Therapy and Medical Management of HIV-Infected Children (2001)

– With dual ARV therapy < 5 fold (0.7 log) decrease from baseline
- Lack of suppression of HIV RNA levels to undetectable by 4 to 6 months
  – However, such suppression is not always achievable in children.
  – Baseline HIV RNA level and the level achieved should be considered when contemplating potential change.
- Repeated detection of HIV RNA in children who initially had undetectable levels in response to ARV
  – Consider more frequent evaluation of HIV RNA.
  – Assess adherence and renew efforts at family education.
- Persistent rise in HIV RNA levels in a child who has had a significant and sustained decrease

8. When changing therapy due to toxicity/intolerance:

- Choose drugs with a different toxicity profile
- Change a single drug or, in certain circumstances, reduce the dose within the therapeutic range

9. Other considerations in changing therapy
   a. Assess adherence as a potential cause of failures.
   b. If the patient is adherent, document the development of drug resistance and change at least two ARVs in the new regimen.
   c. Review all other medications for possible drug interactions with the new regimen.
   d. When changing therapy because of disease progression, consider quality of life issues.

10. The use of ARV drug resistance testing in children
    a. The value of phenotypic or genotypic assays in guiding treatment choices has not been established in children.
    b. HIV-resistance assays may prove useful in guiding initial therapy and in changing failing regimens.
    c. Specific recommendations are not currently available for use of resistance assays in directing ARV choices in children.
    d. Resistance testing should be done while the child is on ARV therapy.
    e. The presence of viral resistance to a particular drug suggests that the drug is unlikely to suppress viral replication, but absence of resistance to a drug does not ensure it will be successful.

11. Special considerations in pediatric antiretroviral therapy
    a. Pharmacokinetic issues
       i. Age-related differences between children and adults in body composition, renal excretion, and liver metabolism affect pharmacokinetics.
       ii. These lead to potential differences in drug distribution, metabolism, and clearance.
       iii. These age-related differences may also affect drug dosing and drug toxicities.
    b. Diagnostic issues
       i. Perinatally acquired HIV disease in infants is primary HIV infection.
       ii. Early diagnosis of infants gives the opportunity for starting ARV therapy during primary/early infection.
    c. Natural history differences
       i. CD_4 T-cell counts in healthy infants are much higher than in adults and slowly decline to adult levels by age 6 years.
       ii. CD_4 percentage may be a better marker for HIV disease progression.
       iii. Age-adjusted CD_4 counts should be used for ARV decisions.

7.4 Adherence to Medical Regimens

1. Unique pediatric/family adherence issues
   a. Not all medications are available in palatable liquid formulations.
   b. Children may refuse strong, unusual tasting or textured medications.
   c. Infants and young children eat more frequently, making it difficult to coordinate medications with or without food.

d. Children are dependent on caregivers for their medications.

e. Secrecy may limit when, where, and who gives the child medications.

2. Psychological issues of adherence

a. HIV infection in children is a family and often multigenerational disease.

   i. A perinatally infected child and mother may both be on antiretroviral therapy.

   ii. A parent may lack parenting skills or be too ill to manage a complex medication regimen.

   iii. Poverty, substance use, denial, secrecy, depression, and mental illness may contribute to an unstable or chaotic home environment, which makes adherence difficult (Gross, Burr, Lewis, Storm, & Boland, 1999).

   iv. Children and adolescents with HIV are often cared for by elderly grandparents struggling with their own chronic illnesses.

3. Developmental issues

a. Giving long-term medications to a toddler is difficult and stressful. A child may refuse or vomit unpalatable medications.

b. Many children are given responsibility beyond their years for their medications (Gross et al., 1999).

c. Adolescents face specific developmental issues.

   i. Adolescents think in concrete terms; when they are asymptomatic, taking medications, particularly if there are side effects, is a problem for them.

   ii. Perinatally infected adolescents are adolescents—they want to be independent and like their peers. A previously compliant child may use medications to rebel when becoming a teenager (Muscari, 1998).

d. Adolescents also have social issues related to adherence.

   i. Adolescents may have unstructured, chaotic lifestyles, which may include homelessness, lack of access to proper nutrition and refrigeration, and lack of family and social support (Martinez et al., 2000).

4. Readiness before prescribing antiretroviral therapy

a. The family needs to be involved in and agree with the treatment plan. Assess family beliefs about medications and treatment, their cultural context, family decision making, (the person bringing the child to visits may not be the decision maker), lifestyle, priorities, and success or problems with past medications (Moloney, Damon, & Regan, 1998). Develop strategies that address past problems. Home visits may help to involve important family members in the plan.

b. Educate the family about HIV, the purpose of antiretroviral therapy, and the importance of adherence. Use multiple strategies, including peer groups, videos, and home visits. Be prepared to repeat information.

c. For youth, a realistic assessment of the support systems they will need to manage adherence must be built into treatment plans.

5. Beginning antiretroviral therapy

a. Prepare the family for problems and common side effects, such as nausea, vomiting, or diarrhea. Many families stop treatment when faced with unexpected side effects. Tell them the plan to help manage these and what to call about, and who, where, and when to call.

b. Prepare the family for the taste or texture of liquid or powder medications. Plan strategies to mask the taste, such as chewing on ice or a flavored ice pop before and after taking the medicine to deaden taste buds or mixing with a small amount of pudding (see additional strategies at www.fxbcenter.org/medicine/medtips.html). Crush pills and use gel caps if the child can swallow pills. Note that crushing should not be done with enteric-coated or time-release pills.

c. Teach pill swallowing. Children as young as 4 years can learn.

d. Develop as simple a schedule as possible that fits the child's and family's life. Taking medicine once a day is ideal; BID is better than TID, especially for children who attend school. Review all medications with the family and discontinue unnecessary ones. Plan for home delivery or mail delivery of medications if available and the family agrees.

e. Employ anticipatory problem solving (e.g., what to do if the child vomits the medication or has diarrhea, if a dose is three hours late, if a trip away from home or weekends change routine).

f. Color-code bottles and syringes to match a written schedule. Use pictures of pills or bottles and a clock, especially for families with low literacy. Plan a trial run for a week (include the weekend) using dummy pills or liquids and a real schedule. Don't use candy for placebos because kids will take candy, and it gives kids the wrong message. If possible, start the first dose under supervision.

g. Be accessible and follow-up with a phone call, a home visit, or both, in the first few days (Reddington et al., 2000). Many problems with medication adherence occur in the first few days of administration.

h. Prepare the family for developmental and behavioral issues, especially for young children. Prevention is always better than trying to fix a difficult situation. Preschool and early school-age children do much better if medication taking is consistent and becomes a ritual. If a child is given responsibility beyond their years for medications, provide supports such as a home health aid, school nurse, or other family member for supervision so that the child can take medications safely. Consult a behavioral psychologist for behavior problems. For very difficult situations in toddlers and young children, a gastrostomy tube may be an option. (Shingadia et al., 2000). Teach the parent/caregiver that a child needs supervision in taking medication, even school-age children who can participate in managing their medications.

6. Assessing family adherence

a. Assessment of adherence should be part of every clinic and home visit. The goals should be to identify problems, provide support, and help the family problem solve so that they can become self-sufficient. Give permission for honesty. Perfect adherence is very difficult for anyone. Families feel guilty if they have missed doses. Further, families who have a history with the child welfare system may fear losing their child if they admit to missing medication doses.

i. Do not assume a family understands their child's medication or regimen. Ask for name, dose, time, and reason for each medication. A small adherence assessment study found that caregivers who could not describe their child's medication regimen were unlikely to be adherent (Katko, Johnson, Fowler, & Turner, 2001).

ii. Display posters of medications and use these in assessment.

iii. Ask specific but open-ended questions such as "Tell me how you are giving the bedtime doses." Asking about problems that led to missed doses may be more successful that simply asking how many doses were missed (Farley, 2002; see www.hivfiles.org for more information).

iv. Home visits, if planned around medication time, are a useful tool in assessing family adherence. Families are more relaxed in their own environment and are able to discuss problems and identify possible solutions.

v. Review medications brought to appointments. Have the caregiver draw up liquid medications when there is possible confusion about the dose.

vi. Methods to assess adherence include self-report and direct observation; prescription refills, pill counts, and bottle checks; electronic pill bottle caps; diaries; and calendars. Each method has limitations when used alone. Viral load may be a good indicator of poor adherence; however, other factors may contribute to treatment failure, such as poor or altered absorption, resistance, concomitant viral or bacterial infections, strain of the virus, and immune functioning.

7. Strategies to support adherence
   a. Use group teaching and family/peer support. Many families are happy to share what works for them and their children.
   b. Use home visits and agencies such as visiting nurses to support adherence (Reynolds, Berrien, Acosta-Glynn, & Salazar, 2001).
   c. Show families how medications are working. A simple chart of falling viral loads and rising CD_4 counts is positive reinforcement.
   d. Involve children in their medications by making calendars, marking syringes, filling pillboxes, and devising reminder strategies.
   e. Use positive reinforcement and realistic incentives/rewards, such as stickers, a favorite meal, a trip to the park, and staying up late to watch TV. Rewards do not have to cost money.
   f. Use contracts with families, school-age children, and adolescents.
   g. Support disclosure to children and to selected family and friends.
      i. Secrecy makes adherence difficult; medications cannot be stored openly or taken in front of others. Disclosure to a family member or friend may provide backup for giving medications to a child and support adherence (Byrne, Honig, Jurgrau, Heffernan, & Donahue, 2002).
      ii. Disclosing to the uncooperative child who can't understand why he or she has to take medicines may help adherence.
      iii. Disclosure to a school nurse may provide a way to give a midday medication. However, most parents are very reluctant to disclose to their child's school

because they fear the child will be treated badly.
   h. Build a trusting relationship and be available and accessible to families (Farley, 2001).
   i. Other supports include visiting nurses, home health aides, substance abuse treatment and mental health services, child life specialists, social workers, and daycare or after-school programs. Pharmacists can be a key resource; they can review medication profiles, discuss potential interactions, serve as a source of information for the family, reinforce instructions, and instruct in masking the taste of unpalatable medications.

References

Abrams, E. (2000). Opportunistic infections and other clinical manifestations of HIV disease in children. *Pediatric Clinics of North America, 47*, 79–108.

Byrne, M., Honig, J., Jurgrau, A., Heffernan, S. M., & Donahue, M. C. (2002). *AIDS Read 12*(4), 151–164.

Centers for Disease Control and Prevention. (1994). Revised classification system for human immunodeficiency virus infection in children less than 13 years of age. *Morbidity and Mortality Weekly Review, 43*, RR-49.

Centers for Disease Control and Prevention. (1995). 1995 revised guidelines for prophylaxis against *Pneumocystis carinii* pneumonia for children infected with or perinatally exposed to human immunodeficiency virus. *Morbidity and Mortality Weekly Review, 44* (R-4), 1–11.

Centers for Disease Control and Prevention. (2001). Prevention and control of influenza: Recommendations of the Advisory Committee on Immunization Practices (ACIP). *MMWR;50*, RR-4.

Connor, E., Sperling, R., Gelber, R., Kiselev, P, Scott, G., O' Sullivan, M., et al. (1994). Reduction of maternal-infant transmission of human immunodeficiency virus type 1 with zidovudine treatment. *New England Journal of Medicine, 33*, 1173–1180.

European Collaborative Study. (2001). Fluctuation in symptoms for human immunodeficiency virus-infected children: The first 10 years of life. *Pediatrics, 108*,116–122.

Farley, J. (2002). *Adherence to HIV therapy in preadolescent children: Where do we go from here?* Retrieved November 18, 2002, from http://www.hivfiles.org/topic2.html

Fowler, M. G., Simonds, R. J., & Roongpisuthipong, A. (2000). Update on perinatal HIV transmission. *Pediatric Clinics of North America, 47*, 21–38.

Gortmaker, S. L., Hugh, M., Cervia, J., Brady, M., Johnson, J. M., Seage, G., et al. (2001). Effect of combination therapy including protease inhibitors on mortality among children and adolescents infected with HIV-1. *New England Journal of Medicine, 345*, 1522–1528.

Gross, E., Burr, C., Lewis, S., Storm, D., & Boland, M. (1999). Medication adherence in pediatric HIV: A provider survey of difficulties and strategies [Abstract]. In *Proceedings of the Association of Nurses in AIDS Care Conference*, 196.

Grubman, S., & Oleske, J. M. (1995). HIV in infants, children, and adolescents. In G. Wormser (Ed.), *A clinical guide to AIDS and HIV*. New York: Raven Press.

Guay, L. A., Musoka, P., & Fleming, T., Bagenda, D., Allen, M., Nakabiito, C., et al. (1999). Intrapartum and neonatal single-dose nevirapine compared with zidovudine for prevention of mother-to-child transmission of HIV-1 in Kampala, Uganda: HIVNET 012 randomized trial. *Lancet, 354*, 795–802.

Katko, E., Johnson, G. M., Fowler, S. L., & Turner, R. B. (2001). Assessment of adherence with medications in human immunodeficiency virus-infected children. *Pediatric Infectious Disease Journal, 20*, 1174–1176.

Laufer, M., & Scott, G. (2000). Medical management of HIV disease in children. *Pediatric Clinics of North America, 47*, 127–154.

Lindegren, M. L., Steinberg, S., & Byers, R. H. (2000). Epidemiology of HIV/AIDS in children. *Pediatric Clinics of North America, 47*, 1–21.

Martinez, J., Bell, D., Camacho, R, Henry-Reid, L. M., Bell, M., Watson, C., et al. (2000). Adherence to antiretroviral drug regimens in HIV-infected adolescent patients engaged in care in a comprehensive adolescent and young adult clinic. *Journal of the National Medical Association, 92*, 55–61.

Mbori-Ngacha, D., Nduti, R., John, G., Reilly, M., Richardson, B., Mwatha, A., et al. (2001). Morbidity and mortality in breastfed and formula-fed infants of HIV-1-infected women: A randomized clinical trial. *Journal of the American Medical Association, 286*, 2413–2420.

Miotti, P. G., Taha, T. E., Kumwenda, N. I. Broadhead, R., Mtimavalye, L., Van der Hoeven, L. et al. (1999). HIV transmission from breastfeeding: A study from Malawi. *Journal of the American Medical Association, 282*, 744–749.

Moloney, C., Damon, B., & Regan, A. M. (1998). Pediatric compliance in combination HIV therapy: Getting it right the first time. *Advance for Nurse Practitioners, 6*, 35–38.

Muscari M. E. (1998). Rebels with a cause: When adolescents won't follow medical advice. *American Journal of Nursing, 98*(12), 26–31.

National Pediatric and Family HIV Resource Center. (2002). *HIV and pregnancy: Managing mother and baby—A curriculum for providers*. Newark, NJ: The National Pediatric & Family HIV Resource Center.

Nduati, R. W., John, G. L., Mbori-Ngacha, D., Richardson, B., Overbaugh J., Mwatha, A., et al. (2000.) Effect of breastfeeding and formula feeding on transmission of HIV-1: A randomized clinical trial of breast feeding and formula feeding. *Journal of the American Medical Association, 283*, 1175–1182.

Nielsen K., & Bryson, Y. J. (2000) Diagnosis of HIV infection in children. *Pediatric Clinics of North America, 47*, 39–64.

Palumbo, P. (2000). Antiretroviral therapy of HIV infection in children. *Pediatric Clinics of North America, 47*, 155–170.

Reddington, C., Cohen, J., Baldillo, A., Toye, M., Smith, D., Kneut, C., et al. (2000). *Pediatric Infectious Disease Journal, 19*, 1148–1153.

Reynolds, E., Berrien, V., Acosta-Glynn, C., & Salazar, J. (2001). *Home based, intense, nursing intervention trial improves adherence to HAART in HIV-infected children*. Paper presented at the Academic Societies Meeting, Baltimore, MD.

Saba, J. (1999, January). *Interim analysis of early efficacy of three short ZDV/3TC combination regimens to prevent mother-to-child transmission of HIV-1: The PETRA trial*. Paper presented at the Sixth Conference on Retroviruses and Opportunistic Infections, Chicago, IL.

Shaffer, N., Chuachoowong, R., Mock, P. A., Bhadrakom, C., Siriwasin, W., Young, N., et al. (1999). Short-course zidovudine for perinatal HIV-1 transmission in Bangkok, Thailand: A randomized controlled trial. *Lancet, 535*, 773–780.

Shingadia, D., Viani, R., Yogev, R., Binns, H., Dankner, W., Spector, S. A., et al. (2000). Gastrostomy tube insertion for improvement of adherence to highly active antiretroviral therapy in pediatric patients with human immunodeficiency virus [Electronic version]. *Pediatrics, 105*, 80–84.

U. S. Public Health Service and Infectious Diseases Society of America & USPHS/ISDA Prevention of Opportunistic Infections Working Group. (2001). *July 2001 draft, 2001 USPHS/ISDA guidelines for the prevention of opportunistic infections in persons infected with human immunodeficiency virus*. Retrieved March 3, 2003, from http://www.hivatis.org/guidelines/other/Ois/OIGNov27.pdf

U. S. Public Health Service Task Force. (2002). *Recommendations for use of antiretroviral drugs in pregnant HIV-1 infected women for maternal health and interventions to reduce perinatal HIV-1 transmission in the United States*. Retrieved March, 3, 2003, from http://www.hivatis.org/guidelines/perinatal/Feb4_02/Perin.pdf

Wade, N. A., Birkhead, G. S., Warren, B. L., Charbonneau T.T., French, P.T., Wang, L., et al. (1998). Abbreviated regimens of zidovudine prophylaxis and perinatal transmission of human immunodeficiency virus. *New England Journal of Medicine, 339*, 1409–1414.

Working Group on Antiretroviral Therapy and Management of Children with HIV Infection. (1998). Antiretroviral therapy and medical management of pediatric HIV infection. *Pediatrics, 102*(Suppl.), 1005–1085.

Working Group on Antiretroviral Therapy and Medical Management of HIV–Infected Children. (2001). *Guidelines for the use of antiretroviral agents in pediatric HIV infection*. Retrieved March, 3, 2003, from http://www.hivatis.org/guidelinesPediatric/Dec12_01/peddec.pdf

Section VIII

Symptomatic Conditions in Infants and Children With Advancing Disease

Thidis section provides comprehensive information about the common conditions experienced by children with HIV/AIDS. Because the disease manifests differently in children than in adults, an entire section is dedicated to the 1994 Pediatric Classification System clinical categories. This expanded emphasis on pediatric infection is necessary as ANAC expands its international efforts and acknowledges that certain areas of the world have not experienced the substantial decline in pediatric infection that the United States has experienced.

Each section discusses the pathophysiology, clinical presentation, diagnostic work-up, and treatments for a particular disorder. Each section concludes with the most important nursing implications. Nurses should use these implications as a guide to tailor their interventions to the specific setting, populations, and scope of practice.

A. SYMPTOMATIC CONDITIONS IN HIV DISEASE

8.1 Anemia

1. Etiology/Epidemiology
   a. Hematologic manifestations may be caused by peripheral destruction of blood elements, adverse effects of medication, HIV replication, poor nutrition, and bone marrow changes related to chronic illness.
   b. Severe thrombocytopenia and anemia are sometimes associated with advanced disease and poor prognosis. Presentations including anemia, neutropenia, lymphopenia, thrombocytopenia, and eosinophilia are common in children with HIV infection.
2. Pathogenesis
   a. Bone marrow damage due to certain cancers, opportunistic infections, or myelosuppressive agents, such as zidovudine, ganciclovir, ribavirin, and vinblastine (Bain, 1999; Coyle, 1997; Levine, 1999), causes decreased erythropoiesis.
   b. Chronic disease is associated with anemia, which is characterized by decreased production of erythropoietin, erythropoietin resistance, abnormalities of iron metabolism, decreased erythrocyte life span, and an increased expression of inflammatory cytokines, which may interfere with erythropoietin production (Abramson, Steinhart, & Frascino, 2000; Bain, 1999; Coyle, 1997).
   c. Iron deficiency anemia results from chronic blood loss or a dietary deficiency (Coyle, 1997; Kreuzer & Rockstroh, 1997; Levine, 1999).
   d. Parvovirus B19 can result in aplastic anemia in immune-compromised patients (Sabella & Goldfarb, 1999).
3. Clinical presentation
   a. Symptoms include fatigue, shortness of breath, a decrease in cognitive function, impairment of activities of daily living, exercise intolerance, amenorrhea, and pallor.
4. Diagnosis
   a. Severity is based on a graded decrease in hemoglobin: mild = 1–1.9 g/dL below normal range; moderate = 2 g/dL below normal range, but > 8.1 g/dL (mild anemia with two or more constitutional symptoms is also considered a moderate anemia); severe = < 8.0 g/dL (Ferri al., 2002).
   b. Physical signs include weight loss, hepatosplenomegaly, guaiac positive stool, mild peripheral edema, and retinal hemorrhages (Hillman, 1998).
5. Prevention/Treatment
   a. During the postneonatal period and in early infancy, children with anemia due to antiretroviral therapy (ART) seldom need cessation of treatment and often respond to erythropoietin if needed (American Academy of Pediatrics, 1998).
   b. In children with erythropoietin levels < 500 IU/L, a trial of erythropoietin at a dose of 100 U/kg/dose, 3 times/week is recommended. Dose may be increased if the response is unsatisfactory (Laufer & Scott, 2000).
6. Nursing implications
   a. Monitor lab work that is suggestive of anemia: complete blood count (CBC), red blood cell count (RBC), hemoglobin (Hbg), hematocrit (Hct), and reticulocyte count.
   b. Educate patients to recognize and report early signs of anemia, such as fatigue, shortness of breath, and amenorrhea.
   c. Provide dietary counseling and nutritional support as needed. Iron is best absorbed from meat, fish, and poultry. Orange juice doubles the absorption of iron from an entire meal, whereas tea or milk reduces absorption to less than one half.
   d. Patients receiving erythropoietin therapy should receive iron supplementation (Laufer & Scott, 2000).

8.2 Cardiomyopathy

1. Etiology/Epidemiology
   a. The cause of cardiomyopathy is not completely understood and may be related to primary HIV disease, infection, or antiretroviral (ARV) medications.
   b. Cardiomyopathy rates in children with HIV infection have been reported to be

as high as 30% among certain cohorts (Abuzaitoun & Hanson, 2000).

2. Pathogenesis
   a. The severity of cardiac disease in children with HIV infection may range from asymptomatic cardiac lesions to fatal disease with severity correlated to the degree of immune suppression (Laufer & Scott, 2000).
   b. Cardiomyopathy has been shown to have an effect on survival in children with HIV infection (Luginbuhl, Orav, McIntosh, & Lipshultz, 1993).

3. Clinical presentation
   a. Most commonly, cardiomyopathy is associated with sinus tachycardia; however, other symptoms including dysrhythmias and blood pressure abnormalities may also be present.
   b. Problems seen in children with HIV infection include cardiomegaly, congestive heart failure, nonbacterial thrombotic endocarditis, cardiac tamponade, conductive disturbances, and sudden death.

4. Diagnosis
   a. Echocardiogram is the most commonly used diagnostic tool for detection of cardiac abnormalities in children.

5. Prevention/Treatment
   a. Medications to improve cardiac output may be prescribed in collaboration with a cardiac specialist.

6. Nursing implications
   a. Patient and family education focuses on the possible cause of the abnormality and any limitations on activity that should be undertaken as well as monitoring needs, such as daily blood pressures or heart rate readings.

8.3 Dermatitis

1. Etiology/Epidemiology
   a. Dermatitis and other mucocutaneous manifestations are commonly seen in children with HIV infection.
   b. Frequency is related to the child's degree of immunosuppression.

2. Pathogenesis
   a. Most skin lesions in HIV-infected children are the result of secondary infections with viral, bacteria, or fungal organisms.
   b. Frequently seen noninfectious skin conditions include seborrheic dermatitis, atopic dermatitis, and eczema. These occur at similar rates to immune-competent patients.

3. Clinical presentation
   a. Infectious skin conditions often present as more severe forms than those seen in healthy children and may be more recalcitrant (Abuzaitoun & Hanson, 2000).

4. Diagnosis
   a. Diagnosis is commonly made by visual inspection of the area and characteristic primary and secondary skin changes.

5. Prevention/Treatment
   a. Treatment is based on etiology. See Section 9.5 for a full discussion of the prevention and treatment of skin lesions.

6. Nursing implications
   a. Nursing care is based on etiology. See Section 9.5 for a discussion of the nursing care required for selected skin lesions.

8.4 Diarrhea, Recurrent or Chronic

1. Etiology/Epidemiology
   a. Infection, noninfectious inflammatory processes, and anatomic abnormalities, as well as antiretroviral therapies, may cause diarrheal illness in HIV-infected children.
   b. In children who are severely immunocompromised, causes may include AIDS-defining illnesses, such as *Cryptosporidium,* cytomegalovirus (CMV), and mycobacterium avium complex (MAC).

2. Pathogenesis
   a. Diarrheal disease in children with HIV infection may be acute, recurrent, or persistent with persistent causes, such as infection with cryptosporidiosis, which may be more likely to cause severe dehydration and weight loss.

3. Clinical presentation
   a. Abdominal pain, distention, frequent watery bowel movements, fever,

dehydration, and weight loss may all be present in children with diarrhea.

4. Diagnosis
   a. Diagnosis is made on the basis of symptoms.
   b. More specific causes of diarrhea are diagnosed with stool collection for culture and sensitivity of suspect organisms.
   c. Ongoing diarrheal illness not caused by medications and in the absence of identified enteric pathogenesis is presumed to be caused by direct HIV infection and replication in the intestinal tract (Abuzaitoun & Hanson, 2000).

5. Prevention/Treatment
   a. Prevention of diarrheal illness includes good nutritional practices, such as a healthy diet and appropriate food preparation techniques.
   b. Immunocompromised patients should also be cautioned about the use of water supplies that may contain infectious organisms.
   c. Treatment measures for diarrheal illness include treating any identifiable underlying infectious causes with appropriate courses of antibiotic therapy.
   d. Treatment can also include bulk-forming diets, antiretroviral (ARV) medication changes or dose adjustments, and short-term use of antidiarrheal agents, such as loperamide.

6. Nursing implications
   a. Caretakers of children with HIV infection should be educated about diarrheal illness and when to report symptoms.
   b. Historical information, such as food intake and illnesses in other members of the household or among school and social contacts, should also be reported.
   c. Parents and children should be informed to anticipate some gastrointestinal symptoms with the initiation of or change in ARV medications.
   d. Antidiarrheal medication may be prescribed in advance when medication regimens are changed so that it can be taken as soon as symptoms begin.

8.5 Hepatitis

1. Etiology/Epidemiology
   a. For discussion of hepatitis A, see Section 3.40; for hepatitis B, see Section 3.41; and for hepatitis C, see Section 3.42.
   b. Successful vaccination of adults and children with HIV makes infection with hepatitis A and B rare.
   c. Hepatitis C is mainly acquired during childhood via true vertical transmission.
   d. The risk of acquiring hepatitis C is related to the presence and amount of RNA for hepatitis C virus (HCV) in mothers at the time of birth. The infection rate for the hepatitis C virus is higher in children from mothers who have tested positive for HIV.
   e. Vertical transmission of HCV is between 5 and 20% but varies according to the presence or absence of certain cofactors (particularly maternal coinfection with HIV) or medical conditions, or both (Lapointe et al., 2002).
   f. The average rate of HCV infection among infants born to women coinfected with HCV and HIV is 14% to 17%, higher than among infants born to women infected with HCV alone.

2. Pathogenesis
   a. Data are limited on the natural history of HCV infection in children. For discussion on the natural history of hepatitis C in adults see Section 3.42.

3. Clinical presentation
   a. There is the absence or paucity of signs and symptoms of this disease in children.

4. Diagnosis
   a. There are two types of tests used in HCV infection evaluation.
      i. Tests measuring serum antibodies: An enzyme-linked immunoassay (EIA) and an immunoblot assay are obtained through genetic recombination (RIBA).
      ii. A test detecting the presence of HCV nucleic acid in plasma (PCR)
   b. For the child 18 months of age or younger, the presence of maternal anti-HCV IgG antibodies in the infant's serum necessitates the use of tests that

detect plasmatic viral RNA with the polymerase chain reaction (PCR) techniques. Due to a very low sensitivity in the newborn period, PCR should be performed after 4 to 6 weeks of age.

c. In children of 18 months of age or older, these tests are diagnostic for current or past infection with HCV, with a sensitivity of 97% and a specificity of 95%. HCV-RNA testing is necessary to confirm active infection.

5. Prevention/Treatment
   a. Testing for hepatitis C virus during pregnancy will also identify infants who require subsequent testing and follow-up.
   b. Antiviral drugs for chronic hepatitis C are not FDA approved for use in children under age 18 years. Therefore, children should be referred to a pediatric hepatologist or similar specialist for management and for determination for eligibility in clinical trials.

6. Nursing implications
   a. Standard precautions should be used on all patients.
   b. Patients with HCV should be screened for hepatitis A and B.
   c. Treatment with INF/ribaviran (if indicated) is associated with many adverse reactions (e.g., injection site reactions, anemia). Educate patients about adverse effects and monitor patient frequently.
   d. Provide patient and family teaching regarding prevention of disease and disease. For discussion of hepatitis A, see Section 3.40; for hepatitis B, see Section 3.41; and for hepatitis C, see Section 3.42.

8.6 Hepatomegaly

1. Etiology/Epidemiology
   a. A common finding in children with HIV infection and can be related to HIV replication, antiretroviral agents, and viral causes such as the hepatotrophic virus
   b. Development of hepatomegaly within the first 3 months of life has been

associated with more rapid disease progression (Diaz et al., 1997).

2. Pathogenesis
   a. Varies according to the etiology

3. Clinical presentation
   a. Typically presents with other findings indicative of lymphoproliferation, such as lymphadenopathy
   b. Palpation of the liver on physical examination may be the only finding in some children.
   c. In some children, abdominal distention and pain may be significant findings.

4. Diagnosis
   a. Initial laboratory testing to determine the cause of hepatomegaly includes liver function tests (LFTs), Epstein-Barr virus (EBV) testing, and hepatitis panels.
   b. Follow-up includes serial LFT monitoring.

5. Treatment
   a. In general, no specific treatment is undertaken for otherwise asymptomatic hepatomegaly.
   b. Treatment may be specific to identified organism.

6. Nursing implications
   a. Nursing interventions primarily focus on patient and family education regarding the possible causes of hepatomegaly and the need for ongoing follow-up of laboratory studies as well as drug toxicity monitoring.

8.7 Herpes Virus

1. Etiology/Epidemiology
   a. Transmission is primarily through oral secretions.
   b. Children living in lower socioeconomic conditions are at higher risk of contracting herpes simplex virus (HSV).
   c. Up to 10% of children with HIV infection will have severe, recurrent episodes of HSV (Whitley & Whitley, 1994).

2. Pathogenesis
   a. After infection, the virus becomes latent and recurs in response to fever, menstruation, sun exposure, or trauma (Czarniecki, Rothpletz-Puglia, & Oleske, 1999).

b. Most commonly seen as herpes labialis, viremia and disseminated disease can develop in the severely immunosuppressed patient (Czarniecki et al., 1999).

3. Clinical presentation
   a. Lesions erupt as painful vesicles evolving to crusted ulcerations.
   b. Patients experience fever, mucosal ulcerations, drooling, pain or burning at lesion site, and anorexia.

4. Diagnosis
   a. The diagnosis is often made on the basis of clinical presentation.
   b. When diagnostic testing is necessary for accurate identification, the techniques to be used are described in Section 3.21.

5. Prevention/Treatment
   a. Treatment: oral, maximum 80 mg/kg/day in 3 to 5 doses; IV: 250 mg/m^2/dose q8h
   b. Secondary prophylaxis for HSV infection: oral, 80 mg/kg/day in 3 to 4 divided doses
   c. Topical (ointment): apply every 3 hours, 6 times/day

6. Nursing implications
   a. Local care of mucocutaneous lesion includes keeping lesions clean and dry by gently cleansing with mild soap and water.
   b. Teach child and parent that frequent hand washing will prevent the spread of infection to others.
   c. Pain can be severe, and analgesia should be administered as needed.

8.8 Leiomyosarcoma

1. Etiology/Epidemiology
   a. In 1994, the Centers for Disease Control and Prevention (CDC) published a revised classification of pediatric AIDS that lists primary brain lymphomas, small noncleaved cell (Burkitt's) non-Hodgkin's lymphoma, immunoblastic or large-cell lymphoma of B-cell or unknown immunologic phenotype, as well as Kaposi's sarcoma (KS) as AIDS-defining events (Category C). Leiomyosarcomas are included in Category B as a sign of a moderately symptomatic stage.
   b. The number of children with HIV infection who develop a malignancy is poorly defined.
   c. Although very rare, leiomyosarcomas are the second leading cancer of children with HIV infection.
   d. A survey conducted by the Children's Cancer Group and the National Cancer Institute identified 64 children (39 boys, 25 girls) with 65 tumors that occurred between July 1982 and February 1997. Forty-two children (65%) had NHL, 11 (17%) had leiomyosarcomas (or leiomyomas), and 3 were diagnosed with KS (Granovsky, Mueller, Nicholson, Rosenberg, & Rabkin, 1998).
   e. Because they are relatively rare in children, much of the information about leiomyosarcoma's natural history and treatment has been derived from studies of adult patients.

2. Pathogenesis
   a. Epstein Barr virus has been demonstrated by in situ hybridization and quantitative polymerase chain reaction, a finding that appears to be unique to tumors from HIV-infected or otherwise immunocompromised (i.e., posttransplant) patients.

3. Clinical presentation
   a. The clinical presentation varies according to the location of the tumor. Unusual localizations, such as spleen, pleural space, adrenal glands, and lungs, have been described, although they present most commonly in the gastrointestinal tract.

4. Diagnosis
   a. The method of diagnosis varies according to the site of tumor.

5. Prevention/Treatment
   a. Smooth muscle tumors are in general not very sensitive to chemotherapy or radiotherapy; local excision, if feasible, is the first line of therapy.
   b. The course of the disease is highly variable, with indolent tumors (more likely leiomyomas) that probably do not necessitate intervention in some children and very aggressive, disseminated tumors in other children.
   c. Intensive and prolonged chemotherapy as used in noninfected patients is rarely

tolerated by HIV-infected children (Mueller, 1999).
6. Nursing implications
   a. Provide education about the disease, specific therapies, and potential side effects and their management.
   b. Emphasize the importance of adequate rest and nutrition. In all diseased states, the body requires adequate rest and nutrition to heal.
   c. A diagnosis of cancer can be distressing to the family and child. Provide emotional support for the patient and the family and significant others.

8.9 Lymphadenopathy

1. Etiology/Epidemiology
   a. High levels of viral replication in the lymphoid tissue associated with perinatally acquired HIV infection make lymphadenopathy a common finding among children with HIV disease.
   b. Lymphadenopathy is typically a direct result of HIV replication but may also be caused by Epstein-Barr virus (EBV), cytomegalovirus (CMV), or mycobacterial infections as well as malignancies.
2. Pathogenesis
   a. Varies according to the etiology
3. Clinical presentation
   a. There are a large number of diseases with which lymphadenopathy can be present; therefore, the detection of lymphadenopathy is common.
   b. Nodes less than 0.5 cm generally are not cause for concern.
   c. If nodes have grown rapidly and are suspiciously large (2 to 3 cm), mildly painful, or fixed, they should be investigated further. Bilateral findings count as one site.
4. Diagnosis
   a. Biposy is the most definitive test to determine the etiology of enlarged lymph nodes.
5. Prevention/Treatment
   a. Meticulous physical examination to detect abnormal lymph nodes is essential.
   b. Treatment varies according to the etiology of enlarged nodes.

6. Nursing implications
   a. See specific implications according to etiology of enlarged nodes.

8.10 Lymphoid Interstitial Pneumonitis (LIP)

1. Etiology/Epidemiology
   a. LIP is considered an AIDS-defining condition, but because it is associated with a relatively benign course, favorable prognosis, and long-term survival, it has been placed in the B category of the Centers for Disease Control and Prevention's (CDC) classification system.
   b. LIP is more commonly seen in children with HIV infection than in adults.
2. Pathogenesis
   a. LIP is a chronic lymphocytic infiltrative disease of the lung, and the cause is poorly understood.
3. Clinical presentation
   a. LIP is often seen in combination with other signs of lymphoproliferation, such as parotitis and hepatomegaly.
   b. It is characterized by its insidious onset, often with persistent cough and tachypnea that over time progresses to dyspnea and hypoxia with resultant finger clubbing.
4. Diagnosis
   a. Though the diagnosis is initially made clinically, serial chest X-rays or chest CT scan, or both, showing a reticulonodular pattern or interstitial infiltrates is used to confirm the diagnosis.
   b. Though biopsy was commonly used for diagnosis in the early years of the HIV epidemic, it is rarely used today.
5. Prevention/Treatment
   a. Prevention of LIP is dependent on controlling HIV viral replication through the use of HAART.
   b. Treatment of symptomatic LIP with hypoxia includes the use of prednisone at 2mg/kg/day for 2 to 4 weeks on a tapering schedule, then continuing at 1 mg/kg/day until oxygen saturation improves. Complete weaning can be undertaken when a satisfactory response is observed.

Repeated courses of steroids may be necessary.

c. Bronchodilators, chest physical therapy, and, in some cases, diuretics may be useful.

6. Nursing implications
   a. Nursing interventions are supportive depending on the severity of the disease.
   b. Patient and family education as to the chronic and persistent nature of LIP and its associated symptoms is essential.

8.11 Nephropathy

1. Etiology/Epidemiology
   a. Prevalence in children ranges from 2 to 10% (Abuzaitoun & Hanson, 2000).
2. Pathogenesis
   a. The pathogenesis of HIV-associated nephropathy is not fully understood but may be associated with autoimmune or immune complex disease (Abuzaitoun & Hanson, 2000).
   b. HIV nephropathy is typically associated with a higher degree of immune suppression and a higher mortality rate.
3. Clinical presentation
   a. May range from an asymptomatic proteinuria to symptomatic renal tubular acidosis, hematuria, and acute renal failure (Abuzaitoun & Hanson, 2000)
4. Diagnosis
   a. In children, diagnosis is made by using the ratio of urine creatinine to protein. A creatinine-protein ratio of more than 0.2 is consistent with nephropathy.
5. Prevention/Treatment
   a. Alkalinizing agents, such as sodium or potassium citrate, in addition to other mineral supplements may be used to correct renal tubular acidosis.
   b. In severe cases, dialysis may be considered.
6. Nursing implications
   a. Dose adjustments on antiretroviral therapy (ART) and other drugs used to treat HIV associated diseases are often necessary.
   b. Nursing interventions focus on supportive care and education.

8.12 Neutropenia

1. Etiology/Epidemiology
   a. In some children, neutropenia represents manifestations of HIV disease and may improve with enhanced suppression of HIV with antiretroviral therapy (ART).
2. Pathogenesis
   a. HIV infection of accessory cells in the bone marrow inhibits production of hematopoietic growth factors (Mitsuyasu, 1999) and induces expression of cytokines that inhibit hematopoiesis (Coyle, 1997).
   b. Myelosuppression related to drugs, concomitant infections, and malignancies (Mitsuyasu, 1999)
   c. HIV-induced apoptosis of lymphocytes (Mitsuyasu, 1999)
3. Clinical presentation
   a. Respiratory tract symptoms, such as cough and sputum production
   b. Urinary tract infection symptoms: frequency, urgency, burning
   c. Fever
4. Diagnosis
   a. Complete blood count (CBC) with differential reveals decreases in white blood cells (WBCs), including neutrophils, lymphocytes, and sometimes monocytes. Atypical lymphocytes may be seen (Doweiko & Groopman, 1998).
5. Prevention/Treatment
   a. If a child is clinically stable, but there is a significant and persistent absolute neutropenia, supportive treatment with Granulocyte Colony Stimulating Factor (G-CSF) or filgastrim should be initiated before modifying ART. The dosage for children is 5–10 mcg/kg/day (IV/SC): a single daily dose for up to 14 days, then titrated to maintain ANC > 1000–2000/mm^3.
   b. If neutropenia does not improve within 1 week of initiating G-CSF, the dose can be increased.
   c. When no alternative etiology is identified and the response to G-CSF is not adequate, then interruption of ART should be considered but for a as brief a period

of time as possible (American Academy of Pediatrics, 1998).

6. Nursing implications
   a. Few HIV-infected children suffer infectious complications of neutropenia. Severe and prolonged fever is suggestive of an infectious complication; thus, teach the patient and family to report high and prolonged fevers immediately.

8.13 Nocardiosis

1. Etiology/Epidemiology
   a. Nocardiosis is primarily a pulmonary disease with systemic and cutaneous manifestations caused by the Gram-positive filamentous bacteria of the genus *Nocardia.* The species commonly pathogenic in humans include *N. asteroides, N. brasiliensis,* and *N. otitidiscaviarum,* formerly *N. caviae.*
2. Pathogenesis
   a. Infection is usually acquired via inhalation of airborne conidia from environmental sources with resultant pneumonitis.
   b. Primary cutaneous or subcutaneous nocardiosis is caused by inoculation of the bacterium as a result of trauma. Immunocompromised are more prone to dissemination from a primary cutaneous site.
3. Clinical presentation
   a. Pulmonary infection is the most common presentation of systemic disease and is frequently associated with dissemination primarily to the central nervous system, kidneys, skin, and subcutaneous tissues; however, any organ system may be involved. Symptoms include fever, cough, dyspnea, and chest pain.
   b. Skin involvement may develop as localized superficial skin infections, including pustules, abscess, cellulitis, paronychia, or granulomas. Cutaneous involvement from disseminated systemic disease is not infrequent. These lesions may remain as localized subcutaneous abscesses or provide a source for further dissemination. Lesions are typically localized to a

single area of the body; however, simultaneous involvement of more than one area has been described.
   c. Regional lymphadenopathy is frequently prominent.
   d. Some patients present with acute fever.
4. Diagnosis
   a. A chest X-ray typically demonstrates an upper lobe process with multiple abnormal findings that mimic tuberculosis.
   b. The organism may be recovered in respiratory secretions
   c. Nonpulmonary infections require the organism to be recovered by biopsy.
5. Prevention/Treatment
   a. Treatment of primary cutaneous and subcutaneous infections without dissemination consists primarily of antimicrobial therapy, although surgical debridement is sometimes required.
   b. Sulfonamides or trimethoprim/sulfamethoxazole are usually satisfactory for localized cutaneous and pulmonary infections. Amoxicillin-clavulanic acid and minocycline are suitable alternatives.
   c. In more aggressive or disseminated infections, multidrug regimens are required. Consult with an infectious disease expert.
6. Nursing implications
   a. Provide education about the disease, specific therapies, and potential side effects and their management.
   b. Emphasize the importance of completing the prescribed regimens because therapy can last 6 months or greater.

8.14 Otitis Media, Recurrent

1. Etiology/Epidemiology
   a. Common finding in children with symptomatic HIV infection
   b. Acute otitis media is much more common in the pediatric HIV-infected patient when compared with noninfected patients.
2. Pathogenesis
   a. Frequency of infections may be related to immunological deficiencies or

eustachian tube dysfunction resulting from lymphoproliferation.

b. The pathogens encountered in recurrent otitis media do not differ from the general population. *Streptococcus pneumoniae, Haemophilus influenzae,* and *Moraxella catarrhalis* predominate.

3. Clinical presentation
   a. Fever and ear pain are the most common presenting symptoms.
   b. Examination of the ear demonstrates marked redness or distinct fullness or bulging of the tympanic membrane.
   c. Hearing loss may be present.
4. Diagnosis
   a. Made on the basis of history and physical examination
5. Prevention/Treatment
   a. Treatment is dependent on suspected or cultured organism.
6. Nursing implications
   a. Families should be educated about the frequency of otitis media in children with HIV infection. Symptoms should be reported promptly, and adherence to antimicrobials is essential to minimize the change of development of resistant organisms.

8.15 Parotitis

1. Etiology/Epidemiology
   a. May occur in up to 15% of children and usually does not require any treatment (Laufer & Scott, 2000)
   b. Although it is the least reported Category A event, parotitis can be difficult to treat and may be associated with life-threatening illnesses.
2. Pathogenesis
   a. Swelling of the parotid gland is generally a benign process associated with lymphoepithelial lesions, but it may also be the result of bacterial infections, malignant processes, or mumps.
   b. *Staphylococcus aureus* is the most common bacterial cause of acute suppurative parotitis and has been cultured in 50% to 90% of cases. Streptococcal species, including *Streptococcus pneumoniae* and

Streptococcus pyogenes (beta-hemolytic streptococcus), as well as *Haemophilus influenzae,* have been recognized as common causes.

3. Clinical presentation
   a. Sudden onset of parotid pain and swelling
   b. Symptoms may be exacerbated by meals.
4. Diagnosis
   a. Physical examination reveals induration, erythema, edema, and extreme tenderness over the cheek and angle of the mandible.
   b. With parotid swelling, the clinician should be suspicious for mumps, and HIV-infected children should be evaluated at appropriate ages (12 months, 4 to 6 years) for MMR (measles, mumps, rubella) immunization.
   c. Malignancy, especially lymphoma, should be considered in the differential diagnosis of rapid, progressive parotid swelling.
5. Prevention/Treatment
   a. Antimicrobial therapy initially is directed toward the Gram-positive and anaerobic organisms identified as common causes.
6. Nursing implications
   a. Attempts must be made to reverse salivary stasis and stimulate salivary flow by application of warm compresses, maximization of oral hygiene and mouth irrigations, and administration of sialogogues, such as lemon drops or orange juice.
   b. External or bimanual massage of the gland both intraorally and externally should be employed if the patient can tolerate these measures.

8.16 Sinusitis, Recurrent

1. Etiology/Epidemiology
   a. Second most commonly diagnosed bacterial infection among HIV-infected children (Abrams, 2000)
2. Pathogenesis
   a. Most infections caused by organisms commonly associated with sinusitis in immune competent hosts.

3. Clinical presentation
   a. Nasal discharge lasting more than 2 weeks, persistent cough, which may be worse at night. Fever and facial pain may or may not be present.
4. Diagnosis
   a. Based on clinical history and examination
   b. Radiographic studies may be useful in producing a definitive diagnosis.
5. Prevention/Treatment
   a. Antimicrobial therapy initially is directed toward the Gram-positive and anaerobic organisms identified as common causes.
6. Nursing implications
   a. Families should be educated about the disease in children with HIV infection.
   b. Symptoms not improved with treatment should be reported promptly to the health care provider.
   c. Adherence to antimicrobials is essential to minimize the change of development of resistant organisms.

8.17 Splenomegaly

1. Etiology/Epidemiology
   a. Splenomegaly is a common manifestation of many underlying diseases.
   b. Splenomegaly is typically a direct result of HIV replication but may also be caused by infections (e.g., Epstein-Barr virus, cytomegalovirus, mycobacterial infections), a hematologic process, neoplasms, cysts, as well as congestion from extrasplenic pathology.
2. Pathogenesis
   a. Varies according to etiology
3. Clinical presentation
   a. A soft, thin spleen may be palpable in 15% of neonates, 10% of normal children, and 5% of adolescents. However, in most individuals, the spleen must be two to three times its normal size before it is palpable.
4. Diagnosis
   a. The diagnostic and laboratory tests vary according to the suspected etiology.
5. Prevention/Treatment
   a. No specific preventative measures are warranted.
   b. Treatment is based on the etiology.

6. Nursing implications
   a. See specific nursing interventions based on etiology.

8.18 Thrombocytopenia

1. Etiology/Epidemiology
   a. Children with undiagnosed and untreated HIV infection may present with thrombocytopenia, initially as a first manifestation that precipitates seeking medical attention. This etiology is more common than thrombocytopenia due to HAART.
2. Pathogenesis
   a. Generally a complication of either an opportunistic infection or opportunistic neoplasm, a side effect of medication, or idiopathic thrombocytopenia purpura.
3. Clinical presentation
   a. Bleeding tendencies: epistaxis, bleeding from gums, petechiae, blood in urine or stool, hemoptysis, and vaginal or rectal bleeding
   b. The potential risk for bleeding is related to the platelet count.
      i. Platelet count < 100,000/mm^3: clinically significant
      ii. Platelet count < 50,000/mm^3: Mild injury may result in bleeding.
      iii. Platelet count < 20,000/mm^3: Patient is at serious risk for a major bleeding episode that may occur spontaneously.
      iv. Platelet count < 10,000/mm^3: Patient is at risk for a life-threatening bleed. Platelet transfusion should be administered.
4. Diagnosis
   a. Identification of certain risk factors, such as recreational drug use, especially heroin
   b. Complete blood count (CBC) with platelet count
   c. Selenium levels below 145 mcg/l are associated with thrombocytopenia.
   d. Platelet-associated antibodies may be detected with HIV-associated idiopathic thrombocytopenia purpura.
5. Prevention/Treatment
   a. Condition may resolve once antiretroviral therapy (ART) is

initiated (American Academy of Pediatrics, 1998).

b. Severely low platelets may be treated with serial high-dose intravenous immune globulin (IVIG) infusions dosed at 1g/kg/day for 2 to 3 consecutive days or a RhoGam injection.

c. A course of corticosteroids may avail if IVIG fails.

6. Nursing implications

a. Teach parent and child the importance of how to prevent bleeding secondary to trauma (e.g., monitored play, avoidance of toys with sharp edges).

b. When platelets are less than 50,000 cells/mm^3, avoid intramuscular injections, rectal temperatures or suppositories, and indwelling catheters.

c. If venipuncture is performed, the site should have pressure held for at least 5 min.

d. Teach parent not to administer over-the-counter medications that contain aspirin or nonsteroidal antiinflammatory agents (NSAIDs).

e. Teach patent to report any signs of mental status changes, acute pain, nose bleeds, or blood in the urine, stool, or sputum.

f. Teach patient to blow nose gently.

g. Teach patient not to strain with bowel movements; stool softeners may be initiated.

8.19 Upper Respiratory Infection, Recurrent

1. Etiology/Epidemiology

a. Upper respiratory infections are common infections and include pharyngitis, sinusitis, epiglottitis, laryngotracheitis, and the common cold.

b. One of the most common diagnoses in children with symptomatic HIV infection

c. May cause significant morbidity, absence from school, and emergency room visits

2. Pathogenesis

a. Typical pathogens (e.g., *S. pneumoniae, H. influenzae, Moraxella catarrhalis*) invade mucosa directly, causing a local inflammatory response. Unusual pathogens, such as *P. aeruginosa*, yeast, and anaerobes, may be present in chronic infections and result in complications, such as invasive sinusitis and mastoiditis.

3. Clinical presentation

a. The most common symptom in pharyngitis is pharyngeal pain that is aggravated by swallowing and may radiate to the ears. Examination usually reveals pharyngeal erythema, pharyngeal or tonsillar exudate, tonsillar enlargement, and tender cervical lymphadenopathy.

b. The most common symptoms in sinusitis are persistent rhinorrhea (which often is purulent), daytime and nighttime cough, foul breath, and (less commonly) fever. Less frequently, high fever, purulent rhinorrhea, and facial tenderness or swelling signal the likely presence of acute sinusitis.

c. Usually, patients affected by epiglottitis are ages 1 to 5 years, and onset is sudden, with sore throat and fever.

d. Children with laryngitis or croup often are noted to bark like seals. Usually, a mild upper respiratory illness with low-grade fever, runny nose, and mild cough occurs for a few days. Hoarseness or loss of voice, sore throat with pain while swallowing, dry cough, a sensation of having a lump in the throat, and a slight fever (sometimes) occur. Swallowing may be difficult, and the person may feel fatigued.

e. Symptoms of the common cold usually begin 2 to 3 days after infection and often include rhinorrhea, obstruction of nasal breathing, sneezing, sore throat, cough, and headache. Fever usually is slight, but the temperature can reach 102°F in infants and young children.

4. Diagnosis

a. Throat culture may be helpful in identifying pathogenic organisms when suspected.

b. Diagnostic tests or examinations generally are not needed but should be considered if the child does not improve

5. Prevention/Treatment

a. Antimicrobial therapy may be indicted when a bacterial infection is suspected.

6. Nursing implications
   a. Teach children the importance of hand washing.
   b. Teach patient to avoid other children who are sick.
   c. Viral illnesses are self-limiting, but parents should be instructed to monitor their sick child carefully. Ensure adequate intake of food and fluid intake.

8.20 Varicella, Disseminated (Complicated Chickenpox)

1. Etiology/Epidemiology
   a. Varicella is a common childhood illness, spread by direct contact as well as through the respiratory route. Children with advanced HIV disease may be at higher risk for recurrent disease or more severe manifestations, but disseminated varicella is unusual.
2. Pathogenesis
   a. Inadequate immune response results in persistent viremia and dissemination of the varicella-zoster virus (VZV) to the lungs, liver, brain, and other tissues.
3. Clinical presentation
   a. Vessicular lesions in varying stages spread over the body. Lesions may be atypical in children with advanced HIV disease.
4. Diagnosis
   a. Made by clinical examination of the characteristic lesions and history of exposure
5. Prevention/Treatment
   a. Prevention of exposure involves minimizing exposure to infectious individuals.
   b. Postexposure prophylaxis should be given within 96 hours of the exposure. Prophylaxis is given with varicella zoster immune globulin 1 vial (1.25 mL)/10 kg (maximum 5 vials) by intramuscular injection (IM).
   c. Treatment for varicella infection: Children with mild VZV may recover without treatment; however, early introduction of acycolvir is recommended. For children with low CD_4 counts, give IV acycolvir 7 to 10 days. In children with good immune function, oral acyclovir (80 mg/kg/day

in 4 divided doses) may be given (Abrams, 2000).
6. Nursing implications
   a. Local care of lesions includes keeping lesions clean and dry, gently cleansing with mild soap and water.
   b. Teach parent and child that noncrusted lesions are infectious, and the child should avoid touching others. Meticulous hand washing should be observed.
   c. Infected children should avoid others who have not been previously exposed to varicella.
   d. Pain can be severe, and analgesia should be administered as needed.

B. AIDS-Defining Conditions in Children With HIV Infection

Bacterial Infections

8.21 Bacterial Infections, Recurrent

1. Etiology/Epidemiology
   a. Pneumonia: Acute pneumonia is a common clinical diagnosis in HIV-infected children, with incidence especially high among children with poorly controlled HIV infection.
   b. Sepsis: Though common organisms are generally the cause of bacteremia, the frequency of these infections in HIV-infected children is significantly higher than that found in their immunocompetent peers.
   c. Sinusitis: Among HIV-infected children, sinusitis is the second most common clinically diagnosed bacterial infection.
2. Pathogenesis
   a. HIV-infected children typically experience bacterial infections with common organisms such as *Streptococcus pneumoniae, Haemophilus influenzae* and *Salmonella* (Bernstein, Krieger, Novick, Sicklick & Rubinstein, 1985).
3. Clinical presentation
   a. Initial presentations of these infections may be atypical. Recurrent or persistent infection is common.
   b. Pneumonia: Most common signs and symptoms of pneumonia are cough, rales, tachypnea, and fever.
   c. Sinusitis: The most commonly reported symptoms related to sinusitis include

persistent nasal discharge and nocturnal persistent cough. If these symptoms are present for more than 2 weeks, consider a diagnosis of sinusitis. Infrequent symptoms include facial pain, periorbital swelling, high fever, and leukocytosis.
  d. In children with HIV infection, sinusitis is often a chronic/recurrent process.
4. Diagnosis
  a. The diagnosis parallels those of non-HIV-infected children, and a thorough history and physical should guide any further diagnostic work-up.
  b. Isolation of causative organisms for definitive diagnosis is preferred.
5. Prevention/Treatment
  a. Prophylaxis: Increasing use of highly active antiretroviral therapy (ART) may have an impact on the frequency and severity of bacterial infections in HIV-infected children.
  b. Appropriate prophylaxis for bacterial infections includes following the guidelines for immunization of HIV-infected children (see Section 7.2 and Table 7.2a).
  c. Prophylaxis with trimethoprim-sulfamethoxazole (TMP-SMX), 150 mg/m^2 divided in 2 daily doses may also aid in the prevention of recurrent bacterial infections.
  d. Treatment for these infections typically follows the principles used for the treatment of bacterial infections in immunocompetent children.
  e. Treatment is determined by the site and source of infection.
  f. A delayed response to treatment may necessitate a longer course of treatment or additional diagnostic tests to exclude complications or secondary pathogens (Abrams, 2000).
6. Nursing implications
  a. See Section 8.19 for implications of upper respiratory infections.

8.22 Mycobacterial Avium Complex (MAC)

1. Etiology/Epidemiology
  a. Typically associated with advanced HIV disease and severe immunosuppression in children with HIV infection
  b. Associated with a poor prognosis and decreased survival
  c. Treatment with highly active antiretroviral (ARV) agents has had a dramatic effect in reducing the incidence of MAC.
2. Pathogenesis
  a. Impaired cell-mediated immunity in children with advanced HIV disease results in uncontrolled replication of the mycobacteria (Abrams, 2000).
3. Clinical presentation
  a. Signs and symptoms can be indolent and slowly progressive.
  b. MAC is the major cause of cervical lymphadenitis in young children.
  c. Other signs and symptoms include fever, weight loss or poor weight gain, abdominal pain, anemia, night sweats, diarrhea, malaise, neutropenia, and possible hepatomegaly.
  d. The symptoms are not specific to *M. avium* and are often attributed to advanced HIV infection (Abrams, 2000).
4. Diagnosis
  a. Diagnosis is made by isolating the organism from the blood or taking a biopsy of bone marrow, lymph nodes, or other tissue.
  b. Identification of MAC in the stool or respiratory secretions indicates colonization but not necessarily disease (American Academy of Pediatrics, 1998).
5. Prevention/Treatment
  a. Prophylaxis of MAC
    i. Indication
      - Children ages 6 years and older: CD$_4$ count $< 50/\mu L$
      - Children ages 2 to 6 years: CD$_4$ count $< 75/\mu L$
      - Children 1 to 2 years of age: CD$_4$ count $< 500/\mu L$
      - Children < 1 year old: CD$_4$ count $< 750/\mu L$
    ii. Clarithromycin 7.5 mg/kg (max 500 mg) po BID or azithromycin 20 mg/kg (max 1,200 mg) po q week (American Academy of Pediatrics, 1998).
  b. Combination therapy with two or more anti-MAC drugs is indicated to

prevent the development of resistant infection.

c. Adverse effects of treatment are common, and lifelong treatment with at least two drugs is presently recommended.

d. Antiretroviral dose adjustments are necessary with the use of several anti-MAC drugs.

6. Nursing implications
   a. Monitor laboratory results (complete blood count with differential) and other indices for side effects, adverse effects, toxicity, and response to therapy.
   b. Perform blood cultures 4 to 8 weeks after initiation of therapy (Bick, 2001; Zwolski & Talotta, 2001).

8.23 Mycobacterial Tuberculosis

1. Etiology/Epidemiology
   a. A resurgence of tuberculosis (TB) was seen during the years corresponding to the beginning of the HIV epidemic.
   b. Estimates place the incidence of tuberculosis in HIV-infected children between 3% and 5%.
   c. Multidrug-resistant TB accounts for a high percentage of these cases.
   d. Children with HIV disease generally develop primary infection as a result of contact with an adult with tuberculosis.

2. Pathogenesis
   a. *M. tuberculosis* is inhaled, organisms penetrate lung parenchyma, and primary infection is established (first time infection). Bacilli are transported to hilar lymph nodes by macrophages, and the macrophages disseminate organisms in blood or wall off infection in granulomas, preventing active disease (latent tuberculosis).
   b. Cell-mediated immunity is activated to halt the infectious process and dissemination; infection can be detected in 2 to 10 weeks with tuberculin skin test. A breakdown of cell-mediated immunity (CD_4 cell count < 200 cells/mm^3) results in reactivation of TB and possibly active disease.

3. Clinical presentation
   a. Commonly reported symptoms in children include fever and cough.

4. Diagnosis
   a. Tuberculin skin tests are commonly negative among children with advanced HIV disease who are among those at highest risk for developing pulmonary and extrapulmonary tuberculosis.
   b. The Mantoux test, 0.1 ml (5TU PPD), should be used when investigating a possible diagnosis. A ≤ 5 mm induration is considered positive in a child with HIV infection.
   c. Diagnosis is typically initiated by the report of a household contact with tuberculosis.
   d. Sputum samples obtained by gastric washings or bronchoalveolar lavage are also important diagnostic tools.
   e. Chest X-rays may not be initially useful because other HIV-related findings and chronic lung changes may complicate the diagnosis.

5. Prevention/Treatment
   a. Children with positive a tuberculin skin test (TST) but no active disease should receive 12 months of isoniazid therapy.
   b. Initial treatment recommendations for tuberculosis disease call for a four-drug regimen of isoniazid, rifampin, pyrazinamide, and ethambutol. Regimen adjustments are made based on obtained sputum sensitivities.
   c. The course of treatment for pulmonary tuberculosis in children with HIV infection is 6 to 12 months, and directly observed therapy is recommended.

6. Nursing implications
   a. Caution must be used in the treatment of tuberculosis because drug–drug interactions with antiretrovirals (ARVs) are common (Abrams, 2000).

8.24 Salmonellosis

1. Etiology/Epidemiology
   a. Salmonellae are potential enteric pathogens and a leading cause of bacterial food-borne illness.
   b. The incidence of salmonellosis in the United States is greatest among children younger than 5 years of age.

2. Pathogenesis
   a. Transmission of salmonellae to a susceptible host usually occurs

by consumption of contaminated foods.

b. The most common sources of salmonellae are beef, poultry, and eggs. Improperly prepared fruits, vegetables, dairy products, and shellfish have also been implicated.

c. Human-to-human and animal-to-human transmission can occur.

3. Clinical presentation

a. Infection with salmonellae usually causes enterocolitis similar to that caused by other bacterial enteric pathogens. In most cases, stools are loose and bloodless. Salmonellae may rarely cause large-volume cholera-like diarrhea or may be associated with tenesmus.

b. Nausea, vomiting, and diarrhea occur within 6 to 48 hours after ingestion of contaminated food or drink.

c. Fever, abdominal cramping, chills, headache, and myalgia are common.

4. Diagnosis

a. Freshly passed stool is the preferred specimen.

5. Prevention/Treatment

a. Prevention efforts include proper sanitation and hygiene as well as the avoidance of insufficiently cooked or mishandled food.

6. Nursing implications

a. Teach children the importance of hand washing.

b. To prevent infection, teach patients to avoid other children who might be sick.

c. Ensure adequate intake of food and fluid intake when patient has diarrhea.

Fungal Infections

8.25 Candidiasis

1. Etiology/Epidemiology

a. Although mucosa and skin infections with fungal agents are relatively common in children, systemic fungal infections continue to be rare.

b. Most commonly, candida albicans is the causative organism.

c. HIV-infected infants may experience more severe or persistent cases of oral candida than their immunocompetent peers.

d. Oral candidiasis is a common finding in healthy infants as well as infants with HIV infection and may be the first clinical indication of HIV infection.

e. Esophageal candidiasis is an AIDS-defining condition in children.

f. Other fungal infections include cryptococcosis, aspergillosis, histoplasmosis, and coccidioidomycosis, which have all been reported in adults but are rare in children.

2. Pathogenesis

a. Any warm, moist part of the body exposed to the environment is susceptible to infection and supports its growth.

3. Clinical presentation

a. Signs and symptoms of candida include weight loss, complaints of substernal pain, and difficulty swallowing, which are often the presenting symptoms of esophageal candidiasis.

b. There are several forms of oral lesions associated with oral candidiasis:

- Thrush/pseudomembranous: Most common are creamy white lesions on the oropharyngeal mucosa, palate, and tonsils.
- Hypertrophic: raised plaques on the lower surface of the tongue, palate, and buccal mucosa
- Erythematous: flat red lesions on the buccal mucosa
- Angular chelitis: red, cracked skin at the corners of the mouth

4. Diagnosis

a. Based on physical findings and symptoms

b. Confirmation of clinical diagnosis can be made by potassium hydroxide (KOH)–stained specimens showing blastospores or pseudohyphae or isolation of candida on culture.

c. Esophageal candidiasis can be diagnosed by endoscopy and biopsy.

5. Prevention/Treatment

a. Primary prophylaxis is not indicated.

b. Secondary prophylaxis may be indicated if the candidiasis recurs frequently or is persistent.

c. Lifelong prophylaxis is considered with recurrent esophageal candidiasis; however, long-term use should be limited due to the risk of resistant organism development.

d. Treatment of oral candidiasis may include topical nystatin suspension or lozenges (100,000–500,000 U po QID for 14 days) or fluconazole (3–6 mg/kg (max 100 mg) po QD for 14 days.

e. Esophageal candidiasis is treated with fluconazole (3–6 mg/kg [max 200 mg]) po QD for 21 days.

6. Nursing implications

a. Good oral hygiene and daily oral debridement may be helpful: wiping the gums, tongue, and palate with a moistened washcloth BID or rinsing with water after eating and drinking (American Academy of Pediatrics, 1998).

8.26 Coccidioidomycosis

1. Etiology/Epidemiology

a. Coccidioidomycosis is a fungal disorder rarely diagnosed in children: One case was reported in 1996 (Centers for Disease Control and Prevention, 1996).

2. Pathogenesis

a. *Coccidioides immitis* is an airborne fungus that enters the respiratory tract and causes pulmonary manifestations.

3. Clinical presentation

a. Most cases of the disease present as an asymptomatic infection.

b. Signs and symptoms are generally nonspecific flulike symptoms or pneumonia. A diffuse erythematous maculopapular rash, erythema multiforme, erythema nodosum, or arthralgias, or all these conditions combined, frequently occur and may be the only clinical manifestations in some children.

c. Disseminated disease occurs in less than 1% of infected persons. The skin, bones and joints, central nervous system (CNS), and lungs are the affected sites.

4. Diagnosis

a. Definitive diagnosis is made by microscopic study or culture of the organism.

5. Prevention/Treatment

a. Antifungal therapy is not indicated for uncomplicated primary infection. Fluconazole and itraconazole have been used successfully to treat nonmeningeal coccidioidomycosis.

b. Secondary prophylaxis is indicated in cases of documented disease.

c. Amphotericin B is the recommended initial therapy for severe progressive disseminated infection not involving the CNS.

6. Nursing implications

a. Encourage patients living in or visiting endemic areas to avoid extensive exposure to soil and dust storms (Centers for Disease Control and Prevention, 1997).

8.27 Cryptococcosis

1. Etiology/Epidemiology

a. Etiologic agent is *Cryptococcus neoformans,* a yeast characterized by distinctive polysaccharide encapsulations that can be divided into serotypic groups A, B, C, and D.

b. Organism is ubiquitous in nature and distributed worldwide. Serotypes A and D are found in pigeon droppings and soil; serotype C has been isolated from fruit and fruit juices.

c. Recurrent disease thought to involve reactivation of initial infection

d. Rare in children with HIV; seen only in children older than 10 years of age with advanced disease

2. Pathogenesis

a. Aerosolized organisms enter the pulmonary tract via inhalation. Most common extrapulmonary site of disease is the central nervous system (CNS) but can also involve skin, bone, and the genitourinary tract.

3. Clinical presentation

a. In children, the disease most commonly presents as a subacute meningitis or meningoencephalitis with nonspecific, subtle symptoms, including fever and headache. Pulmonary involvement occurs in as many as 50% of patients (Abrams, 2000).

4. Diagnosis
   a. Serologic testing for cryptococcal antigen (CRAG) is clinically useful for detecting organisms. Other tests depend on the site of involvement (e.g., lumbar puncture with CNS cryptococcosis).
5. Prevention/Treatment
   a. Amphotericin B (0.7–1.0 mg/kg IV daily) for a minimum of 2 weeks, with or without 5-flucytosine (100 mg/kg orally QID, adjusted for any renal insufficiency development), followed by consolidation therapy of either fluconazole (400 mg orally daily for 8 to 10 weeks) or itraconazole (200 mg orally, twice daily for 8 to 10 weeks).
   b. CNS disease, in the absence of obstructive hydrocephalus, may require serial lumbar punctures to release increased intracranial pressure (ICP). If lumbar puncture is insufficient to manage increased ICP, lumbar drain, ventriculostomy, or placement of a ventricular-peritoneal shunt may be performed.
   c. Suppressive maintenance therapy is lifelong. The usual regimen is fluconazole (200 mg orally daily).
6. Nursing implications
   a. See Section 3.13 Coccidioidomycosis for nursing implications relevant to treatment with amphotericin B, fluconazole, and itraconazole.
   b. For patients treated with 5-flucytosine, frequent monitoring of serum alanine aminotransferase (ALT), alkaline phosphatase, aspartate aminotransferase (AST), bilirubin, creatinine, and blood urea nitrogen (BUN) is indicated.
   c. Ensure lumbar puncture opening pressure is recorded.
   d. Educate patient about prevention and importance of maintenance therapy (see Section 3.13 Coccidioidomycosis for specific interventions).

8.28 Histoplasmosis

1. Etiology/Epidemiology
   a. Histoplasmosis is a fungal infection endemic to the Ohio and Mississippi River valleys as well as Caribbean and Central and South American countries. It is rarely diagnosed in children (one case was reported in 1996; Centers for Disease Control and Prevention, 1996).
2. Pathogenesis
   a. Aerosolized spores enter the pulmonary tract via inhalation. Spores become activated and can spread via the reticuloendothelial system to the liver, spleen, and lymph nodes. Infection is characterized by granuloma formation.
3. Clinical presentation
   a. No data available for children.
   b. In adults, histoplasmosis can appear as a mild, flulike respiratory illness that has a combination of symptoms, including malaise, fever, chest pain, dry or nonproductive cough, headache, loss of appetite, shortness of breath, joint and muscle pains, chills, and hoarseness. Neurologic manifestations, such as meningitis, are reported in 18–20% of cases (Zwolski, 2001).
   c. Skin and mucosal ulcers may be present.
4. Diagnosis
   a. Diagnosis can be difficult secondary to nonspecific presentation, especially in nonendemic areas. Review previous living and travel history to prevent diagnostic delay.
   b. Positive culture from blood or tissue specimens is necessary for definitive diagnosis, which can take up to 3 weeks.
   c. Histopathological evaluation of bone marrow or tissue biopsy is useful for establishing diagnosis in 50% of patients (Zwolski, 2001).
   d. Standard antibody serology test is not useful because it does not distinguish current versus past infection.
   e. Histoplasma specific antigen (HAG) can be assayed in both serum and urine specimens, although urine test is more sensitive. Most diagnoses of disseminated histoplasmosis are now made with this test because of its rapid turnaround time compared with culture.
   f. Diffuse or patchy infiltrates are the most common radiographic abnormality.
5. Prevention/Treatment
   a. Primary prophylaxis is not currently recommended.

6. Nursing implications
   a. Amphotericin B is the recommended acute therapy for severe initial or recurrent disease. Dosage is 0.7–1.0 mg/kg IV daily for 1–2 weeks, followed by itraconazole (200 mg po BID) consolidation therapy for 10–12 weeks. Itraconazole (200 mg po BID) for 3 months can be used for treatment of mild disease.
   b. HIV-infected persons usually require lifelong maintenance therapy for suppression after completion of consolidation therapy. Maintenance therapy is usually itraconazole (200 mg po QD).
   c. See "Nursing Implications" in Section 3.13 Coccidioidomycosis for additional implications.

Protozoal Infections

8.29 Cryptosporidiosis

1. Etiology/Epidemiology
   a. Reported in 3% to 4% of children in the United States; however, it may occur more frequently outside the United States.
   b. Outbreaks have been associated with ingestion of contaminated drinking water in metropolitan areas. Also, person-to-person transmission is common in day care centers.
2. Pathogenesis
   a. Cryptosporidium exists as an oocyst that releases sporozoites that adhere to the surface of the intestinal mucosa.
   b. Following ingestion and attachment, primarily in the small intestine, it is hypothesized that phagocytes are activated, resulting in the release of soluble factors (i.e., histamine, prostaglandins, leukotrienes) that increase the intestinal secretion of water and chloride and also inhibit absorption.
   c. Intestinal epithelial cells are characterized by villus atrophy and crypt hyperplasia. Histological changes are hypothesized to be the result of either direct viral invasion or inflammatory processes (Goodgame, 1996).

3. Clinical presentation
   a. Diarrhea: scant and intermittent or voluminous. Chronic severe diarrhea can develop, resulting in malnutrition, dehydration, and death.
   b. Other gastrointestinal (GI) symptoms: severe abdominal cramping, nausea, and flatulence
   c. Constitutional symptoms: low-grade fever, malaise, and weight loss
4. Diagnosis
   a. Freshly passed stool is the preferred specimen. The finding of oocysts on microscopic examination of stool specimens is diagnostic. Unfortunately, routine laboratory examination of stool for ova and parasites is inadequate to detect *C. parvum,* so health care professionals should ask laboratory personnel to test specifically for *C. parvum.*
5. Prevention/Treatment
   a. Practice hand washing, especially after contact with human or animal feces.
   b. Avoid untreated drinking water and public pools and tubs.
   c. Thoroughly wash fruits and vegetables.
   d. Treatment consists of supportive care consisting of hydration and nutritional supplementation.
   e. There is no proven effective therapy for cryptosporidiosis in HIV-infected persons (American Academy of Pediatrics, 1998).
6. Nursing implications
   a. Teach the patient good hand-washing techniques to prevent transmission of organism.
   b. Encourage water safety and food safety: Use a 0.1–1.0 micron filter on water faucets, boil untreated water, and avoid unpasteurized foods.
   c. Enteric precautions should be initiated for incontinent patients.
   d. Caregivers should use 5% to 10% ammonia or full-strength 70% bleach for cleaning contaminated areas.

8.30 Isosporiasis

1. Etiology/Epidemiology
   a. Common infection in domestic and wild animals; typically found in tropical and subtropical climates

2. Pathogenesis
   a. Advanced HIV disease results in susceptibility to this intestinal parasite.
3. Clinical presentation
   a. Profuse, watery diarrhea, crampy abdominal pain, weight loss, and malaise. Chronic/recurrent infection may result.
4. Diagnosis
   a. Stool studies: ova and parasites; presence of oocyst using a modified acid-fast stain; differentiation from cryptosporidiosis is important.
5. Prevention/Treatment
   a. Treatment: TMP/SMX (TMP 40 mg/kg/day + SMX 200 mg/kg/day orally divided 4 times daily for 10 days (max TMP 640 mg/day, SMX 800 mg/day) then TMP 20 mg/kg/day + SMX 100 mg/kg/day indefinitely (max 320 mg TMP/day, SMX 400 mg/day)
6. Nursing implications
   a. Teach patient to practice good hand washing to avoid infection.
   b. Wash all fresh fruits and vegetables before eating.
   c. Avoid fecal contact during sexual contact.

8.31 *Pneumocystis Carinii* Pneumonia (PCP)

1. Etiology /Epidemiology
   a. PCP is the most common AIDS-defining illness in children.
   b. In the early years of the epidemic, PCP was the presenting problem for many infants and children previously undiagnosed as HIV infected.
   c. New guidelines that include early identification of HIV-infected women and their at-risk infants and prophylaxis for both HIV-exposed and HIV-infected children have made new diagnoses of PCP very rare.
2. Pathogenesis
   a. The organism attaches to type 1 alveolar cells, replicates, and invades the epithelium of the lung.
   b. The immunocompromised host is unable to mount an alveolar macrophage response, resulting in pneumonia and interfering with the transport of fatty acid substrates, an essential component of lung surfactant. Without surfactant, lung distensibility is diminished.
3. Clinical presentation
   a. Children present with clinical findings of tachypnea, dyspnea, cough, and fever.
   b. Physical exam reveals tachycardia, respiratory distress, accelerating tachypnea, and diffuse retractions. Pulmonary auscultation is typically nonspecific.
   c. PCP is characterized by rapidly progressive hypoxia, and arterial blood gas (ABG) reveals decreased arterial oxygen tension (PaO_2) as well as an elevated alveolar-arterial oxygen pressure gradient on room air.
   d. Early radiographic findings may be normal or show hyperinflation with peribronchial thickening. As the disease progresses, the chest X-ray may reveal bilateral alveolar or interstitial infiltrates that are usually spread peripherally to encompass both lung fields.
4. Diagnosis
   a. PCP is diagnosed by the presence of *P. carinii* cysts in sputum from bronchoalveolar lavage during bronchoscopy, induced sputums, or tracheal washings in intubated children (Abrams, 2000).
5. Prevention/Treatment
   a. Routine prophylaxis has resulted in a dramatic decrease in the number of new cases. Trimethoprim-sulfamethoxazole (TMP-SMX) is given twice a day on 3 consecutive days each week at a dose of 75 mg/m^2 per dose. Alternatively, for children with allergy to TMP-SMX, daily dapsone may be given for prophylaxis.
   b. The rapidly progressive nature of PCP in children warrants the initiation of treatment in suspected cases before diagnostic confirmation is obtained.
   c. TMP-SMX is the treatment of choice for PCP. The recommended dosage is 20 mg/kg divided into 4 daily doses for a total of 21 days.

d. Alternately, intravenous pentamidine at a dose of 4 mg/kg once daily for 21 days may be given for children who can not receive or whose therapy with TMP-SMX has failed.

e. Additional components of PCP management include intravenous steroids and intensive respiratory support.

6. Nursing implications

a. Monitor for side effects or adverse effects of medications, such as rash, photosensitivity, peripheral neuropathy, and liver function abnormalities.

b. Patients receiving Bactrim should have their complete blood count monitored every 4 to 6 months because the sulfa component causes thrombocytopenia and neutropenia.

c. Children receiving intravenous infusions of Pentamidine should be monitored for pancreatitis. Monitor the amylase and lipase levels. Hypoglycemia can occur with IV infusions.

d. Children receiving dapsone should be checked for glucose-6-phosphate dehydrogenase (G6PD) deficiency prior to administration. This drug causes hemolysis in the G6PD deficient child.

8.32 *Toxoplasma Gondii*

1. Etiology/Epidemiology

a. A historically common opportunistic infection in adults, which is relatively rare in children

b. Generally pediatric infections are a result of congenital toxoplasmosis.

c. Prevention of congenital toxoplasmosis depends on identification of the infection in pregnant women.

d. Toxoplasmosis is typically a concern for children with severe immune suppression.

2. Pathogenesis

a. After primary exposure, T. gondii can invade and infect contiguous tissue by converting from bradyzoite to tachyzoite form. Cysts can be found in all tissue types and are most common in brain, heart, and striated muscle.

b. There is evidence that cysts rupture and may cause recurrent asymptomatic infections.

3. Clinical presentation

a. Central nervous system (CNS) infection is the most common presentation. The child will present with headache, change in cognitive status, fever, or focal neurologic deficits, such as hemiparesis, ataxia, cranial nerve palsies, and seizures, or they will present with any combination of these conditions (Abrams, 2000).

4. Diagnosis

a. In the United States, routine serologic screening for toxoplasmosis is not recommended; however, it may be performed on HIV-infected children after 12 months of age in high-incidence regions.

b. Diagnosis is usually based on clinical presentation, presence of Toxoplasma IgG antibodies in serum (congenital toxoplasmosis is diagnosed based on presence of specific IgM or IgA serum antibodies), and characteristic findings on imaging studies.

c. Magnetic resonance imaging (MRI) and CT scan will show multiple ring-enhancing lesions in the fontal, basal ganglia, or parietal regions. Cerebral edema is also often present.

d. Cerebral spinal fluid changes are generally nonspecific, ranging from normal to moderate pleocytosis with elevated protein (Abrams, 2000).

5. Prevention/Treatment

a. Prevention of toxoplasmosis in children is accomplished using the same doses of trimethoprim-sulfamethoxazole (TMP-SMX) that are recommended for PCP prophylaxis.

b. Treatment is initiated based on the diagnostic findings. (The diagnosis of toxoplasmosis infection is confirmed if the patient responds to the treatment.) Initial treatment and lifelong suppressive therapy with sulfadiazine, pyrimethamine, and folinic acid have been recommended. An alternative regimen is clindamycin, pyrimethamine, and folinic acid (Abrams, 2000).

6. Nursing implications
   a. Nursing care is supportive and is aimed at maximizing function, assisting with access to necessary rehabilitative therapies, and monitoring for side effects of treatment or further disease progression.

Viral Infections

8.33 Cytomegalovirus Disease (CMV)

1. Etiology/Epidemiology
   a. Historically, CMV infection has been a frequently reported infection among children with HIV.
   b. CMV generally occurs in children with severe immune suppression.
2. Pathogenesis
   a. Commonly reported clinical manifestations in children include chorioretinitis, esophagitis, pneumonitis, and colitis (Abrams, 2000).
3. Clinical presentation
   a. CMV chorioretinitis: visual disturbances such as blurred vision and floaters. Fundoscopic exam shows characteristic lesion—yellowish-white area of retinal necrosis with perivascular exudates and hemorrhage—usually at the periphery of fundus. Children may, however, be asymptomatic until advanced disease gives a significant loss of vision.
   b. CMV pneumonitis: cough, shortness of breath, and progressive hypoxemia. Chest X-ray shows diffuse interstitial infiltrates.
   c. CMV esophagitis: substernal pain, difficulty swallowing, and loss of appetite.
   d. CMV colitis should be a part of the differential diagnosis for children with nonspecific gastrointestinal complaints, such as abdominal pain or diarrhea, and those with significant weight loss.
4. Diagnosis
   a. CMV pneumonitis: Culture shows presence of intracellular inclusions in lung tissue or bronchoalveolar macrophages in the absence of other pulmonary pathogens.
   b. CMV esophagitis: Endoscopy shows small confluent ulcers or erosions.

Mucosal biopsy shows inflammation and CMV inclusion bodies.
   c. CMV colitis: Sigmoid shows diffuse areas of erythema, submucosal hemorrhage, and mucosal ulcerations.
5. Prevention/Treatment
   a. Children with severe immune suppressions should have routine dilated retinal exams with providers familiar with CMV retinitis at least twice yearly.
   b. Discontinuation of prophylaxis has been considered in some cases of children with immune reconstitution.
   c. Treatment of retinitis includes lifelong suppressive therapy and is not curative, but it is preventive of further disease progression.
   d. The treatments for all types of CMV include gancyclovir and foscarnet. Unfortunately, these medications have treatment-limiting side effects in children.
6. Nursing implications
   a. Nursing care is supportive and is aimed at maximizing function, assisting with access to necessary rehabilitative therapies, and monitoring for side effects of treatment or further disease progression.

8.34 Progressive Multifocal Leukoencephalopathy (PML)

1. Etiology/Epidemiology
   a. Caused by a neurotropic polyomavirus known as JC virus (JCV). JCV has a worldwide distribution, and by middle adulthood most individuals have been infected with the virus (Czarniecki, Rothpletz-Puglia, & Oleske, 1999).
2. Pathogenesis
   a. Acute demyelinating disease of the central nervous system with the formation of lesions in the white matter of the brain
3. Clinical presentation
   a. In children, dysarthria, tongue and chin parasthesias, dementia, aphasia, hemiparesis and spastic quadriparesis have been described (Berger, Scott, & Albrecht, 1992).

4. Diagnosis
   a. Diagnosed via white matter lesions on CT scan or magnetic resonance imaging (MRI) or by brain biopsy or postmortem examination
5. Prevention/Treatment
   a. There is no proven effective treatment, but some adult evidence suggests antiretrovirals may bring about remission.
6. Nursing implications
   a. In the early years of the HIV epidemic, a diagnosis of PML was uniformly fatal, usually within 2 to 4 months. Patients were appropriately counseled, and plans for comfort and terminal care were made.
   b. Effective treatment regimens specifically against PML remain elusive. HAART seems prudent, even though clinical trial evidence of other efficacious agents is currently lacking, and cautious optimism may allow nurses to offer hope to patients and their loved ones where before none existed.

Neoplasms

8.35 Malignancies

1. Etiology/Epidemiology
   a. Although the incidence of malignancies in HIV-infected children is significantly higher than that found in immunocompetent children, the types of cancers found in children with HIV infection differs from those typically reported in adults with the disease.
   b. The most common types of cancers found in children with HIV infection include non-Hodgkin's lymphoma, leiomyosarcoma, and leukemia (Granovsky, Mueller, Nicholson, Rosenberg, & Rabkin, 1998).
   c. In children with HIV infection, a strong association between Epstein-Barr virus (EBV) and malignancies has been reported (Jenson et al., 1997).
2. Pathogenesis
   a. Immune suppression and chronic stimulation with oncogenic viruses, such as EBV, human T-lymphotrophic virus-I, cytomegalovirus (CMV), human papillomavirus, and hepatitis B virus (HBV), are thought to contribute to the development of malignant neoplasms.
3. Clinical presentation
   a. Symptoms of lymphoma in children may include fever, weight loss, diffuse adenopathy, jaundice, hepatomegaly, abdominal distention, and pain (Czarniecki, Rothpletz-Puglia, & Oleske, 1999).
4. Diagnosis
   a. The diagnosis of specific malignancies varies according to the disorder. The diagnostic work-up is generally the same in both adults and children. Refer to the specific disorder in the adult section.
5. Prevention/Treatment
   a. Refer to the specific disorder in the adult section.
6. Nursing implications
   a. Counsel regarding course of disease and support decision making about quality of life issues and treatment.

8.36 HIV-Related Wasting Syndrome

1. Etiology/Epidemiology
   a. Wasting syndrome and failure to thrive in HIV infection may result from direct infection of the gastrointestinal (GI) tract with HIV resulting in malabsorption.
2. Pathogenesis
   a. Other organisms infecting the GI tract, including candida, herpes, cryptosporidium, or cytomegalovirus (CMV), may contribute to growth failure and wasting.
3. Clinical presentation
   a. Diarrhea, extreme weight loss, failure to gain weight, and anorexia may be present.
4. Diagnosis
   a. The diagnosis is made when a child's growth rate has declined by 2 major percentiles.
5. Prevention/Treatment
   a. Careful growth assessment at each visit is an essential component of care of the HIV-infected child.
   b. A thorough evaluation of potential causes, including those that are

infectious, behavioral, and environmental, should be conducted.

6. Nursing implications
   a. Nursing interventions may include instruction in appropriate and safe food preparation and maximization of nutrient and caloric intake through improved diet and nutritional supplements.
   b. Enteral or parenteral feedings may all be considered, depending on the severity of the weight loss and the ability of the child to absorb nutrients.

8.37 HIV-Related Encephalopathy

1. Etiology/Epidemiology
   a. In general, no causative organism is identified; however, static and progressive encephalopathy may be a result of HIV, opportunistic infections, inflammatory disease, vascular disease, and neoplastic changes (Laufer & Scott, 2000).
   b. In some cohorts, HIV encephalopathy has been reported in up to 21% of infected children (Abuzaitoun & Hanson, 2000).
2. Pathogenesis
   a. HIV encephalopathy and developmental delay have been associated with poor prognosis and poor outcomes.
   b. HIV-related encephalopathy and developmental delay are commonly seen in children with HIV infection, especially in those with poorly controlled disease as evidenced by immune deficiency and high viral load.
3. Clinical presentation
   a. May include rapid and progressive onset of loss of previously acquired developmental milestones
   b. The findings may be subtler, such as decreased attention span, inability to follow instructions, and difficulties in school performance.
4. Diagnosis
   a. Based on clinical findings as well as brain magnetic resonance imaging (MRI) that may show cortical atrophy, basal gangliar calcifications, or both

   b. Examination by a pediatric neurologist, tests for pathogens, and treatment of other identifiable causes of symptoms may also result in a diagnosis of encephalopathy.
5. Prevention/Treatment
   a. Prevention of HIV-related encephalopathy includes aggressive use of antiretroviral therapy to maintain suppression of viral replication.
   b. Treatment and prophylaxis of organisms, including cryptococcus and mycobacterium, are also indicated.
   c. If acute infectious causes are ruled out and HIV disease progression is the suspected cause, initiation of or changes in antiretroviral therapy (ART) may be beneficial.
   d. Additional supportive measures, including physical therapy or surgery, to address contractures are also indicated.
6. Nursing implications
   a. Nursing care of the child with encephalopathic changes includes identifying strategies and resources to maximize function.
   b. Educate the family and child about the potential benefit of strict adherence to ARV regimens.

References

Abrams, E. J. (2000). Opportunistic infections and other clinical manifestations of HIV disease in children. *Pediatric Clinics of North America, 47*, 79–108.

Abramson, D. I., Steinhart C., & Frascino, R. (2000). Epoetin alfa therapy for anaemia in HIV-infected patients: Impact on quality of life. *International Journal of STD and AIDS, 11*, 659–665.

Abuzaitoun, O. R., & Hanson, I. C. (2000). Organ-specific manifestations of HIV disease in children. *Pediatric Clinics of North America, 47*, 109–125.

American Academy of Pediatrics (1998). Antiretroviral therapy and medical management of pediatric HIV infection. *Pediatrics, 102*(4), 1005–1065.

Bain, B. J. (1999). Pathogenesis and pathophysiology of anemia in HIV infection. *Current Opinion in Hematology, 6*, 89–93.

Berger, J. R., Scott, G., & Albrecht, J. (1992). Progressive multifocal leukoencephalopathy in HIV-1-infected children. *AIDS, 6*(8), 837–841.

Bernstein, L. J., Krieger, B. Z., Novick, B., Sicklick, M. J., & Rubinstein, A. (1985). Bacterial infection in the acquired immunodeficiency syndrome of children. *Pediatric Infectious Disease Journal, 85*, 472.

Bick, J. (2001). Prevention of opportunistic infections (OIs) in those with HIV infection. *HIV and Hepatitis Education Prison Project News, 4*(12), 1–7.

Centers for Disease Control and Prevention (1996). *HIV/AIDS Surveillance Report, 8*(2), 1–39.

Centers for Disease Control and Prevention. (1997). 1997 USPH/IDSA guidelines for the prevention of opportunistic infections in persons infected with human immunodeficiency virus. *Morbidity and Mortality Weekly Report, 46*(RR-12), 1–46.

Coyle, T. E. (1997). Hematologic complications of human immunodeficiency virus infection and the acquired immunodeficiency syndrome. *Medical Clinics of North America, 81,* 449–470.

Czarniecki, L., Rothpletz-Puglia, P., & Oleske, J. (1999). Infants and children: AIDS care management. In P. L. Ungvarski & J. H. Flaskerud (Eds.), *HIV/AIDS: A guide to primary care management* (4th ed., pp. 98–130). New York: W.B. Saunders.

Diaz, C., Hanson, C., Cooper, E. R., Reed, J. S., Watson, J., Mendez, H. A., et al. (1997). Disease progression in a cohort of infants with vertically acquired HIV infection observed from birth: The women and infants transmission study. *Journal of Acquired Immune Deficiency Syndromes and Human Retrovirology, 18,* 221–228.

Doweiko, J. P., & Groopman, J. (1998). Hematologic manifestations of HIV infection. In T.C. Merigan, J. G. Bartlett, & D. Bolognesi (Eds.), *Textbook of AIDS medicine* (2nd ed., pp. 611–627). Baltimore: Lippincott Williams & Wilkins.

Ferri, R., Adinofi, A., Orsi, A., Sterken, D. J., Keruly, J. C., Davis, S., et al. (2002). Treatment of anemia in patients with HIV infection—Part 2: Guidelines for the management of anemia. *Journal of the Association of Nurses in AIDS Care, 1,* 50–59.

Goodgame, R. W. (1996). Understanding intestinal spore-forming protozoa: cryptosporidiosis, microsporidiosis, isospora, and cyclospora. *Annals of Internal Medicine, 124*(4), 429–441.

Granovsky, M. O., Mueller, B. U., Nicholson, H. S., Rosenberg, P. S., & Rabkin, C. S. (1998). Cancer in human immunodeficiency virus-infected children: A case series from the Children's Cancer Group and the National Cancer Institute. *Journal of Clinical Oncology, 16,* 1729–1735.

Hillman, R. S. (1998). Anemia. In A. S. Fauci, J. B. Martin, E. Braunwald, D. L. Kasper, K. J. Isselbacher, S. L. Hauser, et al. (Eds.), *Harrison's principles of internal medicine* (pp. 334–339). New York: McGraw-Hill.

Jenson, H. B., Leach, C. T., McClain, K. L., Joshi, V. V., Pollock, B. H., Parmley, R. T., et al. (1997). Benign and malignant smooth muscle tumors containing Epstein-Barr virus in children with AIDS. *Leukemia and Lymphoma, 27,* 303–314.

Kreuzer, K. A., & Rockstroh, J. K. (1997). Pathogenesis and pathophysiology of anemia in HIV infection. *Annals of Hematology, 75,* 179–187.

Lapointe, N., Martin, S., Pelletier, V., Roberts, E., Schreiber, R., & Smith, L. (2002). *Hepatitis C virus infection.* Retrieved March 8, 2003, from http://www.cps.ca/english/CPSP/Resources/RHepatitis.htm

Laufer, M., & Scott, G. B. (2000). Medical management of HIV disease in children. *Pediatric Clinics of North America, 47,* 127–153.

Levine, A. M. (1999). *Anemia, neutropenia and thrombocytopenia: Pathogenesis and evolving treatment options in HIV-infected patients.* Retrieved July 8, 2002, from http://hiv.medscape.com/Medscape/HIV/ClinicalMgmt/CM.v10/pnt-CM.v10.html

Luginbuhl, L. M., Orav, E. J., McIntosh, K., & Lipshultz, S. E. (1993). Cardiac morbidity and related mortality in children with HIV infection. *Journal of the American Medical Association, 269,* 2869.

Mitsuyasu, R. (1999). Hematologic disease. In R. Dolin, H. Masur, & M. S. Saag (Eds.), *AIDS therapy* (pp. 666–679). New York: Churchill Livingstone.

Mueller, B. (1999). Cancers in children infected with the human immunodeficiency virus. *The Oncologist, 4*(4), 309–317.

Sabella, C., & Goldfarb, J. (1999) *Parvovirus B19 infections.* Retrieved July 8, 2002, from http://www.aafp.org/ afp/991001ap/1455.html

Whitley, R. J., & Whitley, S. J. (1994). Herpes virus infections in children with human immunodeficiency virus. In P. Pizzo & C. Wilfert (Eds.), *Pediatric AIDS: The challenge of HIV infection in infants, children and adolescents* (pp. 346–352). Baltimore: Lippincott Williams & Wilkins.

Zwolski, K. (2001). Fungal infections. In C. Kirton, D. Talotta, & K. Zwolski (Eds.), *Handbook of HIV/AIDS nursing* (pp. 265–270). St. Louis, MO: Mosby.

Zwolski, K., & Talotta, D. (2001). Bacterial infections. In C. Kirton, D. Talotta, & K. Zwolski (Eds.), *Handbook of HIV/AIDS nursing* (pp. 229–253). St. Louis, MO: Mosby.

Section IX

Symptom Management of the HIV-Infected Infant and Child

Symptom management for children living with HIV/AIDS is recognized as an extremely important component of care management because every child experiences symptoms throughout the course of their disease. Many of these symptoms are caused by the disorders associated with HIV; others are caused by the treatments used in HIV. Symptoms may potentially impact the child's growth and development, the ability of the child to learn, and, most important, the ability of the child to adhere to antiretroviral therapy. It is important to note that when the child experiences symptoms, the family may also be impacted in many ways. Consider the parent who may be faced with frequent health care visits or hospitalizations, frequent medication administration and regimen changes, and sometimes the declining health of the child. Changes in the child's clinical condition frequently precipitate a family crisis; thus, frequent family assessments are essential.

This section highlights common issues of children with symptoms seen in HIV/AIDS. Nurses, given their history of diagnosing and treating human responses to illness, are well positioned to manage these common responses to HIV. The authors, a combination of researchers and clinicians, provide clear definitions of the symptoms and the nursing assessment and use a nursing diagnosis as the framework for managing symptoms. The importance of pharmacological and nonpharmacological interventions for management of symptoms has been emphasized as well as the acknowledgement that holistic interventions may be an important part of the care plan.

9.1 Pain

1. Etiology
   a. Advances in the treatment of HIV in children have resulted in a decrease in the incidence of opportunistic infections and other complications that cause pain. However, pain has been reported in children with HIV across the continuum of illness and should be assessed at every patient encounter (Czarniecki, Dollfus & Strafford, 1994; Hirschfeld, Moss & Dragisic, 1996).
   b. Pain results in adverse physiologic effects that can result in increased morbidity and mortality (Pediatric Supportive Care/Quality of Life Committee of the NIAID's Pediatric ACTG, 1995).
   c. Reported adverse effects of pain include biochemical effects similar to the stress response; physiologic changes, such as increased vital signs, autonomic changes, and decreased oxygen saturation; and peripheral blood flow.
   d. Untreated pain in children with HIV can lead to decreased appetite and weight loss, refusal of medications, decreased activity level, and depression (Oleske & Czarniecki, 1999).
   e. Abdominal pain syndromes in the HIV-infected child
      i. Mycobacterium avium causes continuous periumbilical pain. As it advances the pain can become severe. The proliferation of lymph tissue acts like a space-occupying lesion.
      ii. Cryptosporidiosis pain tends to be more intermittent and cramplike.
      iii. Acute pancreatitis has also been a source of abdominal pain.
   f. Oral, throat, and esophageal pain syndromes in children with HIV
      i. Candida, herpes, and cytomegalovirus (CMV) are agents responsible for causing thrush and esophagitis.
      ii. Dental caries, gingivitis, and aphthous ulcers are also sources of pain.
   g. Neurological sources of pain in children
      i. Cryptococcal meningitis causes headache.
      ii. HIV encephalopathy may cause hypertonicity and spasticity.
      iii. Postherpetic neuropathies may cause pain.
      iv. Peripheral neuropathy is secondary to some antiretroviral medications.
      v. Other sources of pain include musculoskeletal pain, chest pain, and total body pain.
   h. Treatment of HIV and procedures also are a source of pain.
      i. Diagnostic tests, such as venipuncture, lumbar puncture, skin testing, biopsies, and other invasive studies, are regular sources of pain for children with HIV.
      ii. Some antiretroviral medications have side effects that cause pain, particularly gastrointestinal discomfort and peripheral neuropathy.
   i. Pain in children with HIV is undertreated for various reasons.
      i. Clinicians caring for children with HIV are focused on controlling the virus, rather than alleviating symptoms.
      ii. HIV subspecialists lack education and training in pain management.
      iii. Pain is difficult to assess and treat in children with a complex disease, such as HIV.
      iv. Pediatric clinicians often believe certain myths about pain in children, which preclude their adequate management of it. These myths include the following:

      - Infants and young children do not experience pain as much as adults. Multiple studies have demonstrated that infants and young children have the physiologic capacity to experience pain.
      - All opioids are dangerous for infants and children. Even premature infants can receive opioids safely as long as doses are titrated carefully and specific physiologic

differences are taken into account.

- Opioids cause addiction. Multiple studies in adults and children have shown that the incidence of addiction from opioids used for pain is less than 1%.
- Children make up pain reports to get attention. Children's reports of pain have been found to be real.
- If a child can play or sleep, he or she has no pain. Children use play as a distraction from pain and, when exhausted, even if in pain, can fall asleep.

2. Nursing assessment
   a. Subjective
      i. Ask the child and caregiver about pain at every encounter. Ask, "Have you had any pain since your last clinic (office, emergency room) visit?"
      ii. Always take the child's report of pain at face value.
      iii. Explain to the child and the caregiver the importance of reporting pain.
      iv. Teach child to use a pain assessment scale and use the scale to assess severity of pain.
         (1) Good scales to use with children include face scales, body charts to color, and, for older children, numerical scales.
         (2) Consider family issues that might affect reports of child's pain (e.g., previous experience with pain in family, culture of family, experience with and fear of addiction).
   b. Objective
      i. Assess child for behavioral signs of pain, such as listlessness; crying; wincing; change in mood, sleep pattern, or activity level; and loss of concentration, playfulness, or interest in things usually enjoyed.
      ii. Consider a trial of pain medication when a patient is unable to report

pain but shows signs and symptoms of pain or has a problem that could be expected to cause pain.

3. Nursing diagnosis
   a. Pain
4. Goals
   a. Reduce incidence and severity of pain using pharmacologic and nonpharmacologic interventions.
   b. Achieve optimal level of patient comfort via the least invasive route.
5. Interventions and health teaching
   a. Nonpharmocological interventions
      i. Nonpharmacological interventions should be used in conjunction with, not instead of, pharmacologic management.
      ii. Nonpharmacological interventions can help children with episodic, chronic, and procedural pain.
      iii. Encourage parents to participate.
      iv. Take the time to teach the child and the caregiver about procedures and the intervention to be employed.
      v. Assess the coping style of the child and family:
         (1) Attenders: those who must know everything that is happening to them. Help them to participate.
         (2) Distractors: those who do not want to know anything and prefer to look away. This is the group for whom nonpharmacologic/behavioral interventions work best.
      vi. Specific intervention types
         (1) Distraction: blow bubbles, read pop-up books, look at "magic wands," sing, tell stories
         (2) Guided imagery: take a mental trip, use a "magic glove," use a mental TV pain knob to turn down pain
         (3) Breathing and relaxation: teach diaphragmatic breathing and muscle relaxation ("being like a rag doll")

(4) Cutaneous stimulation: use superficial heating and cooling, vibration, and massage (efficacy of these modalities has not been scientifically proven, but anecdotal evidence warrants their inclusion as possible options).

b. Pharmacological interventions

   i. General principles

     (1) The backbone of good pain management is pharmacologic treatment (McCaffery & Beebe, 1989).

     (2) The choice of medication is dictated by the cause, type, and severity of pain.

     (3) The dose of medication is determined by the child's weight and severity of pain.

     (4) Predictable, recurrent, or chronic pain is best treated with around-the-clock dosing or continuous administration (preventive approach) as opposed to PRN, allowing a constant blood level to be maintained and thereby decreasing the total amount of medication needed to control pain (Wishnie & Weisman, 1997).

     (5) Injections should be avoided as a route of pain medication administration in children.

     (6) Opioids are safe for infants and young children.

     (7) Monitor and treat side effects aggressively.

   ii. Pain medications: indications

     (1) Mild pain: Use nonopioids, such as acetaminophen or ibuprofen. Some pain may need treatment with a nonanalgesic (e.g., antacid for stomach pain). If pain is not relieved or worsens, add an opioid.

     (2) Moderate pain: Use a nonopioid and add another analgesic, such as codeine. If patient is unresponsive or pain worsens, change to a stronger opioid.

     (3) Severe pain: Begin with a strong opioid, such as morphine.

     (4) Procedural pain: Analgesia and anesthesia should be administered when doing any painful procedure. This minimizes trauma to the patient and prevents future procedure anxiety. The procedure can then be performed safely.

   iii. Use of nonopioids

     (1) Acetaminophen and nonsteroidal antiinflammatory (NSAIDs) relieve more pain than realized. Acetaminophen 325 mg can relieve as much pain as codeine 15 mg.

     (2) There is a ceiling effect on the dose. Higher doses than recommended do not relieve more pain and can cause toxicity.

     (3) When nonopioids no longer relieve pain, add opioids and keep the nonopioids. This can allow for a lower opioid dose because the pain is being targeted at both the peripheral and central levels. Examples of nonopioids include the following:

- Ibuprofen
- Acetaminophen
- Naproxen
- Choline magnesium trisalicylate
- Aspirin

   iv. Use of opioids

     (1) Titrate dose to effect. Can increase by 25–50% to reach pain control. Maintaining a steady level is safer than bolus doses. There is no ceiling on how high opioid doses can go. The dose should be that which relieves pain with the least amount

Table 9.1a   Equianalgesic Conversion Guide

The standard equianalgesic conversion is based on the pain relieving potential of 10 mg of parenteral morphine. To convert from the oral route to another route, or from one opioid to another, find the equianalgesic dose of the present opioid and the opioid you wish to convert to in the chart.
Multiply the 24 hour dose of the current drug by the dose of the new opioid from the equianalgesic conversion guide. Then divide by the dose of the new opioid. This will give you the 24 hour dose of the current opioid.

Drug	Onset (min)	Peak (h)	1 1/2 (h)	Equianalgesic Doses[1]	IV/IM (mg) Oral (mg)
Codeine	10-30	0.5-1	3	120	200
Fentanyl	7-8	ND	1.5-6	0.1	NA
Hydrocodone	ND	ND	3.3-4.5	ND	ND
Hydromorphone	15-30	0.5-1	2-3	1.5	7.5
Methadone	30-60	0.5-1	15-30	10	20
Morphine	15-60	0.5-1	1.5-2	10	60
Oxycodone, PO	15-30	1	ND	NA	30
Oxymorphone	5-10	0.5-1	ND	1	10[2]

ND = no data available; NA = not applicable

1. Based on acute, short-term use. Chronic administration may alter pharmacokinetics and decrease the oral:parenteral dose ratio. The morphine oral:parenteral ratio decreases to 1.5-2.5:1 upon chronic dosing.

2. Rectal.

of undesirable side effects.

(2) Initiate pain control with a short acting preparation to titrate dose. Once pain is stable, switch to a long-acting preparation.

(3) To switch opioids or routes use the equianalgesic chart (see Table 9.1a) (McCaffery & Beebe, 1989, pp. 78–79).

(4) Prevent and treat side effects (nausea, vomiting, itching, constipation) aggressively.

(5) Addiction from use of opioids for pain is a myth. Respiratory depression is a result of dosing errors, and can be prevented with care and knowledge.

(6) Examples of opioids include the following:

- Morphine sulfate
- Codeine
- Hydrocodone
- Oxycodone

- Methadone
- Fentanyl transdermal system

v. Local analgesia: Use local analgesia, such as eutectic mixture of local anesthetic (EMLA) or a mixed solution of tetracaine, adrenaline, and cocaine (TAC) for painful procedures, such as venipuncture and lumbar punctures.

vi. Adjuvants

(1) Adjuvants are medications commonly used for treating something other than pain but that have been found to relieve pain.

(2) Two main types of adjuvants are used: those that prevent or relieve side effects of opioids and those that potentiate opioids.

(3) Tricyclic antidepressants are good for neuropathic pain. Use cautiously in children with cardiac problems.

(4) Anticonvulsants, such as phenytoin, carbamazepine,

and clonazepam are second-line drugs for neuropathic pain.

(5) Anxiolytics, such as benzodiazepines, are good for anxiety but do not relieve pain.

(6) Antihistamines can relieve vomiting and itching and potentiate the pain relief given by opioids. Laxatives can prevent and treat constipation. Patients started on opioids should be started on a bowel program.

c. Alternative/Complementary therapies
   i. Aromatherapy
   ii. Therapeutic touch/Reiki
   iii. Homeopathy

6. Evaluation
   a. Continually reassess the patient's pain to determine the efficacy of nursing and medical interventions.
   b. Adjust doses, routes, and schedules to achieve maximum pain relief.

9.2 Anorexia

1. Etiology
   a. The 1st year of life is critical for adequate physical and psychological growth and development (Pipes, 1996).
   b. The amount of nutrients needed per body weight is greater in infancy than at any other time (Dudek, 2001).
      i Protein, vitamins, and minerals are vital for normal growth and development.
      ii Iron deficiency anemia is the most common nutritional deficiency in children; it is known to cause a delay in mental and physical development and can lower the body's resistance to infection (Pipes, 1996).
   c. Adolescence is a time of rapid growth, physically and psychologically, thus requiring additional nutrients, especially calories, protein, calcium, iron, and zinc (Dudek, 2001).
   d. Loss of appetite can be due to:
      i. Side effects of medications
      ii. Oral candidiasis

      iii. Encephalopathy or discordant swallowing
      iv. Upper gastrointestinal disease or inflammation (Pizzo & Wilfert, 1998)
      v. Depression or psychological stress
      vi. Eating disorder

2. Nursing assessment
   a. Subjective
      i. The parent or child reports loss of appetite, little interest in food, or the child not eating; the parent or child reports abdominal or oral pain or nausea on eating; familial attitude toward weight, thinness, and client's weight may be a factor.
      ii. Medication history, oral lesions, vomiting, diarrhea, flatus, gastrointestinal hypermotility, and change in affect/behavior.
   b. Objective
      i. Nutritional assessment of adolescents should include eating patterns, use of vitamin/mineral supplements—type, amount, and frequency; use of alcohol, tobacco, and other drugs; use of fad diets, methods and patterns of dieting and age client began dieting, and any events associated with eating pattern; and the intensity and frequency of physical activity (Dudek, 2001).

3. Nursing diagnosis
   a. Altered nutrition, less than body requirements.

4. Goals
   a. The child/adolescent's food intake will be sufficient enough to maintain body weight.

5. Interventions and health teaching
   a. Nonpharmacological interventions
      i. A nutritional assessment should be done initially and at each visit.
      ii. If an eating disorder is suspected, appropriate referrals should be made to mental health professional for counseling and treatment.
      iii. Fresh air and activity may also increase or stimulate appetite.

iv. Spicy, sweet, or highly flavored and favorite foods that are ethnically and age appropriate may stimulate the child's appetite.

v. All interventions must consider social and supportive concerns of eating with family and friends, and the child should be encouraged to participate in family and social meal activities.

b. Pharmacological interventions

i. Evaluate all medications; treat oral/esophageal infections or lesions as per standard.

ii. Appetite stimulants (e.g., megestrol acetate) have been used in treating appetite loss with consequent weight gain in children.

6. Evaluation (see following discussion on weight loss)

9.3. Weight Loss

1. Etiology

a. Failure to gain weight is defined as wasting in children and meets the Centers for Disease Control and Prevention's definition of a Class C AIDS–defining condition when one of the following conditions is met:

- Downward crossing of 2 percentile lines on standard weight-for-age growth chart in children > 1 year of age, or
- Persistent 10% loss of baseline body weight, or
- Weight < 5% on growth chart on two consecutive measurements 30 days apart and associated with chronic diarrhea or persistent (30 days) documented fever (Burr, 1996)

b. Anorexia is frequently a cause of weight loss (see Section 9.2)

c. Opportunistic infections (e.g., oral/esophageal candidiasis, mycobacterium avium complex, cryptosporidium, C. *difficile; Salmonella, Shigella, Campylobacter,* and other enteric pathogens)

d. HIV encephalopathy or neurological complications leading to discordant suck and swallowing, inability to chew and swallow, and time demands for feeding

e. Pain associated with oral lesions, poor dental hygiene or significant dental caries, abdominal cramps, and constipation

f. Fullness or discomfort related to organomegaly

g. Poor or inadequate food supply at home

h. Nausea and vomiting, particularly due to medication side effects

i. Fever (persistent, low grade)

j. Diarrhea (persisting > 1 month with ≥ two loose stools daily)

k. Poor absorption secondary to primary HIV infection in the gut

l. Endocrine abnormalities associated with HIV

2. Nursing assessment

a. Subjective

i. The parent or child reports poor or prolonged feedings or that child has difficulty swallowing, has a poor appetite, or refuses food.

ii. History of opportunistic infections, diarrhea, fever, food availability, and medications

b. Objective

i. Accurate serial measurements of height and weight plotted on standard growth curves and assessment of growth in relation to height and age

ii. Anthropometric data, body mass index (BMI), tricep skin-fold measurements (if available), and midarm circumference measurements

iii. Laboratory data, including chemistry panel, liver profile, vitamin B_{12}, fasting glucose and lipids (especially critical in infants and children because weight loss is usually caused by decreased muscle mass rather than body fat; Pizzo & Wilfert, 1998)

iv. Complete physical examination, including abdominal exam for masses or organomegaly, neurological exam, mental state, and oral and dental examination

v. Esophagogastroduodenoscopy to rule out esophagitis, gastritis, or duodenitis (Pizzo & Wilfert, 1998)

3. Nursing diagnosis
   a. Altered nutrition, less than body requirements

4. Goals
   a. The child/adolescent will maintain body weight appropriate to age and development

5. Interventions and health teaching
   a. Nonpharmacological interventions
      i. Refer patient to registered dietitian for full nutritional assessment and recommendations, including enteral or parenteral nutrition, or both.
      ii. Have the family complete a 2-day diet recall to assess caloric intake.
      iii. Evaluate for opportunistic infections that may affect eating or swallowing or the gastrointestinal tract (e.g., esophageal candidiasis, cyptosporidium).
      iv. Evaluate for malabsorption.
      v. Provide nutritional support with high-calorie supplements if gut is functioning.
      vi. Decisions regarding interventions for weight gain and management should have clearly defined short- and long-term goals.
      vii. The family must be involved in the decisions because they will bear the burden and be able to support such highly technical interventions.
   b. Pharmacological interventions
      i. Evaluate, diagnose, and treat opportunistic infections that interfere with oral intake or cause loss of food or fluids through diarrhea or malabsorption.
      ii. Consider use of nasogastric feedings prior (NG) to parenteral intervention.
         (1) NG feedings (bolus or continuous) can provide additional nutritional support or can be used as a main source of nutrition. For older and school-age children, this can be planned as a continuous feeding during sleep.
         (2) In cases of poor absorption, severe diarrhea, or malabsorption, total parenteral nutrition (TPN) should be considered for continued weight loss or during acute medical crises.

6. Evaluation
   a. Perform nutritional assessment, measure weight, review diet and nutritional intake, interview the family and child regarding symptoms and food and eating behaviors, and observe the child eating.
   b. Observe and interview the family and child to determine the extent and effectiveness of interventions.

9.4 Cognitive Impairment and Developmental Delay

1. Etiology
   a. Direct infection of the central nervous system (CNS)
      i. Cognitive, motor, language, and behavioral impairments in HIV-infected children are most often the result of direct infection of the CNS by the virus infecting macrophages and microglia, causing a release of toxic substances into the brain.
      ii. These processes are thought to result in damage to the white matter of the brain, demyelination of nerve tracks, and alterations in the blood brain barrier, which

cause cerebral atrophy; ventricular enlargements; calcifications in the basal ganglia, cerebellum, and subcortical frontal white matter; reduction in white matter; and a process of demyelination (Belman et al., 1988; Mintz, 1999; Mitchell, 2001).

b. Opportunistic infections, secondary to immunodeficiency: Although less common, neurological deficits in children have been shown to be secondary effects of infections such as toxoplasmosis, herpes simplex, and cytomegalovirus (CMV) (Belman et al., 1988; Mintz, 1999; Mitchell, 2001).

c. Neoplasms, strokes, metabolic abnormalities, and sensory impairments due to repeated infections (e.g., hearing loss) (Armstrong, Seidel, & Swales, 1993)

d. HIV progressive encephalopathy
   i. Associated with advanced disease; characterized by cognitive impairment, poor brain growth, abnormalities of motor function and tone, movement disorders, language impairment, and mood and behavioral problems (Belman, 1997).
   ii. Severe form: rapid deterioration and loss of previously acquired milestones; less severe form: developmental plateau or marked delays in acquiring milestones and progressive deterioration (Belman, 1997)

e. Static encephalopathy: characterized by delayed brain development but without deterioration of previously acquired skills; more common than progressive encephalopathy. Cognitive abilities often range from low average to markedly impaired (Belman, 1997).

f. Specific deficits: Many children will not exhibit global deficits or delays in their neurocognitive functioning; however, they can experience specific functional deficits in the areas of memory, processing speed, motor abilities, executive functioning (e.g., problem-solving ability, planning ability), visual-spatial and perceptual-organizational skills, language development, attention, and social-emotional regulation (Bisiacchi, Suppiej, & Laverda, 2000; Tardieu et al., 1995; Wachsler-Felder, & Golden, 2002).

g. Comorbid factors: Other risk factors often seen in HIV-infected children include prenatal drug exposure, poor or no prenatal care, birth complications or prematurity, poor nutrition, limited stimulation during critical periods of development, chronically or terminally ill parents, and maternal death (Armstrong et al., 1993).

2. Nursing assessment
   a. Subjective
      i. Parents report concerns about the child's rate of milestone achievement (e.g., delays in sitting up, crawling, walking, or talking for infants and toddlers); preschoolers not learning age-appropriate skills (e.g., ABCs, letter, number, or color recognition), lack of coordination, gait disturbance when walking, and poor communication skills (e.g., cannot communicate clearly, not using sentences to communicate).
      ii. Parents or school-age children, or both, report difficulty in school or difficulty paying attention in class.
   b. Objective
      i. Many children will exhibit global deficits or delays in their developmental level or neurocognitive functioning. Others experience specific functional deficits in memory, processing speed, motor abilities, executive functioning, visual-spatial and perceptual-organizational skills, language development, attention, and social-emotional regulation.
      ii. Assess physical growth, serial head circumference in young children, viral load and CD_4 count and screen hearing and vision.
      iii. For infants, toddlers, and preschoolers, assess acquisition of motor, language, cognitive, and

social-emotional milestones through observation, Denver Developmental Screen, or parent interview. Observe child walking to assess for gait disturbance, toe walking, hyperreflexia and hypertonicity in lower extremities, spasticity, or clumsiness/poor coordination. Assess language development, including vocabulary, articulation, and clarity of speech. Evaluate current developmental status relative to previously achieved status and assess for deterioration or loss of previously acquired milestones or slowed development of new skills.

    iv. For school-age children and adolescents, ask whether the child is having difficulty keeping up in school or completing class work and homework, failing any classes, or being held back a grade. Assess whether the child is having difficulty concentrating or focusing, sitting still, following directions, or staying on task. Ask the parent if any changes in child's processing speed, attention, memory, judgment, or problem-solving skills have been observed. Also assess for changes in motor functioning, including clumsiness, poor balance, or poor fine motor coordination.

3. Nursing diagnosis
   a. Alteration in growth and development and visual or auditory sensation or perception
   b. Impaired communication and physical mobility related to HIV infection or its complications

4. Goals
   a. Child has been appropriately evaluated by a clinical psychologist, speech pathologist, occupational and physical therapist (OT/PT), and other specialists as indicated to determine current level of developmental and neurocognitive functioning and to determine eligibility for intervention services.
   b. Child is receiving intervention services (e.g., educational intervention, speech therapy, OT/PT) as needed for developmental or neurocognitive delays.
   c. Child's pain has been evaluated and addressed with pain management strategies.
   d. Family has been educated about child's current level of functioning and appropriate expectations for child given any identified deficits.
   e. Child and family have been linked with mental health intervention to help them cope with the child's special needs, compromised physical or mental status, and psychosocial aspects of HIV disease.
   f. Child is receiving regular monitoring and evaluation to ensure that all developmental, behavioral, and emotional needs are being adequately addressed.

5. Interventions and health teaching
   a. Nonpharmacological interventions
      i. Refer to clinical psychologist, speech pathologist, occupational and physical therapist, and other specialists as indicated to determine current level of developmental and neurocognitive functioning and to determine if intervention is needed.
      ii. For intervention services, infants through age 3, refer to early intervention program; for preschoolers, make referrals to special education preschool programs through their local school system; for school-age children and adolescents, refer children to the special education coordinator of their school to develop an Individualized Education Plan to address school interventions. Liaison with the school system and complete a 504 form if the child needs any nonacademic accommodations (e.g., rest periods/shortened day due to fatigue, classes close together to reduce walking, access to elevators, special transportation assistance).

b. Pharmacological interventions
  i. HAART to address declines in functioning
  ii. Pain medications as indicated
  iii. Psychostimulants to address attention problems
c. Alternative/complementary therapies
  i. Behavioral strategies to address attention problems
  ii. After-school programs or supplemental tutoring to address delays
  iii. Educational computer programs or games, workbooks, flashcards, library programs

6. Evaluation
  a. Assess whether child is making gains developmentally or is improving in skills.
  b. Assess whether child is doing better in school with assistance or whether additional accommodations or interventions are needed.
  c. Assess whether child's attention and behavior are being managed or whether additional interventions are needed.
  d. Assess whether child and family's emotional needs are being addressed or whether additional mental health intervention is indicated to help child cope with illness-related stressors and disabilities.
  e. Determine if additional advocacy is needed to assist family in obtaining services for child. If indicated, refer family to child advocacy program for assistance.

9.5 Fever

1. Etiology
  a. Fever is defined as an elevation in normal body temperature, which ranges from 97°F to 99°F orally (36°C to 37.2°C, 1° higher if the temperature is taken rectally).
  b. Equally important is recognizing that hypothermia (rectal temperature of less than 96.8°F or 36.0°C) in infancy can be associated with serious infectious diseases (Baraff et al., 1993).
  c. The evaluation of temperature in an HIV-infected child with an unexplained

fever should be guided by the clinical presentation. Multiple infections may coexist concurrently in the HIV-infected child (Nicholas, 1991, p. S21).
  d. Children with HIV infection are deficient in circulating antibodies. Even in children who are hypergammaglobulinemic, antibodies are not specific and do not function normally (Dorfman, Crain, & Bernstein, 1990).
  e. Some HIV-infected children have fever frequently (daily or several times per week) without any obvious underlying infection other than HIV (Nicholas, 1991, p. S21).
  f. Fever heralds many HIV-related opportunistic infections (OIs), including infections of the respiratory and urinary tract and central nervous system, abscesses, gingivitis, gastroenteritis, drug reactions, and lymphoma, as well as noninfectious processes.

2. Nursing assessment
  a. Subjective
    i. Review of systems: vomiting, diarrhea, lethargy, rashes, cough, congestion, increased irritability, and temperature duration
    ii. Activity level: listlessness, increased sleep, lack of interest in play, and so on
    iii. Elimination patterns: diarrhea, vomiting, fewer wet diapers, and decreased urine output
    iv. Eating habits: decreased oral intake, not waking to eat
    v. Exposure history: infectious diseases, animals (cats, dogs, reptiles, farm animals, birds), molds, day care (large or small), well/city water at home, older/newer home; recent restaurant visits, exposure to anyone from a foreign country, incarceration, residence in a halfway house
    vi. Travel history: outside of the state (which states), outside of the country
    vii. Recent immunizations
    viii. Recent medications

b. Objective
   i. Measure weight, height, temperature, pulse, respiration, and blood pressure (head circumference for children ≤ 12 months).
   ii. Assess general appearance.
   iii. Complete a physical examination.
   iv. Take a complete blood cell count with differential.
   v. Obtain a blood culture (if the child has a central venous catheter or port specimens, blood culture must be obtained from these sites as well).
   vi. Other tests that should be considered include the following (Nicholas, 1991):

   - Chest radiograph
   - Pulse oximetry
   - Urinalysis
   - Urine culture (obtained by suprapubic aspiration or catheterization)
   - Lumbar puncture

3. Nursing diagnosis: include those for which the child/parent/guardian is at risk (Carpenito, 2002)
   a. Anxiety
   b. Risk for imbalanced body temperature
   c. Impaired comfort
   d. Risk for infection
4. Goals
   a. Stabilize patient clinically.
   b. Identify source of fever.
   c. Communicate test results and plan of care in a timely fashion to patient/parent/guardian.
5. Interventions and health teaching
   a. Nonpharmacological interventions
      i. The principle rationale for treating fever is relief of discomfort, and there is no general level of temperature that requires treatment (Whaley & Wong, 1993).
      ii. Cooling procedures such as sponging or tepid baths have been shown to be ineffective in treating fever, either alone or in combination with antipyretics, and they inflict considerable discomfort on the child.

   iii. Repeat cultures to verify sterility and if fever persists or clinical deterioration occurs.
   iv. Collect lab specimens and evaluate need for other diagnostic procedures.
   v. Guidelines for parents of HIV-infected child with fever (Whaley & Wong, 1987, p. 1119): Call your primary care provider immediately if:

   - Child is < 6 months of age
   - Fever is > 101°F for more than 24 hours
   - Child is crying inconsolably
   - Child is difficult to awaken
   - Child is confused or delirious
   - Child has had a seizure
   - Child has a stiff neck
   - Child has purple spots on the skin
   - Breathing is difficult and the child does not feel better after the nose is cleared
   - Child is acting very sick

b. Pharmacological interventions
   i. Empirical treatments are best avoided but may be acceptable when both the clinical suspicion of infection is high and the risk from a delay in starting treatment is significant (Dorfman, Crain, & Berstein, 1990; Nicholas, 1991).
   ii. Acetaminophen for discomfort
   iii. Organism specific antibiotics
c. Alternative/complementary therapies
   i. Reiki therapy: Universal life force energy is facilitated through the practitioner's hand and naturally goes to the places in the recipient's body in which it is needed. Universal life force energy is connected to the body's innate power of healing and promotes physical, mental, emotional, and spiritual self-healing (Nield-Anderson & Ameling, 2001, p. 42).
   ii. Touch therapy: used to promote relaxation, reduce pain, and accelerate the healing process

(Wardell & Engebretson, 2001, p. 439)

6. Evaluation
   a. Evaluate patient's response to the febrile symptoms and their treatment.
   b. Criteria for hospital admission (Nicholas, 1991, p. S22)
      i. Temperature > 105°F (40.5°C)
      ii. Marked leukocytosis (white blood cell count > 25,000 cells/mm³)
      iii. Marked immature neutrophils
      iv. The diagnostic procedures used to work up the patient depend on the presenting symptoms (Nicholas, 1991).
   c. Evaluation in the febrile HIV-positive child with focal findings
      i. Meningeal signs: lumbar puncture
      ii. Severe oral thrush: consider a barium esophagram
      iii. Respiratory distress: chest radiograph, pulse oximetry, or arterial blood gas; depending on the severity, consider gallium scan, bronchoalveolar lavage
      iv. Diarrhea: stool smear for white blood cells, stool culture for bacteria, examination for ova and parasites
      v. Dehydration: serum electrolytes
      vi. Bone or joint pain: consider bone scan, radiographs, bone or joint aspirations
   d. Expand the diagnostic evaluation when a child's condition deteriorates or when the frequency or pattern of fever noticeably changes (Nicholas, 1991, p. S23).

9.6 Skin Lesions

1. Etiology
   a. Pathogenesis of cutaneous manifestations (Torre, Zeroli, Fiori, Ferraro, & Speranza, 1991, p. 197)
      i. Immune system deficiencies
         (1) The incidence, multiplicity, and severity of cutaneous manifestations are related to the level of immunosuppression (CD$_4$ cells < 100 cells/mm³).
         (2) Children with CD$_4$ counts of < 500 cells/mm³ commonly have skin lesions, oral candidiasis, molluscum contagiosum, recurrent aphthous ulcers, seborrheic dermatitis, ichthyosis, and xerosis.
      ii. Nutritional deficiencies: zinc, niacin, and ascorbic acid
      iii. Drug reactions and hypersensitivity: trimethoprim-sulfamethoxazole
   b. Cutaneous manifestations associated with HIV infection in children
      i. Neoplasm (very rare): Kaposi's sarcoma, lymphoma
      ii. Infectious manifestations
         (1) Viral: herpes simplex, varicella-zoster virus, molluscum contagiosum, and condyloma acuminata (venereal warts)
         (2) Bacterial: skin abscesses, cellulitis, persistent folliculitis, impetigo, and mycobacterium avium-intracellulare infection
         (3) Fungal: candida albicans, cheilitis, cryptococcus, tinea faciale, tinea corporis, and onychomycosis
      iii. Vascular lesions: seborrheic dermatitis, atopic dermatitis, and drug reactions
      iv. Other infectious agents: sarcoptes scabiei (scabies)
      v. Other cutaneous manifestations: nonspecific rashes
      vi. Nutritional deficiencies: zinc and vitamin C deficiencies
2. Nursing assessment
   a. Subjective
      i. Review of systems (birthmarks, rashes, skin type), current illness, current medications, allergies (type of reaction), and recent immunizations.
      ii. Exposure to infectious diseases, animals, and sick contacts
      iii. Travel history
   b. Objective
      i. Complete, careful inspection of the entire cutaneous surface

    ii. Identification and description of primary lesion and secondary changes

    iii. Color, arrangement, distribution, location, and associated symptoms

3. Nursing diagnosis
   a. Disturbed body image
   b. Impaired comfort
   c. Risk for infection
   d. Impaired skin integrity

4. Goals
   a. Prevent secondary infection
   b. Relieve pruritus
   c. Identify the rash or associated disease process

5. Interventions and health teaching
   a. Nonpharmacological interventions
      i. Oral candidiasis: Plaques cannot be removed with a moistened swab; call immediately if infant refuses liquids; diaper rash may occur concomitantly.
      ii. Molluscum contagiosum: Although highly contagious, lesions are benign.
      iii. Aphthous ulcers: Recurrences are usually irregular, several months apart; healing occurs in 7 to 10 days, without scarring.
      iv. Seborrheic dermatitis: Use bland shampoos (Selsun Blue, Head & Shoulders), leaving on for 10 to 15 minutes and then rinsing; continue treatment for several days after lesions disappear.
      v. Ichthyosis: Hydrate the skin twice daily (Aquaphor, Lubriderm, fragrance-free Eucerin cream).
      vi. Xerosis: Limit daily bath or shower to 5 to 10 minutes. Use warm water and mild soaps. Apply emollients 2 to 3 times per day (Aquaphor, Lubriderm), and consider need to restrict diet (dairy products, eggs, citrus).
      vii. Herpes simplex: Recurrences are common at the same site, preceded by a burning or tingling sensation; transmission occurs through direct contact.
      viii. Varicella zoster: Recommend baking soda or Aveno oatmeal bath; call if child develops a high fever, a stiff neck, a headache, cough, or dyspnea or if the child exhibits vomiting, listlessness, hyperirritability or breaks out with new lesions after 7 days.
      ix. Impetigo: Remove crusts by gently washing with warm water and an antiseptic soap (phisoHex, Dial, Betadine); call primary care provider immediately if dark-colored urine, decreased urinary output, or edema is noted.
      x. Tinea corporis (ringworm): transmitted by direct/indirect contact; thrives in moist areas; generally takes 1 to 3 weeks for effective cure
      xi. Scabies: acquired by close personal contact; launder with hot water and detergent, use hot dryer
      xii. Nutritional deficiencies
         (1) Zinc: important for cellular metabolism, growth, and repair; signs of deficit include anorexia, growth retardation, skin changes, and immunological abnormalities.
         (2) Vitamin C: essential for collagen formation and function, promotes growth and tissue repair, enhances iron absorption, improves wound healing; signs of deficit include scurvy, cracked lips, bleeding gums, slow wound healing, and easy bruising.
   b. Pharmacological interventions
      i. Oral candidiasis (thrush)
         (1) Topical agents
            (a) Infants and young children: Nystatin oral suspension (200,000 to 800,000 U/day in 4 divided doses). Treat for 14 days.
            (b) Older children: Nystatin oral pastilles (200,000 U/day or 2 oral pastilles 5 times daily) or Clotrimazole oral troches (10 mg, 1 tablet 5 times daily). Treat for 14 days.

(2) Systemic antifungal therapy: Reserved for children who do not improve after 5 to 7 days of topical therapy and those with severe lesions interfering with normal hydration and nutrition

    (a) Fluconazole 6 mg/kg (vs. ketoconazole) is preferred for its more reliable gastrointestinal absorption, fewer medication interactions, and less-common hepatotoxicity. A short course: Five to 7 days of systemic therapy usually suffices, with completion of a longer course of topical therapy.

(3) Relapses and recurrences are common and may require prophylactic or maintenance therapy: nystatin 100,000 to 400,000 U daily by mouth twice daily), clotrimazole 10 mg by mouth twice daily, or fluconazole administered either daily or weekly.

ii. Molluscum contagiosum: Satisfactory therapy is unavailable; cryotherapy and curettage have been used in persons with relatively few lesions; local irritants (e.g., cantharidrin, podophyllin, or tretinoin) also can be used (dangerous around the eye).

iii. Recurrent aphthous ulcers usually resolve spontaneously, use oral analgesics, topical anesthetics, antibacterial mouth rinses with chlorhexidine (0.12%), or topical steroids if severe.

iv. Seborrheic dermatitis: Use 1% hydrocortisone cream BID or TID for lesions other than scalp; should see improvement in 10 to 14 days.

v. Herpes simplex: acyclovir 10 mg/kg orally 4 to 5 times per day.

    (1) Children with severe lesions or an inability to take oral liquids should be treated intravenously (10 mg/kg every 8 hours).

    (2) Frequently recurring cutaneous or oral herpetic lesions may require prophylactic oral acyclovir (10 mg/kg 2 to 3 times daily).

vi. Varicella-zoster virus

    (1) Uncomplicated chickenpox or herpes zoster: oral acyclovir (20 mg/kg 4 times daily; maximum dose, 800 mg 4 times daily)

    (2) Severe disease, evidence of visceral dissemination, inability to take oral liquids: intravenous acyclovir (10 mg/kg every 8 hours)

    (3) Chronic disease that does not respond to acyclovir therapy and suggests drug resistance may respond to foscarnet.

vii. Condyloma acuminata (Starr, 2000b, p. 1053): No treatment eradicates this disease.

    (1) Patient applied: Podofilox 0.5% solution or gel twice a day for 3 days, no treatment for 4 days, for a total of 4 cycles (contraindicated in pregnancy); imiquimod 5% cream applied with finger at bedtime 3 times a week for up to 16 weeks.

    (2) Provider applied: cryotherapy (liquid nitrogen or cryoprobe every 1 to 2 weeks); podophyllin resin 10% to 25% in benzoin (washed off in 1 to 4 hours to decrease local irritation, repeated weekly contraindicated in pregnancy); trichloroacetic acid; bichloroacetic acid, surgical removal

viii. Staphylococcal infections (Nelson & Bradley, 2000)

    (1) Skin abscesses: cephalexin 50 to 75 mg/kg/day PO divided q 8 hours or cloxacillin 50 mg/kg/day q 6 hours; × 5 to 10 days

(2) Folliculitis: if superficial, may be treated with topical kerolytics, such as benzoyl peroxide gels; systemic therapy is Dicloxacillin 15 to 50 mg/kg/day PO q 6 hours for 7 to 10 days.

(3) Cellulitis (Nelson & Bradley, 2000): oxacillin 150 mg/kg/day IV q 6 hours or cefazolin 100mg/kg/day IV q 8 hours, then cephalexin 50 to 75 mg/kg/day q 8 hours or cloxacillin 50 mg/kg/day PO q 6 hours; × 7 to 10 days

ix. Impetigo (Boynton, Dunn, & Stephens, 1988)

(1) Apply topical antibiotic ointment (Neosporin/ Bacitracin).

(2) Nonbullous impetigo: penicillin VK 250 mg PO QID for 10 days (if allergic to penicillin, give erythromycin 250 mg PO QID for 10 days)

(3) Bullous impetigo: dicloxacillin 250 mg PO QID for 10 days or erythromycin 250 mg PO QID for 10 days

x. Tinea corporis

(1) Topical antifungals (Boynton, Dunn, & Stephens, 1988): clotrimazole (Lotrimin, Myclex 1%) tid, miconazole TID until 1 to 2 weeks after tinea is resolved, a minimum of 4 weeks

(2) Extensive infection unresponsive to topical treatment (Starr, 2000a, p. 1080): griseofulvin for 4 to 8 weeks

xi. Onychomycosis (Nelson & Bradley, 2000): itraconazole 200 mg PO BID or terbinafine 500 mg daily, treat for 1 week per month × 3 months for hands; 1 week per month × 6 months for toes

xii. Scabies (Starr, 2000a, p. 1095): permethrin 5% cream (Elimite)

(1) Apply a thin layer of scabicide to the entire body, excluding the eyes. Apply for 8 to 14 hours and rinse. Should be reapplied in 7 days on all symptomatic patients.

(2) Areas of special importance are under the fingernails, on the scalp, behind the ears, in all folds and creases, and on the feet and hands.

c. Alternative/complementary therapies

i. Atopic dermatitis (Blosser, 2000, p. 1334)

(1) Herbal treatment approach: Evening primrose oil (use 4 to 12 weeks for benefit). Infants and children: 4 caps/day (300 grams) PO; adolescents: 8 to 12 caps/day PO

(a) Benefit: decreased scaling, itching, and general severity; contains high amounts of fatty acid that children with eczema are thought to have a defect in metabolizing

(b) Side effects: very safe; rare, mild gastrointestinal (GI) effects, headache

ii. Skin irritation and diaper rash

(1) Herbal treatment approach: aloe vera. For all ages, use pure gel form and apply topically several times daily (Blosser, 2000, p. 1347).

(a) Benefit: antibacterial effects; accelerates healing. Possible side effects: contact dermatitis

(2) Nutritional treatment approach: Zinc (infants 10 mg/day for formula-fed infants with a history of yeast diaper rashes)

(a) Benefit: may help prevent yeast diaper rash in infants

6. Evaluation

   a. Determine whether the child has had an allergic condition or a previous skin disease.

   b. Determine when the lesion or symptom first became apparent as well as whether it is related to ingestion of a food or other substance, any medication that the child is taking, or activity such as contact with plants, insects, or chemicals.

   c. Rule out possibility of the condition being related to a systemic disease.

   d. Diagnostic modalities include microscopic examination, cultures, skin biopsy, cytodiagnosis, complete blood count with differential, and sedimentation rate (ESR).

   e. Document improvement of rash with current therapy (if no improvement, reevaluate or consult dermatologist).

   f. Measure and mark affected areas and examine for resolution or continued spread.

   g. Have patient disrobe completely; use good light and magnification if needed.

   h. Counsel the family about whom to call if rash worsens or shows no signs of resolution in expected time frame (depends on the rash).

References

Armstrong, F. D., Seidel, J. F., & Swales, T. P. (1993). Pediatric HIV infection: A neuropsychological and educational challenge. *Journal of Learning Disabilities, 26*, 92–103.

Baraff, L., Bass, J., Fleisher, G., Klein, J., McCracken, G., & Powell, K., et al. (1993). Practice guidelines for the management of infants and children 0–36 months of age with fever without source. *Pediatrics, 93*, 1–12.

Belman, A. L. (1997). Pediatric neuro-AIDS. *Neuroimaging Clinics of North America, 7*(3), 593–613.

Belman, A. L., Diamond, G., Dickson, D., Horoupian, D., Llena, J., Lantos, G., et al. (1988). Pediatric acquired immunodeficiency syndrome. Neurologic syndromes. *American Journal of Diseases of Children, 142*, 29–35.

Bisiacchi, P. S., Suppiej, A., & Laverda, A. (2000). Neuropsychological evaluation of neurologically asymptomatic HIV-infected children. *Brain and Cognition, 43*, 49–52.

Blosser, C. (2000). Complementary medicine. In C. Burns, M. Brady, A. Dunn, & N. Starr (Eds.), *Pediatric primary care: A handbook for nurse practitioners* (pp. 1310–1351). Philadelphia: W.B. Saunders.

Boynton, R., Dunn, E., & Stephens, G. (1988). *Manual of ambulatory pediatrics.* Glenview, IL: Scott Foresman.

Burr, C. K. (1996). Clinical management of pediatric patients. In K. McMahon Casey, F. Cohen, & A. M. Hughes (Eds.), *ANAC's core curriculum for HIV/AIDS nursing* (pp. 389–391). Philadelphia: Nursecom.

Carpenito, L. (2002). *Handbook of nursing diagnosis.* Philadelphia, PA: Lippincott.

Czarniecki, L., Dollfus, C., Strafford, M. (1994). Children with pain and HIV/AIDS. In D. Carr & R. Addison (Ed.), *Pain in HIV/AIDS.* Washington DC: France-USA Pain Association.

Dorfman, D., Crain, E., & Bernstein, L. (1990). Care of febrile children with HIV infection in the emergency department. *Pediatric Emergency Care, 6*, 305–310.

Dudek, S. G. (2001). *Nutrition essentials for nursing practice.* Philadelphia: Lippincott, Williams & Wilkins.

Hirschfeld, S., Moss, H. Dragisic, K., et al. (1996). Pain in pediatric human immunodeficiency virus infection: Incidence and characteristics in a single-institution pilot study. *Pediatrics, 98*(3), 449–456.

McCaffery, M., & Beebe, A. (1989). *Pain. Clinical manual for nursing practice.* St. Louis, MO: Mosby.

Mintz, M. (1999). Clinical features and treatment interventions for human immunodeficiency virus-associated neurologic disease in children. *Seminars in Neurology, 19*, 165–176.

Mitchell, W. (2001). Neurological and developmental effects of HIV and AIDS in children and adolescents. *Mental Retardation and Developmental Disabilities Research Review, 7*, 211–216.

Nelson, J., & Bradley, J. (2000). *Nelson's pocket book of pediatric antimicrobial therapy.* Philadelphia: Lippincott Williams & Wilkins.

Nicholas, S. (1991). Management of the HIV-positive child with fever. *Journal of Pediatrics, 119*, S21-S24.

Nield-Anderson, L., & Ameling, A. (2001). Reiki: A complementary therapy for nursing practice. *Journal of Psychosocial Nursing, 39*, 42–49.

Oleske, J., & Czarniecki, L. (1999). Continuum of palliative care: Lessons from caring for children infected with HIV-1. *The Lancet, 354*, 1287–1291.

Pediatric Supportive Care/Quality of Life Committee of the NIAID's Pediatric ACTG. (1995). Enhancing supportive care and promoting quality of life: Clinical practice guidelines. *Pediatric AIDS and HIV Infection: Fetus to Adolescent, 6*(4), 187–203.

Pipes, P. (1996). Nutrition during infancy. In B. S. Worthington-Roberts & S. Rodwell Williams (Eds.), *Nutrition throughout the life cycle* (pp. 236–237). New York: McGraw-Hill.

Pizzo, P. A., & Wilfert, C. M. (1998). *Pediatric AIDS—The challenge of HIV infection in infants, children, and adolescents* (pp. 516–531). Baltimore: Lippincott Williams & Wilkins.

Starr, N. (2000a). Dermatological diseases. In C. Burns, M. Brady, A. Dunn, & N. Starr (Eds.), *Pediatric primary care: A handbook for nurse practitioners* (pp. 1059–1133). Philadelphia: W. B. Saunders.

Starr, N. (2000b). Gynecological conditions. In C. Burns, M. Brady, A. Dunn, & N. Starr (Eds.), *Pediatric primary care: A handbook for nurse practitioners* (pp. 1022–1058). Philadelphia: W. B. Saunders.

Tardieu, M., Mayaux, M. J., Seibel, N., Funck-Bretano, I., Straub, E., Teglas, J. P., et al. (1995). Cognitive assessment of school-age children infected with maternally transmitted human immunodeficiency virus type 1. *Journal of Pediatrics, 126,* 375–379.

Torre, D., Zeroli, C., Fiori, G., Ferraro, G., & Speranza, F. (1991). Dermatologic manifestations of AIDS in children. *Pediatrician, 18,* 195–203.

Wachsler-Felder, J. L., & Golden, C. J. (2002). Neuropsychological consequences of HIV in children: A review of the current literature. *Clinical Psychology Review, 22*(3), 441–462.

Wardell, D., & Engebretson, J. (2001). Biological correlates of Reiki touch healing. *Journal of Advanced Nursing, 33,* 439–445.

Whaley, L., & Wong, D. (1987). *Nursing care of infants and children.* St. Louis, MO: Mosby.

Whaley, L., & Wong, D. (1993). *Nursing care of infants and children.* St. Louis, MO: Mosby.

Wishnie, E., & Weisman, S. J. (1997). Children with AIDS. Pain syndromes and unique issues of assessment and management. *Child and Adolescent Psychiatric Clinics of North America, 6*(4), 863–878.

Section X

Psychosocial Concerns of the HIV-Infected Infant and Child and Their Significant Others

A child with a chronic illness has multiple ongoing needs, including interventions to mitigate the multiple psychosocial responses to illness. Questions about disclosure, schooling, friendships, dating, and death are appropriate and must be incorporated in the plan of care. Section X is a collection of experts in this field who provide important conceptual and practical information when approaching the child and family who have psychosocial concerns related to HIV infection.

10.1 Decision Making and Family Autonomy

1. Decision-making styles vary among individuals, within and between groups (e.g., medical team vs. family) and may significantly impact the outcome of treatment. Therefore, be aware of decision-making styles and use them in assessing the effectiveness of a treatment plan.
2. Styles of decision making
   a. Autocratic or authoritarian (top-down): One individual makes all decisions without input from others.
      i. This style may fail to anticipate potential conflicts, impediments, or factors that can negatively impact treatment.
      ii. With one primary decision maker in a family, it is helpful to offer alternative viewpoints that may need to be considered. Suggest the inclusion of others who are perceived as helpful or supportive (a second in command).
   b. Inclusive: An individual seeks input, assigns members to research issues prior to final decision making, attempts to identify problems, and suggest solutions before implementing a plan.
      i. Limited agreement (not necessarily consensus) is usually a goal.
      ii. There is potential for too much input, which can delay a needed decision. An identified primary person or consensus is needed.
   c. Passive: An individual succumbs to outside influences (e.g., individuals, policies, money) without exploring resources or the impact those influences may have on treatment. This style can lead to feelings of ineffectiveness and may delay a decision until a crisis forces one.
3. Types of decisions common to HIV care
   a. Testing
      i. Often families learn that siblings need testing when one child in the family is diagnosed.
      ii. Decisions regarding testing include which tests to perform; communication decisions related to staff, family members, child welfare agencies, or all three; informed consent; and sharing of results and the meaning of those results.
      iii. Families need time to process how positive test results may impact their lives, and they need simple, clear, and practical written information about what to expect. The prospect of caring for a potentially ill child can be overwhelming; some caregivers are reluctant to take on this role.
   b. Treatment
      i. Families with an HIV-infected child need to make decisions about available treatment options and whether those options are helpful given the health status of the child and the family supports.
      ii. Single-parent households may need help identifying their support system or need assistance navigating institutional systems.
      iii. Factors that affect treatment decisions may include the caregivers' HIV status, their health beliefs, the support or resources available to them, and their sense of trust or mistrust of the clinician or team.
      iv. Supports and resources can be family members, friends, hospital personnel, and clergy, who provide emotional, financial, physical, and concrete assistance when needed. The assistance may include attending clinic visits and providing or arranging transportation, food assistance, respite, or help with entitlement applications.
   c. Antiretroviral therapy and other treatments
      i. Families and clinicians struggle with when and if to start antiretroviral medications, particularly when the child is asymptomatic.

ii. Families may be reluctant to burden their child who appears healthy with daily medicines and possible side effects.

iii. Respect family reluctance and acknowledge their confusion while educating them (in understandable terms) about disease progression and treatment options.

    (1) Explore beliefs about taking medication. Disagreements between clinician and family on starting treatment early may result in nonadherence and the development of viral resistance, which can compromise future treatment. Does the family have the resources (financial, emotional, etc.)? Is the household disorganized and chaotic with little structure for getting routine tasks done? Does the caregiver have a backup plan for giving medicine if they are unavailable? Would they be willing to involve a school nurse or extended family members?

    (2) Families must know when a medication is required (e.g., PCP prophylaxis) and the consequences of not adhering.

d. Quality of life issues

i. HAART has lessened the burden of HIV disease on children and caregivers. However, the dilemma for many families is the benefit of suppressing viral load versus side effects, daily struggles with the child, and disruption of family life.

e. Enrollment in study protocols

i. The Tuskegee Syphilis Study has made African Americans and others wary of medical research and medical practitioners (Gamble, 1997).

ii. Families may be concerned that their children are being used as guinea pigs in studies. Open discussion of these concerns is critical for gaining the trust the family.

iii. Families have the right to refuse to participate in studies and must be reassured that their refusal will not affect their child's care.

f. Complementary treatments

i. Many families use alternative or complementary medicines and therapies. This should be acknowledged early in the treatment relationship. Families should be encouraged to discuss what, if any, alternative treatments they use so that the effects of both treatments and possible interactions can be assessed.

g. Disclosure

i. One of the most difficult decisions for parents/guardians is that of disclosure. The stigma of HIV/AIDS exists. Many parents fear that their child will be isolated, ostracized, made fun of, or discriminated against (see Section 10.5).

h. End of life issues

4. Family autonomy

a. Families need to have the sense of being capable of independent action, the ability to provide for ones own needs.

b. Families need independence from control of others (Barker, 1995).

c. Most families have a sense of autonomy. They determine what they need and make decisions without input from nonfamily members; decisions are made by the parent or parents. However, for families who receive care for chronic illness it is quite easy for decision-making boundaries to be blurred. The nature of chronic illness requires that decisions be made on many issues. New treatments, medications, referrals to agencies, and each intervention are perceived as helpful, but each comes with loss of privacy and independence.

d. Decision-making assistance

i. Boundaries

    (1) Many families rely on the advice of the clinician for

medical decisions and social concerns.

(a) It is not the provider's job to dictate treatment but to provide all available information in a way that is understandable, so the family can determine what is in their best interest.

(b) Boundaries help define roles for both the family and the provider. For a family to maintain as much autonomy as possible, providers need to recognize boundaries. Providers who become too friendly in building rapport place undo burden on families. When a family feels that their provider is their friend, they may agree to things they would not normally agree to and may not be truthful to avoid disappointing the provider.

ii. Child welfare system issues

(1) If and when it is necessary for a provider to inform the child protective agency of (suspected) physical, mental, or sexual abuse or neglect, the method of reporting can sustain or damage the rapport that has been established with the family. Families often feel angry and resentful about this interference in their life.

(2) The family should be told that the referral was made out of concern for the child's well-being. Often when families see that providers are genuinely concerned about their child, an effective working relationship can be rebuilt. Document all attempts to educate families, make referrals, or provide assistance for needed services and the family's response. Document the physical and emotional state of the child at each visit as well as any missed appointments.

iii. Obstacles to good decision making

(1) Caregivers' mental state

(a) Emotional and mental problems may block good parental decision making. Guardians suffering from depression or anxiety may have difficulty making decisions concerning their child. Recognize signs and symptoms of depression, anxiety, or other mental illness and make referrals to the appropriate mental health professional.

(2) Effective communication

(a) Failure in communication usually involves a clinician who is too hurried or authoritarian or an explanation that is too long or technical.

(b) Ask questions and get feedback from the patient and family to verify their understanding of what has been communicated.

(c) Stress interferes with learning. A person who has just been told that their child has a life-threatening illness will remember little else. Be prepared to repeat basic information and answer questions previously answered. Education of patients and family members is an ongoing process.

(3) Substance abuse

(a) Recognize signs and symptoms of drug or alcohol abuse and address these with the child's guardian. If a child is solely in the care of a person demonstrating signs and symptoms of drug or alcohol abuse, it may be necessary to contact child protection services.

(b) Document the behavior and what assistance was offered (e.g., referral to a rehabilitation center and any follow-up provided).

(c) Decisions regarding the child's care should to be discussed when the family member is not under the influence of any substances.

(4) Need for support systems

(a) Identify what supports the primary caregiver has. Invite the caregiver to bring other family members to the clinic to learn more about the disease and caring for the child.

iv. Rapport building with families

(1) Inquire about family/caregiver goals and expectations for their child's treatment.

(2) Identify family/caregiver needs and assist them in getting them met. Listen and reflect on their thoughts and concerns. With each family, identify the best ways, and sometimes the best staff, to relay information.

(3) Be patient; rapport building can take time. Families need to trust the clinician.

(4) Respect and understand cultural differences and religious beliefs.

(5) Be honest, genuine, and consistent. People need to know what to expect from their clinician and agency.

(6) Work with the family in partnership.

v. Empowerment of families

(1) Empowerment is a gift for any person or family. HIV, like other chronic illnesses, leaves people feeling disempowered.

(a) Help families recognize the opportunities to make decisions that can have a positive impact in their lives.

(b) Help them realize that they do not need to have someone else do everything for them. Empowerment directs them to find resources for themselves and become responsible caregivers for themselves and their children.

(c) Families who feel that they are legitimate partners in the decision-making process are more likely to work with the treatment team to develop creative solutions for solving problems. This includes the right to say something is not working.

vi. Case conference

(1) The case conference is a very powerful tool in the decision-making process. It is used for anticipating difficulties, exploring options, and cooperatively implementing a treatment plan. Multidisciplinary discussions allow input and perspectives from each professional, providing exploration of various facets of a patient's life.

vii. Provision of resources

(1) In urban areas or areas with a high HIV/AIDS incidence, numerous agencies provide support and assistance to families dealing with HIV.

(2) In rural or low-incidence areas, HIV-specific resources may be organized on a regional basis. Examples of this assistance include federally funded HIV drug-assistance programs, housing for people with HIV/AIDS, and support groups for caregivers. A social worker should be knowledgeable about these resources.

10.2 Stress Reduction and Pediatric HIV Infection

1. Psychological and emotional ramifications of chronic illness
   a. Typical responses (American Psychiatric Association, 1991)
      i. Cognitive: distressing dreams, poor attention span, and disorientation
      ii. Emotional: helplessness, frustration, feeling of abandonment, feeling of isolation, grief, irritability, numbness, and feelings of inadequacy
      iii. Interpersonal/social: child—lack of close peer group, loss of ability to participate in activities, ostracism by others, loss of family members or friends due to illness, activities only focused on illness; parent–child interactions— intrusive, overprotective, avoidant
      iv. Behavioral: withdrawn, excessive humor, and emotional outbursts
   b. Atypical response (American Psychiatric Association, 1991)
      i. Mood disorders: depressed, elevated, expansive, or irritable mood, possibly caused by general medical condition
      ii. Anxiety disorders: symptoms of anxiety and fear avoidance
2. Stressors in children with HIV infection
   a. Chronic illness of a parent
   b. Increased instability of a child's world due to multiple losses, family disruption and separation, and changing roles of family members

c. HIV effects on cognition and physical development
3. Stress response according to developmental stage (Gaynard, Wolfer, Goldberger, Thompson, Redburn, & Laidley, 1990)
   a. Infant: increased crying, lethargy, elevated heart rate, tactile hypersensitivity, feeding issues, failure to thrive, emesis
   b. Toddler: temper tantrums, noncompliance, irritability, demanding behavior, attachment, separation issues, refusal to eat
   c. Preschool child: regression of toilet training; attachment issues; increased tantrums; reckless play; development of new fears or nightmares; misconceptions with treatments and care; stranger fear, especially with medical staff; language difficulty
   d. School-age child: noncompliance, disruption in school routine or formal learning, avoidance of school, need for information, misconceptions, regression of social behaviors, refusal of treatment, withdrawal
   e. Preteen child: separation from peer group, loss of independence, depression or withdrawal, coping with changes in physical appearance or abilities, risk-taking behavior, fear of peer rejection, aggressive behavior
   f. Teenager/adolescent: body image issues; withdrawal from peer group; loss of privacy; risk-taking behavior, such as substance abuse; psychosomatic complaints; sleep disturbances; increased dependence on parents
4. Strategies for helping families deal with the stress of having an HIV-positive child
   a. Assess support system during initial visit and at each consecutive visit.
   b. Tell the child about their disease.
      i. Infected child: Discussion needs to be developmentally appropriate. Be sensitive to parental guilt. Teach personal responsibility in relationship to containing blood, having safe sex, and informing potential sexual partners. Regarding disclosure, remember the importance of not telling

everyone (Nehring, Lashley, & Malm, 2000). Help the child understand HIV and treatment effects.

   ii. Affected siblings: Discussion needs to be developmentally appropriate. Anticipate questions and help the family come up with creative solutions.

c. Support family members in changing roles.

d. Keep family intact as much as possible.

   i. Involve children in gradual transition to extended family situation.

   ii. Permanency planning is the process of anticipating the complexity of caregiver issues, including a discussion of who cares for the child if the caregiver is hospitalized or dies. If the parents are still alive, discuss guardianship issues prior to crisis situations (Ledlie, 2001).

e. Review with parent/guardian developmentally appropriate behavior in relationship to their child (expected vs. unexpected).

f. Discuss the importance of adherence to medication regimes and acknowledge the complexity of treatment regimens.

g. Acknowledge and discuss the complexities of raising an adolescent with HIV: relationship issues, dating, intimacy (e.g., help to develop scripts for future relationships), secrecy about their illness, realistic expectations for their future, asserting their need for independence with full knowledge of the consequences.

h. Acknowledge the impact of parental guilt.

   i. Administering a child's medication is a constant reminder of a child's illness.

   ii. Parents struggling to come to terms with their child's illness may conveniently forget to give the medication.

   iii. Failure to adhere to antiretrovirals may occur because of the complexity of the treatment regimens and because the child hates the way the medicine tastes (i.e., not wanting to fight with the child).

   iv. Parents may deny their own health needs, resulting in exhaustion, lack of nutrition, lack of adherence to their own antiretroviral regime, and hospitalization.

   v. The synergy of guilt and shame provide for more isolation than encountered with most other conditions.

   vi. Refer parents for counseling if the parents think it would be helpful to discuss their own personal guilt issues.

i. Recognize the complexities of disclosure.

   i. Discuss the difference between honesty and complete disclosure.

   ii. Support a family's choice to limit disclosure (Nehring, Lashley, & Malm, 2000).

   iii. Discuss the social stigma that is still attached to HIV/AIDS.

   iv. When a child discloses his or her HIV status, he or she may have to deal with the cruelty of classmates.

   v. Taking medications for HIV at school can be difficult for the child.

     (1) Taking medication singles the child out as different.

     (2) Lack of trained personnel to administer complex medication regimens might cause difficulties.

     (3) Children might have a difficult time dealing with what to say to classmates who inquire about medications.

j. Providing formal education for the HIV-infected child, while being sensitive to his or her needs.

   i. Tailor education to the needs of the child (e.g., special education classes, tutoring, homebound teachers) for extended illnesses.

   ii. Understand that absences may occur due to illness, clinic visits, or hospitalization.

iii. Encourage participation in team sports. The American Academy of Pediatrics (1999) recommends that children be allowed to participate in competitive sports to the extent that their health permits. Children with bleeding tendencies should be encouraged to choose sports other than high-contact sports, such as wrestling, boxing, and football (Dominguez, 2000).

k. Use complementary therapies, such as massage, creative visualization, Reiki, drumming, puppets, art therapy, and acupuncture (Nield-Anderson & Ameling, 2001; Wardell & Engebretson, 2001).

10.3 Isolation and Stigmatization

1. Social isolation refers to the lack of interaction with other people, usually outside of the immediate family. Social isolation, stigma, and disclosure issues are tightly entwined, for both families and children affected by HIV and adults. Factors promoting social isolation include the following:

   - The illness, with its associated lack of energy, and changes in appearance, which interfere with social interactions
   - The unpredictable course of the illness, with long absences or frequent interruptions in schooling and other activities outside the family
   - Concerns about stigma and disclosure of HIV status, such as the following:

     - Fear of social rejection
     - Secrecy about HIV, making social interactions feel inauthentic, less satisfying
     - Preference for social isolation over having to be dishonest about HIV-status disclosure

2. Consequences of social isolation include the following:

   - Loneliness
   - Interference with developmental progress in socialization (at all ages), which is needed for development of intimate friendships and social skills
   - Interference with development of a healthy self-concept and self-esteem
   - Diminished resources for social support
   - Isolation related to having HIV, which may be compounded by other problems that often affect families with HIV, including poverty, unstable living situations, multiple infected family members, multiple losses

3. Social isolation affects all members of the family, but with different emphases.

   a. For children with HIV, social isolation interferes with the following:

      - Development of social skills, including the ability to form intimate friendships and attachments
      - Formation of self-concept and self-esteem
      - Development of autonomy in relating to the outside world

   b. For adolescents, the lack of a peer group and close friendships can exacerbate feelings of not belonging. Concerns about being rejected may also be more intense for adolescents.

   c. For healthy siblings, the social isolation of the family as a whole can decrease their access to social interaction outside the family. Healthy children may also feel isolated within the family because of the amount of attention required by their ill sibling.

   d. For parents, the burden of care may absorb energy that would otherwise go toward generating social interactions. Concerns about protecting their children from stigma may dominate any considerations of social activities. Fear of infection may keep the family from engaging with others.

4. A stigma is a trait, attribute, or characteristic that society defines as highly undesirable (Goffman, 1963). Having such a trait makes a person vulnerable to stigmatization, which can cause the following:

   - Changes in how the person is viewed by others (social identity)
   - Social rejection or decreased acceptance in social interactions

- Limitation of opportunities (e.g., in housing, jobs, access to health care)
- Feelings of shame and self-hatred if the person shares society's evaluation of what the trait means about its possessor
- Significant erosion of a person's quality of life

a. The types of traits that can be stigmatizing include physical deformities, moral flaws (e.g., dishonesty or weak will), and tribal stigma, such as race, religion, or nationality. Stigma arising from having HIV can be influenced by all three of these categories.

b. The intensity of the stigma produced by a trait is modulated by various factors (Jones et al., 1984), three of which are highly pertinent to HIV:

  - How well the trait can be concealed from others
  - Who is responsible or who is to blame
  - The perceived danger of being around someone with the trait

c. Stigmatization occurs when the undesirable meanings of the trait become attached to a person who possesses the trait. In addition to being stigmatized by others (enacted stigma), the person with HIV may stigmatize or denigrate himself or herself (felt stigma), resulting in feelings of self-blame or disempowerment.

d. Interactions are often anxiety provoking for people with HIV because it is difficult to predict how others will respond once they know a person has HIV.

e. Courtesy stigma, or associative stigma, occurs when the stigma applied to the person with the trait is also applied, though sometimes to a lesser extent, to those who are related to or associated with the person, even though they do not themselves possess the trait. Courtesy stigma related to HIV has been applied to family members, friends, health care providers, and volunteers and can affect the amount of social support available to these people as well.

5. Managing stigma generally means avoiding or minimizing enacted stigma.
  a. HIV status is undisclosed; the person with HIV may pass (i.e., present oneself as not having HIV). This may involve disguising symptoms or hiding HIV medications, which can interfere with medication adherence. Passing can require considerable effort and energy (Ingram & Hutchinson, 1999). Many parents and families avoid disclosing that their child has HIV so that the child can pass and continue to be treated as a "normal" child.
  b. If others know a person has HIV, the infected person may attempt to minimize enacted stigma by covering (i.e., making HIV-related symptoms or actions less noticeable or less obtrusive).
  c. Avoiding social situations—limiting the circle of people that the person meets and interacts with—is another approach to managing stigma. The result is often social isolation and loneliness.

6. Prevalence of HIV-related stigma
  a. The prevalence and intensity of HIV-related stigma varies from country to country and, within a particular society, from group to group (Herek et al., 1998). Surveys in the United States and Europe of the general public (Centers for Disease Control and Prevention, 2000) and nurses (Surlis & Hyde, 2001) continue to demonstrate stigmatizing attitudes toward people with HIV, although the proportion of people who stigmatize has decreased. Stigmatization of people with HIV is also widely reported in Africa and Asia.
  b. Rejection related to stigma is a pervasive theme in research on the psychosocial effects of HIV infection and includes subtle distancing as well as ostracism and discrimination.
  c. The proportion of people with HIV who experience stigma is not known. Many people with HIV are not stigmatized, but many others are to devastating effect.
  d. The risk of experiencing HIV-related stigma can vary according to the following:

- The imputed mode of transmission
- Possession of other stigmatizing traits (e.g., homosexuality, injecting drug use)
- Presence of visible physical changes that suggest HIV infection
- The degree of anticipated physical contact
- Individual characteristics of either party in the interaction (gender, cultural background, level of knowledge about HIV)
- Geographical location (country, urban/suburban/rural location)

7. The experience of stigma for patients and families
   a. The degree to which having HIV can be concealed and the results of initial disclosures will influence the person's experience of stigma.
   b. For families affected by HIV, stigma is a group experience, which often includes social isolation.
   c. The potential for stigmatization may negatively affect many aspects of health care delivery, including confidentiality, willingness to be tested for HIV, and adherence to therapy.
8. Assessing the child and family for HIV-related stigma
   a. Individuals with HIV-related stigma may experience psychological sequelae, including depression, loneliness, anxiety, withdrawal, suicidal thoughts, and anger.
   b. HIV-related stigma for individuals and families can include the following:
      - Discrimination in job, housing, schools, health care, and insurance
      - Social isolation due to rejection, withdrawal, or both
      - Less-satisfying relationships due to lack of self-disclosure and increased social conflict
      - Loss of relationships that might have provided material support
      - Physical violence
   c. Nurses should ask directly about the following:
      - Any changes in relationships or living situation since diagnosis

- Problems at home, school, place of worship, or work
- Unpleasant incidents, including physical or verbal assaults
- Experiences or concerns about disclosing HIV status

9. Interventions for the child and family with HIV-related stigma include the following:
   a. Counseling
      i. Anticipatory counseling about issues of disclosure, possible discrimination and stigma, and social isolation should occur in conjunction with HIV testing and in treatment settings.
      ii. Tailor counseling individually.
   b. Recognition of the ongoing tension between wanting to disclose and fear of rejection and discrimination
   c. Discussion about ways to test the water with others (e.g., asking "How did you feel when you heard [name of someone famous] had HIV?")
   d. Exploration of previous experiences with stigma (related to sexual orientation or other traits); can strategies used previously be applied to managing HIV-related stigma?
   e. Education of patients, families, and partners about the following:

   - Actual risk of transmission and safety of household members
   - The potential for HIV-related stigma
   - The importance of maintaining and developing new social contacts for all members of the family

   f. Referrals
      i. Ongoing counseling for the individual, the family, or both
      ii. Support groups, which may offer practical tips for managing or avoiding stigma in addition to chances for social interaction in a less-threatening situation

10.4 Surrogate Caregivers

1. Why Surrogates?
   a. Many children with HIV have been left without parents due to parental illness and death, incarceration, severe

dysfunction related to drug abuse, or abandonment.

b. Families of children perinatally infected with HIV by definition have mothers who have HIV infection, whereas the fathers may or may not be infected.

c. A large percentage of HIV-involved families are headed by single parents (Burr & Lewis, 2000).

d. Many abandoned infants in hospital nurseries and children in foster care have been exposed to HIV and require screening (Child Welfare League of America, 2002; HIV/AIDS Treatment Information Service, 2001).

    i. Child welfare concerns

      (1) Research has demonstrated that on measures of health and psychological and social well-being, children fare better in small family-like groupings rather than in institutional care (Bowlby, 1951; Frank, Klass, Earls, & Eisenberg, 1996; Kaler & Freeman, 1994).

      (2) Recent child welfare reforms in the United States mandated that the states first attempt to reunite children with their biological families and, failing reunification within a specified time frame, attempt to locate extended family to care for the child (Adoption and Safe Families Act of 1997, P. L. 105–89). Although such efforts are made, children may be placed in foster care. Should these efforts fail (again, within a legally mandated time frame), the children must be legally cleared for adoption. Many states have adopted a dual track, where simultaneous case plans are developed for reunification with immediate family and adoption. If reunification fails, adoption can be expedited.

2. Concept of family

a. The nuclear family, consisting of a mother, a father, and their biological offspring, is only one of many possible examples of family.

b. Other types of families include a child and his or her grandparents; a mother (or father), a stepfather (or stepmother), and several half-siblings; an aunt, uncle, and cousins; a single parent or two same-sex parents with an older sibling and the younger children.

c. Respecting and supporting the family that is caring for the patient is essential in developing a relationship of trust with a pediatric patient.

3. Who are the surrogate caregivers or guardians?

a. Some surrogates may be family members (e.g., grandparents, aunts/uncles, older siblings, cousins).

b. Minority families are more likely to provide surrogate care for their relatives' children rather than allowing the children to enter the child welfare system (Groce, 1995).

c. Other surrogates may be foster or adoptive parents.

d. The caregiver may be a friend of the family designated by the parent(s) but without any legal status in relation to the child. Every family has its unique history, style of coping, strengths, and weaknesses.

e. Severely ill parents should be encouraged to create a legal document stating their wishes concerning custody and guardianship of their children after consultation with those named.

4. Extended family

a. An extended family may consist of grandparents, aunts, uncles, older siblings, cousins, or more distant relatives and is the most common placement for children requiring surrogate caregivers.

b. The extended family may voluntarily take children in or may be identified and approached by the local child welfare agency.

c. The extended family may offer psychological and cultural benefits to the child but may present problems as well.

d. Some families may have a cross-generational history of addictions, child neglect, or both. Extended family members may not be competent in caring for a chronically ill child.

   e. Members of the family often hold within their possession the precious but sometimes problematic gift of history. They know the biological parents and may know how HIV was contracted. They have formed opinions about the parents and have feeling and beliefs about this child and his or her parents that may impact on the child's care. They also have ideas about what it means to be sick, and these feelings need to be explored.

   f. Some families believe that it is important to keep the family together at all costs and may be financially overburdened, emotionally and mentally fatigued or bereft, or simply inundated with too many of their own family struggles.

   g. Many family members will not prevent children from having contact with the biological parents, even if the courts deny it.

   h. It is important to educate families about HIV and its treatment and transmission, so the child does not become isolated or ostracized out of fear of contamination. Having witnessed family members die of HIV, many families have strong beliefs about HIV treatment (e.g., some will refuse zidovudine) and may struggle to carry out the last wishes of a deceased parent.

   i. Some families see HIV as a conspiracy created in a lab to eliminate African Americans, and such beliefs may impair the provider–patient relationship. The provider must work hard to gain and maintain the family's trust and offer examples of successful treatment rather than confront this issue directly (Klonoff & Landrine, 1999).

5. Foster families

   a. Fostering is a legal relationship sanctioned by the child welfare agency.

   b. Foster parents may undergo specialized training to care for children with chronic medical conditions and HIV.

   c. Occasionally a family friend or other individual with some relationship to the child provides foster care (e.g., a teacher or nurse). Such individuals should be encouraged to formalize the relationship through legal guardianship or adoption where possible.

   d. Foster parents must be told the child's diagnosis prior to accepting the child for placement to ensure that appropriate medical care is provided. Clinicians who become aware that this information was omitted prior to placement should contact the child welfare agency immediately to facilitate appropriate disclosure.

6. Adoptive family

   a. Extended family members may choose to adopt the child they are caring for, but more often adoption involves a new, unrelated family for the child.

   b. Adoptive parents need to know the child has HIV infection or is HIV exposed to determine whether they can provide for the child's needs and can cope with the uncertainties of having a child with a chronic and life-threatening illness.

   c. In unrelated adoptions the prospective parents are most often White couples seeking a healthy, White infant. Therefore, children with HIV may be at the bottom of the list in terms of adoptability (Clark & Shute, 2001). When they do occur, such adoptions are often transracial. Gentle education about culture-specific needs (such as hair and skin care for African American children) and respect for the child's culture of origin is appropriate.

7. Fost-adopt

   a. Historically, foster parents were barred from adopting their charges and were even discouraged from forming strong attachments to the children. Increasingly children are placed in foster families who may be willing to adopt them when and if they become legally cleared for adoption.

   b. This minimizes disruption in the child's relationships and provides the continuity now recognized as the foundation of healthy personality development.

8. Family constellation
   a. In any family situation there may be additional caregivers other than the legally designated ones who assist with daily care and medication administration.
   b. Good practice dictates determining who those other caregivers are and inviting them to attend clinic visits for education regarding the disease and its management.
   c. Although the child's specific medical needs must first be met, many families benefit from education concerning the notion that the child is not an AIDS patient but first a child, who happens to have HIV.
   d. Placing the disease in the proper perspective enables families to better attend to the business of being families, such as making sure children go to school, setting aside time for recreation, providing appropriate guidance to all of the children in the household, and so on.
9. Understanding family history
   a. It is extremely useful for all clinicians to draw a genogram or family tree when encountering a new patient (Moore Hines & Boyd-Franklin, 1982).
   b. A genogram gives the clinician a snapshot of who is infected, identifies family members, which siblings may need to be screened, and which human resources are available for the family.
   c. Asking about medical history of extended family members, including alcoholism and drug dependence, will yield useful information.
   d. Ask about prior experiences in coping with stress and crises to gain a fuller picture of family functioning.
10. Contact with biological parents
   a. When biological parents are not the immediate caregivers, they may still have significant contacts with the child, and children may be aware of the health status of their parents.
   b. Some extended families (and even some foster and adoptive families) are able to gracefully incorporate the biological parents into their lives.

   c. Clinicians may be surprised to see a parent assumed absent at a clinic visit.
   d. Pediatric patients routinely scrutinize clinicians' responses, and any display of disrespect toward the child's family will be noted and may jeopardize the clinician–patient relationship.
11. Supporting the child within the surrogate family includes the following:

   - Educating the surrogate family concerning the disease and the management required for the individual patient
   - Normalizing the developmentally appropriate tasks and conflicts that caring for a child entail (e.g., some families may attribute any misbehavior to bad genes and may need to be educated about the power struggles inherent in the toddler and teen years)
   - Discussion of any disagreements with caregivers' management of the child's illness outside of the hearing of the child, especially if they are under the age of 12
   - Encouraging teens to be part of the discussion because they will increasingly need to assume responsibility for their own care
   - Assessing the child's well-being within the surrogate family
   - Recognizing when the child's needs (medical, psychological, or other) are not being met within the surrogate family and attempting to educate the surrogate family concerning the child's needs, referring the family to social services or the child protection authority, or both; documenting interactions, which is important in protecting and advocating for the child

10.5 Disclosure to the Child

1. Disclosure is the process of informing the child or youth of disease diagnosis, health changes, and opportunities that involve education, risks, benefits, adaptation, therapies, and

responsibilities as they happen in the life continuum.

2. Common to other chronic illness disclosure is the perspective of illness and disability—the less-than-perfect child, the invalid, and the helpless one—which are similar to other chronic illnesses, such as cystic fibrosis, cerebral palsy, and sickle cell anemia. HIV shares the threat of terminal illness with cancer and the stigma of generational responsibility related to genetic disorders. Each of these chronic illnesses involves disclosure to the child at a developmentally appropriate level chosen by family and health providers, with the family as active partners in the child's health decisions.

3. Among children diagnosed with other illnesses, including cancer, the literature suggests that failure to provide age-appropriate disclosure of diagnosis results in depression, poor self-esteem, acting out behaviors, and poor family social interactions. Clinicians routinely encourage families to start the disclosure process early, but families affected by HIV continue to be reluctant to disclose (Instone, 2000; Ledlie, 1999).

4. Family issues related to disclosure
    a. Disclosure is often discussed from the parental perspective, including factors that impact the decision to disclose of HIV diagnosis. However, despite delaying disclosure, 45% of the children in one sample reported that they were not surprised when they were told of their diagnosis. In this study, the median age of children in the sample who knew their diagnosis was 7.5 years (Wiener, Battles, Heilman, Sigelman, & Pizzo, 1996).
    b. Families are reluctant to tell the diagnosis for the following reasons: perception that the child is not ready to hear the diagnosis; burden of knowledge and loss of innocence; unreadiness of parent/caregiver to reveal his or her own diagnosis; guilt and shame related to acquisition and transmission of HIV; fear of social rejection should the child tell others; and social, financial, and housing discrimination.

    c. Factors that prompt families to disclose include death of other family members; school problems; medicine adherence problems; child's direct question; spiritual issues; health care team partnership with family; and unexpected disclosure by family member, friend, or staff.

5. Children's issues related to disclosure
    a. Children are not small adults. Their concepts of health and illness may be different from their developmental or chronological age. Their concepts are first based in their experiences. It is with education and experience as well as cognitive development that they understand illness, its causes, and the effects. An 8-year-old may think that catching a cold occurs randomly with cold mornings; the relationship between germ, cold, and medicine will not be understood. On the other hand, an 11-year-old will know from educational experience the effect of a germ causing an infection that produces the symptoms of a cold.
    b. Literature does not fully address the adaptation and functioning of the child after disclosure of the diagnosis of HIV, but in a recent small qualitative research study (Donohoe, 2002) the following factors were identified:

        - Feelings of being different from peers
        - Trusting to tell friends who will not tell
        - Sadness related to taking medicines
        - Need to ask questions of family members and health care providers for better understanding
        - Identifying self with new label—HIV/sick (see Figure 10.5a)

6. Specific approaches for disclosure in child's environment
    a. Family—Families may enlist the help of the health care team when sharing the diagnosis. Illness or death of a parent or grandparent caregiver may require disease disclosure to other family members.

Figure 10.5a *"Being Told" Model*

When children participating in a pilot focus group described their feelings when they were told they had HIV, they talked of sadness related to the number of medications, side effects, fatigue, trusting friends, and their perceived differences from other children. The study identified the child's development as a key to adaptation to diagnosis disclosure. Themes evolved after the transcription, coding, and analysis of focus group tapes. Themes were collapsed to three major responses that led to the identification that the children developed their own ways of coping to build self-esteem fostered by those who care for the children—family and medical providers. Families may find this model reassuring when considering disclosing the diagnosis of HIV because children perceive themselves as stronger after being told of diagnosis (Donohoe, Steele, Hinds, & Dillard, 2002).

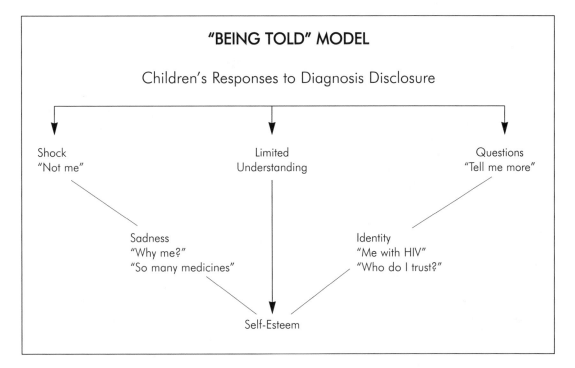

b. School—Except for Illinois and South Carolina, parents do not have to disclose the child's HIV diagnosis to the school or school district. Children or teens may need special educational resources for academic achievement, and the disclosure of the disease would facilitate the acquisition of resources. Disclosure to the school can be limited to the principal, school nurse, and carefully selected others, with confidentiality stressed and laws maintained.

c. Church—The child or family's decision to disclosure to a pastor or church members is an individual decision. More churches are offering health ministries and promoting understanding of HIV/AIDS.

d. Community—HIV/AIDS awareness is growing in communities, but there is still discrimination. Families are often the best judge of disclosure acceptance in their communities. More community agencies are addressing the needs of families affected by HIV. Multidisciplinary teams can provide the families with social agency referrals and local resources throughout the continuum of health care.

7. Specific approaches to the child when disclosure is delayed

a. Until disclosure of the name of the disease takes place and the child understands why medicines are taken, clinic visits are made and no one talks about what is "wrong." Several interval interventions can be incorporated in the disclosure process. Using a multidisciplinary team that includes the health care provider/clinic staff, social worker, child life specialist, and psychologist, these interventions can educate the child on a developmentally appropriate level.

b. Play therapy techniques

   - Drawing virus (bad guys), drawing T-cells (good guys) and medicines (destroyers of bad guys and helpers of the good guys)
   - Medical play for painful procedures
   - Support groups for families, children, teens that provide safe environments for role playing

c. Assessment of parental/ caregiver knowledge about HIV to build confidence in dealing with issues of disclosure

d. Assessment of familial cultural beliefs that may affect the child's understanding and acceptance of the disease

8. Nursing implications in the disclosure process

   a. Assess parent/caregiver plans for disclosure.

   b. Identify perceived risks and benefits of disclosure for the family.

   c. Assess child's developmental level and understanding of health and illness, which may be unrelated.

   d. Assess cultural beliefs and spirituality.

   e. Assess social support within the family and in the community.

   f. Develop a plan from a partnership meeting with the family and the multidisciplinary team that identifies the disclosure process, including a disclosure event date.

   g. Monitor postdisclosure coping of the child and family.

h. Establish time intervals to assess the child's and family's understanding of disease diagnosis after the disclosure event—6 months or yearly.

i. Update the child's understanding of disease diagnosis as the child develops and matures.

10.6 Multiple Hospitalizations

1. Pediatric hospitalizations

   a. Over the last 20 years the average frequency and length of stay of hospital admissions has significantly decreased.

   b. With the advent of combination therapies and better medications for the treatment of opportunistic infections available to children, there have been fewer admissions and subsequently fewer deaths.

2. Treatment decisions

   a. Parents are expected to make decisions about various tests and procedures, as well as understand the results and their implications to the child.

   b. It is essential to know who the legal guardian is and who has the legal right to consent for medical treatments.

      i. In nuclear or adoptive families, usually both mother and father have the right to consent for treatment.

      ii. In extended families it is important to identify the legal guardian and to have a copy of the custody papers in the medical record. If child protective services is involved, ascertain if the biological parents' rights are terminated or intact by contacting the case manager. If they have been terminated, determine who is authorized to consent for treatment.

      iii. Identify the family decision maker or primary contact. This may not be the same person. Clarify with the family who should be contacted to discuss all necessary procedures. Include all involved parties on medical decisions. If a guardian depends on guidance from a grandmother, aunt, or other family member, involve that person in these discussions because it is likely that the guardian will discuss any concerns with that person before making a decision.

3. Effects of multiple or prolonged hospitalizations
   a. Parental concerns
      i. Parents need to know the reason the child is hospitalized. They should be told the current diagnosis, the body system affected, the anticipated course of treatment, and how it will affect their child's overall health. Factors that can interfere parents' interpretation of information include the following:

      - Fatigue and frustration with long waits
      - Discomfort and disorientation because most of the medical personnel treating their child are strangers
      - Sudden or unexpected crises, which increase anxiety and prevent people from being able to fully grasp what is happening; strategies to address this issue include the following steps:

      (1) Approach the parents with concrete and essential information. Gather more details after the initial crisis is over.
      (2) Give the diagnoses and explain possible causes in laymen's terms.
      (3) Allow ample time with the family to answer any questions.
   b. Child concerns
      i. Following these steps when sharing the hospital diagnosis with a child:
      (1) Discuss with the child or adolescent their somatic complaints according to their cognitive age and understanding.

(2) Reassure the child that the staff and the medicine and treatments are meant to help.
(3) Many young children and some adolescents may not know their HIV diagnosis. To avoid inadvertently disclosing the diagnosis to the child, or his or her family and friends, document what the child knows (or that they do not know the diagnosis) in the chart and communicate this to staff. Restrict discussion about HIV to those who know the diagnosis.

      ii. Children and adolescents have worries and fears about what is happening to them. They need to know what to expect from tests and procedures (e.g., where they have to go, what will be done, whether their parent can go with them), so they are less afraid. Following are guidelines to appeasing children's fears:
      (1) Explain what to expect before, during, and after each procedure. Educate children using dolls. Allow them to talk to other children who had a similar experience.
      (2) Always reassure children that a painful procedure is being done to help them, not to punish them.
      (3) Assess depression, which is often a sign of pain in young children, and determine the need for pain medications or sedation. Provide a positive experience for them for getting through a test or procedure (e.g., give stickers or a favorite dessert, allow them to play with a favorite game or toy, take a trip to the child life room).
      iii. Death is commonly an unspoken fear for both children and adolescents who are hospitalized frequently or for prolonged periods. They fear they will not

get to realize their hopes and dreams. They also worry they will be forgotten. Following are guidelines for dealing with children's fears:

(1) Some children are afraid to verbalize their fears. It may be helpful to vocalize their fears for them and give them voice. Ask them what they are most fearful of, such as specific tests or procedures or dying.

(2) Assess the family's thinking about care and treatment. Some families tell children and adolescents if they do not take their medication, they will die. It is a scare tactic used to gain compliance. Extended or frequent hospital stays may reinforce this notion. Address these statements with the child and family (i.e., does the child/adolescent feel he or she has brought this admission on themselves because he or she didn't take medicines or listen to guardians, and is the child afraid he or she will die because of this).

(3) Provide reassurance about their specific condition.

iv. Some children express their fears by acting out behaviorally. Others may be reserved and withdrawn. If a child is particularly anxious or depressed, get a consult from a mental health professional.

v. The following techniques are useful for children and adolescents who become anxious and panicked by tests, procedures, or going to the doctor or hospital. They require practice, and not all patients find them helpful. Find a therapist certified in specific techniques (McKay, Davis, & Fanning, 1997, pp. 58–63.).

(1) Hypnotherapy is the use of guided imagery to help a patient reduce anxiety, particularly about testing or procedures. It is a process by which a patient incorporates deep breathing and visualizes a calm, safe, and peaceful place to reduce anxiety. The goal is for the patient to visualize actually being in that place, not just picturing themselves there. They should focus on what they see, hear, smell, and feel in that place.

(2) Relaxation techniques include abdominal breathing. Abdominal breathing involves slow, deep inhalations that fill the lungs and lower the diaphragm before they are slowly exhaled. This technique is helpful in preventing hyperventilation.

(3) Muscle relaxation is the process of tightening the muscles and then quickly releasing them to relieve the tension. The patient pays attention to how relaxed they feel after releasing the muscle. They are encouraged to focus on the relaxed state.

(4) Cue-controlled relaxation is a combination of abdominal breathing and muscle relaxation. The patient associates the cue of "inhaling" and "exhaling" with the release of tension. At each exhale they become more relaxed.

vi. The school-age child

(1) If a child is going to be hospitalized for a long period of time, or will spend time at home recuperating, it is important to arrange tutoring services with the Board of Education.

(2) For shorter stays encourage families to get school assignments for the child to complete to prevent the child from falling behind.

(3) Allow patients as much autonomy as is possible, given the hospital setting.

(4) Patients may find the following helpful in expressing their feelings: journaling, creative writing, poetry, or arts and crafts.

c. Family concerns

i. Be aware of the strain of multiple admissions on the whole family. Families with more than one child may find frequent or prolonged hospitalizations stressful and disruptive to family routine.

(1) Parents/guardians often have problems with child care arrangements or transportation, in addition to many other decisions.

(2) Chores, homework, and other responsibilities may fall to older siblings or may be left unattended while a parent is at the hospital.

ii. Siblings have a range of emotions and experiences as well.

(1) Some siblings find themselves feeling jealous of the attention, gifts, and perks associated with being hospitalized and may feel excluded.

(2) The aftereffects of jealousy and envy could be guilt, especially if the hospitalized child's condition deteriorates.

(3) Some siblings worry that their sibling will die. Often they wish to share or take away the pain.

(4) Explain to the siblings, at their cognitive level, what is happening to the hospitalized child. Give voice to their fears and feelings. Encourage them to write, paint, or draw about how they feel about their sibling being in the hospital.

4. Religious beliefs

a. Families often find emotional and spiritual strength through their beliefs. Acknowledging a family's spiritual strength is essential. Assist them in having clergy or spiritual leaders present during hospital stays.

5. Empowering families in the inpatient setting

a. Encourage them to use resources (family, friends, clergy, colleagues, time, money, transportation, etc). If necessary help them identify those resources.

b. If parents have limited resources, refer them to the appropriate service, agency, or professional.

c. Encourage parents to make the connections on their own or to use as many of their own resources as possible.

d. Avoid providing for every need all the time. This will allow families to have a sense of self-sufficiency and increased confidence and will reduce enabling.

e. Inform them of the services within the hospital setting that will make their stay more comfortable (child life for their child, the chapel, a cot for the parent at night, meal vouchers for those who need it, etc.).

10.7 Community-Based Care Issues

1. The community is the base setting for the child and family. Individuals define community in many ways, and the definition is often influenced by culture and individual needs. The child and family can negotiate their individual community because of their knowledge and experience within their community. Their confidence in their own community decreases transitions to new agencies if the agencies are community based. Community-based care and social service systems respond to the individual needs identified by the community and attempt to draw on the resources of the community (American Public Health Association, 1991; Courtney, Ballard, Fauver, Gariota, & Holland, 1996).

2. The child's own family is the first community for a child. It is within the family that the child learns to navigate progressively larger complex social systems (Tannen, 1996).

a. The basis for a child's social system is the parent/caregiver, who forms a supportive, nurturing environment for growth, development, social interaction, and education (Erikson, 1964; Lidz, 1976).

b. Family has varying defining characteristics. Kinship groups involving grandparents, aunts, uncles, cousins, and sometimes siblings may be the primary caregivers for the child with HIV.

c. Socioeconomic factors may define or limit the abilities of the child's family to provide health care and appropriate educational and social resources (Green, 1994).

3. Beyond family, community expands to the locale where the child and family reside.

4. Within the locale, there may be supports and barriers to accessing care, securing resources, and receiving supportive services. Communities are able to provide varying levels of support for children and families affected by HIV through governmental and nongovernmental agencies and social services (American Academy of Pediatrics, 1999).

5. Ryan White Care Act funding, Maternal Child Health Bureau (MCHB) grants, AIDS Education and Training Center (AETC) and private foundations, as well as philanthropic and local social groups offer options for support services that can be tailored by the community to meet specific needs.

6. Coordination of community care often requires the nurse, multidisciplinary team facilitator, or case manager to partner with the family to develop a plan that can be more easily managed within the child's immediate community (Jackson & Vessey, 1996).

7. Community-based services for the HIV-infected child

a. State, county, and city laws, policies, and resources establish the basic design for educational and health resources available to a child and family with a chronic illness or disability.

b. Social welfare systems (public and private) provide the health care support, respite care, and guidance for families caring for medically fragile children.

c. The MCHB, a bureau of the Health Resources and Services Administration, U.S. Department of Health and Human Services, administers Title V of the Social Security Act, assuring the health of mothers and children. This agency promotes the development of community projects that increase the information, education, multidisciplinary care, and services needed by the child with HIV and his or family (Austin & Donohoe, 1996). The MCHB endorses care that is family centered, coordinated, comprehensive, culturally sensitive, and developed through collaboration with the child and family (Grayson & Guyer, 1994).

d. Each child and family should have a case management plan that reflects the needs and strengths of the child within his or her community and that includes the following (American Academy of Pediatrics, 1999; Jackson & Vessey, 1996):

- Primary health care with ongoing health coordination and continuity of primary health care provider
- Referral to specialty services for medical, therapeutic, and other developmental or vocational services
- Care coordination by case manager in collaboration with the caregiver of the child
- Interdisciplinary team identification and review of child's strengths and family strengths as well as challenges faced by the child and family at home and in the community
- Assessment and access to counseling and social supports as necessary
- Assessment and access to financial resources as needed
- Inclusion and referral of child and family to appropriate educational services
- Interagency collaboration to provide services that meet the individual priorities of the child and family
- Communication and exchange of information among agencies, professionals, and the child's family

e. The nurse partner performs a community assessment (Broome & Rollins, 1999).

    i. Thoughtful interest and assessment by the nurse promotes a bond of trust with the family and promotes confidence when referrals to other agencies are necessary.

    ii. The nurse's awareness of and coordination with local community resources and agencies providing further services demonstrates and reaffirms the family's ability to successfully care for their child.

    iii. Development of a coordinated community-based plan empowers the child and family to achieve success in their community.

    iv. A community assessment includes the following:

- Assessment of the neighborhood and the home
- Assessment of the family's cultural/ethnic influences on care
- The expectations of children by adult family members, which vary in different cultures. The role of the child may differ by age, gender, culture, and mental/physical health of the child's caregiver(s). For example, a grandmother may expect a school-age child as young as 7 years old to self-administer medication without supervision (Farley, Hines, Musk, Ferrus, & Tepper, in press; Leininger, 1996).
- Location of the home and its safety, limited finances, exposure to violence, availability of transportation, and barriers to health care and other services, which may indirectly influence a family's ability to be an equal partner in a care plan for the child (Fry-Bower, 1997)

- Ongoing assessment of family changes, housing, finances, support of extended family, and access to a telephone are necessary for follow-up care management.

8. Significant variables may prevent the client (caregiver or child) from seeking out community.

a. State laws for HIV testing, confidentiality, reporting and mother-baby follow-up may pose barriers to care. Continuity of care and safety within the child's community are necessary for the health, growth, and development of the child with HIV. Referrals to existing community programs benefit the child, preserve the family, and protect the child from medical neglect and abuse.

b. Substance abuse of the child's caregiver may affect the child's care and lead to a referral to child protective services for medical neglect (Haack & Budetti, 1993).

c. Prenatal identification of risk of drug exposure may require the removal of the newborn from the mother's custody at birth and impair maternal bonding (Robbins & Mills, 1993).

d. Fear of stigma and discrimination in the neighborhood from accidental disclosure (Forehand et al., 1998)

e. Lack of comprehensive community-based care for substance-abusing women caring for children

f. Child's exposure to domestic and environmental violence

    i. Children in urban areas witness more acts of violence than children in suburban and rural areas (Fry-Bower, 1997).

    ii. Behavioral problems are a known consequence of exposure to violence.

    iii. Developmental neuropsychological assessments identify strengths of the child and the confounding factors of disease, socioeconomic influences, and family environment.

    iv. Ongoing assessment is necessary for the safety and development of the child and family.

9. Spiritual referrals to supportive community faith-based ministries can provide a dimension to the caring for the whole person that often medical and social resources are not prepared to fulfill. Acknowledging the need for spiritual support promotes interpersonal bonding and respect (O'Neill & Kenny, 1998).

10. Referrals to existing resources in the community, whether social services, day care, respite care, housing, food, or spiritual support, enables the family to access resources that are designed by community advocates to provide the child with a safe, nurturing environment. This builds on the strengths of the child and family (Grayson & Guyer, 1994; Jeppson & Thomas, 1995).

10.8 End of Life Issues

1. Definition: End of life occurs when the physical body ceases all function as a result of acute illness or chronic deterioration of the body related to HIV or other accident or unexpected illness. End of life can also be marked by when family and friends say good-bye to a child who will not return to his or her active, daily life.

2. Disclosure of diagnosis to dying child
   a. Disclosure of terminal status: Elisabeth Kübler-Ross (1983), in *On Children and Death*, describes how children and parents cope with terminal as well as sudden illness and provides insight into the inner world of the dying child, affirming the positive nature of disclosure of the terminal diagnosis to the child. Some families may differ in their acceptance of disclosure of the terminal nature of the illness, which may be due to previous experiences with death, cultural norms, issues with loss, fear that it will frighten the child, or other reasoning. Dottie Ward-Wimmer (1997), in *Working with and for Children*, describes working with a child whose parent had refused disclosure. She discusses how she allowed the child to ask questions, and, although she did not

answer them directly, she encouraged him to communicate his feelings and fantasies. This was acceptable to the parent and appeared to help the child have a peaceful end to his life and to help his mother live at peace with her decision.

b. Disclosure of HIV: Some children die without knowing that their illness is related to HIV. Although disclosure of HIV status to the child is often described as preferable, some parents and caregivers do not choose this option. In working with children, it is possible to discuss dying without discussing HIV status. Often caregivers will allow discussion of organ failure (e.g., "Your heart is not working well."). If there are more questions, it is important to work with the family on acceptable reasons that are as truthful as possible.

c. Assessment of child and family needs regarding unfinished tasks
   i. When appropriate, discuss the level of comfort with death with the family and the child.
   ii. The child may need to write a will. The child may have specific toys or items he or she wishes to leave to someone specific. If the child is afraid of being forgotten, he or she can be given control of memories that will be left behind.
   iii. The family may need assistance in deciding how they want to say good-bye. It can be helpful to explore their unfinished business.

d. Interventions for dying child
   i. Decision making
      (1) Do not resuscitate (DNR) versus medical interventions: Some people believe that discussing end of life decisions will hasten death. It may be helpful if the practitioner discusses death as part of the natural course of life. For those children and adolescents mature enough to do so, living wills can be a helpful tool in deciding the child's and family's wishes.

(2) It is important to clarify what the medical staff is telling the child and family.

(3) Clarify staff, family, and the child's beliefs regarding the child's condition and whether or not it can be reversed with interventions.

(4) If the family or child disagrees with the health care provider, explore the basis for the alternate viewpoint (e.g., previous experiences, health belief, and culture).

(5) Parent and child disagreement on health care issues may require the intervention of the health care team.

(6) An ethics committee intervention may be warranted if there is a disagreement. These meetings can be helpful for practitioners to work through their own thoughts regarding the situation.

ii. Home hospice versus institutional care

(1) Hospice

(a) Some families are unable to have the child die at home. Previous experiences with death are a common reason for this. Some may be afraid of the reactions of the other children or people in the home. Counseling regarding fears and expectations of what death may look like can be helpful. Knowledge can often decrease fear.

(b) Explore whether hospice agencies in your area have experience with children who are dying. If they do not, they may need more support from the HIV care provider regarding issues specific to children.

(c) A home assessment by a hospice provider is often useful to determine if the home is adaptable for a terminally ill person.

(d) If the family's support network is not in agreement with this plan, arrangements can be made so that they are not disruptive to the process.

(2) Death in the hospital, nursing home, or other institution

(a) If a family decides that the child cannot die at home, plans can be put in place for a peaceful death in an institution.

(b) Hospice care can be provided in an institution, if acceptable by that institution.

(c) Discussions regarding invasive procedures and DNRs need to be conducted early in the process. This is often helpful in reducing the child's and the family's chance of the choice becoming a crisis. However, it is important for families to know that up until the time of death there is always the possibility of changing one's mind. Some families may decide to take their loved one home right before death. Others may choose to bring their loved one into the hospital. Flexibility is helpful in assisting with the dying process. Although there are guidelines, very rarely are two deaths the same. Children and families are as different as their unique life experiences.

e. Comfort care

    i. Complementary therapies: These techniques may be learned by the practitioner, or other professionals may be called in to assist the child. They may also be helpful to the child's caregivers as routes of support and coping mechanisms. It is imperative that those choosing to do these therapies be appropriately trained.

    ii. Pain management: Pharmacological pain management may be used in conjunction with alternative therapies (see Section 9.1).

    iii. Behavioral health services: It is helpful to assess how the child and caregivers view behavioral health services and what types of providers may be acceptable to them. Sometimes home services may be more appropriate, depending on the family situation. Some families may prefer to have a social worker visit their home; they may not want to attend therapy. This will depend on the individualized goals for the child and family.

References

American Academy of Pediatrics. (1999). Issues related to human immunodeficiency virus transmission in schools, child care, medical settings, the home, and community. *Pediatrics, 104*, 318–324.

American Psychiatric Association. (1991). *Diagnostic and statistical manual of mental disorders* (4th ed.). Washington, DC: Author.

American Public Health Association. (1991). *Healthy communities 2000: Model Standards. Guidelines for community attainment of the Year 2000 National Health Objectives.* Washington, DC: Author.

Austin, J. R. D., & Donohoe, M. (1996). *Continuing educational needs for nurses caring for children with special health care needs.* Washington, DC: Georgetown University and National Center for Education in Maternal and Child Health.

Barker, R. L. (1995). *The social work dictionary* (3rd ed.). Washington, DC: NASW Press.

Bowlby, J. (1951). *Maternal care and mental health* (Monograph No. 2). Geneva: World Health Organization.

Broome, M. E. & Rollins, J. A. (1999). *Core curriculum for the nursing care of children and their families.* Pittman, NJ: Jannetti Publications.

Burr, C., & Lewis, S. (2000). *Making the invisible visible: Services for families living with HIV infection and their affected children.* Newark, NJ: National Pediatric & Family HIV Resource Center, University of Medicine and Dentistry.

Centers for Disease Control and Prevention. (2000). HIV-related knowledge and stigma—United States, 2000. *Morbidity and Mortality Weekly Report, 49*, 1062–1064.

Child Welfare League of America. (2002). *Factsheet: The health of children in out-of-home care.* Retrieved November 18, 2002, from http://www.cwla.org/programs/health/healthcarecwfact.htm

Clark, K., & Shute, N. (2001, March 12). The adoption maze. *U.S. News & World Report, 130*, 60–69.

Courtney, R., Ballard, E., Fauver, S., Gariota, M., & Holland, L. (1996). The partnership model: Working with individuals, families and communities toward a new vision of health. *Public Health Nursing, 13*(3), 177–186.

Dominguez, K. L. (2000). Management of HIV-infected children in the home and institutional settings. In M. Rogers (Ed.), *HIV/AIDS in infants, children, and adolescents. Pediatric clinics of North America, 47.* Philadelphia: W.B. Saunders.

Donohoe, M., Steele, R., Hinds, P., & Dillard, M. (2002). *Child responses to being told the diagnosis of HIV.* Unpublished manuscript.

Erikson, E. (1964). *Insight and responsibility.* New York: Norton.

Farley, J., Hines, S., Musk, A., Ferrus, S., & Tepper, V. (in press). Assessment of adherence to antiretroviral therapy in HIV-infected children using Medication Event Monitoring System (MEMSTM), pharmacy refill, provider assessment, caregiver self-report, and appointment keeping. *Journal of Acquired Immune Deficiency Syndromes.*

Forehand, R., Steele, R., Armistead, L., Morse, E., Simon, P., & Clark, L. (1998). The Family Health Project: Psychosocial adjustment of children whose mothers are HIV infected. *Journal of Consulting and Clinical Psychology, 66*(3), 513–520.

Frank, D. A., Klass, P. E., Earls, F., & Eisenberg, L. (1996) Infants and young children in orphanages: One view from pediatrics and child psychiatry. *Pediatrics, 47*, 569–578.

Fry-Bower, E. K. (1997). Community violence: Its impact on the development of children and implications for nursing practice. *Pediatric Nursing, 23*(2), 117–127.

Gamble, V. N. (1997). Under the shadow of Tuskegee: African Americans and health care. *American Journal of Public Health, 87*(11), 1773–1778.

Gaynard, L., Wolfer, J., Goldberger, J., Thompson, R., Redburn, L., & Laidley, L. (1990). *Psychosocial care of children in hospitals: A clinical practice manual from the ACCH child life research project.* Rockville, MD: Child Life Council.

Goffman, E. (1963). *Stigma: Notes on the management of spoiled identity.* New York: Simon & Schuster.

Grayson, H. A., & Guyer, B. (1994). *Assessing and developing primary care for children: Reforms in health systems.* Arlington, VA: National Center for Education in Maternal and Child Health.

Green, M. (1994). *Bright futures: Guidelines for health supervision of infants, children, and adolescents.* Arlington, VA: National Center for Education in Maternal and Child Health.

Groce, N. E. (1995). Children and AIDS in a multicultural perspective. In S. Geballe, J. Gruendel, & W. Andiman (Eds.), *Forgotten children of the AIDS epidemic* (pp. 95–106). New Haven, CT: Yale University Press.

Haack, M. R. & Budetti, P. P. (1993). An analysis of resources to aid drug exposed infants and their families. *Addictions Nursing Network, 5,* 107–114.

Herek, G. L., Mitnick, L., Burris, S., Chesney, M., Devine, P., Thompson Fullilove, M., et al. (1998). Workshop report: AIDS and stigma: A conceptual framework and research agenda. *AIDS and Public Policy Journal, 13*(1), 36–47.

HIV/AIDS Treatment Information Service. (2001). *Guidelines for the use of antiretroviral agents in pediatric HIV infection.* Retrieved November 18, 2002, from http://www.hivatis.org/guidelines/Pediatric/Dec12_01/peddec.pdf

Ingram, D., & Hutchinson, S. A. (1999). HIV-positive mothers and stigma. *Health Care for Women International, 20,* 93–103.

Instone, S. (2000). Perception of children with HIV infection when not told for so long: Implications for diagnosis disclosure. *Journal of Pediatric Health Care, 14,* 235–243.

Jackson, P. L., & Vessey, J. A. (1996). *Primary care of the child with a chronic condition.* St. Louis: Mosby.

Jeppson, E. S., & Thomas, J. (1995). *Essential allies: Families as advisors.* Bethesda, MD: Institute for Family-Centered Care.

Jones, E. E., Farina, A., Hastorf, A. H., Markus, H., Miller, D. T., Scott, R. A., et al. (1984). *Social stigma: The psychology of marked relationships.* New York: W. H. Freeman.

Kaler, S. R., & Freeman, B. J. (1994). An analysis of environmental deprivation: Cognitive and social development in Romanian orphans. *Journal of Child Psychiatry and Psychology and Allied Disciplines, 35,* 769–781.

Klonoff, E. A., & Landrine, H. (1999). Do Blacks believe that HIV/AIDS is a government conspiracy against them? *Preventive Medicine, 28*(5), 451–457.

Kübler-Ross, E. (1983). *On children and death.* New York: Macmillan.

Ledlie, S. (1999). Diagnosis disclosure by family caregivers to children who have perinatally acquired HIV disease: When the time comes. *Nursing Research, 48*(3), 141–149.

Ledlie, S. (2001). The psychosocial issues of children with perinatally acquired HIV disease becoming adolescents: A growing challenge for providers. *AIDS Patient Care and STDs, 15,* 231–236.

Leininger, M. (1996). Cultural theory, research, and practice. *Nursing Science Quarterly, 9*(2), 71–78.

Lidz, T. (1976). *The person: His or her development throughout the life cycle.* New York: Basic Books.

McKay, M., Davis, M., & Fanning, P. (1997). *Thoughts and feelings: Taking control of your moods and your life.* Oakland, CA: New Harbinger Publications.

Moore Hines, P., & Boyd-Franklin, N. (1982). Black families. In M. McGoldrick, J. K. Pearce, & J. Giordano (Eds.), *Ethnicity and family therapy* (pp. 8–107). New York: Guilford Press.

Nehring, W., Lashley, F., & Malm, K. (2000). Disclosing the diagnosis of pediatric HIV infection: Mother's view. *Journal of the Society of Pediatric Nurses, 5,* 5–14.

Nield-Anderson, L., & Ameling, A. (2001). Reiki: A complementary therapy for nursing practice. *Journal of Psychosocial Nursing, 39,* 42–49.

O'Neill, D. P., & Kenny, E. K. (1998). Spirituality and chronic illness. Image. *Journal of Nursing Scholarship, 30*(3), 275–280.

Robbins, L. N., & Mills, J. L. (Eds.). (1993). Effects of in utero exposure to street drugs. *American Journal of Public Health, 83*(Suppl.), 1–32.

Surlis, S., & Hyde, A. (2001). HIV-positive patients' experiences of stigma during hospitalization. *Journal of the Association of Nurses in AIDS Care, 12*(6), 68–77.

Tannen, N. (1996). *Families at the center of development of a system of care.* Washington, DC: Maternal and Child Health Bureau of the Health Resources and Services Administration.

Wardell, D., & Engebretson, J. (2001). Biological correlates of Reiki touch healing. *Journal of Advanced Nursing, 33,* 439–445.

Ward-Wimmer, D. (1997). Working with and for children. In M. Winiarski (Ed.), *HIV mental health for the 21st century* (pp. 190–205). New York: New York University Press.

Wiener, L. S., Battles, H. B., Heilman, N., Sigelman, C. K., & Pizzo, P. A. (1996). Factors associated with disclosure of diagnosis to children with HIV/AIDS. *Pediatrics AIDS and HIV Infection: Fetus to Adolescent, 7*(5), 310–324.

Section XI

Nursing Management Issues

This section highlights three important issues germane to HIV/AIDS nursing practice. Section 11.1 describes HIV nursing case management in which the nurse functions as the facilitator, coordinator, and manager of patient care services and expected outcomes for those infected. Nursing case managers provide important and vital services to the individual, groups, and, in some cases, communities. This section describes the benefits and the limitations of case management systems.

As we learn more about HIV disease and continue to shape clinical practice and initiate policies, we are often confronted with ethical and legal dilemmas. Nurses caring for persons infected and affected by HIV must be aware of these ethical principles when evaluating their own actions and the actions of others. The authors provide nurses with the important questions nurses should ask when faced with such impasse.

The last section discusses important infection-control principles that protect the health of the infected, the health care worker, and other people cared for by nurses. Important to this discussion is the treatment of postexposure interventions for health care workers who have been exposed to potentially infected body fluids.

11.1 Case Management

1. Definitions of case management
   a. "A process of consumer support in which clients are assisted in negotiating for the services and supports they want for themselves" (Anthony, Cohen, Farkas, & Cohen, 1988, p. 220)
   b. Based on the recognition that a trusting and empowering direct relationship between the client and the case manager is essential to expedite the client's use of services along a continuum of care and to restore or maintain the client's independent functioning to the fullest extent possible (Sowell & Meadows, 1994)
   c. A service delivered by a discipline-specific provider with knowledge and experience that enables patients to have available options and services needed to meet their physical, mental, and emotional health needs (National Case Management Task Force, Case Management Society of America, 1995)
   d. A dynamic and systematic collaborative approach to providing and coordinating health care services to a defined population; a participative process to identify and facilitate options and services for meeting individuals' health needs, while decreasing fragmentation and duplication of care and enhancing quality, cost-effective clinical outcomes; uses a framework consisting of five components: assessment, planning, implementation, evaluation, and interaction (American Nurses Association Task Force on Case Management, 1988)
   e. A collaborative process that assesses, plans, implements, coordinates, monitors, and evaluates the options and services required to meet an individual's health needs, using communication and available resources to promote quality, cost-effective outcomes (Commission for Case Manager Certification, 1996)
2. A case manager is someone who has knowledge of the disease process, human nature, and the health care delivery system (U.S. Department of Health and Human Services , Health Resources and Services Administration, HIV/AIDS Bureau, 2001)
3. Case management models
   a. Nursing model
      i. Nursing case management uses the nursing process and an RN as the case manager; the RN functions as the facilitator, coordinator, and manager of patient care services and expected outcomes. Rather than providing direct patient care, the RN focuses on using assessment skills and disease-specific knowledge to plan care according to the identified patient needs (Cesta, Tahan, & Fink, 1998).
      ii. Nursing case management uses a holistic approach to planning care for the patient, the significant other, and the family—as well as their interaction in the community—and is used in the following settings: ambulatory care, acute care, home care, long-term care, rehabilitation, and managed care.
      iii. Nursing case management leads to a decrease in duplication of services and an increase in economic savings and extensions of available benefits over the disease continuum.
   b. Medical model
      i. The medical model uses a medical provider (e.g., a physician, advanced nurse practitioner, or physician assistant) as the coordinator/gatekeeper of patient care services (medical care).
      ii. Potential deficiencies of this model are fragmentation of care and duplication of services. Additionally, because this model is provider driven, aspects of care other than the presenting medical problem may not be addressed due to a lack of knowledge of available services and resources.
   c. Community-based/public health models

i. These models are focused on primary care and primary prevention and are predominately focused on well and at-risk individuals or those who have a potential need for health care services.

ii. Goals of these models are to support individuals to minimally maintain their present physical condition through use of disease-prevention methods and to empower them to maximize their optimal level of wellness through the use of community resources.

d. Diagnosis-related/population-based model

  i. This model focuses on a group of patients with a specific diagnosis. The management of the selected diagnosis may need improvement in the areas of cost and quality of care, or it may be at high risk for financial loss or have potential for revenue.

  ii. Criteria to be considered when deciding which population to case manage could include volume of the patient population, cost and complexity of care, the need for multiple services, and the length of stay in an acute care facility (Tahan & Cesta, 1995).

e. Psychosocial model

  i. Social work case management is a method of providing services in which a professional social worker assesses the needs of the client and the client's family, when appropriate, and arranges, coordinates, monitors, evaluates, and advocates for a package of multiple services to meet the specific client's complex needs (Case Management Standards Work Group, National Association of Social Workers, 1992). Services provided may include the following:

    • Assessing housing and food needs of the client

    • Assisting the client in preparing a do not resuscitate order, medical power of attorney, durable power of attorney, and advance directives

    • Investigating all sources of funding for medical care and entitlement programs that may provide coverage for medications, such as AIDS drug assistance programs (ADAP), drug studies, and vendor drug and compassionate use programs

4. Benefits of case management in the HIV epidemic

  a. Access to care

    i. Definition: ability and ease of patients to obtain health care when needed

    ii. Issues related to access to and quality of care:

      • Locating quality case management that is convenient for the service user

      • Maintaining a central location, with both private and public transportation access

      • Creating one system that provides both medical and comprehensive/psychosocial case managers

      • Providing specific cultural needs, such as translation

      • Providing staff members of both genders who are ethnically diverse

  b. Continuity of care

    i. Definition: seamless system of care over the disease continuum, which supports the best patient outcomes

    ii. Involves use of an interdisciplinary team approach, including medical providers, nurses, social workers, nutritionists, pharmacists, client advocates, pastoral care, and others as needed. The primary goal of the team is to evaluate the effectiveness of a patient-supported plan of care. The team approach allows for communication exchanges among disciplines to appropriately evaluate and update the care plan as needed, without missing important data.

c. Decreased fragmentation of care and decreased duplication of services
   i. With continual assessment of the patient's plan of care, the case manager is able to observe the progress of the plan and, with the patient, decide when the patient is ready to access services; with the patient in agreement, the possibility of a positive outcome is increased.
   ii. Communication is a tool used by the case manager to involve clients in the plan of care and allow them to decide which outcomes are appropriate for them.

d. Support
   i. Many locales have established specific HIV support groups. However, because needed services may not be directly related to the HIV diagnosis, clear care goals are needed to address areas of the patient's life that need support. With a holistic approach to care, assessment helps determine the type of support needed and allows the case manager to appropriately direct care and resources.
   ii. Follow-up is necessary to be sure the patient has followed through and actually accessed the service; encouragement and referral to services are provided by the case manager as new needs are identified.

e. Education
   i. Education and knowledge empower clients and allow them to be active participants in their own plan of care.
   ii. Client education is often needed on the following topics:

      • Adherence techniques to enhance outcomes of drug regimens and medical treatment
      • Nutritional assessment and dietary counseling on implications of increased caloric requirements and on potential food–drug interactions
      • Effective navigation of the health care delivery system
      • Eligibility requirements for entitlement programs
      • Other needs, such as visual screening, stress management, and self-care and wellness strategies

5. Limitations of case management
   a. Access and quality of care issues
      i. Barriers to care may include difficulty in finding an educated provider; issues related to funding sources (e.g., third-party source/insurance, Medicare/Medicaid, managed care or public finding) or the health care system delivery; and social stigmatization.

6. Development of standards and protocols for case managers
   a. Education level and experience are key to quality of care for patients.
   b. Case managers should identify both strengths and weaknesses of the systems within their service area.
   c. Development and ongoing evaluation of all external referral sources across a wide network of services and providers should be conducted.

11.2 Ethical and Legal Concerns

1. Since the early days of the HIV/AIDS epidemic, ethical and legal issues have raised questions and concerns in relation to HIV/AIDS care; these issues have been due, in part, to the characteristics of HIV disease, the nature of the epidemic, and the nature of the populations infected and affected by HIV.

2. Four principles are commonly used by health care professionals in dealing with ethical and legal issues in HIV care (Beauchamp & Childress, 2001):

   • Nonmaleficence (avoiding harm or injury to others)

- Beneficence (promoting the good or welfare of others)
- Respect for autonomy (respecting the liberty, privacy, and self-determination of others)
- Justice (treating others fairly)

3. Other relevant principles include fidelity (keeping promises, contracts) and veracity (telling the truth).
4. Nurses caring for persons infected and affected by HIV must be aware of these ethical principles when evaluating their actions and those of others. Decision making may also be guided by state and federals laws; thus, ethics and legal issues are closely related.
5. Two common approaches to ethical decision making in health care include:

- A rights-based approach (actions grounded in understandings of individual rights)
- A duty-based approach (a willingness or an obligation to act on behalf of others)

6. Specific ethical issues in HIV care
   a. Individual choice: Autonomy and self-determination
      i. Individual choice is based on the ethical principle of respect for autonomy; autonomy deals with one's right to self-determination.
      ii. Autonomy incorporates the concepts of confidentiality, informed consent, the right to accept and to refuse medical treatment, privacy, and disclosure.
      iii. Autonomous individuals are free to choose and to self-govern.
      iv. Within the context of health care, informed consent assists a person to voluntarily choose a course of action.
      v. Other elements of informed consent are information that is understandable by the person and that the person freely and without coercion accepts the plan of care and mutually participates in decision making and does not merely sign a form.
      vi. Autonomy requires a person to be competent to have decision-making capacity.
      vii. Health care providers are obligated to protect persons with diminished capacity as well as those who have never had the capacity for decision making.
   b. Inequitable access to care
      i. Disparity has been noted in the United States in relation to access to care, research participation, and experimental therapies.
      ii. Many HIV-infected patients rely on Medicaid; others have no health care insurance, which has a major impact on their ability to get necessary care and therapies.
      iii. Managed care may also complicate the ability of patients who need complex or expensive treatment to get adequate care.
      iv. All states participate in AIDS Drug Assistance Programs (ADAP), which provide health care services, including medications, to patients; nurses are in an excellent position to advocate for access to these entitlements and clinical trials for their patients.
      v. Minority patients in the United States may not have equal access to HIV clinical drug trials (Jones, Messmer, Charron, & Parns, 2002).
      vi. Ninety-five percent of people with AIDS live in developing countries; HIV/AIDS is now the leading cause of death in sub-Saharan Africa and the fourth cause of death worldwide (UNAIDS, 2002).
      vii. HIV has placed an additional financial burden on economically deficient health care systems in underdeveloped countries.
      viii. Antiretroviral therapy is extremely expensive, and global issues have emerged regarding cost and availability of HIV drug therapy.
   c. Privacy, confidentiality, and disclosure
      i. Protecting the privacy of patients and safeguarding information, which should remain confidential, is central to maintaining

autonomy and avoiding nonmaleficence.

ii. The following questions are designed to help health care providers consider the best ways to strike an appropriate balance between beneficence, nonmaleficence, justice, and autonomy:

- What approaches to teaching risk reduction or avoidance behavior respect the patient's autonomy and privacy?
- Does anyone besides the person being tested have a right or need to know the results?
- How does one reconcile the duty to warn with the duty to maintain privacy and confidentiality?
- Should results be disclosed only with the consent of the person being tested?
- What criteria are used for overriding confidentiality (not all ethical models will support all criteria)?
- What safeguards protect the confidentiality of patient information?
- How does a health care worker maintain privacy within the context of third-party notification policies? mandatory testing? mandatory names reporting laws? partner notification requirements?
- What ethical models/principles can be used to establish that partners have a right to information about a person's HIV status if the infected person doesn't want them to know?
- What ethical models/principles would make it difficult to establish such rights?
- How is partner notification accomplished?
- How does duty to warn compare with privilege to warn (consequences of warning others may include violence)?

- How does disclosure violate the principle of justice in these situations?

d. Discrimination and worker protection
   i. The incidence of HIV/AIDS is disproportional among minority and disenfranchised groups.
   ii. HIV/AIDS still carries a stigma not attached to many other serious diseases.
   iii. To protect against or minimize discrimination, nurses must be aware of persons and groups who remain most vulnerable to obvious forms of discrimination.
   iv. Nurses must consider the following about groups of HIV-infected patients:

   - Which groups are most likely to suffer a significant loss of autonomy in the health care system?
   - Which remain the most vulnerable to discrimination and thus the injustices involving privacy and confidentiality?
   - Which are the most vulnerable to discrimination and thus the injustices involving privacy and confidentiality?
   - Which tend to be excluded from clinical trials and access to experimental therapies?
   - Which are most likely to face significant discrimination in the workplace?

e. Estate, will, and advance directive planning
   i. Planning for the future entails paying attention to one's future health care needs, to a time when autonomous decision making is no longer possible, as well as to the disposition of one's tangible assets.
   ii. Estate and will planning are appropriately carried out with the assistance of an attorney.
   iii. Future care of dependent children needs advance consideration;

standby guardianship and custody arrangements for minors are legal proceedings, and some patients may require volunteer legal services if unable to afford legal costs.

   iv. Advance directive planning, enabled by the Patient Self-Determination Act of 1991, includes assigning a surrogate decision maker for health care decisions, called a health care proxy or durable power of attorney for health care, as well as providing directions for types of care desired, called a living will or do not resuscitate order (Ulrich, 1999).

   v. Some states require that a person provide advance instructions about withholding or withdrawing artificial food and hydration; a proxy decision maker in these states may not make decisions about these medical treatments.

   vi. A do not resuscitate order (DNR) is another form of treatment directive, which authorizes withholding cardiopulmonary resuscitation (CPR) in the event of cardiopulmonary arrest.

   vii. In many terminally-ill AIDS patients, a DNR order is completely appropriate, and a focus on comfort care and palliation of symptoms is often desired by patients and families at the end of life.

   viii. HIV patients may be wary of signing advance directives because of a mistrust of the medical system (Jones, Messmer, Charron, & Parns, 2002).

f. Ethical issues and the public health

   i. The goal of prevention and public health campaigns includes HIV-positive and HIV-negative persons and focuses on keeping the whole community healthy. When considering public health interventions, one must ask the following:

- What approaches to teaching risk reduction or avoidance behavior respects autonomy and privacy?
- What ethical reasoning is used to support the provision of clean needles to drug users or condoms to teenagers?
- What ethical reasoning is used to oppose such programs?
- What are the issues that face risk reduction programs for children?
- What risk reduction approaches are supported by research?

   ii. Nurses and other health care professionals may encounter HIV-infected individuals who continue with unsafe behaviors:

- How should health care professionals respond to those who practice unsafe behaviors that put others in jeopardy?
- How can respecting autonomy and culture be used to justify a minimalist approach to intervention?
- How can the utilitarian framework ("the rightness of an action based on consequences") be used to justify a more interventionist approach?
- Is there a role for compulsory testing for those who engage in unsafe behaviors? When might compulsory testing be protective of public health? What are the negative implications of this? In what instances is it more political than scientific?

   iii. Testing of childbearing women and newborn infants

   iv. Reasoned ethical positions can produce contradictory answers to questions.

   v. What information and which ethical model/principles support your positions on the following questions? What information and which ethical model/principles would support contrary positions?

- What advice should an HIV-positive woman receive about pregnancy?
- With data that demonstrate the effectiveness of prenatal AZT in reducing the rate of transmission of HIV from mother to fetus, should all pregnant women be HIV-antibody tested?
- Should HIV testing be mandatory or voluntary?
- If the HIV antibody test is positive, is there an obligation to provide the patient with access to AZT?
- Is there an obligation for a mother to take AZT?

g. Ethical issues related to clinical trials
  i. Disparity has been noted in access to research participation and experimental therapies.
  ii. People with HIV infection are often willing to take the risks of unproven therapies, including participation in underground buyers' clubs, expanded access programs, and clinical trials.
  iii. The exclusion of certain groups from research has been seen as discrimination rather than protection; access to clinical trials is generally seen as a benefit.
  iv. AIDS activists have challenged attitudes and some regulations regarding research participation and access to experimental therapies as too restrictive and discriminatory.
  v. Nurses are in an excellent position to advocate for access to care and to clinical trials for their patients.
  vi. In addition, trial design, rigid exclusion criteria, the use of placebos, double blinding, and clinical endpoints have been challenged by AIDS activists, researchers, alternative practitioners, and some pharmaceutical companies.

  vii. Scientific conflicts of interest, scientific integrity, competition in HIV research, and the role of economics in research have become important areas of concern.
  viii. The demand for quicker results, more effective clinical trials, and scientific integrity have led to stricter oversight by safety monitoring boards.
  ix. Community representatives have become more involved in decisions about research through community advisory boards.
h. Obligation to provide care
  i. According to the American Nurses Association's (2001) first provision of the *Code of Ethics for Nurses,* "the nurse, in all professional relationships, practices with compassion and respect for the inherent dignity, worth and uniqueness of every individual, unrestricted by consideration of social or economic status, personal attributes, or the nature of health problems."
  ii. The Association of Nurses in AIDS Care (1999, August) "recognizes . . . the moral, legal, and professional responsibility of all nurses to care for persons with HIV infection."
  iii. An ethic of care emphasizes caring for others and their significant relationships and recognizing the special obligations toward and a willingness to act on behalf of people with whom one has a relationship (Gordon, Benner & Noddings, 1996).
i. Protecting health care workers
  i. If standards of practice include universal precautions, are health care workers protected by knowledge of a patient's HIV status?
  ii. What changes in purchasing practices would better protect health care workers from occupational exposure to infections?

iii. What infectious agents are most responsible for occupational morbidity and mortality among health care workers?

j. Euthanasia, assisted suicide, and suicide

   i. Euthanasia refers to the deliberate administration of medication to end a life (Quill, 2001).

   ii. Suicide refers to the deliberate taking of one's own life.

   iii. Euthanasia (except in the situation of capital punishment) and suicide are illegal acts in the United States.

   iv. Assisted suicide is about providing patients with the means to end their life should they choose to do so.

   v. Assisted suicide has been a passionately debated topic in recent years and is currently legal only in Oregon; the right to die is not constitutionally guaranteed.

   vi. The American Nurses Association (ANA) condones neither active euthanasia (1994a) nor assisted suicide (1994b).

   vii. The Association of Nurses in AIDS Care (ANAC) encourages nurses (1997) to "carefully weigh one's right to conscientious objection with the professional obligations to patient advocacy, respect and non-abandonment."

   viii. Both ANA and ANAC encourage pursuit of palliative care practices, which include aggressive attention to pain management and psychosocial and spiritual care (Ferrell & Coyle, 2001).

   ix. Expert, compassionate care at the end of life is now recognized as a critical component of the wellness-illness continuum (Lynn, Schuster & Kabcenell, 2000).

11.3. Preventing Transmission of HIV in Patient Care Settings

1. Infection control

  a. Infection control is necessary to help ensure a safe environment for patients and health care workers (HCW).

b. When caring for patients, infection control practitioners recommend a two-tiered system of isolation precautions, using both standard precautions and transmission-based precautions.

   i. Standard precautions

    (1) All body fluids are to be treated as if they are potentially infected with HIV, hepatitis B (HBV) and hepatitis C (HCV).

    (2) Emphasizes use of appropriate hand-washing techniques, barrier equipment, and engineering controls or devices to reduce blood-borne pathogen transmission to HCWs and clients.

    (3) Standard precautions are used in situations where exposure to blood or potentially infectious body fluids is anticipated; may be combined with transmission-based precautions if the hospitalized patient has or is suspected of having a highly transmissible disease.

   ii. Transmission-based precautions

    (1) Designed to care for patients with known or suspected infections that can be transmitted by airborne, droplet, or contact modes

     (a) Droplet precautions are used when the organism is transmitted by infected droplets, which could come in contact with HCWs' eyes or mucous membranes; HCWs are to wear gloves and a regular mask and gown.

     (b) Airborne precautions are used to prevent transmission from airborne infectious agents, such as tuberculosis (TB) and require patient placement in a private room with negative airflow; HCWs must wear N-95-type respirator masks.

    (c) Contact precautions are used when the organism is transmitted by direct contact and require patient placement in a private room with disposable medical supplies; HCW should wear gloves, a mask, and a gown.

  c. Hand washing is one of the most effective methods to prevent transmission of blood-borne pathogens.

2. Postexposure prophylaxis

  a. Transmission of blood-borne pathogens, especially HIV, HBV, and HCV, is a concern for HCWs and patients; the diseases differ in modes of transmission, development of disease, and disease progression.

  b. All hospitals should have procedures for HCWs to report occupational exposures to blood and other body fluids. These procedures should include counseling and testing for potentially infectious diseases and, when appropriate, offering medications for the disease.

  c. Transmission HIV, HBV, and HCV

    i. HIV, HBV, and HCV from a hollow bore needle to the HCW is reported to occur 0.3%, 5%, and 1.8%, respectively (Centers for Disease Control and Prevention, 2001).

    ii. In the United States, there are 56 documented HIV seroconversions from occupationally related injuries. The Centers for Disease Control and Prevention (CDC) is investigating 138 other episodes of reported HCWs' HIV seroconversion from an occupational exposure (Centers for Disease Control and Prevention, 2001).

    iii. Factors that assist in determining risk of infection from an exposure include mode of transmission (whether the injury occurred with a percutaneous device or with a sharp or blunt instrument) and contact with skin or mucous membrane.

    iv. Assessment of percutaneous/ sharp injury includes determining the quantity of blood involved, the type of needle or sharp instrument (hollow-bore/solid/size), the depth of the puncture (did wound bleed?), whether the device came from a vein or an artery, whether the source patient is in early HIV seroconversion or has advanced AIDS, and whether the viral load is high.

    v. Contact to nonintact skin exposures has not been documented with precise estimates.

    vi. Mucous membrane exposure is estimated to be 0.09%.

  d. Considerations and recommendations for postexposure prophylaxis (PEP) for HIV

    i. Early pathogenesis of HIV infection may theoretically be prevented by the administration of antiretroviral therapy within a few hours following exposure.

    ii. The risks and benefits of PEP must be thoroughly explained to the HCW. The use of PEP after an occupational exposure is not 100% effective in preventing HIV seroconversion (Centers for Disease Control and Prevention, 2001; Jones, 2002).

    iii. Antiretroviral therapy: Medications from three classes of drugs are available to treat occupational exposure: nucleoside reverse transcriptase inhibitors (NRTIs), nonnucleoside reverse transcriptase inhibitors (NNRTs), and protease inhibitors (PIs). Drug selection depends on several factors: the type of injury and device, the source patient's HIV viral load, and, where possible, the source patient's past and current regimens and resistance tests.

iv. Nearly 50% of HCWs taking PEP have experienced adverse symptoms, and about 33% stop taking PEP because of adverse symptoms; a higher discontinuation rate was associated with triple combination therapy versus a two-drug regimen; reported symptoms included nausea, malaise, headache, and anorexia (Centers for Disease Control and Prevention, 2001).

v. PEP may be prescribed to pregnant women, except for efavirenz (Sustiva), which has caused teratogenic effects in primates.

vi. The use of rapid testing (which will yield results in 15 min) of the source patient's blood helps in the decision whether or not to initiate PEP and prevents unnecessary side effects from drug therapy.

e. PEP for HBV transmission

i. Risk of infection is related to the HCW's degree of contact with blood in the workplace, the hepatitis B e antigen (HbeAg) status of the source person, and the vaccination status of the HCW (Centers for Disease Control and Prevention, 2001, 2002).

ii. Percutanous injury is the most noted route of exposure, but HBV can survive in dried blood at room temperature for 1 week; many HCWs who have tested positive do not recall having a percutaneous injury (Centers for Disease Control and Prevention, 2001).

iii. It is now mandated by Occupational Safety and Health Administration (OSHA) that HCWs with job placements in blood-borne areas be offered the HBV vaccine prior to job placement; declines in the incidence of acute HBV have occurred among highly vaccinated populations; from 1983 to 1995, the rate of HBV infection in HCWs declined 95% and is now lower than the rate of infection in the general population (Centers for Disease Control and Prevention, 2002).

iv. From 1982 to 2002, an estimated 70 million infants, children, and adults have received the HBV vaccine; side effects are minimal and include pain at the injection site and postinjection mild to moderate fever. HBV vaccine and hepatitis B immune globulin (HBIG) may be given to pregnant and lactating women. The vaccine should always be administered in the deltoid muscle; if indicated, HBIG can be given at the same time as the HBV vaccine, but at a separate site.

v. A vaccine responder is a person with adequate levels of serum antibody to hepatitis B surface antigen (HbsAg), demonstrated as serum levels for antibody to HbsAg (anti-HBs) at or less than 10 mIU/mL; a vaccine nonresponder is a person with inadequate response to vaccination, with serum anti-HBs greater than 10 mIU/mL (Centers for Disease Control and Prevention, 2001).

vi. PEP is not needed for previously vaccinated HCWs who have responded to the vaccine (Centers for Disease Control and Prevention, 2001).

vii. PEP for unvaccinated HCWs: If source patient is HbsAg positive, administer one dose of HBIG (0.06 mL/kg IM) and initiate the HB vaccine series; if source patient is HbsAg negative or status is unknown or unavailable, initiate the HB vaccine series (Centers for Disease Control and Prevention, 2001).

viii. PEP for vaccinated nonresponders: No treatment is required if the source patient is HbsAg negative; if the source patient is HbsAg positive, and the exposed HCW has not completed a second three-dose vaccine series, administer one dose of HBIG and initiate revaccination. If the exposed HCW previously completed a second vaccine series but failed to respond, immediately give one dose of HBIG and one month later give a second dose. If the source patient's status is unknown or unavailable, but the patient is a high-risk source, treat as if the source were HbsAg positive (Centers for Disease Control and Prevention, 2001).

ix. PEP for previously vaccinated but unknown antibody response: No treatment is required if the source patient is HbsAg negative. If the source is HbsAg positive, test the exposed person for anti-HBs. If they are adequate, no treatment is required; if they are inadequate, administer one dose of HBIG and a vaccine booster. If the source is unknown or unavailable, test the exposed person for anti-HBs. If adequate, no treatment is required; if inadequate, administer vaccine booster and recheck titer in 1 to 2 months (Centers for Disease Control and Prevention, 2001).

f. PEP for HCV transmission

i. HCV transmission from a hollow-bore needle and a known positive source is documented at 1.8%. Data are limited as to the length of time HCV survives in the environment. More than 3.5 million Americans are estimated to be HCV positive due to transmission from unsterilized medical equipment, sharing of drug tools, and sexual transmission.

ii. There is no vaccine against HCV because of the rapid progression and natural mutations of the virus; vaccine development is pending.

iii. Immune globulin and antiviral agents are not recommended at this time for PEP (Centers for Disease Control and Prevention, 2001).

iv. Although interferon and ribavirin are approved for the treatment of HCV, they are not FDA approved for HCV PEP.

v. Because there is no approved PEP regimen, recommended management consists of early detection of chronic disease and then evaluation of treatment options.

3. OSHA regulations

a. The incidence of occupationally acquired HIV infection created a need for the government to mandate safety programs in medical settings to protect HCWs and patients. In 1991, OSHA required all hospitals and medical facilities in the private setting to develop a blood-borne pathogen plan to educate HCWs in the differences in transmission of blood-borne pathogens, communicate to HCWs how to practice safely, use protective equipment, introduce and evaluate engineering controls, and provide medical care and follow-up for an injured employee.

b. Blood-borne pathogen plans include engineering controls (devices and tools) and work practice controls (policies and procedures) to reduce exposures.

i. Engineering controls: person protective equipment (PPE) must be made available, including gloves, gowns, and eye and foot protection to help prevent exposures. PPE must be the proper size for the employee. N-95-type respirator masks must be worn in areas where TB is presumed or diagnosed.

ii. Work practice controls are written policies and procedures that inform HCWs as to what type of PPE should be worn and the type of device necessary to perform care duties.

iii. Sharp disposal units must be puncture resistant, identified with the biohazard logo, and placed in convenient locations for HCWs. It is recommended that all boxes be no higher than 51 in. from the ground, within 6 ft of the treatment area, stabilized to prevent falling over, and replaced when three fourths full.

iv. Patient placement is based on patient diagnosis. HIV/AIDS diagnosis by itself is not reason for isolation or placement in a private room; patients with communicable diseases, such as TB, require a private room with negative airflow.

v. There are no restrictions for food delivery to patient's rooms; reusable dishes and silverware can be used; however, appropriate washing and drying of dishes should be performed to kill any pathogens.

vi. Laboratory specimens should be placed in plastic tubes and containers and then placed in a labeled, biohazard, plastic leak-proof bag. Minimal handling of specimens is recommended. During transportation to the lab, specimens should be placed in a covered leak-proof container.

vii. Cleaners and disinfectants should be Environmental Protection Agency (EPA) approved and should be bactericidal, fungicidal, and tuberculocidal. In the home setting, patients may use diluted bleach or over-the-counter cleansing agents.

viii. Medical waste is disposed of differently from general waste; depending on state regulations, medical waste should be placed in a red bag with a biohazard logo; these bags are designed to be thicker for protection against splitting.

ix. Biohazard labels must be placed on containers of blood, utility room doors, waste containers, and any other area or containers that contain blood or body fluids.

x. Linens are treated as infectious. Gloves must be worn while changing linen; linens are then placed in an impervious laundry bag. Industrial washing will remove potentially infectious material.

xi. Medical emergencies should be assessed, documented, and treated by the employer; PEP may be necessary, as well as HBV vaccine and immunoglobulins; and the process of patient and employee serial testing will be outlined and prescribed. The employer pays all costs.

xii. Employers will educate their staff initially, and then annually, regarding the blood-borne pathogen plan and newly approved engineering controls and work practice controls. Employees hired into a position that places them in direct or indirect care of patients or body fluids must be offered the HBV vaccine within 10 days of employment.

References

American Nurses Association. (1988). *American Nurses Association Task Force on Case Management.* Kansas City, MO: American Nurses Association.

American Nurses Association. (1994a). *Position Statements: Active euthanasia.* Retrieved January 26, 2003, from http://www.nursingworld.org/readroom/position/ethics/eteuth.htm

American Nurses Association. (1994b). *Position Statements: Assisted suicide.* Retrieved January 26, 2003, from http://www.nursingworld.org/readroom/position/ethics/etsuic.htm

American Nurses Association. (2001). *Code of ethics for nurses: Provisions.* Retrieved January 26, 2003, from http://www.nursingworld.org/ethics/chcode.htm

Anthony, W. A., Cohen, M., Farkas, M., & Cohen B. F. (1988). Case management—More than a response to a dysfunctional system. *Community Mental Health Journal 24*(3), 219–228.

Association of Nurses in AIDS Care. (1997). *Resolution: Role of the HIV/AIDS nurse in assisted suicide.* Retrieved January 26, 2003, from http://www.anacnet.org/about/policy.htm#Suicide

Association of Nurses in AIDS Care. (1999). *Position statement: Duty to care.* Retrieved January 26, 2003, from http://www.anacnet.org/about/policy.htm#Duty

Beauchamp, T. L., & Childress, J. F. (2001). *Principles of biomedical ethics* (5th ed.). New York: Oxford University Press.

Case Management Standards Work Group, National Association of Social Workers. (1992). *NASW standards for social work case management.* Washington, DC: Author.

Centers for Disease Control and Prevention. (2001). Updated U. S. public health service guidelines for the management of occupational exposures to HBV, HCV, and HIV and recommendations for postexposure prophylaxis. *MMWR, 50*(RR-11), 1–42.

Centers for Disease Control and Prevention. (2002). Hepatitis B vaccination—United States, 1982–2002. *MMWR, 51*(25), 549–552.

Cesta, T. G., Tahan, H. A., & Fink, L. F. (Eds.). (1998). *The case manager's survival guide: Winning strategies for clinical practice.* St. Louis, MO: Mosby.

Commission for Case Manager Certification. (1996). *CCM certification guide.* Rolling Meadows, IL: Author.

Ferrell, B. R., & Coyle, N. (2001). *Textbook of palliative nursing.* New York: Oxford University Press.

Gordon, S., Benner, P. E., & Noddings, N. (1996). *Caregiving: Readings in knowledge, practice, ethics, and politics.* Philadelphia: University of Pennsylvania Press.

Jones, S. G. (2002). The other side of the pill bottle: The lived experience of HIV+ nurses on HIV combination drug therapy. *Journal of the Association of Nurses in AIDS Care, 13*(3), 22–36.

Jones, S. G., Messmer, P. R., Charron, S. A., & Parns, M. (2002). HIV-positive women and minority patients' satisfaction with inpatient hospital care. *AIDS Patient Care and STDs, 16*(3), 127–134.

Lynn, J., Schuster, J. L., & Kabcenell, A. (2000). *Improving care for the end of life: A sourcebook for health care managers and clinicians.* New York: Oxford University Press.

National Case Management Task Force, Case Management Society of America. (1995). *Standards of practice for case management.* Little Rock, AR: Author.

Quill, T. E. (2001). *Caring for patients at the end of life: Facing an uncertain future together.* New York: Oxford University Press.

Sowell, R., & Meadows, T. (1994). An integrated case management model: Developing standards, evaluation, and outcomes. *Nursing Administration Quarterly, 18*(2), 53–64.

Tahan, H. A., & Cesta, T. G. (1995). Developing case management plans using a quality improvement model. *Journal of Nursing Administration, 24*(12), 49–58.

Ulrich, L. P. (1999). *The Patient Self-Determination Act: Meeting the challenges in patient care.* Washington, DC: Georgetown University Press.

UNAIDS. (2002). *AIDS epidemic update 2002.* Retrieved January 26, 2003, from http://www.unaids.org

U. S. Department of Health and Human Services, Health Resources and Services Administration, HIV/AIDS Bureau. (2001). *Outcomes evaluation technical assistance guide: Case management outcomes, Titles I and II of the Ryan White CARE Act.* Washington, DC: Author.

Appendix A

Public Health Service Revised Classification System for HIV Infection (Adolescents and Adults)

1993 Revised

The following material contains the most important aspects of the report published by Centers for Disease Control and Prevention (CDC).[1] The complete document may be found as cited.

The classification system for HIV infection among adolescents and adults has been revised to include the CD_4 lymphocyte count as a marker for HIV-related immunosuppression. This revision establishes mutually exclusive subgroups for which the spectrum of clinical conditions is integrated with the CD_4 lymphocyte count. The objectives of these changes are to simplify the classification of HIV infection, to reflect current standards of medical care for HIV infected people, and to categorize more accurately HIV-related morbidity.

The revised CDC classification system for HIV-infected adolescents and adults[2] categorizes people on the basis of clinical conditions associated with HIV infection and CD_4 lymphocyte counts. The system is based

on three ranges of CD_4 lymphocyte counts and three clinical categories and is represented by a matrix of nine mutually exclusive categories (Table A1). This system replaces the classification system published in 1986, which

---

[1]*Notes:* From "1993 Revised Classification System for HIV Infection and Expanded Surveillance Case Definition for AIDS Among Adolescents and Adults," by Centers for Disease Control and Prevention, 1992, *MMWR, 41*(RR-17), 1-9.

[2]Criteria for HIV infection for people ages $\geq$ 13 years: (a) repeatedly reactive screening tests for HIV antibody (e.g., enzyme immunoassay) with specific antibody identified by the use of supplemental tests (e.g., Western blot, immunofluorescence assay); (b) indirect identification of virus in host tissues by virus isolation; (c) HIV antigen detection; or (d) a positive result on any other highly specific licensed test for HIV.

Table A1   1993 Revised Classification System for HIV Infection and Expanded AIDS Surveillance Case Definition for Adolescents and Adults*

	Clinical Categories		
CD4 T-Cell Categories	*(A)* *Asymptomatic, Acute (Primary) HIV or PGL[†]*	*(B)* *Symptomatic, Not (A) or (C) Conditions*	*(C)* *AIDS-Indicator Conditions*
(1) $\geq$ 500/mm³	A1	B1	C1
(2) 200–499/mm³	A2	B2	C2
(3) < 200/mm³ AIDS-indicator T-cell count	A3	B3	C3

* The shaded cells illustrate the expanded AIDS surveillance case definition. People with AIDS-indicator conditions (Category C) as well as those with CD4 T-lymphocyte counts < 200/mm³

[†] PGL (persistent generalized lymphadenopathyl). Clinical Category A includes acute (primary) HIV infections.

351

included only clinical disease criteria and which was developed before the widespread use of CD_4 T-cell testing.

CD₄ Lymphocyte Categories

The three CD_4 lymphocyte categories are defined as follows:

- Category 1: ≥ 500 cells/mm³
- Category 2: 200–499 cells/mm³
- Category 3: < 200 cells/mm³

These categories correspond to CD_4T lymphocyte counts per microliter of blood and guide clinical and therapeutic actions in the management of HIV-infected adolescents and adults. The revised HIV classification system also allows for the use of the percentage of CD_4T lymphocytes.

HIV-infected people should be classified based on existing guidelines for the medical management of HIV-infected people. Thus, the lowest accurate, but not necessarily the most recent, CD_4T lymphocyte count should be used for classification purposes.

Clinical Categories

The clinical categories of HIV infection are defined as follows:

Category A

Category A consists of one or more of the conditions listed below in an adolescent or adult (≥ 13 years) with documented HIV infection. Conditions listed in Categories B and C must not have occurred.

- Asymptomatic HIV infection
- Persistent generalized lymphadenopathy
- Acute (primary) HIV infection with accompanying illness or history of acute HIV infection

Category B

Category B consists of symptomatic conditions in an HIV-infected adolescent or adult that are not included among conditions listed in clinical Category C and that meet at least one of the following criteria: (1) the conditions are attributed to HIV infection or are indicative of a defect in cell-mediated immunity or (b) the conditions are considered by physicians to have a clinical course or to require management that is complicated by HIV infection. Examples of conditions in clinical Category B include, but are not limited to the following:

- Bacillary angiomatosis
- Candidiasis, oropharyngeal (thrush)
- Candidiasis, vulvovaginal; persistent, frequent, or poorly responsive to therapy
- Cervical dysplasia (moderate or severe)/ cervical carcinoma in situ
- Constitutional symptoms, such as fever (38.5°C) or diarrhea lasting > 1 month
- Hairy leukoplakia, oral
- Herpes zoster (shingles), involving at least two distinct episodes or more than one dermatome
- Idiopathic thrombocytopenic purpura
- Listeriosis
- Pelvic inflammatory disease, particularly if complicated by tubo-ovarian abscess
- Peripheral neuropathy

For classification purposes, Category B conditions take precedence over those in Category A. For example, someone previously treated for oral or persistent vaginal candidiasis (and who has not developed a Category C disease) but who is now asymptomatic should be classified in clinical Category B.

Category C

Category C includes the clinical conditions listed in the AIDS surveillance case definition (Table A2). For classification purposes, once a Category C condition has occurred, the person will remain in Category C.

Equivalences for CD₄ Lymphocyte Count and Percentage of Total Lymphocytes

Compared with the absolute CD_4 lymphocyte count, the percentage of CD_4 T-cells of total

Table A2   Conditions Included in the 1993
AIDS Surveillance Case Definition

- Candidiasis of bronchi, trachea, or lungs
- Candidiasis, esophageal
- Cervical cancer, invasive*
- Coccidioidomycosis, disseminated or extrapulmonary
- Cryptococcosis, extrapulmonary
- Cryptosporidiosis, chronic intestinal (> 1 month's duration)
- Cytomegalovirus disease (other than liver, spleen, or nodes)
- Cytomegalovirus retinitis (with loss of vision)
- Encephalopathy, HIV-related
- Herpes simplex: chronic ulcer(s) (> 1 month's duration) or bronchitis pneumonitis, or esophagitis
- Histoplasmosis, disseminated or extrapulmonary
- Isosporiasis, chronic intestinal (> 1 month's duration)
- Kaposi's sarcoma
- Lymphoma, Burkitt's (or equivalent term)
- Lymphoma, immunoblastic (or equivalent term)
- Lymphoma, primary, of brain
- *Mycobacterium avium* complex of *M. kansasii*, disseminated or extrapulmonary
- *Mycobacterium tuberculosis,* any site (pulmonary* or extrapulmonary)
- *Mycobacterium,* other species or unidentified species, disseminated or extrapulmonary
- *Pneumocystis carinii* pneumonia
- Pneumonia, recurrent*
- Progressive multifocal leukoencephalopathy
- *Salmonella* septicemia, recurrent
- Toxoplasmosis of brain
- Wasting syndrome due to HIV

---

* Added in the 1993 expansion of the AIDS surveillance case definition

lymphocytes (or CD_4 percentage) is less subject to variation on repeated measurement. However, data correlating natural history of HIV infection with the CD_4 percentage have not been as consistently available as data on absolute CD_4 lymphocyte counts. Therefore, the revised classification system emphasizes the use of CD_4T lymphocyte counts but allows for the use of CD_4 percentages (Table A3).

Table A3   Equivalences for Absolute Numbers of CD_4 Lymphocytes and CD_4 Percentage

CD_4 T-Cell Category	CD_4 T-Cells/mm^3	CD_4 Percentage (%)
(1)	≥ 500	≥ 29
(2)	200–499	14–28
(3)	< 200	< 14

Expansion of the CDC Surveillance Case Definition for AIDS

In 1991, CDC, in collaboration with the Council of State and Territorial Epidemiologists (CSTE), proposed an expansion of the AIDS surveillance case definition. This proposal was made available for public comment in November 1991 and was discussed at an open meeting on September 2, 1992. Based on information presented and reviewed during the public comment period and at the open meeting, CDC, in collaboration with CSTE, expanded the AIDS surveillance case definition to include all HIV-infected people with CD_4 lymphocyte counts of < 200 cells/mm^3 or a CD_4 percentage of < 14. In addition to retaining the 23 clinical conditions in the previous AIDS surveillance definition, the expanded definition includes pulmonary tuberculosis, recurrent pneumonia, and invasive cervical cancer. This expanded definition requires laboratory confirmation of HIV infection in people with a CD_4 lymphocyte count of < 200 cells/mm^3 or with one of the added clinical conditions. This expanded definition for reporting cases to CDC became effective January 1, 1993.

In the revised HIV classification system, people in subcategories A3, B3, and C3 meet the immunologic criteria of the surveillance case definition, and people with conditions in subcategories Cl, C2, and C3 meet the clinical criteria for surveillance purposes.

Appendix B

Selected Laboratory Values

Type of Test	Normal Value/Range	Comments
Enzyme immunoassay (EIA or ELISA) for HIV antibodies	Nonreactive	The test has sensitivity and specificity rates of > 98% (Mylonakis, Paliou, Lally, Flanigan, & Rich, 2000; Sloand, Pitt, Chiarello, & Nemo, 1991). HIV-antibody screening test; if reactive, is confirmed with a Western Blot. False negatives are usually due to testing in the window period; the interval from infection to reactive EIA averages 10 to 14 days with new test reagents (Morens, 1997; Mylonakis et al., 2000). Seroconversion may take 3 to 4 weeks, but virtually all individuals seroconvert within 6 months (Mylonakis et al., 2000).
Western Blot (WB)	Negative: No bands	HIV antibody used to confirm a reactive EIA; a positive WB shows reactivity to bands gp41+ gp120/160 or p24 + gp120/160. An indeterminate test occurs when there is the presence of any band pattern that does not meet criteria for positive results (see above). False-positive EIA and WB in low-prevalence populations are very rare and are most often due to technical errors.

Rapid HIV Tests

Type of Test	Normal Value/Range	Comments
Single use diagnostic system (SUDS); Murex Diagnostics/ Abbott	Nonreactive	Only FDA-approved (10/17/00) rapid test for HIV and is commercially available in the United States. Comparable in accuracy to the EIA and is 99.9% sensitive and the specificity is 99.6% (Irwin, Olivo, Schable, Weber, Janssen, & Ernst, 1996); results reported in 10 to 15 minutes. It is recommended that a negative result be reported as definitive but that positive results be confirmed with standard serology.
OraQuick Rapid HIV-1 Test	Nonreactive	First FDA-approved (11/17/02) rapid, point-of-care test designed to detect

OraSure Technologies/ Abbott Diagnostics		antibodies to HIV-1 within approximately 20 minutes. Has reported sensitivity of 99.6% and specificity of 100% using finger stick whole-blood specimens. A reactive (preliminary positive) must be confirmed.

Urine and Salivary HIV-1 Tests

Type of Test	Normal Value/Range	Comments
Orasure Test; Epitope Co.	Nonreactive	FDA-approved device for collecting oral mucosal transudate (OMT), which contains antibodies from the blood vessels of the mucous membranes. The pad is then placed in preservative and sent to a clinical laboratory for testing with an initial EIA test for HIV antibody, and, if reactive, the WB confirmatory assay is performed. May be anonymous or confidential and results are available by phone or fax within 3 days. Sensitivity and specificity are comparable to standard serology (Gallo, George, Fitchen, Goldstein, & Hindahl, 1997).
Urine test Calypte HIV-1 Urine EIA	Nonreactive	FDA approved urine screening EIA. Reported sensitivity is 99% and specificity is 94% (Desai, Bates, & Michalski, 1991; Urnovitz, Sturge, Gottfried, & Murphy, 1999). Positive results require confirmation by a standard serologic test.

Virological and Immunologic Markers in HIV Infection

Type of Test	Normal Value/Range	Comments
DNA PCR assay	No DNA detected	The most sensitive qualitative measure to detect cell-associated proviral DNA as low as 1 to 10 copies. Sensitivity is > 99% depending on stage of disease and test technique, and specificity is 98%. Not considered sufficient for diagnosis due to low levels of false positives but is more sensitive than the p24 antigen; will need confirmation with standard antibody testing. Test is not FDA approved for HIV diagnosis (Owens et al., 1996). Useful in documenting neonatal infection, primary infection, and indeterminate serologic tests.
HIV RNA PCR	No RNA detected	Qualitative measure of cell-free or cell-associated viral RNA. Sensitivity is between 95% and 98%, depending on stage of disease and test technique and assumes no ARV therapy.

		Not considered sufficient for diagnosis due to low levels of false positives; will need confirmation with standard antibody testing. Test is not FDA approved for HIV diagnosis.
PBMC (peripheral blood mononuclear cell culture)	Negative	Measures infectious, cell-associated virus. Expensive, labor-intensive process which lasts 28 days. Sensitivity is between 95% and 100% Quantitative results correlate with stage of HIV disease.

Quantitative Plasma HIV RNA (viral load)

Type of Test	Normal Value/Range	Comments
• RT-PCR (Roche): – Standard detection: 400 to 750,000 copies/ml – Ultrasensitive detection: 50 to 75,000 copies/ml • bDNA (Bayer): 100 to 500,000 copies/ml • Nuclisens HIV-1 QT (Organon): 40 to 10,000,000 copies/ml	Undetectable	Quantitative measure of HIV viral load in plasma. Useful in the diagnosing of acute HIV infection, predicting progression in chronically infected individuals, risk of transmission with nearly any type of exposure, and for therapeutic monitoring. Assays should be obtained at times of clinical stability, at least 4 weeks after immunizations or intercurrent infections, and with use of the same lab and same technology.
CD_4 cell count	Normal adult values are 800 to 1,050 cells/mm^3, with a range representing two SD of about 500 to 1,400 cells/mm^3	CD_4 cells are a primary target of HIV infection. As HIV infection advances, the number declines progressively. Test is used to stage the disease, provide guidelines for differential diagnosis of patient complaints, and dictate therapeutic decisions about antiviral treatment and prophylaxis of opportunistic disease. It is a prognostic indicator and complements the viral load assay. Individual variability in results up to 15% can be seen in the course of 1 day. Small variations in the number of WBCs or in the percentage of lymphocytes greatly influences CD_4 counts. Additional factors affecting the CD_4 cell count include seasonal and diurnal variation; the use of corticosteroids; intercurrent illness; coinfection with HTLV-1; as well as inter- and intralaboratory variation.
CD_4 Lymphoctye percentage	> 29%	Measures the percentage of total lymphocytes with the CD_4 marker. Is less subject to variation based on the CBC and differential and preferred as

a measure of the degree of immunosupression

A CD_4 % < 20 correlates with immunosuppression.

A CD_4 % < 14 meets the criteria for an AIDS diagnosis.

Resistance Testing

Type of Test	Normal Value/Range	Comments
		An in vitro method of measuring virus resistance to antiretroviral agents. Aids in the selection of antiretroviral drugs. Limitations of resistance testing: — Measure only the dominant species at the time the test was performed; therefore, resistant variants that may comprise less than 20% of the total viral population may not be detected due to being in reservoirs (CNS, latent CD_4 cells, genital tract, lymph nodes). — Individual must have a sufficient viral load to do the test ($\geq$ 500–1,000 copies/ml). — Genotypic assays are hard to interpret because multiple mutations are required for ARV agents and cross-resistance. — Phenotypic assays are hard to interpret due to the thresholds used to define susceptibility. — Individuals must be tested while on the ARV agents being questioned.
Genotypic assays		Methodology involves (1) amplification of the reverse transcriptase (RT), protease (Pr) gene, or both by RT PCR; (2) DNA sequencing of amplicons generated for the dominant species; (3) reporting of the mutations for each gene using a letter-number-letter standard. Updated information on resistance testing can be found at http://www.viral-resistance.com
Phenotypic assays		This assay is comparable to conventional in vitro tests of antimicrobial sensitivity, in which the microbe is grown in serial dilutions of antiviral agents. Insertion of the RT and Pr genes from the patient's strain into the backbone of the laboratory clone by cloning or by recombination Replication is monitored at various drug concentrations and compared to a reference wild type virus. Results are reported as the IC_{50} for the test strain relative to that of the reference or wild type strain.

Formerly, interpretation of resistance was based on a fourfold change greater than the reference strain. The newer method is to individualize by drug.

Hepatitis B Serology

Type of Test	Normal Value/Range	Comments
Hepatitis B core antibody (HbcAb)	Nonreactive (no core antibodies detected)	USPHS/IDSA guidelines recommend screening for hepatitis B core antibody (Centers for Disease Control and Prevention, 1999) with HBV vaccination of those who are susceptible. HBV seroprevalence is 3% to 14% in the general population, 35% to 80% for gay men, 60% to 80% for IDUs, and 5% to 20% in heterosexuals with multiple partners. Positive marker will appear between 6 and 14 weeks after exposure and remain in serum for a longer time; together with HbsAb represents the convalescent stage; indicates past infection.
Hepatitis B surface antibody (HbsAb)	Nonreactive (no surface antibodies detected)	CDC recommends postvaccination serology with anti-HBs in individuals with HIV infection at 1 to 6 months after the third dose of vaccine to confirm antigenic response. Positive marker indicates previous exposure, clinical recovery, immunity to hepatitis B; the marker for permanent immunity to hepatitis B. Positive marker appears 4 to 10 months after infection or vaccination.
Hepatitis B surface antigen (HBsAg)	Negative (no surface antigen detected)	Recommended for suspected acute and chronic viral hepatitis. HBsAg usually becomes detectable 2 weeks to 2 months before clinical symptoms, and as little as 2 weeks after infection. It is usually present for 2 to 3 months. Five to 10 percent of patients will have persistent HBsAg levels beyond 6 months (chronic carrier, chronic hepatitis). The EIA test will detect 100 pg/mL or more of HBsAg. All positive HBsAg are further tested using the HBsAg confirmation test. About 5% of positive HBsAg's are false positives and will not neutralize in the confirmatory assay.
Hepatitis B virus antigen (HBeAg)		Useful to monitor chronic HBV infection. The HBeAg appears in close association with HBsAg, but normally does not persist as long. Its presence is generally associated with higher infectivity, but it is of limited usefulness diagnostically.

Hepatitis B virus antibody (Anti-HBe)		The development of anti-HBe coincides with the disappearance of e antigen. This is usually after the appearance of anti-HBc and before that of anti-HBs. Anti-HBe often disappears, but its persistence has been associated with chronic hepatitis and the chronic carrier state. It does not confer protection.
Hepatitis B virus DNA ultra sensitive quantitative PCR		A molecular test useful for monitoring the response to treatment in chronically infected HBV patients.

Hepatitis C Serology

Type of Test	Normal Value/Range	Comments
		The 2001 USPHS/IDSA guidelines recommend screening for HCV because some HIV-positive individuals (IDUs and those with hemophilia) are at increased risk for HCV infection and related disease and because knowledge of HCV status is important for management of all HIV-positive individuals to interpret and manage elevated LFTs.
Anti-HCV EIA	Nonreactive (no antibodies detected)	Screening method for HCV antibodies using enzyme immunoassays (EIAs) licensed for detection of antibody to HCV in blood. Detects $\geq$ 97% of infected persons but does not distinguish if they are acute, chronic, or resolved Positive anti-HCV results should be verified with additional testing (RIBA or HCV RNA). Anti-HCV may be negative with acute HCV infection and with severe immunosuppression (CD_4 cell count < 100 cells/mm^3).
HCV RIBA™ recombinant immunoblot assay	Negative	Used to confirm anti-HCV positive result.
RT-PCR for HCV RNA	Negative	Used to confirm anti-HCV positive result HCV RNA (quantitative or qualitative) is required to confirm chronic HCV infection.
Quantitative HCV PCR	Negative	Quantitative tests show a threshold of detection of 100–1,000 c/ml and are less sensitive than qualitative RT-PCR; may be useful in predicting response to therapy but not yet useful in therapy monitoring.
HCV genotype	HCV is grouped into six major genotypes, which are subtyped according to sequence characteristics and are designated as 1a, 1b, 1c, 2a, 2b, 2c, 3a, 3b, 4a–h, 5a, and 6a.	Genotype assay identifies six genotypes and > 90 subtypes. Genotype 1 accounts for 70% of HCV-infected persons in the United States and is associated with the poorest response to therapy when compared with genotypes 2 and 3.

Syphilis Serology VDRL or RPR	Nonreactive Weakly reactive Reactive N. B. weakly reactive and reactive results are titered.	Performed at baseline and repeated annually due to the high rates of coinfection with HIV and *Treponema pallidum*. False positives are not uncommon and can be excluded with a confirmatory fluorescent treponemal antibody test.
Toxoplasma gondii antibodies, IgG	Negative antibodies = no latent infection Positive antibodies = latent infection	HIV-positive people with evidence of latent toxoplasmosis infection may be candidates for prophylactic therapy; in those with CNS symptoms, evidence of latent infection assists in the development of differential diagnoses. HIV-positive people without evidence of latent infection may be counseled to avoid unnecessary exposure. It is estimated that 20% to 50% of HIV-positive toxoplasma-seropositive patients will develop toxoplasmic encephalitis; therefore, seropositive patients should receive prophylaxis against toxoplasmosis after their CD_4 cell count falls below 100 cells/mm^3.
Cytomegalovirus antibodies, IgG	Negative antibodies = no latent infection Equivocal = repeat testing Positive antibodies = latent infection	Now recommended by the USPHS/IDSA guidelines, especially in those at lower risk for CMV infection (other than gay men and IDUs). Even though prevalence is high in HIV-positive individuals, identification of CMV-infected patients allows for the use of CMV- or leukocyte-reduced blood products when transfusions are needed, thus reducing the risk of iatrogenic CMV infection.
Glucose-6-phosphate dehydrogenase (G-6-PD)	4.6–13.5 U/g hemoglobin (Hgb)	G-6-PD deficiency is a genetic condition that predisposes individuals to hemolysis following exposure to oxidant drugs, especially dapsone, primaquine, and sulfonamides. Routine screening for G-6-PD deficiency is sometimes recommended in patients with appropriate genetic background. These include men with the following ancestry: African American, Italian, Sephardic Jew, Arab, and those from India and Southeast Asia.
Lactate	17 years of age and older: 0.5–2.2 mmol/L	Lactic acidosis is characterized by an elevated venous lactate level. A confirmed lactate level about 5 mmol/1 in the presence of signs and symptoms associated with lactic acidema should be used to establish the diagnosis of NRTI-associated lactic acidema.

References

Centers for Disease Control and Prevention. (1999). 1999 USPHS/IDSA guidelines for the prevention of opportunistic infections in persons infected with human immunodeficiency virus. U.S. Public Health Service (USPHS) and Infectious Diseases Society of America. *MMWR, 48*(RR-10), 41.

Desai, S., Bates, H., & Michalski, F. J. (1991). Detection of antibody to HIV-1 in urine. *Lancet, 337,* 183–184.

Gallo, D., George, J. R., Fitchen, J. H., Goldstein, A. S, & Hindahl, M. S. (1997). Evaluation of a system using oral mucosal transudate for HIV-1 antibody screening and confirmatory testing. OraSure HIV Clinical Trials Group. *Journal of the American Medical Association, 277,* 254–258.

Irwin, K., Olivo, N., Schable, C. A., Weber, J. T., Janssen, R., & Ernst, J. (1996). Performance characteristics of a rapid HIV antibody assay in a hospital with a high prevalence of HIV infection. CDC-Bronx-Lebanon HIV Serosurvey Team. *Annals of Internal Medicine, 125,* 471–475.

Morens, D. M. (1997). Serological screening tests for antibody to human immunodeficiency virus—The search for perfection in an imperfect world. *Clinical Infectious Diseases, 25,* 101–103.

Mylonakis, E., Paliou, M., Lally, M., Flanigan, T. P., & Rich, J. D. (2000). Laboratory testing for infection with the human immunodeficiency virus: Established and novel approaches. *American Journal of Medicine, 109,* 568–576.

Owens, D. K., Holodniy, M., Garber, A. M., Scott, J., Sonnad, S., Moses, L., et al. (1996). Polymerase chain reaction for the diagnosis of HIV infection in adults. A meta-analysis with recommendations for clinical practice and study design. *Annals of Internal Medicine, 124*(9), 803–815.

Sloand, E. M., Pitt, E., Chiarello, R. J., & Nemo, G. J. (1991). HIV testing. State of the art. *Journal of the American Medical Association, 266,* 2861–2866.

Urnovitz, H. B., Sturge, J. C., Gottfried, T. D., & Murphy, W. H. (1999). Urine antibody tests: New insights into the dynamics of HIV-1 infection. *Clinical Chemistry, 45,* 1602–1613.

Appendix C

Treatment of Tuberculosis (TB in Adult and Adolescent Patients Coinfected With the Human Immunodeficiency Virus [HIV])

This is intended as a convenient reference for health-care providers managing adult and adolescent HIV-infected patients who have drug-susceptible TB. It is not intended as a complete reference for treatment of TB in HIV coinfected patients, and readers are referred to the references listed on page 367.

Table C1 Treatment Strategies for Adult and Adolescent TB Patients Coinfected With HIV

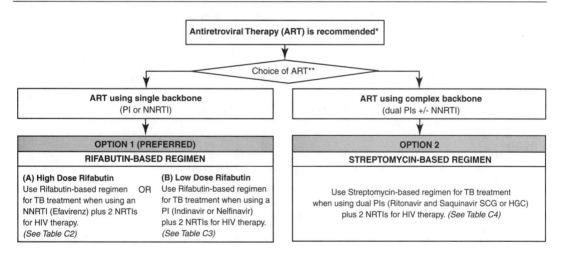

* In those rare circumstances when antiretroviral therapy is not recommended, use a standard 6-month rifampin-based regimen.

** HIV antiretroviral therapy described here only includes strongly recommended DHHS regimens.

Table C2   Option 1A: Rifabutin-Based Regimen, High Dose, TB Treatment Regimens for Adult and Adolescent Patients Receiving Antiretroviral Therapy With an NNRTI[a,b] (Efavirenz) and Two NRTIs[c]

Six-month RFB[d]-based therapy (may be prolonged to 9 months[e])

Induction Phase		Duration	Continuation Phase		Duration
Drugs		**Duration**	**Drugs**		**Duration**
INH[f]	5mg/kg up to maximum of 300mg PO or IM		INH[f]	5mg/kg up to maximum of 300mg PO or IM	Daily for 4 months (18 weeks)
RFB[d]	450-600mg PO or IV	Daily for 2 months (8 weeks)		450-600mg PO or IV	
PZA[d]	15-30mg/kg up to maximum 2mg PO				
EMB[d]	15-25mg/kg up to maximum 1600mg PO		**OR**		
or					
SM[h]	15mg/kg up to maximum 1gm M or IV		INH[f]	15mg/kg up to maximum of 900mg PO or IM	Twice weekly for 4 months (18 weeks)[i]
			RFB[d]	600 PO or IV	

Abbreviations for TB Medications

EMB: Ethambutol; INH: Isoniazid; PZA: Pyrazinamide; RIF: Rifampin; RFB: Rifabutin; SM: Streptomycin

a. The recommended dose for Efavirenz is 600 mg once daily.

b. Nevirapine is an alternative NNRTI in the treatment of HIV but is given a lower ranking. See DHHS reference. Delavirdine should not be used concurrently with a Rifamycin.

c. Currently five NRTIs are approved, of which four are recommended, for the treatment of HIV infection and are divided into two categories; thymidine analogues, Stavudine (d4T, Zerit) and Zidovudine (ZDV, Retrovir) and nonthymidine analogues, didanosine (ddI, Videx), lamivudine (3TC, Epivir) and zalcitabine (ddc, Hivid). NRTI therapy should include one thymidine analogue (ZDV or d4T) plus a nonthymidine analogue (ddI or 3TC).

d. RFB normally given in a dose of 5 mg/kg/d (maximum 300 mg/d PO or IV). In patients receiving Efavirenz, the dose of RFB is increased from 300 mg to either 450 mg–600 mg daily or 600 mg twice weekly.

e. Duration of treatment should be prolonged 4 to 6 months after culture conversion of sputum if there is a delayed response to therapy. Criteria for delayed response include lack of sputum culture conversion from positive to negative within 3 to 4 months or lack of resolution of signs or symptoms of TB.

f. Pyridoxine (Vitamin B6) 25–50 mg/d or 50–100 mg twice weekly should be given to all HIV-infected patients receiving INH.

g. Continue PZA and EMB for the total duration of the induction phase (8 weeks).

Table C3   Option 1B: Rifabutin-Based Regimen, Low Dose, TB Treatment Regimens for Adult and Adolescent Patients Receiving Antiretroviral Therapy With a PI [j,k] (Indinavir, or Nelfinavir) and Two NRTIs[c]

Six-month RFB[l]-based therapy (may be prolonged to 9 months[e])

Induction Phase			Continuation Phase		
Drugs		**Duration**	**Drugs**		**Duration**
INF[f]	5mg/kg up to maximum of 300mg PO or IM		INF[f]	5mg/kg up to maximum of 300mg PO or IM	
RFB[l]	150mg PO or IV	Daily for 2 months	RFB[d]	150mg PO or IV	Daily for 4 months
PZA[g]	15-30mg/kg up to maximum 2gm PO	(8 weeks)			(18 weeks)
EMB[g]	15-25mg/kg up to maximum 1600mg PO				
or			**OR**		
SM[h]	15mg/kg up to maximum 1gm IM or IV		INF[f]	15mg/kg up to maximum of 900mg PO or IM	Twice weekly for 4 months
			RFB[d]	300mg PO or IV	(18 weeks)[i]

h. SM contraindicated in pregnancy.

i. All intermittent TB drug dosing should be directly observed.

j. The usual prescribed dose of indinavir is 800 mg q 8h, and the dose of nelfinavir is 750 mg TID; when coadministered with RFB increase indinavir and nelfinavir to 1000 mg q 8h PO respectively. Periodic assessment for decreased anti-HIV drug activity should be monitored by measuring viral load.

k. Amprenavir with reduced dose of RFB (150 mg) is an alternative PI based treatment option but is given a lower ranking.[4]

l. RFB normally given in a dose of 5 mg/kg/d (maximum 300 mg/d PO or IV). In patients receiving a PI, the dose of RFB is decreased from 300 mg to 150 mg OD. The twice weekly dose of RFB (300 mg) remains unchanged. Patients should be monitored carefully for RFB drug toxicity (arthralgia, uveitis, leukopenia).

Table C4   Option 2: Streptomycin-Based Regimen, TB Treatment Regimens for Adult and Adolescent Patients Receiving Antiretroviral Therapy With a Backbone of Dual PIs[a]

Nine Month SM-based therapy (may be prolonged to 12 months[b])

Induction Phase		Continuation Phase	
Drugs	**Duration**	**Drugs**	**Duration**
INH[c] 5mg/kg up to maximum of 300mg PO or IM SM[d] 15mg/kg up to maximum 1gm IM or IV PZA 15-30mg/kg up to maximum 2gm PO EMB 15-25mg/kg up to maximum 1600mg PO	Daily for 2 months (8 weeks)	INH[c] 15mg/kg up to maximum of 900 mg PO or IM SM[d] 25-30mg/kg up to 1.5gms IM or IV PZA 50-70mg/kg up to 3.5gms PO	2-3 times per week for 7 months (30 weeks)[e]
OR		**OR**	
INH[c] 5mg/kg up to maximum of 300mg PO or IM SM[d] 15mg/kg up to maximum 1gm IM or IV PZA 15-30mg/kg up to maximum 2gm PO EMB 15-25mg/kg up to maximum 1600mg PO	Daily for 2 weeks and then 2-3 times per week for 6 weeks (at the intermittent dose)	INH[c] 15mg/kg up to 900 mg PO or IM SM[d] 25-30mg/kg up to 1.5gms IM or IV PZA 50-70mg/kg up to 3.5gms PO	2-3 times per week for 7 months (30 weeks)[e]

a. Treatment with two PIs amplifies the complexity of drug interactions when Rifamycins are also coadministered. When combinations of PIs or NNRTIs are prescribed the use of anti-TB regimens containing no Rifamycins should be considered. It may also be used for other complex ART regimens (e.g., PI + NNRTI + 2NRTIs) that are given a lower ranking.

b. Duration of treatment should be prolonged if there is a delayed response to therapy. Criteria for delayed response should be assessed at the end of the 2-month induction phase and include lack of sputum culture conversion from positive to negative or lack of resolution of signs or symptoms of TB. Treatment should be prolonged for at least 6 months after culture conversion of sputum. The NJMS National TB Center cautions that these anti-TB regimens have not been studied in HIV positive patients. It has been our policy to treat TB in these patients with a non-Rifamycin-containing regimen for 18–24 months.

c. Pyridoxine (Vitamin B6) 25–50 mg/d or 50–100 mg twice weekly should be given to all HIV-infected patients receiving INH.

d. SM is contraindicated in pregnancy. Every effort should be made to continue SM for the total duration of treatment. When SM cannot be used for the recommended 9 months, EMB should be added to the regimen and treatment duration extended from 9 months (38 weeks) to 12 months (52 weeks).

e. All intermittent TB drug dosing should be directly observed.

Treatment Information

- The management of TB in adult and adolescent patients who are coinfected with HIV should be undertaken by health care providers who are experienced in TB/HIV care. TB treatment regimens should be directly observed to assure patient adherence, and therapy should be prolonged if there is a delay in clinical or bacterial response. Patients should also be closely monitored for both TB- and HIV-treatment failures, paradoxical reactions, and adverse drug effects.
- Drug interactions make TB treatment in HIV coinfected patients taking NNRTIs and PIs more difficult. NNRTIs induce and PIs inhibit CYP450 hepatic enzymes causing, respectively, reductions and elevations of Rifamycin serum levels. The rifamycins discussed here (RIF, RFB) induce CYP450 hepatic enzymes that accelerate the metabolism of PIs and NNRTIs and may significantly decrease serum levels of these drugs. RIF, the most potent member of the rifamycins in this regard, is generally not used when treating TB in HIV coinfected patients who are also talking PIs or NNRTIs and is substituted with RFB.
- Although the principles of treatment are similar for children and adults, there are unique treatment considerations that must be followed when treating TB in an HIV coinfected child. HIV-infected children who are suspected of having TB should be treated without delay. However, consultation with a specialist who has experience in managing HIV-infected children with TB is advised because indications for antiretroviral therapy, dosing of medications, and optimal length of therapy in children can vary.

References

1. CDC. Prevention and Treatment of TB among Patients Infected with Human Immunodeficiency Virus: Principles of Therapy and Revised Recommendations. *MMWR* 1998;47 (No. RR-20).
2. CDC. Updated Guidelines for the Use of Rifabutin or Rifampin for the Treatment and Prevention of TB among HIV-infected Patients Taking Protease Inhibitors or Nonnucleoside Reverse Transcriptase Inhibitors. *MMWR* 2000; 49 (No. 9).
3. American Academy of Pediatrics. TB. In: Pickering LK, ed. *2000 Red Book:* R George.
4. DHSS. *Guidelines for the Use of Antiretroviral Agents in HIV-infected Adults and Adolescents. Panel on Clinical Practices for Treatment of HIV Infection* 2000.
5. NJMS National TB Center. *Treatment of TB: Standard Therapy for Active Disease* 2000.

SOURCE: *Treatment of Tuberculosis (TB) in Adult and Adolescent Patients Co-infected with the Human Immunodeficiency Virus (HIV)*, New Jersey Medical School, National Tuberculosis Center, 2001.

Appendix D

Medications

HIV Antiretroviral Therapy

Please refer to a pharmacological text for more detailed information.

Dosages listed are usual doses; dosages may be individualized according to specific patient parameters.

Because dosages, indications, and adverse effects may change over time, neither the author nor ANAC can be held responsible for new dosage recommendations, unforeseen adverse effects, and new indications.

Legend

NRTI: Nucleoside reverse transcriptase inhibitor

NA: Nucleotide analog

NNRTI: Nonnucleoside reverse transcriptase inhibitor

PI: Protease inhibitor

FI: Fusion inhibitor

OD: Once daily

BID: Twice daily

TID: Three times daily

QOD: Every other day

Trade Name (Generic)	Category	Usual Dosage	Side Effects/Drug–Drug and Drug–Food Interactions	Comments
Agenerase (amprenavir)	PI	Adult/adolescent dose: > 50 kg: 1,200 mg BID (capsules), 1,400 mg BID (oral solution); < 50 kg: 20 mg/kg BID (capsules), maximum 2,400 mg daily total, 1.5 mL/kg BID (oral solution), maximum 2,800 mg daily total Pediatric/Adolescent dose (< 50 kg): For children 4–12 years of age or 13–16 years olds weighing less than 50 kg: Oral Solution: 22.5 mg/kg BID or 17 mg/kg TID (maximum daily dose 2,800 mg). Capsules: 20 mg/kg BID or 15 mg/kg TID (maximum daily dose 2,400 mg). Supplied as 50 mg, 150 mg capsules; oral solution: 15 mg/mL,	*Side Effects:* Rash, gastrointestional (GI) intolerances (e.g., nausea, vomiting, diarrhea), abdominal pain, mood alterations, perioral paresthesia; hemolytic anemia *Drug–Drug Interactions:* **AVOID THESE MEDICATIONS WITH THIS AND ALL PI DRUGS:** Zocor (simvastatin); Mevacor (lovastatin); Versed (midazolam); Halcion (triazolam); Hismanal (astemizole); Seldane (terfenadine); Propulsid (cisapride); St. John's wort; Migranal (dihydroergotamine) & Cafergot (ergotamine) Take agenerase 1 hour apart from ddI or antacids Do not take with Vasocor (bepridil) or Rifadin, Rimactane (rifampin)	Because of the potential risk of toxicity from large amounts of the propylene glycol in Agenerase oral solution, it is contraindicated in the following patient populations: children age < 4 years, pregnant women, patients with renal or hepatic failure, patients treated with disulfiram or metronidazole. Oral solution should be used only when Agenerase capsules or other protease inhibitors cannot be. Monitor blood glucose levels with all PIs; PI drugs are associated with hypo- and hyperglycemia, insulin resistance, and new onset diabetes. Monitor cholesterol and triglyceride levels with all

Trade Name (Generic)	Category	Usual Dosage	Side Effects/Drug–Drug and Drug–Food Interactions	Comments
		contains propylene glycol as an inactive ingredient	Birth control pills: levels decreased, use alternative birth control method *Food considerations:* Avoid taking with a high-fat meal *Other considerations:* Dose adjustment: decrease rifabutin to 150 mg OD or 300 mg 2–3x/week Methadone: Coadministration can decrease plasma levels of methadone, dosage of methadone may need to be increased, or another antiretroviral agent considered. Coadministration of Agenerase and ketaconazole raises the levels of both drugs; this combination is currently under investigation.	PIs because the PI agents have been associated with fat redistribution and elevated cholesterol and triglyceride levels. Establish baseline weight, hip-to-waist ratio, and breast size to monitor lipodystrophy. Monitor CBC for anemia. Coadministration with anticonvulsant agents may substantially decrease Agenerase levels; monitor anticonvulsant levels. Coadministration with Viagra (sildenafil) increases Viagra levels; caution patients not to exceed 25 mg in a 48-hour period. Contains Vitamin E; advise clients that they do not need to take additional Vitamin E to meet daily Vitamin E requirements.
Combivir (lamivudine 150 mg and zidovudine 300 mg)	Combination NRTI	Adult/adolescent dose: one tablet BID Supplied as 300 mg zidovudine and 150 mg lamivudine per tablet	*Side effects:* Anemia, neutropenia, rash, headache, malaise, fever, chills, GI symptoms (nausea, vomiting, diarrhea, anorexia), abdominal pain/cramps, neuropathy, insomnia, dizziness; lactic acidosis with hepatic steatosis is a rare but potentially life-threatening toxicity with the use of NRTIs. *Food considerations:* Take with or without foods	Monitor all clients on NRTIs for symptoms suggestive of mitochondrial toxicity; fatigue, tachycardia, abdominal pain, weight loss, peripheral neuropathy, and exercise-induced dypsnea. Hyperlactemia may also be seen but is not always detected in mitochondrial toxicity Check CBC every 3 months for all clients on ZDV because a common side effect is anemia; may need therapy with epoetin alpha to maintain stable hemoglobin level; also watch for leukopenia and thrombocytopenia. Explain to client that one tablet of this drug contains two medications and that they should not take additional doses of zidovudine or lamivudine.
Crixivan (indinavir sulfate)	PI	Adult/adolescent dose: 800 mg every 8 hours Supplied as 200, 333, 400 mg capsules	*Side effects:* Kidney stones (may present as flank pain and/or hematuria), GI	Explain to client the importance of drinking at least 1.5 liters of water daily to avoid

Trade Name (Generic)	Category	Usual Dosage	Side Effects/Drug–Drug and Drug–Food Interactions	Comments
			intolerances (nausea, diarrhea, vomiting), abdominal pain, headache, insomnia, blurred vision, altered or metallic taste, dizziness, generalized weakness, rash, asymptomatic hyperbilirubinemia, alopecia, thrombocytopenia, hyperglycemia, fat redistribution and lipid abnormalities, possible increased bleeding episodes in patients with hemophilia *Drug–Drug Interactions:* See agenerase for PI interactions Take at least 1 hour apart from ddI Avoid rifampin and carbamazepine *Food considerations:* Take 1 hour before or 2 hours after meals; may take with skim milk or low-fat meal; drink at least 1½ quarts of water a day. If combined with ritonavir, no food restriction *Other considerations:* Dose adjustment: decrease rifabutin to 150 mg OD or 300 mg 2–3x/week and increase indinavir to 1,000 mg TID	nephrolithiasis; if excessive sweating due to environment (at the beach, summertime, exercising at the gym), more water needs to be taken. Explain that capsules are sensitive to moisture and should not be kept in bathroom; keep in original container (has desiccants). Advise lactose-intolerant clients because drug contains lactose; clients should take Lactaid tablets before taking drug. Caution patients that coadministration with Viagra (sildenafil) raises Viagra levels; do not exceed 25 mg in a 48-hour period.
Epivir (lamivudine; 3TC)	NRTI	Adolescent/Adult dose: Body weight > 50 kg: 150 mg BID < 50 kg: 2 mg per kg of body weight BID Neonatal dose (infants age < 30 days): 2 mg per kg of body weight BID Pediatric dose: 4 mg per kg of body weight BID Supplied as 150 mg tablets and 10 mg/mL oral solution	*Side effects:* Peripheral neuropathy, pancreatitis, fever, chills or sore throat, skin rash, headache, GI (e.g., nausea, diarrhea), malaise, insomnia, dizziness, muscle and joint pain; lactic acidosis with hepatic steatosis is a rare but potentially life-threatening toxicity with the use of NRTIs. *Food considerations:* Take with or without food	Monitor all clients on NRTIs for symptoms suggestive of mitochondrial toxicity, fatigue, tachycardia, abdominal pain, weight loss, peripheral neuropathy, and exercise-induced dypsnea. Hyperlactemia may be seen but is not always detected in mitochondrial toxicity. Monitor for signs of peripheral neuropathy (tingling, burning, numbness or pain in the hands, arms, feet or legs). Monitor for signs of pancreatitis (nausea, vomiting, severe abdominal or stomach pain).

Trade Name (Generic)	Category	Usual Dosage	Side Effects/Drug–Drug and Drug–Food Interactions	Comments
Fortovase (saquinavir)	PI	Adult/adolescent dose: 1,200 mg TID Supplied as a 200-mg soft gel capsule	*Side effects:* GI intolerances (nausea, diarrhea, dyspepsia, abdominal discomfort/ pain), rash, weakness, headache; elevated transaminase enzymes; fat redistribution and lipid abnormalities; hyperglycemia; possible increased bleeding episodes in patients with hemophilia *Drug–Drug Interactions:* See agenerase for PI interactions Avoid rifampin and rifabutin *Food considerations:* Levels increase sixfold when taken with food, so take with large meal or up to 2 hours after eating *Other considerations:* Dose adjustment needed if concurrently taking rifabutin, saquinavir, and ritonavir; will need to change rifabutin dose to 150 mg 2–3x/week; if taking rifampin, ritonavir and saquinavir, then use rifampin 600 mg OD or 2–3x/week	Advise that if Viagra (sildenafil) is prescribed for erectile dysfunction, a lower starting dose of 25 mg of sildenafil should be used. Explain that grapefruit juice increases saquinavir levels, whereas dexamethasone decreases levels.
Fuzeon (T-20; enfuvirtide)	FI	Adults: 90 mg SC BID Children 6 years of age: 2 mg/kg SC BID (max of 90 mg BID)	*Side Effects:* Almost all patients have experienced mild to moderate injection site reactions (ISRs) (pruritus, erythema, pain, tenderness, induration, nodules, cysts); bacterial pneumonia; hypersensitivity reactions (rash, fever, shortness of breath, nausea, vomiting, chills, rigors, hypotension, elevated tranaminases); eosinophilia (Lalezari, 2003) *Drug-Drug Interactions:* Not an inhibitor or inducer of CYP enzymes; no significant drug interactions expected	Comparable absorption with SC injection in abdomen, thigh or arm Most patients will have an ISR with erythema at some point, which can last from 20 minutes to 24 hours; nodules also frequently occur, which become smaller and will disappear over time, but presence of multiple nodules may limit available injection sites (Glutzer, 2003). Techniques to minimize ISRs include rotating injection sites, using a 27-gauge needle, injecting slowly, avoiding intramuscular (IM) injection, injecting in areas with thicker adipose tissue, and gently massaging the site after injection; no benefit of

Trade Name (Generic)	Category	Usual Dosage	Side Effects/Drug–Drug and Drug–Food Interactions	Comments
				topical treatments has been observed (Glutzer, 2003).
				Key components of patient education include need for adherence to regiment, importance of rotating sites to prevent ISRs (fewer ISRs are observed with injections in the arm, but this site is harder to self-inject; teaching family and friends how to assist with injections; helping the client overcome "needle phobia" (anxiety over self-injecting); integrating bid injections into routines of daily life; allowing sufficient time to reconstiture T-20; management of ISRs; proper drug storage; sterile technique for injection; organization of necessary equipment and proper disposal; and travel planning (Glutzer, 2003).
				Reconstitution: Two doses can be reconstituted at one time; vial should be gently rotated and tapped to help crystals dissolve, but not shaken (avoid foaming)(Glutzer, 2003)
				Available patient education materials and injection equipment: T-20 injection kit includes 1 vial of T-20 and 1 vial of sterile water at room temperature, one 3-cc safety syringe with 25-gauge needle for reconstitution, one 1-cc safety syringe with 27-gauge needle for injection; starter kits include introductory leaflet, educational booklet, written injection instructions, a videotape, a practice injection device, a site rotation planner, a preparation mat listing instructions for each injection, and a sharps container. Travel

Trade Name (Generic)	Category	Usual Dosage	Side Effects/Drug–Drug and Drug–Food Interactions	Comments
				pack includes a week's supply of T-20, pocket for oral medications, and certificate of medical need (remind patients to carry with them and to not pack in luggage that will be checked and stored). Training materials can also be ordered for nursing staff (Glutzer, 2003). Clients with a history of injection drug use should be closely supported and counseled to limit any risks to sobriety (Glutzer, 2003)
Hivid (zalcitibine; ddC)	NRTI	Adult/adolescent dose: 0.75 mg TID Pediatric usual dose: 0.01 mg per kg of body weight every 8 hours Supplied as 0.375, 0.75 mg tablets	*Side effects:* Pancreatitis, peripheral neuropathy, abdominal pain, GI (nausea, vomiting), rash, fever, sore throat, headache, fatigue, muscle pain, oral ulcers, difficulty swallowing, arthralgia *Drug–Drug Interactions:* Avoid taking with aluminum/magnesium containing antacids Avoid combining the "d" drugs (ddi, ddC, d4T) due to overlapping toxicities *Food considerations:* Take with or without food	Teach client that the tablets can be swallowed whole with a large amount of water. Monitor liver function tests; rare cases of hepatic failure and death have been reported in patients taking ddC with underlying hepatitis B infection. Monitor for signs of peripheral neuropathy (numbness, tingling, burning and pain in lower extremities). Monitor for signs of pancreatitis (nausea, vomiting, severe abdominal or stomach pain). Monitor for anemia and granulocytopenia if also on ZDV.
Invirase (saquinavir)	PI	Adult/adolescent dose: 400 mg BID with ritonavir; Invirase not recommended otherwise Supplied as a 200-mg capsule	*Side effects:* Same as for Fortovase *Drug–Drug Interactions:* See agenerase for PI interactions *Food considerations:* No food effect when taken with ritonavir	Same as for Fortovase
Kaletra (lopinavir/ ritonavir)	Combination PI	Adult/adolescent dose: 400 mg lopinavir/ 100 mg ritonavir (three capsules or 5 mL) BID Pediatric dose: 6 months to 12 years of age (without NVP or EFV): 7 to < 15 kg: 12 mg	*Side effects:* GI intolerances (nausea, vomiting, diarrhea), weakness, elevated transaminase enzymes; hyperglycemia; fat redistribution and lipid abnormalities; possible increased bleeding	Explain to client that one tablet contains two medications and that they should not take additional doses of ritonavir. Monitor for signs of pancreatitis (abdominal pain, nausea, vomiting).

Trade Name (Generic)	Category	Usual Dosage	Side Effects/Drug–Drug and Drug–Food Interactions	Comments
		per kg lopinavir/3 mg per kg ritonavir BID; 15–40 kg: 10 mg per kg lopinavir/2.5 mg per kg ritonavir BID; > 40 kg: same as adult Supplied as a soft gel capsule containing 133.3 mg of lopinavir and 33.3 mg of ritonavir; liquid has 80 mg lopinavir + 20 mg ritonavir per mL oral solution	episodes in patients with hemophilia *Drug–Drug Interactions:* See agenerase for PI interactions Avoid Tambocor (flecainide), Rythmol (propafenone), Orap (pimozide), Rifadin (rifampin) Take ddI 1 hour before or 2 hours after birth control pills: levels decreased, use additional or alternative method *Food considerations:* Take with food *Other considerations:* Dose adjustment: decrease rifabutin to 150 mg qod; increase methadone dose	Advise patients that oral solution contains 42% alcohol. Caution patients taking sildenafil that coadministration may result in increased sildenafil levels; do not exceed 25 mg in a 48-hour period.
Norvir (ritonavir)	PI	Adult/adolescent dose: 600 mg BID Pediatric usual dose: 400 mg per m^2 of body surface area q12h; to minimize nausea/vomiting, initiate therapy starting at 250 mg per m^2 of body surface area q12h and increase stepwise to full dose over five days as tolerated. Supplied as 100 mg soft-gel capsules; liquid is 600 mg/7.5 mL	*Side effects:* GI intolerances (nausea, vomiting, diarrhea, loss of appetite) abdominal pain, taste alterations, headache, dizziness, sleepiness and tingling sensation or numbness around the lips, hands or feet, fatigue, weakness; fat redistribution and lipid abnormalities; possible increased bleeding episodes in patients with hemophilia; hyperglycemia; lab: triglycerides increase > 200%, transaminase elevation, elevated CK and uric acid *Drug–Drug Interactions:* See agenerase for PI interactions Avoid Cordarone (amiodarone); quinidine; Tambocor (flecainide); Rythmol (propafenone); Vascor (bepredil); Orap (pimozide); Clozaril (clozapine) Do not exceed 200 mg ketoconazole daily Birth control pills: levels decreased; use additional or alternative method	To minimize nausea/vomiting, initiate therapy starting at 300 mg BID and increase stepwise to full dose over 5 days as tolerated. Explain to client that the capsules should be refrigerated; the oral solution should not be refrigerated. Monitor theophylline levels. Advise clients taking sildenafil that sildenafil levels are increased; do not exceed 25 mg in a 48-hour period.

Trade Name (Generic)	Category	Usual Dosage	Side Effects/Drug–Drug and Drug–Food Interactions	Comments
			Food considerations: Take with food *Other considerations:* Dose adjustment: decrease rifabutin to 150 mg QOD or 3x/week; increase dose of methadone; reduce desipramine dose	
Rescriptor (delavirdine mesylate)	NNRTI	Adult/adolescent dose: 400 mg TID Supplied as 100 and 200 mg tablets	*Side effects:* Arthralgia, rash, GI intolerances (nausea, diarrhea), insomnia, changes in dreams, headache, fatigue, increased liver enzymes; rare cases of Stevens-Johnson syndrome have been reported with all NNRTIs. *Drug–Drug Interactions:* Avoid using rifampin, rifabutin, Zocor (simvastatin), Mevacor (lovastatin), Versed (midazolam), Halcion (triazolam), Hismanal (astemizole), Seldane (terfenadine), Propulsid (cisapride); ergot medications, H2 blockers and proton pump inhibitors Take one hour apart from antacids and ddI May increase levels of dapsone, warfarin, and quinidine *Food considerations:* Take with or without food *Other considerations:* Dose adjustment: clarithromycin if renal failure present	Teach client that 100 mg tablets can be dispersed in > 3 oz water to produce slurry for ease in swallowing. Advise sildenafil users not exceed 25 mg in a 48-hour period.
Retrovir (zidovudine; ZDV; AZT)		Adult/adolescent dose: 200 mg TID or 300 mg BID Neonatal dose (infants aged < 90 days): Oral: 2 mg per kg of body weight q6h; IV: 1.5 mg per kg of body weight q6H Pediatric usual dose: Oral: 160 mg per m^2 of body surface area every 8 hours.	*Side effects:* Bone marrow suppression (anemia and/or neutropenia), GI intolerances, headache, insomnia, weakness; lactic acidosis with hepatic steatosis is a rare but potentially life-threatening toxicity with the use of NRTIs. *Drug–Drug Interactions:* Avoid ribavirin,	Monitor CBC for anemia, neutropenia; ZDV may be associated with hematologic toxicities, including granulocytopenia and severe anemia, particularly in advanced HIV patients. Prolonged zidovudine use has been associated with symptomatic myopathy

Trade Name (Generic)	Category	Usual Dosage	Side Effects/Drug–Drug and Drug–Food Interactions	Comments
		Intravenous (intermittent infusion): 120 mg per m² of body surface area q6h; continuous IV infusion: 20 mg per m² of body surface area per hour Supplied as 100 mg capsules; 300 mg tablets; 10 mg/mL IV solution and 10 mg/mL oral solution	inhibits phosphorylation of ZDV *Food considerations:* May be taken with or without food Take with food to decrease nausea but avoid high-fat meal, which may impair absorption	
Sustiva (efavirenz)	NNRTI	Adult/adolescent dose: 600 mg OD Pediatric dose: Administered once daily. Body weight 10 to < 15 kg: 200 mg; 15 to < 20 kg: 250 mg; 20 to < 25 kg: 300 mg; 25 to < 32.5 kg: 350 mg; 32.5 to < 40 kg: 400 mg > 40 kg: 600 mg Supplied as 50, 100, 200 mg capsules	*Side effects:* Rash (may become serious); central nervous system symptoms (drowsiness, insomnia, trouble concentrating and unusual dreams); symptoms tend to go away after 2 to 4 weeks); in a small number of patients, severe psychiatric symptoms (severe depression, strange and suicidal thoughts, angry behavior); rare cases of Stevens-Johnson syndrome have been reported with all NNRTIs; increased transaminase levels; may cause a false positive cannabinoid (marijuana) test *Drug–Drug Interactions:* Avoid Hismanal (astemizole); Propulsid (cisapride); Versed (midazolam); Halcion (triazolam) and ergot medications such as Wigraine and Cafergot *Food considerations:* Avoid taking with a high-fat meal *Other considerations:* Dose adjustments: Increase rifabutin dose to 450–600 mg OD or 600 mg 2–3x/week Dose changes may be needed with the following medications: indinavir, saquinavir, methadone, birth control pills, and clarithromycin	Advise bedtime dosing for the first weeks of therapy due to CNS side effects. Tell clients that Sustiva can be swallowed with water, juice, milk, or soda. Explain to clients that CNS symptoms may be worsened if Sustiva is taken with alcohol or mood-altering illegal drugs (street drugs or party drugs, such as ecstasy). Advise women not to become pregnant; birth defects were seen in animals treated with Sustiva.

Trade Name (Generic)	Category	Usual Dosage	Side Effects/Drug–Drug and Drug–Food Interactions	Comments
Trizivir (lamivudine 150 mg and zidovudine 300 mg and abacavir 300 mg)	Combination NRTI	Adult/adolescent dose: one tablet BID Supplied as 300 mg zidovudine, 150 mg lamivudine, and 300 mg abacavir per tablet	Chills; bone pain; loss of appetite; trouble sleeping/sleeplessness; hypersensitivity reaction, including abdominal or stomach pain; cough; diarrhea; fever; headache; nausea; numbness or tingling of face, feet, or hands; pain in joints; pain in muscles; shortness of breath; skin rash; sore throat; swelling of feet or lower legs; unusual feeling of discomfort or illness; unusual tiredness or weakness; or vomiting Also see Retrovir, Epivir, and Ziagen	Do not coadminister with zalcitabine; take with or without food.
Videx (didanosine; ddI)	NRTI	Adult/adolescent dose: > 60 kg: 200 mg BID or 400 mg OD; (buffered tablets), 250 mg BID (buffered powder); < 60kg: 125 mg BID or 250 mg OD (buffered tablets), 167 mg BID (buffered powder) Neonatal dose (infants aged < 90 days): 50 mg per m^2 of body surface area q12h Pediatric usual dose: in combination with other antiretrovirals: 90 mg per m^2 of body surface area every 12 hours Supplied as 25, 50, 100, 150, 200 mg chewable/dispersible buffered tablets 100, 167, 250 mg buffered powder for oral solution Pediatric powder for oral solution, when reconstituted, yields 10 mg/mL	Side effects: Pancreatitis, peripheral neuropathy, rash, visual problems, anxiety, headache, irritability, inability to sleep, restlessness, dry mouth, nervousness, rash; lactic acidosis with hepatic steatosis is a rare but potentially life-threatening toxicity with the use of NRTIs. Drug–Drug Interactions: Coadministration of tenofovir with ddI should be undertaken with caution; monitor closely for didanosine-related toxicities; suspend tenofovir if signs or symptoms of pancreatitis, symptomatic hyperlactemia, or lactic acidosis develop. Coadministration of ribavirin with ddI should be undertaken with caution; monitor closely for didanosine-related toxicities; discontinue ddI if signs or symptoms of pancreatitis, symptomatic hyperlactemia, or lactic acidosis develop. Take 2 hours apart from dapsone Avoid combining the "d" drugs (ddI; ddC; d4T)	Teach client how to take drug; tablets need to be chewed or dispersed in water but cannot be taken with acidic liquids, such as citrus juices; tablets contain a buffering agent, which helps prevent degradation but causes stomach upset in some patients and is associated with a bitter and chalky taste. Monitor for signs of pancreatitis (abdominal pain, nausea, vomiting); cases of fatal and nonfatal pancreatitis have occurred in treatment-naive and treatment-experienced patients during therapy with ddI or in combination with other drugs, particularly d4T or d4T + hydroxyurea. Monitor for signs of peripheral neuropathy (numbness, tingling, burning, and pain in lower extremities). Pregnant women may be at increased risk for lactic acidosis and liver damage when treated with the combination of stavudine and ddI; this combination should be used in pregnant women only when the potential

Trade Name (Generic)	Category	Usual Dosage	Side Effects/Drug–Drug and Drug–Food Interactions	Comments
			due to overlapping toxicities *Food considerations:* Take at least 30 minutes before or 2 hours after a meal Avoid acid or acidic liquids, which quickly degrades the drug *Other considerations:* Increase ddl dose if on methadone	benefit clearly outweighs the potential risk.
Videx EC (didanosine release capsules)	NRTI	Adult/adolescent dose: Body weight > 60 kg: 400 mg OD; body weight < 60 kg: 250 mg OD Supplied as a 400 mg enteric-coated (EC) capsule containing enteric-coated beadlets of didanosine	*Side effects:* Same as for Videx *Drug–Drug Interactions:* Same as for Videx *Food considerations:* Take on an empty stomach	Teach client how to take capsule, which must be swallowed whole, not chewed; do not open capsule; do not sprinkle beadlets into water or onto food. Monitor for vision changes and signs of neuropathy.
Viracept (nelfinavir mesylate)	PI	Adult/adolescent dose: 750 mg (3 tablets) tid or 1,250 mg (5 tablets) BID Pediatric: 20 to 30 mg per kg of body weight TID Supplied as a 250 mg tablet; oral powder is 50 mg per one level gram scoop (200 mg per one level teaspoon)	*Side effects:* GI intolerances (diarrhea, flatulence, nausea), abdominal pain, generalized weakness, rash, fat redistribution and lipid abnormalities, hyperglycemia, possible increased bleeding episodes in patients with hemophilia *Drug–Drug Interactions:* See Agenerase for PI interactions Birth control pills: levels decreased; use additional or alternative method *Food considerations:* Take with food *Other considerations:* Dose adjustment: give rifabutin 150 mg OD or 300 mg 2–3x/week and change the nelfinavir dose to 1,000 mg TID; Dose adjustment: increase methadone dose	Anticipate diarrhea and advise client to have Imodium readily available to take to decrease diarrhea
Viramune (nevirapine)	NNRTI	Adult/adolescent dose: 200 mg OD × 14 days, then 200 mg BID Pediatric dose: 120–200 mg/m^2 q12h; initiate therapy	*Side effects:* Rash, fever, nausea, headache, abnormal liver function tests, hepatitis, stomatitis, numbness, muscle pain; rare cases of Stevens-Johnson	Monitor for signs of hepatitis (yellow skin, diarrhea, nausea, headache); advise patients to seek medical evaluation immediately if signs and symptoms of hepatitis

Trade Name (Generic)	Category	Usual Dosage	Side Effects/Drug–Drug and Drug–Food Interactions	Comments
		with 120 mg/m^2 (maximum 200 mg) given once a day for 14 days, then increase to full dose; or 7 mg/kg q12h < 8 years of age, 4 mg/kg q12h > 8 years of age Supplied as a 200 mg tablets; 50 mg/5 mL oral suspension	syndrome have been reported with all NNRTIs. *Drug–Drug Interactions:* Avoid rifampin *Food considerations:* Take with or without food *Other considerations:* Dose adjustment may be needed with methadone and birth control pills	occur. Severe, life-threatening hepatotoxicity, including fulminant and cholestatic hepatitis, hepatic necrosis, and hepatic failure, have been reported. Monitor for signs of skin reactions; severe, life-threatening, and even fatal skin reactions, including Stevens-Johnson syndrome, toxic epidermal necrolysis, and hypersensitivity reactions characterized by rash, constitutional findings, and organ dysfunction, have occurred with nevirapine treatment; a 14-day lead-in period with nevirapine 200 mg daily must be strictly followed; patients should be monitored intensively during the first 12 weeks of nevirapine therapy to detect potentially life-threatening hepatotoxicity or skin reactions; nevirapine should not be restarted after severe hepatic, skin, or hypersensitivity reactions.
Viread (tenofovir disoproxil; fumarate)	Nucleotide analog	300 mg OD for patients with creatinine clearance > 60 mL/min; not recommended if creatinine clearance < 60 mL/min Supplied as 300 mg tablet	*Side effects:* GI intolerances (nausea, vomiting, diarrhea, flatulence), headache, weakness *Drug–Drug Interactions:* Coadministration of tenofovir with ddl should be undertaken with caution. *Food considerations:* Take with food	Closely monitor patients taking ddl and tenofovir; monitor for ddl-related toxicities; suspend tenofovir if signs or symptoms of pancreatitis, symptomatic hyperlactemia, or lactic acidosis develop.
Zerit (stavudine; d4T)	NRTI	Adult/adolescent dose: > 60 kg: 40 mg BID; < 60 kg: 30 mg BID Pediatric dose: 1 mg per kg of body weight every 12 hours (up to weight of 30 kg) Supplied as 15, 20, 30, 40 mg capsules; 1mg/mL for oral solution	*Side effects:* Pancreatitis; peripheral neuropathy; GI intolerances (nausea, vomiting, diarrhea); muscle, joint, and back pain; loss of strength or energy; insomnia; anxiety; loss of appetite; headache; chills/fever; dizziness; nervousness;	Monitor for signs of peripheral neuropathy (tingling, burning, pain, numbness of hands, feet) Monitor for signs of pancreatitis (abdominal pain, nausea, vomiting); cases of fatal and nonfatal pancreatitis have occurred in treatment-naive and

Trade Name (Generic)	Category	Usual Dosage	Side Effects/Drug–Drug and Drug–Food Interactions	Comments
			lactic acidosis with hepatic steatosis is a rare but potentially life-threatening toxicity with the use of NRTIs. *Drug–Drug Interactions:* Avoid combining the "d" drugs (ddl; ddC; d4T) due to overlapping toxicities *Food considerations:* Take with or without food	treatment-experienced patients during therapy with ddl, d4T, or d4T plus hydroxyurea. Pregnant women may be at increased risk for lactic acidosis and liver damage when treated with a combination of stavudine and didanosine; this combination should be used in pregnant women only when the potential benefit clearly outweighs the potential risk.
Zerit XR (d4T XR)	NRTI	100 mg OD for persons weighing at least 60 kg and 75 mg OD for persons under 60 kg; supplied as individual	See Zerit	Take with or without food; mix with applesauce for patients who have difficulty swallowing
Ziagen (abacavir sulfate)	NRTI	300 mg BID Pediatric/Adolescent dose: 8 mg/kg of body weight BID, maximum dose 300 mg BID Supplied as 300 mg tablets; 20 mg/mL oral solution	*Side effects:* Headache; nausea; vomiting; malaise; diarrhea; hypersensitivity reaction (can be fatal): fever, rash, nausea, vomiting, malaise, or fatigue; loss of appetite; and respiratory symptoms may also be component (sore throat, cough, shortness of breath); lactic acidosis with hepatic steatosis is a rare but potentially life-threatening toxicity with the use of NRTIs. *Food considerations:* Take with or without food	Caution client to report any signs of a hypersensitivity reaction; patients who develop signs or symptoms of hypersensitivity (which may include fever, rash, fatigue, nausea, vomiting, diarrhea, and abdominal pain) should discontinue abacavir as soon as a hypersensitivity reaction is suspected; abacavir should not be restarted, because more severe symptoms will recur within hours and may include life-threatening hypotension and death.

References

Glutzer, E. (2003, March). Patient care management. *The AIDS Reader, 13* (3-Special Supplement), S14-S16.

Lalezari, J.P. (2003, March). Clinical safety and efficacy of enfuvirtide (T-20), a new fusion inhibitor. *The AIDS Reader, 13* (3-Special Supplement), S9-S13.

Panel on Clinical Practices for the Treatment of HIV, Department of Health and Human Services & the Henry J. Kaiser Family Foundation. (2002). *Guidelines for the use of antiretroviral agents in HIV-infected adults and adolescents.* Retrieved February 4, 2002, from www.aidsinfo.nih.gov

The Working Group on Antiretroviral Therapy and Medical Management of HIV-Infected Children, National Pediatric and Family HIV Resource Center (NPHRC), The Health Resources and Services Administration (HRSA), & The National Institutes of Health (NIH). (2001). *Guidelines for the use of antiretroviral agents in pediatric HIV infection.* Retrieved December 14, 2001, from www.aidsinfo.nih.gov

Nonantiretroviral Medications Commonly Used in HIV/AIDS Treatment/Palliative Care

Please refer to a pharmacological text for more detailed information.

Dosages listed are usual doses (see AIDSInfo, www.aidsinfo.nih.gov; Centers for Disease Control and Prevention, 2002a); dosages may be individualized according to specific patient parameters.

There are many drug interactions between HAART medications and other drugs used in HIV care. Please refer to the HAART table for specific drug–drug interactions.

Because dosages, indications, and adverse effects may change over time, neither the author nor ANAC can be held responsible for new dosage recommendations, unforeseen adverse effects, and new indications.

Generic Name (Trade)	Indications	Dosage	Side Effects	Comments
acyclovir (Zovirax)	Herpes simplex virus infection (HSV), varicella-zoster virus infection (VZV), Epstein-Barr virus (EBV) infection (oral hairy leukoplakia)	*HSV (treatment)* Adults (PO): 400 mg TID up to 800 mg 5 times/day; (IV): 15–30 mg/kg/day for at least 7 days Children (PO): Maximum 80 mg/kg/day in 3–5 doses; (IV): 250 mg/m²/dose q8h *Varicella/Herpes zoster treatment* Adults (PO): 800 mg 5 times/day; (IV) 30 mg/kg/q 8h Children (PO): 20 mg/kg/dose up to 800 mg/dose; (IV) 10/mg/kg q8h *Secondary prophylaxis for HSV infection* Adults (PO): 200 TID or 400 mg BID. Children (PO): 80 mg/kg/day in 3–4 divided doses (only if subsequent episodes are frequent or severe) *Topical (ointment)* Adults/Children: apply every 3 hours 6 times/day	Nausea, diarrhea, vomiting, abdominal pain, headache	Oral forms may be taken with or without food. Capsules and tablets should not be crushed or opened. Maintain adequate hydration/urine output. IV infusion should be administered over at least 1 hour; monitor IV site for pain, swelling, or redness at injection site.
alitretinoin (Panretin)	Kaposi's sarcoma	*Topical* Apply sufficient gel to cover lesions BID; increase to 3–4 times daily if tolerated	Itching and rash	Nursing instructions to patients should include the following (Rhoads, 2001): Avoid use if pregnant; potential fetal harm Use gel exactly as prescribed without altering dosage Clean skin lesions before applying gel Dry 3–5 minutes before covering with clothes; do not cover with occlusive dressing

Generic Name (Trade)	Indications	Dosage	Side Effects	Comments
				Avoid applying to unaffected skin or to mucosal areas May cause photosensitivity; to prevent serious sunburn, avoid sun exposure and sun lamps Avoid insect repellants with DEET (potential for increased toxicity) Decrease frequency of application if irritation occurs; temporarily discontinue if severe reactions occur
amitriptyline (Elavil, Endep)	Depression, neuropathic pain	*Depression* Adults (PO): initially 25 mg BID or QID may increase to 150 mg/day Children (PO): 10–30 mg/day in 2 divided doses *Neuropathic pain* Adults (PO): initially 10–25 mg at bedtime, may increase to 75 mg at bedtime Children (PO): initially, 0.1 mg/kg at bedtime, may increase to 0.5–2 mg/kg at bedtime	Blurred vision, constipation, dizziness, drowsiness, headache, increased appetite, altered taste, nausea, vomiting	May take with food to decrease gastric irritation; avoid alcohol May cause drowsiness, dry mouth Avoid discontinuing abruptly Interacts with MAO inhibitors, cimetidine, drugs metabolized by cytochrome p450 2D6, SSRIs, ethchlorvynol, sympathomimetic and anticholinergic agents; may block antihypertensive action of guanethidine; may potentiate the effects of alcohol, barbiturates, and other CNS depressants
amphotericin B (Fungizone)	Aspergillosis, esophageal or disseminated candidiasis, coccidioidomycosis, cryptococcosis, histoplasmosis	Adults (IV): 0.25 mg/kg initially, then gradually increased to maintenance dose of 0.25–1 mg/kg/ day (maximum daily dose); infuse at a rate of 0.2–0.4 mg/kg/hr Children (IV): 0.25 mg/kg initially, increased to maintenance dose of 0.25–1 mg/kg/day Test dose should be administered first. *Secondary prophylaxis for cryptococcus neoformans* Children (IV): 0.5–1.0 mg/kg 1–3x/week (alternative regimen) *Secondary prophylaxis for histoplasmosis, coccidioides*	Unusually tired, weak, irregular heartbeat, muscle cramps or pain, fever or chills, nausea, vomiting, diarrhea, headache, altered urination, pain at injection site, loss of appetite, stomach pain	To reduce side effects, premedicate with agents such as ibuprofen or acetaminophen, steroids, antihistamine, and/or meperidine When administered concurrently, corticosteroids, corticotropin (ACTH), or potassium-depleting diuretics may potentiate amphotericin B–induced hypokalemia, which may lead to digitalis toxicity. Need to closely monitor if receiving any combination of nephrotoxic drugs. Avoid concurrent or sequential use of drugs with similar nephrotoxic effects (e.g., aminoglycosides, vancomycin, cyclosporine, and pentamidine).

Generic Name (Trade)	Indications	Dosage	Side Effects	Comments
		Children (IV): 1.0 mg/kg a week (alternative regimen)		Concomitant administration with zidovudine can lead to increased myelotoxicity and nephrotoxicity. amphotericin B combined with antineoplastic agents may enhance renal toxicity, bronchospasm, and hypotension. Concurrent use of bone marrow–depleting medications or radiation therapy may increase anemia or other hematologic effects.
amphotericin B, lipid-based (Abelcet, lipid complex) (Amphotec, colloidal dispersion) (AmBisone, liposome)	See amphotericin B	Adults/Children (IV): For empiric therapy, the usual dose for lipid preparations is 3 mg/kg/day. Aspergillosis: Recommendation for all lipid preparations is 5 mg/kg/day.	Fever, chills, headache, nausea, vomiting, diarrhea, loss of appetite, unusually tired or weak, sore throat, unusual bleeding/bruising	The lipid complex preparations of amphotericin permit delivery of high doses with less nephrotoxicity but cost more than nonlipid amphotericin B. The IV infusion time for amphotericin B lipid compounds (ABLC) is 2 hours versus 4 hours with conventional (nonlipid) amphotericin B (Weissman, 1999).
atovaquone (Mepron)	Pneumocystis carinii pneumonia (PCP), toxoplasmosis	Primary prophylaxis for PCP Adults (PO): 1,500 mg/day (alternative regimen) Children (PO): 1–3 months and > 24 months: 30 mg/kg OD; 4–24 months, 45 mg/kg OD Secondary prophylaxis for PCP Adults/children: Same as primary Treatment: Adults (PO): atovaquone 750 mg suspension with meal BID × 21 days (alternative regimen) Primary prophylaxis for toxoplasmosis Adults (PO): 1,500 mg/day with or without pyrimethamine 25 mg/d + leucovorin 10 mg/day (alternative regimen)	Skin rash, fever, cough, headache, inability to sleep, nausea, vomiting, diarrhea, increased liver enzymes	Take with food (increases absorption). Store in cool, dry place (avoid freezing).

Generic Name (Trade)	Indications	Dosage	Side Effects	Comments
		Children (PO): 1–3 months and > 24 months: 30 mg/kg OD; 14–24 months: 45 mg/kg OD (alternative regimen) *Secondary prophylaxis for toxoplasmosis* Adults (PO): 750 mg q6–12h with or without pyrimethamine 25 mg/d + leucovorin 10 mg/d (alternative regimen)		
azithromycin (Zithromax)	MAC	*Primary prophylaxis for MAC* Adults (PO): 1,200 mg/week, or 1,200 mg/week + rifabutin 300 mg/day Children (PO): 20 mg/kg (maximum 1,200 mg) once a week; alternative regimen: 5 mg/kg (maximum 250 mg) OD *Treatment of MAC* Adults (PO): 500 mg/day plus ethambutol 15 mg/kg OD with or without rifabutin 300 mg OD Children (PO): 10–20 mg/kg/d once daily. Maximum: 40mg/kg *Secondary prophylaxis for MAC* Adults (PO): 500 mg/day + ethambutol 15 mg/kg/day with or without rifabutin 300 mg/day *Alternative children regimen* 5 mg/kg (maximum 250 mg) OD + ethambutol 15 mg/kg (maximum 900 mg) OD, with or without rifabutin 5 mg/kg (maximum of 300 mg) OD	Abdominal pain, nausea, vomiting, diarrhea	Aluminum and magnesium-containing antacids may decrease the amount of azithromycin in the blood, which may decrease its effects; take azithromycin at least 1 hour before or at least 2 hours after antacids. Take capsules and pediatric oral suspension 1 hour before meals or 2 hours after meals; ·tablets and powder packet may be taken without regard to food.
Bleomycin (Blenoxane)	Kaposi's sarcoma	Refer to individual protocols	Erythema, rash, striae, vesiculation, hyperpigmentation, and tenderness of the skin; hyperkeratosis, nail changes, alopecia,	Antineoplastic agent: refer to oncology text for specific information on administration and care. Interactions of bleomycin have been reported with

Generic Name (Trade)	Indications	Dosage	Side Effects	Comments
			pruritus, and stomatitis; fever, chills, vomiting, anorexia, and weight loss; infrequently, pain in tumor site, phlebitis, and other local reactions; pulmonary fibrosis/toxicity is serious adverse effect.	general anesthetics, other antineoplastics, cisplatin, vincristine, and with radiation therapy. Give IV slowly over at least 10 minutes.
carbamazepine(Tegretol)	Seizures, neuropathic pain	*Seizures* Adults (PO): initially, 100 mg 4 times/day, increase up to maintenance dose of 800–1,200 mg/day Children (PO): (6–12 years) initially, 50 mg 4 times/day, increase up to maintenance dose of 400–800 mg/day; (< 6 years) initially, 10–20 mg/kg/day in 2–3 divided doses, increase up to maintenance of 250–350 mg/day *Neuropathic pain* Adults (PO): initially, 100 mg BID, increasing to 800 mg/day	Blurred vision, skin rash, itching, hives, diarrhea, confusion, clumsiness, nausea, vomiting, loss of appetite, dry mouth, irritation of tongue, mouth, unusually tired, weak	Take with food (decreases GI irritation); avoid alcohol. May cause drowsiness. Avoid sun due to increased sensitivity of skin to sunlight.
chlorhexidine (Peridex)	Oral candidiasis, gingivitis, prevention of thrush	Adults, children (PO): 15 ml BID (after brushing/ flossing teeth)	Change in taste; increased tartar in teeth; increased staining of teeth, mouth, tooth fillings, or dentures; swollen glands on side of face or neck; irritation to mouth and tip of tongue; superficial desquamative lesions (mouth irritation) reported mainly in children ages 10 to 18 (the lesions are transient and may be painless).	Use after brushing/flossing, rinsing toothpaste completely from mouth before using; swish in mouth for 30 seconds, then spit out; do not swallow. Do not eat or drink for several hours after using. May cause staining and increase in tartar, change in taste.
cidofovir (Vistide)	Cytomegalovirus retinitis	Adults (IV): induction dose is 5 mg/kg weekly × 2; maintenance dose is 5 mg/kg every other week (reduce dosage with renal impairment) Intraocular: 20–40 mcg by intraocular injection. *Secondary prophylaxis* Adult (IV): 5 mg/kg every other week with probenecid (PO)	Nausea, vomiting, fever, generalized weakness, rash, diarrhea, headache, loss of hair, chills, loss of appetite, dyspnea, abdominal pain, renal failure, infection, unusually tired or weak, pneumonia, decrease in intraocular pressure	Contraindications: Serum creatinine > 1.5 mg/dL, a calculated creatinine clearance of < 55 mL/min, or a urine protein > 100 mg/dL; history of severe hypersensitivity to cidofovir, probenecid, or other sulfur-containing medications. Pre- and postinfusion care: stop nephrotoxic drugs at least 7 days before starting therapy.

Generic Name (Trade)	Indications	Dosage	Side Effects	Comments
		2 grams (PO) 3 hours before the dose, followed by 1 gram (PO) 2 hours after the dose, and 1 gram (PO) 8 hours after the dose (total of 4 grams of probenecid)		Give probenecid (refer to probenecid); antihistamines, acetaminophen, or antiemetics may be given to reduce probenecid hypersensitivity. Infuse 1 L of N/S over 1–2 hours prior to starting cidofovir infusion; if able to tolerate, infuse second L over 1–3 hours at start (or end) of cidofovir infusion. If breathing problems occur with N/S infusion, try splitting dose and giving 500 ml 1 hour prior to infusion and the second 500 ml over an hour after completion of cidofovir (Dodge, 1999). Do not give with other drugs with potential renal toxicity (foscarnet, amphotericin, pentamidine, NSAIDs). Teach client to call health care provider for signs and symptoms of kidney damage: chills, fever, or sore throat; decreased urination; or increased thirst and urination.
clarithromycin (Biaxin)	Mycobacterium avium complex (MAC), pharyngitis, sinusitis, otitis, pneumonitis, skin and soft tissue infections	*Primary prophylaxis for MAC* Adults (PO): 500 mg BID Children (PO): 7.5 mg/kg (max 500 mg) BID *Treatment of infection* Adults (PO): 500 mg BID Children (PO): 15–30 mg/kg/day in 2 divided doses. maximum: 1 g/day *Secondary prophylaxis for MAC* Adults (PO): 500 mg BID plus ethambutol 15 mg/kg/day with or without rifabutin 300 mg/day Children (PO): 7.5 mg/kg (max 500 mg) BID plus ethambutol 15 mg/kg (maximum	Abnormal taste, nausea, vomiting, diarrhea, dyspepsia, abdominal pain/discomfort and headache; rare cases of ventricular arrhythmias	May take without regard to food; may take with milk. Avoid crushing or breaking tablets. Contraindications: hypersensitivity to clarithromycin, erythromycin, or any of the macrolide antibiotics. Interacts with theophylline, carbamazepine, digoxin, anticoagulants, ergotamine, triazolam, cyclosporine, hexobarbital, phenytoin, warfarin, antiinfective agents and drugs metabolized by the cytochrome P450 system. Increases terfenadine plasma levels threefold; decreases zidovudine bioavailability.

Generic Name (Trade)	Indications	Dosage	Side Effects	Comments
		900 mg) OD, with or without rifabutin 5 mg/kg (maximum 300 mg) OD		
clindamycin (Cleocin, Dalacin C)	Toxoplasmosis	*Secondary prophylaxis for toxoplasmosis* Adults (PO): clindamycin 300–450 mg q 6–8 hr + pyrimethamine 25–50 mg/day + leucovorin 10–25 mg/day (alternative regimen) *Alternative children regimen* clindamycin 20–30 mg/kg/day in 4 divided doses OD + pyrimethamine 1 mg/kg OD + leucovorin 5 mg every 3 days	Fever, myalgia, diarrhea, abdominal pain, nausea, vomiting, esophageal irritation, loss of taste, leukopenia, skin rashes	Administer capsules with full glass of water to prevent esophagitis.
clotrimazole (Mycelex, Gyne-Lotrimin)	Vulvovaginal, oropharyngeal candidiasis	*Vulvovaginal candidiasis* Adults/children (vaginal) (> 12 years): one vaginal tablet (100 mg) at bedtime for 7 days or 2 tablets (200 mg) at bedtime for 3 days or 1 tablet (500 mg) once; vaginal cream: one full applicator at bedtime for 7–14 days *Oropharyngeal candidiasis* Adults/children (buccal) (>3 years): 10 mg troches 3–5 times/day for 7–14 days	*Vaginal application:* Vaginal burning, itching, vaginal discharge *Oral administration:* Abdominal or stomach cramping or pain, nausea, vomiting, diarrhea	Vaginal tablet/cream: Use vaginal applicator, inserting high into vagina. Troches: Dissolve in mouth over 15–30 min and swallow saliva; do not chew or swallow whole.
cytarabine (Cytosar)	Used primarily in combination with other drugs for the treatment of acute myelocytic leukemia Under investigation for treatment of progressive multifocal leuko-encephalopathy (PML)	Refer to individual protocols	Loss of appetite, nausea, vomiting, headache, dizziness, drowsiness, itching, loss of hair, fever, chills, painful urination, sore in mouth or on lips, unusual bleeding, bruising, pinpoint red spots on skin, unusual fatigue, numbness, joint pain, swelling of feet or lower legs, and tingling in fingers, toes, face Main toxic effect: bone marrow suppression with anemia, leukopenia, and thrombocytopenia	Antineoplastic agent; refer to oncology text for specific information on administration and care. There is no antidote for overdose; overdose can result in irreversible central nervous system toxicity and death. May decrease digoxin absorption; gentamicin and fluorocytosine activity may also be inhibited.

Generic Name (Trade)	Indications	Dosage	Side Effects	Comments
dacarbazine (DTIC; DTIC-Dome; Imidazole Carboxamide)	Hodgkin's disease	Refer to individual protocols	Pain, redness, swelling at injection site, fever, chills, cough, lower back pain, painful urination, unusual bleeding, bruising, pinpoint red spots on skin, nausea, diarrhea, loss of appetite, loss of hair, joint or muscle pain May interact with allopurinol, blood dyscrasia–causing medications, bone marrow depressants or radiation therapy, hepatic enzyme inducers, killed-virus vaccines, or live-virus vaccines	Antineoplastic agent; refer to oncology text for specific information on administration and care. Refrigerate, protect from light. Avoid sunlight exposure. Try to restrict food intake for 4–6 hours prior to dose (decreases vomiting).
daunorubicin hydrochloride liposome (DaunoXome)	Kaposi's sarcoma	Adult (IV): 40 mg in D5W infused over 30 minutes, once every 2–3 weeks for as long as client responds satisfactorily and can tolerate treatment	Besides usual side effects of chemotherapy, severe side effects can include cardiac toxicities, myelosuppression, and palmar-plantar erythrodysethesia (reddish appearance to palms and soles)	Antineoplastic agent; refer to oncology text for specific information on administration and care. Infuse slowly and monitor for acute infusion-related reactions (which may be related to liposome): flushing, shortness of breath, facial swelling, headache, chills, back pain, chest or throat tightness, and hypotension. Reactions usually resolve in 1 day and are usually limited to first dose.
dapsone (Avlosulfone)	Pneumocystis carinii pneumonia (PCP), toxoplasmosis	Primary prophylaxis for PCP Adults (PO): 50 mg po BID or 100 mg/day, or dapsone 50 mg/d + pyrimethamine 50 mg/week + leucovorin 25 mg/wk, or dapsone 200 mg/week + pyrimethamine 75 mg/week + leucovorin 25 mg/week (alternative regimens) Children (PO): (> 1 month) 2 mg/kg/day (maximum 100 mg) or 4 mg/kg (maximum of 200 mg) every week Treatment PCP	Back, leg, or stomach pain; loss of appetite; pale skin; unusual fatigue, weakness; fever; bluish fingernails, lips, or skin; skin rash; difficulty breathing; nausea Most common adverse effect: dose-related hemolysis; expect a decrease of hemoglobin (1–2 g), an increase in reticulocytes (2–12%), shortened red cell life span, and increased methemoglobin; may also cause agranulocytosis, aplastic anemia, and other blood dyscrasias Peripheral neuropathy with motor loss is a definite but unusual complication seen in nonleprosy patients. Discontinue if muscle weakness appears.	May take with or without food. Do not give with antacids (may decrease absorption). Give 2 hours before or after didanosine. Use with caution in patients with glucose-6-phosphate dehydrogenase deficiency receiving or exposed to other drugs or agents that are capable of inducing hemolysis (e.g., nitrite, aniline, phenylhydrazine, naphthalene, niridazole, nitrofurantoin, primaquine). Concurrent use of a folic acid antagonist (e.g., pyrimethamine): Increased risk of hematologic adverse effects.

Generic Name (Trade)	Indications	Dosage	Side Effects	Comments
		Adults (PO): 100 mg/day for 21 days plus trimethoprim 15 mg/kg/day *Secondary prophylaxis for PCP* Adults (PO): same as primary Children (PO): (>1 month) 2 mg/kg/day (maximum 100 mg) or 4 mg/kg (maximum of 200 mg) every week *Primary prophylaxis for toxoplasmosis* Adults (PO): 50 mg/day + pyrimethamine 50 mg/week + leucovorin 25 mg/week, or dapsone 200 mg/week + pyrimethamine 75 mg/week + leucovorin 25 mg/week (alternative regimens) Children (PO): (≥ 1 month) 2 mg/kg or 15 mg/m² (maximum 25 mg) daily + pyrimethamine 1 mg/kg OD + leucovorin 5 mg every 3 days (alternative regimen)		Rifampin may decrease serum dapsone concentrations. Trimethoprim may increase plasma dapsone concentrations, potentially may increase risk of adverse effects.
desipramine (Norpramin)	Depression, neuropathic pain	*Depression* Adults (PO): initially, 75 mg/day in divided doses (maximum 300 mg/day) Children (PO) (> 12 years): initially, 25–50 mg/day; maximum: 150 mg/day Children (PO) (6–12 years): initially, 1–3 mg/kg/day; maximum: 5 mg/kg/day *Neuropathic pain* Adults (PO): initially, 25 mg at bedtime, increasing to 100–150 mg/day (maximum 300 mg/day)	Blurred vision, constipation, dizziness, drowsiness, headache, increased appetite, altered taste, nausea, vomiting	Take with food to decrease GI irritation; avoid alcohol. May cause drowsiness; may increase appetite. May cause urine to change to blue-green color

Generic Name (Trade)	Indications	Dosage	Side Effects	Comments
diphenoxylate/ atropine (Logen, Lomotil)	Diarrhea	Adults (PO): 15–20 mg/day in 3–4 divided doses/day Children (PO) (8–12 years): 2 mg 5 times/day; (5–8 years) 2 mg 4 times/day; (2–5 years) 2 mg 3 times/day.	Blurred vision, constipation, dry skin, mouth, fever, loss of appetite, stomach pain, nausea, vomiting, dizziness, drowsiness, depression	May give with food (decreases GI irritation); avoid alcohol.
doxepin (Adapin, Sinequan)	Depression, neuropathic pain	*Depression* Adults, children (> 12 years) (PO): initially, 25 mg TID and increased gradually (maximum daily dose 150 mg) *Neuropathic pain* Adults (PO): initially, 25 mg at bedtime up to 150 mg (maximum single dose 150 mg)	Blurred vision, constipation, dizziness, drowsiness, headache, increased appetite, altered taste, nausea, vomiting	May give with food to decrease GI irritation; avoid alcohol. May cause drowsiness, dry mouth. May increase appetite. Avoid exposure to sunlight.
doxorubicin (Adriamycin)	Lymphoma	Refer to individual protocols	Fever, chills, cough or hoarseness, lower back pain, difficult urination, sores in the mouth and on the lips, shortness of breath, swelling in feet and lower legs, pain at injection site, unusual bruising or bleeding, nausea, vomiting, diarrhea, loss of hair	Antineoplastic agent; refer to oncology text for specific information on administration and care. Give slow IV over 3–5 min or IV infusion over 1–4 hours. Transient red/orange urine discoloration. Teach client to notify health care provider if fever, sore throat, bleeding, or bruising occurs and to report any stinging at injection site.
doxorubicin hydrochloride liposome (Doxil)	Kaposi's sarcoma	Adults (IV): 20 mg/m^2 over 30 min, once q 3 weeks	Nausea, fatigue, headache, loss of appetite, abdominal pain, diarrhea, vomiting, cough, fever, allergic reaction (skin rash or itching), sweating, loss of hair, sores in the mouth and on the lips, fever, chills, cough or hoarseness, lower back pain, painful or difficult urination Serious adverse effect: cardiac toxicity Principle dose-limiting toxicity in HIV has been myelosuppression.	Antineoplastic agent; refer to oncology text for specific information on administration and care. Refer to daunorubicin for liposomal reaction. To ease nausea and vomiting (common side effect), administer parenteral antiemetics 30–45 min prior to therapy and around the clock for 24 hours posttherapy as needed. Monitor closely for signs or symptoms of cardiac toxicity, may be acute and transient or late onset (1–6 months later).

Generic Name (Trade)	Indications	Dosage	Side Effects	Comments
				Vesicant drug: monitor injection site; discontinue IV and restart in another vein if extravasation occurs.
dronabinol (Marinol)	HIV-related weight loss	Adults (PO): initially, 2.5 mg BID (before lunch and supper) for a total of 5 mg/day; if not tolerated, decrease to 2.5 mg as single evening or bedtime dose; may increase to 5 mg BID (maximum: 20 mg/day)	Dizziness, abnormalities in thinking, drowsiness, nausea, vomiting, changes in mood, fast or pounding heartbeat, altered vision	May cause drowsiness; patient should use caution in performing hazardous tasks. May cause dry mouth. Avoid alcohol.
EMLA brand for lidocaine and prilocaine	To prevent procedural pain (IVs starts, spinal taps, dressing changes)	Adults/children > 3 months (topical): apply thick layer to intact skin, cover with occlusive dressing at least 1 hour before procedure	At application site, burning feeling, swelling, itching, skin rash, very white or red skin	Avoid contact with eyes, lips or mouth; do not apply to open wounds, burns, broken or inflamed skin. Apply thick layer, and cover with occlusive dressing; the longer EMLA is left on, the deeper the penetration and anesthetic effect.
epoetin alfa (Epogen, Procrit)	Anemia related to HIV infection (serum erythropoietin level < 500 mU/ml)	Adults (SC/IV): initially, 100 units/kg/dose 3 times/wk for 8 weeks, then dose adjusted by 50–100 units/kg to a maximum of 300 units/kg 3 times/week	Chest pain, swelling of face/fingers/ankles/feet, increased weight, headache, increased blood pressure, altered vision, bone pain, muscle weakness, nausea, diarrhea, fatigue, dizziness. Contraindicated in patients with uncontrolled hypertension, known sensitivity to mammalian cell-derived products, and known hypersensitivity to human albumin	Do not shake vial. Refrigerate multidose vial. Single-use vial (1 ml/vial) must be discarded (does not contain a preservative).
ethambutol (Myambutol)	*Mycobacterium tuberculosis, mycobacterium avium complex*	Adults (PO): 15–25 mg/kg/d as single daily dose (maximum 2.5 gm/day or 50 mg/kg/dose), 2 times/week (maximum 2.5 gm/dose) Children (PO): 15–25 mg/kg/day as single daily dose (maximum 2.5 gm/day) *Secondary prophylaxis for MAC*	Optic neuritis, acute gouty arthritis (chills, pain, and swelling of joints especially the toes, ankle or knee, hot skin over affected joint), confusion, disorientation, abdominal pain, nausea, vomiting, loss of appetite, headache	Contraindicated in patients with optic neuritis. Take with food to prevent GI upset. Teach client to report any visual changes, numbness, tingling in hands or feet, rash, fever or chills. May cause elevated serum uric acid levels, possibly resulting in precipitation of acute gout. Abnormal liver function tests also have been noted.

Generic Name (Trade)	Indications	Dosage	Side Effects	Comments
		Adult (PO): clarithromycin 500 mg bid + ethambutol 15 mg/kg/day with or without rifabutin 300 mg/day (rifabutin dosage adjusted for clarithromycin, concurrent PI, NNRTI) *Alternative adult regimen* Adult (PO): azithromycin 500 mg/day + ethambutol 15 mg/kg/day with or without rifabutin 300 mg OD Children (PO): Clarithromycin 7.5 mg/kg (max 500 mg) BID plus ethambutol 15 mg/kg (maximum 900 mg) OD, with or without rifabutin 5 mg/kg (maximum 300 mg) OD *Alternative children regimen* azithromycin 5 mg/kg (maximum 250 mg) OD + ethambutol 15 mg/kg (maximum 900 mg) OD, with or without rifabutin 5 mg/kg (maximum of 300 mg) OD		
etoposide (Etopophos (phosphate salt); Toposar, VePesid)	Kaposi's sarcoma	Refer to individual protocols PO: 50 mg/d for 7 days every other week; may dose escalate up to 100 mg/d IV: give slowly over a minimum of 30–60 minutes	Fever, chills, cough, hoarseness, lower back pain, painful or difficult urination, unusual bleeding or bruising, nausea, vomiting, loss of appetite, loss of hair Use caution in presence of bone marrow depression, hepatic function impairment, general infection, renal function impairment, and in presence of previous cytotoxic drug therapy and radiation therapy	Antineoplastic agent; refer to oncology text for specific information on administration and care. Contraindicated in the presence of chicken pox or existing or recent herpes zoster. Teach client to notify health care provider if fever, sore throat, painful/burning urination, bruising, bleeding, or shortness of breath occurs. Dental work during etoposide therapy is discouraged due to the bone marrow depressant effects, which may

Generic Name (Trade)	Indications	Dosage	Side Effects	Comments
				result in an increased incidence of microbial infection, delayed healing, and gingival bleeding.
famciclovir (Famvir)	Herpes simplex virus infection, varicella-zoster virus infection	*Herpes simplex* Adults (PO): 250 mg TID for 5 days *Herpes zoster* Adults (PO): 500 mg q8h for 7 days	Headache, nausea	May take with or without food; give with food to decrease GI upset. Only recommended for immunocompetent individuals; use in immunosuppressed persons is under study.
fluconazole (Diflucan)	Oropharyngeal, esophageal, vaginal candidiasis, cryptococcosis, histoplasmosis.	*Primary prophylaxis (not routinely recommended; indicated for use only in unusual cases)* Adults (to prevent candidiasis, cryptococcosis) (PO): 100–200 mg daily Children (to prevent cryptococcus neoformans) (PO): 3–6 mg/kg daily *Treatment* *Oropharyngeal candidiasis* Adults (PO): 200 mg on first day, then 100 mg/day (up to 400 mg) Children (PO/IV): 6–12 mg/kg daily (maximum 200 mg/day). *Esophageal candidiasis* Adults (PO/IV): 200 mg on first day, then 100 mg/day (up to 400 mg) Children (PO/IV): 6–12 mg/kg daily (maximum 200 mg/day) *Vaginal candidiasis* Adults (PO): 150 mg one-time dose *Cryptococcus meningitis* Adults (PO/IV): 400 mg on first day, then 200–400 mg daily until cultures are negative Children (PO/IV): 6–12 mg/kg daily (maximum 200 mg/day)	Fever, chills, rash, itching, dizziness, drowsiness, headache, constipation or diarrhea, nausea, vomiting, loss of appetite, abdominal pain	*Candida:* Teach clients signs and symptoms of mucosal candidiasis, necessity for adherence to prescribed antifungal therapies, potential drug interactions, and signs and symptoms of liver toxicity (Thomas, 1998). Drug interactions: cisapride, terfenadine, zidovudine, warfarin, oral hypoglycemic agents, theophylline, phenytoin, carbamazepine, cyclosporine, tacrolimus, rifampin, and rifabutin. Co-administration with cisapride is contraindicated. When fluconazole is given in doses of 400 mg or greater, administration with terfenadine also is contraindicated. Patients taking fluconazole and warfarin concomitantly may have an increased prothrombin time. Fluconazole can increase the plasma concentrations of oral hypoglycemic agents, such as tolbutamide, glyburide, or glipizide, resulting in hypoglycemia. Plasma concentrations of theophylline, phenytoin, carbamazepine, cyclosporine, and tacrolimus can also increase, leading to possible toxicity. Rifampin increases the metabolism of fluconazole, which may

Generic Name (Trade)	Indications	Dosage	Side Effects	Comments
		Secondary prophylaxis Adults (PO): for cryptococcosis: 200 mg daily; for coccidioidomycosis, histoplasmosis: 400 mg daily; for vaginal or esophageal candidiasis in severe cases: 100–200 mg daily Children (PO): for cryptococcus neoformans: 3–6 mg/kg daily; for coccidioides immitis: 6 mg/kg daily; for candidiasis in severe cases: 3–6 mg/kg daily		necessitate an increase in fluconazole dose. There have been reports of uveitis in patients taking rifabutin and fluconazole.
flucytosine (Ancobon, 5-FC)	Used with amphotericin B for treating acute cryptococcal meningitis, severe candidiasis, cryptococcosis	Adults/children (PO): 25.0–37.5 mg/kg PO q6h (100–150 mg/kg/day), usually 100 mg/kg/day in 4 doses	Unusually tired or weak, yellow eyes or skin, skin rash, redness, or itching, fever, sore throat, unusual bruising or bleeding, increased sensitivity of skin to sunlight, abdominal pain, diarrhea, loss of appetite, nausea, vomiting, headache, drowsiness, dizziness or lightheadedness	Drug interactions: norfloxacin, cytarabine, and drugs which impair glomerular filtration
fomivirsen (Vitravene)	Cytomegalovirus (CMV) infection	*Secondary prophylaxis, alternative regimen* 330 mcg (1 vial) injected into the vitreous, then repeated every 2–4 weeks	Ocular inflammation (uveitis), increased intraocular pressure	Monitor light perception and optic nerve head perfusion after injection. Monitor intraocular pressure. Suspend treatment if there is unacceptable inflammation.
foscarnet (Foscavir)	Cytomegalovirus (CMV) infection, acyclovir-resistant herpes simplex virus (HSV) and varicella-zoster virus (VZV) infection	*Treatment of CMV retinitis and other sites* Adults/children (IV): initially, 60 mg/kg q 8 h or 90 mg q12h for 14–21 days, then, 90–120 mg/kg/day as single daily dose Children (> 3 months) (IV): 2–5 mg/kg/dose q8h or 5 mg/kg/dose q12h *Treatment of acyclovir-resistant HSV or VZV infection* Adults (IV): 40 mg/kg q 8 h or 60 mg/kg q12h up to 3 weeks or until lesions heal *Secondary prophylaxis* Adults/children (IV): 90–120 mg/kg daily	Abdominal pain, loss of appetite, nausea, vomiting, anxiety, confusion, dizziness, fatigue, headache, either decreased urination or increased thirst and urination, peripheral neuropathy (tingling, burning, numbness or pain in fingers or feet), penile ulcers, seizures (related to renal failure or hypocalcemia) Use with caution in patients with a history of renal impairment; must adjust dosage based on renal function Major toxicity: renal failure	Give by IV infusion over 2 hours. Report any symptoms of hypocalcemia: numbness or tingling in extremities, perioral paresthesia. Possible interaction with IV pentamidine causing hypocalcemia. Avoid use with potentially nephrotoxic drugs, such as aminoglycosides, amphotericin B, and IV pentamidine. Administered locally via sustained-release intravitreal implant

Generic Name (Trade)	Indications	Dosage	Side Effects	Comments
ganciclovir (Cytovene)	Cytomegalovirus (CMV) retinitis and CMV disease	*Primary prophylaxis (not routinely recommended; indicated for use only in unusual cases)* Adults (PO): 1 gm TID Children (PO): 30 mg/kg TID *Treatment of CMV retinitis* Adults/children (> 3 months) (IV): 5 mg/kg q12h for 14–21 days *Secondary prophylaxis* Adults (IV): 5 mg/kg/day daily 5–7 days/week or (PO) 1 gm TID; or sustained release implant every 6–9 months + PO ganciclovir 1.0–1.5 grams TID Children (IV): 5 mg/kg daily; alternative regimen for retinitis: sustained release implant every 6–9 months + PO ganciclovir 30 mg/kg TID	Fever, sore throat, unusual bruising or bleeding, tiredness or weakness, headaches, seizures, confusion Concurrent use of bone marrow depressants and ganciclovir may increase bone marrow toxicity. Nephrotoxic medications used with ganciclovir may increase the chance of renal function impairment, decreasing clearance of ganciclovir, leading to toxicity.	Take capsules with food to maximize bioavailability. Administer IV over 2 hours. Neutropenia may require coadministration of filgrastim. Solutions of ganciclovir are alkaline (pH 11). Direct contact with the skin or mucous membranes of capsule powder of parenteral solutions should be avoided. Should be handled and disposed of according to guidelines issued for cytotoxic drugs. Probenecid may decrease clearance of ganciclovir. Use of zidovudine with ganciclovir may cause severe hematologic toxicity in some patients. Combined therapy with imipenem-cilastatin and ganciclovir has resulted in generalized seizures. Intravitreal implant is designed to release ganciclovir over a period of 5 to 8 months.
granulocyte colony-stimulating factor (G-CSF) (filgrastim, Neupogen)	Neutropenia (absolute neutrophil count (ANC) < 500–750/mm^3)	Adults/children (IV/SC): 5–10 mcg/kg/day as single daily dose for up to 14 days then titrated to maintain ANC >1000–2000/mm^3 *Primary prophylaxis, neutropenia in bacterial infection, not routinely indicated* Adult (SC): 5–10 mcg/kg qd × 2–4 weeks	Redness or pain at injection site, headache, skin rash or itching, pain in joints and muscles, lower back, or pelvis	Use nonnarcotic analgesics to assist with management of medullary bone pain.
granulocyte macrophage colony-stimulating factor (GM-CSF, sargramostim) (Leukine, Prokine)	Neutropenia in bacterial infections	*Primary prophylaxis, neutropenia in bacterial infection, not routinely indicated* Adult (SC, IV): 250 mcg/m^2 × 2–4 weeks	Lethargy, malaise, headache, fatigue, hypotension, tachycardia, anemia, thrombocytopenia, bone pain, myalgia, arthralgia, fever, diarrhea, anorexia, rash, pruritus	Monitor for first-dose reaction: hypotension, tachycardia, fever, rigors, flushing, nausea, vomiting, diaphoresis, back pain, leg spasms, dyspnea. Monitor for respiratory symptoms during and immediately after infusion, especially in clients with preexisting pulmonary problems.

Generic Name (Trade)	Indications	Dosage	Side Effects	Comments
				Peripheral edema, pleural or pericardial effusion has occurred postadministration; reversible with dose reduction. Use corticosteroids and lithium with caution. Should not be administered within 24 hours preceding or following chemotherapy or within 12 hours preceding or following radiotherapy.
human growth hormone (Serostim)	HIV-related wasting syndrome and weight loss	Adults (SC) (based on weight): > 55kg, 6 mg daily; 45–55 kg, 5 mg daily; 35–45 kg, 4 mg daily	Muscle and joint pain, tissue swelling, discomfort, fever, increased tissue turgor, diarrhea, neuropathy, nausea, headache, abdominal pain, fatigue	Reconstituted solution should be refrigerated and must be used within 24 hours after reconstituting. Do not shake vial. Rotate injection sites. Concomitant antiretroviral therapy is required (may potentiate HIV replication).
imipramine (Tofranil, Tipramine)	Depression, neuropathic pain	*Depression* Adults (PO): initially, 25 mg 3–4 times/day, increase gradually to 300 mg/day maximum Children (PO): initially, 1.5 mg/kg/day, increase by 1 mg/kg q3–4 days up to maximum of 5 mg/kg/day in 1–4 divided doses *Pain* Adults (PO): same as for depression Children (PO): initially, 0.2–0.4 mg/kg at bedtime, increase by 50% q2–3 days up to maximum of 1–3 mg/kg/dose	Blurred vision, constipation, dizziness, drowsiness, headache, increased appetite, altered taste, nausea, vomiting, dry mouth	Take with food to decrease gastric irritation. Avoid alcohol. Teach patient to avoid excessive sunlight (may have photosensitivity). Contraindicated with the concomitant use of MAO inhibiting compounds (may result in hyperpyretic crises or severe convulsive seizures) and during acute recovery period post-MI. Use caution with clients on thyroid medications or receiving methylphenidate hydrochloride; in clients receiving anticholinergic drugs (including anti-Parkinsonism agents), the atropine-like effects may become more pronounced (e.g., paralytic ileus).
immune globulin (IVIG) (Gamimune N, Gammagard, Iveegam, Sandoglobulin, Venoglobulin)	Invasive bacterial infections	Children (IV): 400 mg/kg every 2–4 weeks; this dosage is used for secondary prophylaxis only if subsequent episodes are frequent or severe.	Trouble breathing, fast or pounding heartbeat, burning sensation in hand, fatigue, wheezing, pain, backache, headache, joint pain, malaise, muscle pain, vomiting, facial flushing, sweating, rash, dizziness	May require premedication with a corticosteroid. IV administration: Give in a rate-escalating manner (increasing flow rate gradually) based on vital signs and clinical response; have epinephrine available for hypersensitivity reactions.

Generic Name (Trade)	Indications	Dosage	Side Effects	Comments
				May interfere with body's immune response to MMR vaccine. Administration of vaccines containing measles virus vaccine live should be deferred for at least 8–10 months following administration of IVIG for replacement therapy of immunodeficiencies or treatment of idiopathic thrombocytopenic purpura.
interferon alfa 2a (Roferon A)	Kaposi's sarcoma, hepatitis, Non-Hodgkin's lymphoma	Adults (IM/SC): 36 million units/day for 10–12 weeks, then 3 times/wk or 20 million units/m^2/day for 4 weeks then 3 times/wk	Fever, chills, flulike symptoms, nausea, vomiting, loss of appetite, altered taste or metallic taste, diarrhea, dizziness, dry mouth, liver toxicity	Rotate SC injection sites. Advisable to stay with same brand. Refrigerate; do not shake. Best given at bedtime (because of flulike symptoms after injection). Teach client to inform health care provider of any mental status changes. Alpha interferons may cause or aggravate fatal or life-threatening neuropsychiatric, autoimmune, ischemic, and infectious disorders. Discontinue therapy if persistently severe or worsening signs and symptoms of these conditions; may resolve after drug stopped. Closely monitor with periodic clinical and laboratory evaluations.
interferon alfa 2b (Intron A)	Kaposi's sarcoma, cervical cancer, non-Hodgkin's lymphoma	Adults (IM/SC): 30 million units/m^2 3 times/wk	Fever, chills, flulike symptoms, nausea, vomiting, loss of appetite, altered taste or metallic taste, diarrhea, dizziness, dry mouth, liver toxicity	Refer to interferon alfa 2a
interferon alfa n1 (Wellferon)	Kaposi's sarcoma, hepatitis, non-Hodgkin's lymphoma	Adults (IM/IV): 20 million units/m^2 daily for 2 months	Fever, chills, flulike symptoms, nausea, vomiting, loss of appetite, altered taste or metallic taste, diarrhea, dizziness, dry mouth, liver toxicity	Refer to interferon alfa 2a
isoniazid (INH, Isotamine, Laniazid, Teebaconin, Nydrazid)	*Mycobacterium tuberculosis*	*Primary TB prophylaxis* Adult (PO): 300 mg + pyridoxine 50 mg qd × 9 months, or 900 mg + pyridoxine 100 mg twice a week × 9 months	Anorexia, nausea, vomiting, diarrhea, malaise, jaundice, peripheral neuropathy, bleeding, bruising, sore throat, rash, pain at injection site, arthralgia, seizures,	Once- or twice-weekly therapy with INH and a rifamycin appears to increase the risk of acquired rifamycin resistance among TB patients with advanced

Generic Name (Trade)	Indications	Dosage	Side Effects	Comments
		Children (PO): INH-sensitive: 10–15 mg/kg (maximum 300 mg) qd × 9 months, or 20–30 mg/kg (maximum 900 mg) twice a week × 9 months *Treatment* Adults (PO): 300 mg daily or 900 mg 2–3 times a week Children (PO/IM): 10–20 mg/kg daily (maximum 300 mg) or 20–30 mg/kg (maximum 900 mg) 2–3 times/week	depression, blurred vision with or without eye pain Peripheral neuritis is the most common toxic effect; INH hepatitis may occur at any time during therapy.	HIV disease (Centers for Disease Control and Prevention, 2002b). Assess monthly for clinical signs of hepatitis; monitor liver function tests; discontinue if alanine transaminase rises to or above 5x the upper normal limits. Take with pyridoxine to help prevent neurotoxic effects of INH-induced Vitamin B_6 depletion. May be taken with or without food; taking alcohol with INH increases potential for hepatitis. Take INH at least 1 hour before taking antacids containing aluminum. Due to its MAO-inhibiting activity, there is a risk of serotonin syndrome when given with SSRIs or other serotonergic medications. Advise patients that eating tyramine-containing foods (such as Swiss or Cheshire cheese or smoked fish) or histamine-containing foods (tuna, skipjack, sauerkraut juice, yeast extracts) may cause redness or itching of the skin, fast heartbeat, sweating, chills, headache, and lightheadedness.
itraconazole (Sporanox)	Aspergillosis, candidiasis (esophageal, oropharyngeal, vaginal), cryptococcosis, histoplasmosis, dermatophytic infections	*Primary prophylaxis for cryptococcosis, histoplasmosis (not routinely recommended; indicated for use only in unusual cases)* Adults (PO): 200 mg daily Children (PO): 2–5 mg/kg q12–24h *Treatment Aspergillosis* Adults (PO): 200 mg BID *Esophageal or vaginal candidiasis* Adults (PO): 100–200 mg TID	Fever, chills, rash, itching, dizziness, drowsiness, headache, constipation or diarrhea, nausea, vomiting, loss of appetite, abdominal pain	Take with food; requires gastric acid; best taken with orange juice, cola drinks, ginger ale. Do not give with antacids or H-2 antagonists. Coadministration of itraconazole and drugs primarily metabolized by the cytochrome P450 3A4 enzyme system may result in increasedplasma concentrationsof the drugs. Severe hypoglycemia has been reported in patients receiving concomitant

Generic Name (Trade)	Indications	Dosage	Side Effects	Comments
		Thrush Adults (PO): 100–200 mg BID × 1 day or 100–200 mg daily for 2–3 days *Histoplasmosis* Adults (PO): initially, 300 mg q12h for 3 days, then 200 mg q12h *Cryptococcosis* Adults (PO): 200 mg TID × 3 days, then 200 mg BID *Dermatophytic infections* Adults (PO): 100 mg daily *Secondary prophylaxis to prevent recurrent cryptococcosis, histoplasmosis, coccidioidomycosis* Adults (PO): 200 mg BID Children (PO): 2–5 mg/kg q12–48h *Secondary prophylaxis for esophageal candida (only if subsequent episodes are frequent or severe)* Children (PO solution): 5 mg/kg qd (alternative regimen)		administration of itraconazole and oral hypoglycemic agents; tinnitus and decreased hearing with concomitant itraconazole and quinidine; edema with concomitant itraconazole and dihydropyridine calcium channel blockers. Monitor prothrombin time when taking itraconazole with coumadin-like drugs.
kaolin-pectin (Kaopectate)	Diarrhea	Adults (PO): 60–120 ml after each loose bowel movement Children (PO): (> 12 years) 45–60 ml/dose; (6–12 years) 30–60 ml; (3–6 years) 15–30 ml	Constipation (usually mild, transient)	Do not use if diarrhea accompanied by fever or by blood or mucus in stool; notify physician if diarrhea not controlled within 48 hours.
ketoconazole (Nizoral)	Candidiasis (esophageal, oropharyngeal, vaginal)	*Treatment* *Esophageal candidiasis* Adults (PO): 200–400 mg BID Children: PO: 5–10 mg/kg/day in divided doses *Thrush* Adults (PO): 200 mg 1–2 times/day Children (PO): 5–10 mg/kg/day in divided doses	Fever, chills, rash, itching, dizziness, drowsiness, headache, constipation or diarrhea, nausea, vomiting, loss of appetite, abdominal pain	Give with food to minimize GI irritation, nausea, vomiting. Give 2 hours before antacids or H2 antagonists. Avoid alcohol. Requires gastric acid; best taken with orange juice, cola drinks, ginger ale. May interact with the following: antacids, cimetidine, ranitidine, rifampin, isoniazid,

Generic Name (Trade)	Indications	Dosage	Side Effects	Comments
		Vaginal candidiasis Adults (PO): 200–400 mg/day for 7 days or 400 mg/day for 3 days *Secondary prophylaxis for frequent or severe episodes* Adults (PO): 200 mg OD		acyclovir, vidarabine, norfloxacin; coumadin anticoagulants; cyclosporine; phenytoin; theophylline; terfenadine and astemizole; loratadine; corticosteroids; alcohol; cisapride, triazolam, oral sulfonylurea antidiabetic agent, and paclitaxel.
leucovorin (folinic acid, Wellcovorin)	Prophylaxis and treatment of toxicity related to use of folic acid antagonists (methotrexate, pyrimethamine, trimethoprim, trimetrexate)	*Primary prophylaxis for toxoplasmosis (alternative regimens)* Adults (PO): atovaquone 1,500 mg/day with or without pyrimethamine 25 mg/d + leucovorin 10 mg/day, or dapsone 50 mg/day + pyrimethamine 50 mg/week + leucovorin 25 mg/week, or dapsone 200 mg/week + pyrimethamine 75 mg/week + leucovorin 25 mg/week Children (PO): (≥ 1 month) dapsone 2 mg/kg or 15 mg/m^2 (maximum 25 mg) daily + pyrimethamine 1 mg/kg OD + leucovorin 5 mg every 3 days *Secondary prophylaxis for toxoplasmosis* Adults (PO): sulfadiazine 500–1000 mg QID + pyrimethamine 25–50 mg/day + leucovorin 10–25 mg/day *Alternative adult regimens* Adults (PO): clindamycin 300–450 mg q 6–8 hr + pyrimethamine 25–50 mg/day + leucovorin 10–25 mg/day, or atovaquone 750 mg q6–12h with or without pyrimethamine 25 mg/day + leucovorin 10 mg/day	May cause allergic reactions	Leucovorin may interact with barbiturate or hydantoin anticonvulsants, primidone, and central nervous system depressants. May enhance the toxicity of fluorouracil. Leucovorin is a specific antidote ("rescue drug") for the hematopoietic toxicity of methotrexate. Administer 24 hours after the first methotrexate dose; must be given on time to avoid potentially fatal methotrexate toxicity (Kirton, 2001).

Generic Name (Trade)	Indications	Dosage	Side Effects	Comments
		Children (PO): sulfadiazine 85–120 mg/kg/day in 2–4 divided doses + pyrimethamine 1 mk/kg or 15 mg/m² (maximum 25 mg) OD + leucovorin 5 mg every 3 days *Alternative children regimen* Clindamycin 20–30 mg/ kg/day in 4 divided doses qd + pyrimethamine 1 mg/kg OD + leucovorin 5 mg every 3 days *Primary prophylaxis for PCP* Adults (PO): dapsone 50 mg/day + pyrimethamine 50 mg/week + leucovorin 25 mg/week, or dapsone 200 mg/week + pyrimethamine 75 mg/ week + leucovorin 25 mg/week (alternative regimens) *Secondary prophylaxis for PCP* Same as primary		
loperamide (Imodium)	Treatment of diarrhea	Adults (PO): initially, 4 mg, then 2 mg after each loose bowel movement; Maximum: 16 mg/day Children (PO) (2–11 years): 0.08–0.25 mg/kg/day in 2–3 divided doses; Maximum: 2 mg/dose	Rare: skin rash, bloating, constipation, loss of appetite, severe stomach pain, nausea, vomiting, dizziness, drowsiness, dry mouth	Do not use if diarrhea accompanied with fever or blood/mucus in stool. Maintain adequate fluid intake.
megestrol acetate (Megace)	HIV-related wasting syndrome, weight loss	Adults (PO): 80 mg QID up to 800 mg/day Children (PO): 8 mg/kg/day, titrated to achieve weight gain	Diarrhea, impotence, rash, increased blood pressure, generalized weakness, inability to sleep, nausea, headache, possible drug-induced diabetes	Should not be used when hyperglycemia and weight loss develop as a result of protease inhibitor therapy.
methadone (Dolophine)	Pain, treatment for opiate addiction	*Pain* Adults (PO): 5–20 mg q4–8h (maximum 120 mg/day); (SC/IM): 2.5–10 mg q6–8h Children (PO): 0.2 mg/kg q4–8h; (IV) 0.1mg/kg q4–8h *Opiate addiction in adults* Individualized	Confusion, constipation, decreased blood pressure, increased heart rate, sweating, redness, flushed face, trouble breathing, decreased urination, stomach pain or cramps, dizziness, lightheadedness, unusually tired or weakness, drowsiness, dry mouth, headache	Teach client to avoid getting up suddenly and to lie down if lightheadedness, nausea, vomiting, or dizziness occurs. Use sugarless gum or candy for relief of dry mouth. Half-life of methadone is 72 hours; cumulative effects may develop. Interacts with many HAART agents. Use with caution and in reduced dosage in patients concurrently

Generic Name (Trade)	Indications	Dosage	Side Effects	Comments
				receiving other narcotic analgesics, general anesthetics, phenothiazines, other tranquilizers, sedative-hypnotics, tricyclic antidepressants, and other CNS depressants (including alcohol) because respiratory depression, hypotension, and profound sedation or coma may result.
methotrexate (MTX, Folex, Mexate, Rheumatrex)	Kaposi's sarcoma; mixed drug therapy for lymphoma	Refer to individual protocols	GI ulceration, bleeding, diarrhea, stomach pain, fever, chills, cough, hoarseness, lower back pain, painful urination, unusual bleeding or bruising, pinpoint red spots on skin, sores in mouth or on lips, loss of appetite, nausea, vomiting, skin rash, itching, loss of hair	Antineoplastic agent; refer to oncology text for specific information on administration and care. Avoid alcohol. Teach client to report any fever, sore throat, bleeding, bruising, shortness of breath, painful urination. Potential for toxicity is usually dose related. Large doses may cause convulsions.
metformin (Glucophage, Glucophage XR)	Antihyperglycemic; used in HIV for treatment of metabolic disturbances (fat redistribution, insulin resistance, and hyperinsulinemia) associated with HIV lipodystrophy syndrome	Adult (PO): 500 mg BID; extended-release tablets: 500 mg OD with evening meal	GI disturbances, usually transient and dose-related; diarrhea, abnormal stools, nausea, vomiting, abdominal bloating or cramping, flatulence, and taste disorder; hypoglycemia (more common in patients on other antidiabetic drugs or insulin), myalgia, lightheadedness, headache, dyspnea, nail disorder, rash, increased sweating, chest discomfort, chills, flu syndrome, flushing, and palpitation. Lactic acidosis is a rare, but serious, metabolic complication that can occur as a result of metformin accumulation.	Dose reduction, administration with meals, or both, may improve GI side effects. Risk of metformin accumulation and lactic acidosis increases with HIV infection, degree of renal function impairment, and age of patient. Lactate levels in patients taking metformin and NRTIs must be carefully monitored. Combined use of metformin and excessive alcohol can increase risk of lactic acidosis. Cationic drugs (e.g., amiloride, digoxin, morphine, procainamide, quinidine, quinine, ranitidine, triamterene, trimethoprim, and vancomycin) have potential for interaction.
metronidazole (Flagyl)	Bacterial vaginosis, gingivitis, amebiasis, trichomoniasis, diarrhea due to C. difficile	Adults (PO): 250–500 mg QID Children (PO): 20–35 mg/kg/day divided q6h	Headache, dizziness or lightheadedness, diarrhea, loss of appetite, nausea, vomiting, stomach pain or cramps, altered taste, metallic/sharp taste, dry mouth, dark urine,	Take with food to decrease gastric irritation. Teach patient that alcohol should not be consumed during and for at least 3 days following therapy. Disulfiram-like reactions, including flushing,

Generic Name (Trade)	Indications	Dosage	Side Effects	Comments
			numbness, tingling, pain or weakness in hands or feet, seizures with high doses	sweating, headache, nausea, vomiting, and abdominal cramps, may occur.
miconazole (Monistat)	Vaginal candidiasis	Adults (vaginal): (suppository): 200 mg OD for 3 days or 100 mg OD for 7 days; (cream): one full applicator at bedtime for 7 days	Vaginal burning, itching	Teach patient to take full course of therapy; can be continued during menstrual cycle. Instruct on application: Insert high into the vagina at bedtime, remain recumbent for 30 minutes postinsertion; sanitary napkins may be used to avoid staining bed linen.
mitoxantrone (Novantrone)	Kaposi's sarcoma, Non-Hodgkin's lymphoma	Refer to individual protocols	Cardiotoxicity, cough, shortness of breath, GI bleeding, fever, chills, painful urination, decreased urination, fast or irregular heartbeat, swelling of feet and lower legs, yellow eyes and skin, seizures, unusual bleeding, bruising, pinpoint red spots on skin, diarrhea, nausea, vomiting, headache, loss of hair	Antineoplastic agent; refer to oncology text for specific information on administration and care. May cause blue-green color in urine or in whites of eyes. Possibly interacts with allopurinol, colchicine, probenecid, sulfinpyrazone, blood dyscrasia–causing medications, bone marrow depressants, radiation therapy, daunorubicin, doxorubicin, killed or live virus vaccines, and previously administered anthracycline.
nandrolone (Durabolin)	HIV-related muscle wasting	Adults (IM): 25–100 mg/week	Chills, diarrhea, feeling of stomach fullness, altered libido, muscle cramps, trouble sleeping; in men: acne, decreased sex ability	Important to have diet high in protein and calories while taking this drug. Anabolic steroid; can interact with anticoagulants, adrenocorticoids (especially those with significant mineralocorticoid activity), sodium-containing medications or foods, or hepatotoxic medications.
nortriptyline (Aventyl, Pamelor)	Depression, neuropathic pain	*Depression* Adults (PO): initially 10–25 mg at bedtime, increasing to 50–100 mg at bedtime or 25 mg TID or QID *Neuropathic pain* Adults (PO): 10–25 mg at bedtime increasing over a 2 to 3–week period to a maximum of 75 mg at bedtime	Dry mouth, dizziness, blurred vision, constipation, urinary hesitancy, orthostatic hypotension, sedation, decreased libido, weight gain	Teach client to avoid getting up suddenly and to lie down if dizziness, nausea, vomiting, or lightheadedness occur. Use sugarless gum or candy for relief of dry mouth.

Generic Name (Trade)	Indications	Dosage	Side Effects	Comments
nystatin (Mycostatin, Nilstat)	Oropharyngeal candidiasis	*Solution* Neonates (PO): 100,000 units QID or 50,000 units to each side of mouth QID Infants (PO): 200,000 units QID or 100,000 units to each side of mouth QID Adults/children (PO): 400,000–600,000 units QID *Lozenges* Adults, children (PO): (> 5 years) 200,000–400,000 units QID *Vaginal tablets* Adults (vaginal): 100,000 units 1–2 times/day	Stomach pain, nausea, vomiting, diarrhea	Shake suspension well prior to administration. Place and hold suspension in mouth or swish throughout mouth as long as possible before swallowing or spitting out. For neonates/infants: paint suspension into recesses of mouth. Allow lozenges to dissolve slowly; do not chew or swallow whole.
octreotide (Sandostatin)	Diarrhea associated with *cryptosporidiosis, microsporidiosis*	Adults (SC/IV): 50–500 mcg TID at 1 mcg/hour Children (SC): 1–10 mcg q12h.	Abdominal pain or discomfort; nausea; diarrhea; vomiting; pain, burning, stinging, redness, or swelling at injection site; dizziness; lightheadedness; swelling of feet or lower legs; headache; fatigue; red or flushed face; weakness	Give by subcutaneous injection; rotate injection sites. Assess frequency of stools and bowel sounds throughout therapy. Administer between meals and at bedtime to decrease GI side effects.
ondansetron (Zofran)	Nausea, vomiting	Adults/children (IV): (> 11 years) 4 mg/dose (PO): 8 mg TID Children (IV): (4–11 years) 0.15 mg/kg/dose (PO): 4 mg TID	Constipation, diarrhea, headache, fever, abdominal pain, stomach cramps, dizziness, drowsiness, dry mouth, rash, unusual fatigue or weakness	Report to health care provider if vomiting persists.
oxandrolone (Oxandrin)	HIV-related wasting syndrome and weight loss	Adults (PO): 2.5 mg 2–4 times/day; range: 2.5–20 mg/day Children (PO): 0.25 mg/kg/day in 2–4 divided doses	Chills, diarrhea, feeling of stomach fullness, altered libido, muscle cramps, trouble sleeping; men: acne, decreased sex ability	It is important to have diet high in protein and calories while taking this drug.
paclitaxel (Taxol)	Kaposi's sarcoma	Adults (IV): 135 mg/m^2 every 3 weeks or 100 mg/m^2 every 2 weeks	Fever, chills, unusual bleeding or bruising, muscle pain, joint pain, numbness in the feet or lower legs, nausea, vomiting, diarrhea, unusual fatigue or weakness	Antineoplastic agent; refer to oncology text for specific information on administration and care. Infused slowly over 3 hours.
para-amino-salicylate (PAS)	*Mycobacterium* tuberculosis	Adults (PO): 3.3–4 gm q8h or 5–6 gm q 12h (maximum 20 gm/day)	Fever, joint pain, skin rash, itching, unusual fatigue or weakness, lower back pain, pain while urinating,	Take with or after meals to decrease gastric irritation.

Generic Name (Trade)	Indications	Dosage	Side Effects	Comments
		Children (PO): 50–75 mg/kg q6h or 67–100 mg q8h	abdominal pain, loss of appetite, nausea, diarrhea, vomiting, yellow eyes or skin	
paromomycin (Humatin)	Crypto-sporidiosis	Adults (PO): 500–750 mg QID for 21 days	Headache, vertigo, rash, diarrhea, nausea, abdominal cramps, loss of appetite, steatorrhea, ototoxicity, hematuria	Take with food. Report ringing in ears, dizziness, loss of hearing.
peginterferon alfa-2a (Pegasys)	Chronic hepatitis C virus	Adult Dose: peginterferon alfa-2a 1.5 mcg/kg per week and ribavarin (Copegus) 800 mg/d (dosage range may vary according to patient's response)	Musculoskeletal pain, fatigue, inflammation at injection site, flulike symptoms, rigors, fever, weight loss, viral infection, headache, depression, anxiety, emotional lability, irritability, insomnia, dizziness, nausea, anorexia, diarrhea, abdominal pain, pharyngitis, alopecia, pruritus, dry skin	Use with ribavirin: refer to ribavirin. Contraindications: auto-immune hepatitis, decompensated hepatic disease (Child-Pugh class B and C); neonates and infants due to benzyl alcohol content, hypersensitivity to peginterferon or any of its components, or to ribavirin (Copegus); in women who are pregnant; men whose female partners are pregnant; and patients with hemoglobinopathies (e.g., thalassemia major, sickle-cell anemia). Alpha interferons may cause or aggravate fatal or life-threatening neuropsychiatric, autoimmune, ischemic, and infectious disorders. Monitor closely with periodic clinical and laboratory evaluations. Therapy should be withdrawn in patients with persistently severe or worsening signs or symptoms of these conditions.
pentamidine (NebuPent, Pentam-300)	Pneumocystis carinii pneumonia	*Primary prophylaxis* Adults (inhalation): 300 mg once a month via Respigard II™ nebulizer Children (inhalation): > 5 years: 300 mg once a month via Respigard II™ nebulizer *Treatment* Adults/children (IV): 3–4 mg/kg daily × 21 days (usually reserved for severe cases)	*Aerosol:* Chest pain or congestion, cough, difficulty breathing, burning pain or dryness in the throat, difficulty swallowing, skin rash, wheezing, bitter or metallic taste *Parenteral:* Sudden rash or itching, anemia, unusual fatigue, fever or chills, cough or hoarseness, lower back pain, painful or difficult urination, unusual bruising or bleeding,	Report fever, cough, shortness of breath; avoid alcohol; maintain adequate fluid intake. IV administration stimulates the release of histamine, so hypotension can occur during infusion; give IV over 60 minutes. Sterile abscess may occur with IM injections.

Generic Name (Trade)	Indications	Dosage	Side Effects	Comments
		Secondary prophylaxis Adults/children: Same as primary	pinpoint red spots on skin, diarrhea, headache, loss of appetite, nausea, vomiting, skin rash	
primaquine	*Pneumocystis carinii* pneumonia	Adults (PO): 26.3–52.6 mg (15–30 mg base) daily for 21 days	Back, leg, or stomach pain; dark urine; loss of appetite; fever; unusual fatigue or weakness; bluish fingernails, lips, or skin; dizziness or lightheadedness; difficulty breathing; nausea; vomiting; abdominal pain	Take with meals or antacids to decrease GI irritation.
probenecid	Given with cidofovir for CMV	Cidofovir infusion: give probenecid (PO) 2 g (PO) 3 hours before the dose of cidofovir, followed by 1 g (PO) 2 hr after the dose, and 1 g (PO) 8 hr after the dose (total of 4 of Probenecid)	Flushing, dizziness, fever, headache, nausea, vomiting, anorexia, anemia, exacerbations of gout, uric acid kidney stones	Minimize GI adverse effects by giving after meals, with food, or with milk. Give with a full glass of water.
prochlor-perazine (Compazine)	Nausea, vomiting	Adults (PO): 5–10 mg 3–4 times/day (maximum 40 mg/day); (extended release) 15–30 mg once daily or 10 mg q12h (maximum 40 mg/day) Children (PO): (syrup) (9–13 kg) 2.5 mg 1–2 times/ day (maximum 7.5 mg/day); (14–17 kg) 2.5 mg 2–3 times/ day (maximum 10 mg/day); (18–39 kg) 2.5 mg 3 times/ day or 5 mg 2 times/day (maximum 15 mg/day)	Constipation, dizziness, drowsiness, dry mouth, nausea, vomiting, stomach pain, decreased sweating	Take with food to decrease gastric irritation. Do not chew extended release capsules; take whole.
pyridoxine (Vitamin B6)	Treatment/ prevention of neuropathy due to isoniazid (INH) therapy; management of INH overdose	*Primary prophylaxis TB* Adults (PO): INH 300 mg/day + pyridoxine 50 mg/day × 9 months, or INH 900 mg + pyridoxine 100 mg 2 × week × 9 months *INH toxicity* Adults (IV): administer 4 g IV followed by 1 g IM every 30 min	Clumsiness; numbness of hands or feet (with large doses)	Use caution when coadministered with levodopa (Parkinson's disease); interferes with therapeutic response to levodopa. May cause false elevation in urobilogen lab concentrations If extended-release capsule is too large to swallow, may mix capsule contents with jam or jelly and swallow without chewing.

Generic Name (Trade)	Indications	Dosage	Side Effects	Comments
pyrazinamide (PZA)	Mycobacterium tuberculosis	Primary prophylaxis TB, alternative regimen Adults (PO): PZA 15–20 mg/kg qd × 2 months + either rifampin 600 mg po OD or rifabutin 300 mg po OD × 2 months	Pain/swelling of joint especially big toe, ankle, and knee; hot skin over affected joints; loss of appetite; unusual fatigue or weakness; yellow eyes or skin; itching; skin rash	Stop rifabutin-PZA combination if symptomatic and increased ALT, or ALT increased over 5X upper limits of normal, or an increase in bilirubin.
pyrimethamine (Daraprim)	Toxoplasmosis, Pneumocystis carinii pneumonia	Primary prophylaxis for toxoplasmosis (alternative regimen) Adults (PO): atovaquone 1500 mg/day with or without pyrimethamine 25 mg/d + leucovorin 10 mg/day, or dapsone 50 mg/day + pyrimethamine 50 mg/week + leucovorin 25 mg/week, or dapsone 200 mg/week + pyrimethamine 75 mg/week + leucovorin 25 mg/week Children (PO): (≥ 1 month) dapsone 2 mg/kg or 15mg/m^2 (maximum 25 mg) daily + pyrimethamine 1 mg/kg OD + leucovorin 5 mg every 3 days (alternative regimen) Treatment Adult (PO): 100–200 mg loading dose, then 50–100 mg/day + folinic acid 10 mg/day + sulfadiazine for at least 6 weeks Secondary prophylaxis for toxoplasmosis Adults (PO): Sulfadiazine 500–1000 mg qid + pyrimethamine 25–50 mg/day + leucovorin 10–25 mg/day Alternative adult regimen Adults (PO): Clindamycin 300–450 mg q 6–8 hr + pyrimethamine 25–50 mg/day + leucovorin 10–25 mg/day, or	Pain, burning, or inflammation of the tongue; change or loss of taste; fever; sore throat; unusual fatigue or weakness; unusual bruising or bleeding; high doses may cause loss of appetite, nausea, vomiting, or diarrhea.	Give with meals to decrease GI side effects. Report rash, sore throat, pallor, glossitis (pain, burning, inflammation of tongue, change in taste). Give with folinic acid (leucovorin).

Generic Name (Trade)	Indications	Dosage	Side Effects	Comments
		atovaquone 750 mg q6–12h with or without pyrimethamine 25 mg/d + leucovorin 10 mg/day Children (PO): sulfadiazine 85–120 mg/kg/day in 2–4 divided doses + pyrimethamine 1 mk/kg or 15 mg/m^2 (maximum 25 mg) qd + leucovorin 5 mg every 3 days *Alternative children regimen* clindamycin 20–30 mg/ kg/day in 4 divided doses OD + pyrimethamine 1 mg/kg OD + leucovorin 5 mg every 3 days *Treatment of toxoplasmosis* Adults (PO): 100–200 mg loading dose, then 50–100 mg/day with leucovorin and sulfadiazine or trisulfapyrimidine Children (PO): 1–2 mg/kg/day daily for 1–3 days, then 0.5–1mg/kg daily *Primary prophylaxis for PCP* Adults (PO): dapsone 50 mg/d + pyrimethamine 50 mg/week + leucovorin 25 mg/wk, or dapsone 200 mg/week + pyrimethamine 75 mg/week + leucovorin 25 mg/week (alternative regimens) *Secondary prophylaxis for PCP* Same as primary *Treatment of PCP* Adults: 50 mg weekly with dapsone and leucovorin		
ribavirin (Copegus)	Used in combination with peginterferon alpha-2a	Adult: peginterferon alfa-2a 1.5 mcg/kg per week and ribavarin 800 mg/d (dosage range may vary	Feelings of tiredness, nausea and appetite loss, rash and itching and cough	Use with Pegasys: refer to peginterferon alfa-2a. Take with food. Advise patients to avoid alcohol (including beer,

Generic Name (Trade)	Indications	Dosage	Side Effects	Comments
	for hepatitis C	according to patient's response)	Significant adverse effects: severe depression and suicidal ideation, hematolytic anemia (primary toxicity), bone marrow suppression, autoimmune and infectious disorders, pulmonary dysfunction, pancreatitis, and diabetes	wine, and liquor) due to its effect on liver disease. Refer to didanosine (Videx) for caution when using in combination (Food and Drug Administration, 2002). Advise patients not to drive or operate machinery if feeling tired, dizzy, or confused. Advise to call health care provider right away for following signs and symptoms: trouble breathing, hives or swelling, chest pain, severe stomach or lower back pain, bloody diarrhea or stools, bruising or unusual bleeding, vision change, high fever, worsening of psoriasis, or depression and suicidal feelings. Monotherapy with ribavarin is not effective for treatment of chronic hepatitis C. Patients with a history of significant or unstable cardiac disease should not be treated with ribavarin due to the side effect of anemia that may worsen cardiac disease and lead to MI. Ribavarin has significant teratogenic and/or embryocidal effects and is contraindicated in women who are pregnant and in the male partners of women who are pregnant; extreme care must be taken to avoid pregnancy during therapy and for 6 months after completion of treatment in both female patients and in female partners of male patients who are taking ribavirin. Females taking Copegus or female sexual partners of male patients taking Copegus must have a pregnancy test before treatment begins, every month during treatment, and for

Generic Name (Trade)	Indications	Dosage	Side Effects	Comments
				6 months after treatment ends to make sure that there is no pregnancy.
rifabutin (Mycobutin)	*Mycobacterium avium complex (MAC), Mycobacterium tuberculosis (TB)*	*Primary prophylaxis for MAC, alternative regimens* Adults (PO): 300 mg/day, or 300 mg/day + azithromycin 1,200 mg/week Children (PO): age 6 years, 300 mg OD *Treatment for MAC* Adults (PO): 300–600 mg/day Children (PO): 10–20 mg/kg/day *Secondary prophylaxis for MAC* Adults (PO): Clarithromycin 500 mg BID + ethambutol 15 mg/kg/day with or without rifabutin 300 mg/day (rifabutin dosage adjusted for clarithromycin, concurrent PI, NNRTI) *Alternative adult regimen* Azithromycin 500 mg/day + ethambutol 15 mg/kg/day + rifabutin 300 mg/day (rifabutin dosage adjusted for clarithromycin, concurrent PI, NNRTI) Children (PO): clarithromycin 7.5 mg/kg (max 500 mg) BID plus ethambutol 15 mg/kg (maximum 900 mg) OD, with or without rifabutin 5 mg/kg (maximum 300 mg) OD *Alternative children regimen* Azithromycin 5 mg/kg (maximum 250 mg) OD + ethambutol 15 mg/kg (maximum 900 mg) OD, with or without rifabutin 5 mg/kg (maximum of 300 mg) OD	Skin rash; nausea; vomiting, reddish-orange to reddish-brown discoloration or urine, feces, saliva, skin, sputum, sweat, tears; may also discolor soft contact lenses	Stop rifabutin-PZA TB combination if symptomatic and increased ALT, or ALT increased over 5X upper limits of normal, or an increase in bilirubin. Take on an empty stomach or with food if gastric irritation occurs. Mix contents of capsules with applesauce if swallowing capsule is difficult. Rifabutin dose modifications: With indinavir 100 mg q8h, nelfinavir 1,250 mg bid, or amprenavir 1,200 mg bid, use rifabutin 150 mg daily or 300 mg 2–3 times a week; with ritonavir/saquinavir 400/400 mg, use rifabutin 150 mg 2–3 times a week; with lopinavir/ritonavir 400/100, use rifabutin 150 mg qod; with nevirapine 200 mg bid, use rifabutin 300 mg/day; and with efavirenz 600 mg hs, use rifabutin 600 mg 2–3 times a week

Generic Name (Trade)	Indications	Dosage	Side Effects	Comments
		Primary prophylaxis for TB Adult (PO): INH-sensitive or INH-resistant: 300 mg po OD × 4 month, or 300 mg OD + PZA 15–20 mg/kg/day × 2 months		
rifampin (Rifadin, Rimactane)	*Mycobacterium tuberculosis*	*Primary TB prophylaxis, INH sensitive* Adults (not on HAART) (PO): 600 mg/day × 4 months, or 600 mg/day + pyrazinamide 15–20 mg/kg/day × 2 months (alternative regimen) Children (PO): 10–20 mg/kg (maximum 600 mg) OD × 4–6 months *Primary TB prophylaxis, INH-resistant* Adult (PO): (not on HAART): 600 mg po qd × 4 months; alternative regimen: 600 mg qd + pyrazinamide 15–20 mg/kg qd × 2 months *Treatment* Adults (PO): 10 mg/kg/day once daily or 2–3 times a week (maximum 600 mg/day) Children (PO): (up to 1 month) 10–20 mg/kg/day or 2–3 times/week Children (PO): (> 1 month) 10–20 mg/kg/day or 2–3 times/week (maximum 600 mg/day)	Stomach cramps; diarrhea; reddish-orange to reddish-brown discoloration of urine, feces, saliva, skin, sputum, sweat, tears; may also discolor soft contact lenses	Best given 1 hr before or 2 hr after meals. Give with food to decrease GI upset. May mix contents of capsules with applesauce.
spiramycin	Respiratory tract infections, toxoplasmosis in pregnant women	Adults and teenagers (PO): 1 to 2 g (3,000,000 to 6,000,000 International Units [IU]) BID, or 500 mg to 1 g (1,500,000 to 3,000,000 IU) TID. For severe infections, the dose	Skin rash and itching; unusual bleeding or bruising; with injection, pain at site of injection; diarrhea; chest pain; fever; heartburn; irregular heartbeat; nausea; recurrent fainting; stomach pain and tenderness; vomiting; yellow eyes or skin	Best taken on an empty stomach. Do not store the tablet form of spiramycin in the bathroom, near the kitchen sink, or in other damp places; heat or moisture may cause the medicine to break down.

Generic Name (Trade)	Indications	Dosage	Side Effects	Comments
		is 2 to 2.5 g (6,000,000 to 7,500,000 IU) BID. Children weighing 20 kilograms (kg) (44 lb) or more (PO): Dose is based on body weight. The usual dose is 25 mg (75,000 IU) per kg (11.4 mg per lb) of body weight BID, or 17 mg (51,000 IU) per kg (7.7 mg per lb) of body weight TID. Adults and teenagers (IV): 500 mg (1,500,000 IU) injected slowly into a vein every 8 hours. For severe infections, the dose is 1 g (3,000,000 IU) injected slowly into a vein every 8 hours. Adults and children 12 years of age and older (rectal): Two or three 750 mg (1,950,000 IU) suppositories per day Children up to 12 years of age (rectal): Two or three 500 mg (1,300,000 IU) suppositories per day Newborns (rectal): Dose is based on body weight. The usual dose is one 250 mg (650,000 IU) suppository per 5 kg (250 mg suppository per 11 pounds) of body weight once a day.		
streptomycin	*Mycobacterium tuberculosis*	Adults (IM): 15 mg/kg/ day daily (maximum 1 g) Children (IM): 20–40 mg/kg/day daily (maximum 1 g)	Urinary frequency, increased thirst, loss of appetite, nausea, vomiting, twitching, numbness, seizures, tingling, loss of hearing, ringing or buzzing in ears, fullness in ears, dizziness, nausea, vomiting, clumsiness, burning of face or mouth, itching, redness, rash or swelling, any loss of vision	Inject deep IM into large muscle mass. Do not exceed concentration of 500 mg/ml.

Generic Name (Trade)	Indications	Dosage	Side Effects	Comments
sulfadiazine	Toxoplasmosis	*Secondary prophylaxis for toxoplasmosis* Adults (PO): sulfadiazine 500–1000 mg qid + pyrimethamine 25–50 mg/day + leucovorin 10–25 mg/day Children (PO): 85–120 mg/kg/day in 2–4 divided doses + pyrimethamine 1 mk/kg or 15 mg/m² (maximum 25 mg) OD + leucovorin 5 mg every 3 days *Treatment* Adults (PO): 2–8 g/day divided q6h (with pyrimethamine and folinic acid) Children (PO): 120–200 mg/kg/day divided q6h (with pyrimethamine and folinic acid)	Dizziness, headache, lethargy, nausea, vomiting, diarrhea, loss of appetite, fever, itching, skin rash, increased sensitivity to sunlight	Give on an empty stomach (with 8 oz of water). Take several extra glasses of water daily to prevent kidney stones. Avoid large amounts of vitamin C or acidifying agents (e.g., cranberry juice) to prevent crystalluria. Report rash, sore throat, fever, arthralgia, shortness of breath.
terconazole (Terazol)	Vulvovaginal candidiasis	Adults (vaginal): 1 tablet at bedtime for 3 days or 1 full applicator at bedtime for 7 days or 0.8% cream for 3 days	Vaginal burning, itching, discharge, irritation; headache; abdominal or stomach cramps or pain	Use at bedtime.
testosterone (Testosterone cypionate, Testosterone enanthate)	Hypogonadism and HIV-related wasting	Adult men (IM): 100–200 mg every 2 weeks Adult men (transdermal): 4–6 mg patch changed every day	Bladder irritability, urinary tract infection, edema, nausea, vomiting, diarrhea, acne, irritation at site of injection, gynecomastia, irritation at site of transdermal patch	Patch must be applied to dry, shaved scrotum.
thalidomide (Thalomid)	Severe aphthous ulcers, HIV-related wasting	*Aphthous ulcers* Adults (PO): 100–200 mg/day, with increases up to 400–600 mg/day if unresponsive *Wasting* Adult (PO): initial dose is 100 mg PO OD with increases up to 200 mg/day	Drowsiness, dizziness, altered mood, constipation, xerostomia, increased appetite and weight, headache, decreased libido, nausea, itching, loss of hair, fever, chills, dry skin, rash, numbness, tingling, burning of hands and feet, swelling of face, hands, and legs	Teratogenic effects: Any woman of childbearing potential should not receive thalidomide unless great precautions are taken to prevent pregnancy (pills and barrier protection). Because thalidomide may be present in semen, condom use is recommended for men.
trimethoprim	*Pneumocystis carinii pneumonia (PCP)*	Adult (PO): (with SMX as TMP-SMX or with dapsone): 5 mg/kg PO tid or qid (usually 300 mg tid or qid) × 21 days	Pruritis and skin rash, GI intolerance, marrow suppression (anemia, neutropenia, thrombocytopenia)	Refer to trimethoprim-sulfamethoxazole. Increased activity of phenytoin (monitor levels) and procainamide Levels of both dapsone and TMP are increased when given concurrently.

Generic Name (Trade)	Indications	Dosage	Side Effects	Comments
trimethoprim-sulfamethox-azole (Bactrim, Septra, TMP-SMX)	*Pneumocystis carinii* pneumonia (PCP), toxoplas-mosis	*Primary prophylaxis for PCP* Adults (PO): one double-strength or single-strength tablet/day; alternative regimen: one double-strength tablet 3 times a week Children (PO): 150/750mg/m^2/day in 2 divided doses 3 times a week on consecutive days *Alternative regimen* PO: Single dose 3 times a week on consecutive days, 2 divided doses qd, or 2 divided doses 3 times a week on alternate days *Treatment PCP* Adults (PO/IV): TMP 15 mg/kg/day/SMX 75 mg/kg/day PO or IV × 21 days in 3 to 4 divided doses (typical oral dosage is 2 DS TID) *Alternative regimen* TMP 15 mg/kg/day PO + dapsone 100 mg/day PO × 21 days Children: (PO/IV): TMP 15–20 mg/kg/day + SMX 75–100 mg/kg/day in 3–4 divided doses/day *Secondary prophylaxis for PCP* Adults (PO): Same as primary Children (PO): 150/750mg/m^2/day in 2 divided doses 3 times a week on consecutive days, or single dose 3 times a week on consecutive days, or 2 divided doses OD, or 2 divided doses 3 times a week on alternate days *Primary prophylaxis for toxoplasmosis* Adults (PO): one double-strength tablet/day (preferred) or one single-strength tablet/day (alternative regimen)	Dizziness, headache, feeling of lethargy, nausea, vomiting, diarrhea, loss of appetite, fever, itching, skin rash, increased sensitivity to sunlight	Oral: Administer on empty stomach (with 8 oz water) and drink several extra glasses of water daily. IV: Infuse over 60 to 90 minutes; rapid infusion can cause severe nausea. Cautious use with impaired liver or kidney function, severe allergy or bronchial asthma, G6PD deficiency, hypersensitivity to sulfonamide derivative drugs. Not recommended for infants under 2 months of age.

Generic Name (Trade)	Indications	Dosage	Side Effects	Comments
		Children (PO): 150/750 mg/m^2/day in 2 divided doses qd *Secondary prophylaxis for Salmonella bacteremia* Children (PO): 150/750 mg/m^2/day in 2 divided doses for several months *Secondary prophylaxis for invasive bacterial infections (not routinely recommended; indicated for use only in unusual cases)* Children (PO): 150/750 mg/m^2/day in 2 divided doses		
trimetrexate (NeuTrexin)	*Pneumocystis carinii* pneumonia	Adults (IV): 45 mg/m^2 daily + folinic acid 20 mg/m^2 PO or IV q6h.	Fever, sore throat, unusual fatigue or weakness, mouth sores or ulcers, skin rash or itching, unusual bruising or bleeding, blood in urine or stool, pinpoint red spots on skin, confusion, nausea, vomiting, stomach pain	Infuse IV over 60 to 90 minutes. Leucovorin (folinic acid) must be given concurrently and again at 72 hours following last dose trimetrexate.
valacyclovir (Valtrex)	Herpes zoster virus infection, genital herpes simplex (HSV)	Adults (PO): HZV: 1 g TID HSV: 1 g BID	Nausea, headache, dizziness, fatigue, constipation, diarrhea, loss of appetite, stomach pain, vomiting	Take with meals. Only recommended for immunocompetent individuals; use in immunosuppressed persons is under study.
valganciclovir (Valcyte)	Cytomegalovirus	Secondary prophylaxis 900 mg po/day (alternative regimen)	Fever, headache, insomnia, peripheral neuropathy, diarrhea, nausea, vomiting, abdominal pain, neutropenia, anemia	Not recommended for persons on hemodialysis Hold drug and notify physician for the following: ANC < 500 cells/mm^3, platelet count < 25,000 mm^3, hemoglobin < 8 g/dL, declining creatinine clearance.
vancomycin (Vancocin, Vancoled)	*Clostridium difficile* colitis	Adult (PO): 125–500 mg q6h Children (PO): 40 mg/kg/d divided q6h (maximum 2 g/day)	Ototoxicity, neurotoxicity, hypersensitivity reactions, nausea	Assess hearing (ototoxic); tinnitus (ringing in the ears) and high-pitched hearing loss may precede deafness; serum levels of 60–80 mcg/mL are associated with ototoxicity.
vinblastine (Velban)	Kaposi's sarcoma	Refer to individual protocols	Fever, chills, cough, hoarseness, lower back pain, painful/difficult urination, muscle pain, nausea, vomiting, joint pain, loss of hair, sores in the mouth or on the lips,	Antineoplastic agent; refer to oncology text for specific information on administration and care. For IV administration only Report fever, sore throat, bleeding, bruising.

Generic Name (Trade)	Indications	Dosage	Side Effects	Comments
			pain, redness at injection site, swelling of the feet or lower legs	
vincristine (Oncovin)	Kaposi's sarcoma	Refer to individual protocols	Constipation, stomach cramps, dizziness or lightheadedness, joint pain, lower back or side pain, diarrhea, loss of weight, nausea, vomiting, skin rash, loss of hair, pain or redness at injection site, blurred vision or double vision, pain or numbness in the fingers or toes	Antineoplastic agent; refer to oncology text for specific information on administration and care. For IV administration only Report fever, sore throat, bleeding, bruising or shortness of breath.

References

Bartlett, J. G., & Gallant, J. D. (2001). Management of opportunistic infections and other complications of HIV infection. In J. G. Bartlett & J. D. Gallant(Ed.), *Medical management of HIV*. Retrieved March 31, 2003, from http://www.hopkins-aids.edu/publications/book/ch5.html

Centers for Disease Control and Prevention. (2002a). Guidelines for preventing opportunistic infections among HIV-infected persons, 2002: Recommendations of the U.S. Public Health Service and the Infectious Diseases Society of America. *Morbidity and Mortality Reports, 51*(RR08), 1–46.

Centers for Disease Control and Prevention. (2002b). Notice to readers: Acquired rifamycin resistance in persons with advanced HIV disease being treated for active tuberculosis with intermittent rifamycin-based regimens. *Morbidity and Mortality Reports, 51*(10), 214–215.

Dodge, R. (1999). A case study: The use of cidofovir for the management of progressive multifocal leukoencephalopathy. *Journal of the Association of Nurses in AIDS Care, 10*(4), 70–74.

Food and Drug Administration. (2002). *New safety information for Videx (didanosine, ddI) used with ribavarin–FDA announcement*. Retrieved September 25, 2002, from http://aidsinfo.nih.gov/other/videx.asp

Kirton, C. A. (2001). Oncological conditions. In C. A. Kirton, D. Talotta, & K. Zwolski (Eds.), *Handbook of HIV/AIDS nursing*. St. Louis, MO: Mosby.

Rhoads, J. (2001). Alitretinoin (Panretin) gel 0.1%. *Journal of the Association of Nurses in AIDS Care, 12*(5), 86–91.

Thomas, C. J. (1998). Triazole therapy for mucocutaneous candidiasis in HIV-infected patients. *Journal of the Association of Nurses in AIDS Care, 9*(5), 36–44.

Weissman, A. C. (1999). Treatment of fungal infections with ABLC in the home-care setting. *Journal of the Association of Nurses in AIDS Care, 10*(3), 43–52.

Index

AA. *See* Alcoholics Anonymous
Abacavair (Ziagen, 1592), 52
Access to care, defined, 339
ACE (AIDS Counseling and
      Education) program, 201
Acetaminophen, 296
Acute renal failure, 274
Acute stress disorder, 168
Acute T-cell Leukemia (ATL), 22
Acyclovir, 382
ADAP. *See* AIDS Drug Assistance
      Program
ADC. *See* AIDS dementia complex
Addiction, defined, 221
Adherence to medical regimens,
      infant and child
   adherence strategies
      build trusting
            relationship, 264
      group teaching, family/
            peer support, 264
      home visits, agencies, 264
      involve children, 264
      positive reinforcement, 264
      support disclosure, 264
      use contracts, 264
   beginning therapy
      anticipate problems, 263
      color coding, 263
      developmental, behavioral
            issues, 263
      follow-up, 263
      masking taste
            strategies, 262
      pill swallowing skills, 262
      prepare family for
            problems, 262
      schedule simplicity,
            262–263
   developmental issues
      child refusal, 262
      independence, peer
            pressure, 262
   family adherence assessment
      assessment methods,
            263–264

identify problems, 263
      problem solving aid, 263
      provide support, 263
   family readiness issues, 262
   pediatric, family issues
      caregiver dependence, 262
      eating schedule
            difficulties, 261
      liquid formulations
            availability, 261
      patient refusal, 261
   psychological adherence issues
      grandparent caregiver
            factor, 262
      multigenerational
            factor, 262
      parent illness, 262
      parent lifestyle factors, 262
      parenting skills, lack of, 262
   social issues, 262
ADIs. *See* AIDS-defining illnesses
Adjuvant therapy, 145, 297–288
Adolescent community
   access to care, treatment,
         research, 177–178
   community care approaches
      adolescent models as guide,
            178–179
      condom distribution, 178
      counseling, testing, 178
      education, 178
      group involvement, 178
      individual involvement, 178
      outreach avenues, 178
   community description
      definitions, 176
      demographics, 176
   health issues, 176
   individual care approaches
      assessment, 178
      communication, negotiation
            skills, 178
      condom distribution, 178
      counseling, testing, 178
      education, 178
      trust, confidentiality, 178

long-term success, 35
   transmission, risk behaviors,
         prevention issues
      alcohol, substance use, 177
      knowledge, 176
      prevention programs,
            barriers to, 177
      sexual activity statistics,
            176–177
      STDs, 177
      transmission modes, 176
   See also Antiretroviral therapy
         management; Baseline
         assessment; Health care
         follow-up;
         Immunizations,
         adolescent and adult;
         Teaching for health
         promotion, wellness and
         transmission prevention
Adoptive families, 322
Advanced disease, symptomatic
      conditions in. *See* Bacterial
      infections; Bartonellosis,
      adolescent and adult;
      Comorbid complications,
      adolescent and adult; Fungal
      infections, adolescent and
      adult; Fungal infections,
      infant and child; Herpes
      zoster (varicella-zoster virus,
      VZV), adolescent and adult;
      Human papillomavirus
      (HPV) infection; Idiopathic
      thrombocytopenia purpura
      (ITP), adolescent and adult;
      Listeriosis; Neoplasms; Oral
      hairy leukoplakia;
      Peripheral neuropathy;
      Protozoal infections; Viral
      infections
Advisory Committee on
      Immunization Practices
      (ACIP), 40
AFDC (Aid to Families with
      Dependent Children), 195

Africa
    AIDS in, 2
    HIV incidence, 9, 10–11, 12
    life expectancy rates, 11
African American community
    access to care, treatment,
            research
        barriers to care, 212–213
        discrimination, 212–213
        health insurance
                factors, 213
        research mistrust, 213
        research under-
                representation, 213
        social determinants, 212
        stigma factor, 213
        therapy inferiority, 213
    community care approaches
        AIDS-conspiracy theories
                factor, 214
        faith-based
                intervention, 214
        social support, 214
    community description
        census statistics, 211
        West African
                descendants, 211
    health issues
        cancer, 211
        diabetes, 211
        heart disease, 211
        mental disorders, 211–212
        stroke, 211
        women's health care,
                211, 229
    individual care approaches
        cultural assessment, 213
        racism acknowledgment, 213
        risk education,
                interventions, 214
        testing efforts, 213–214
    transmission, risk behaviors,
            prevention issues
        anemia, 212
        statistics regarding, 212
        STDs reporting, 212
        subgroup statistics, 212
        testing age, 212
    See also African Americans
African Americans
    adolescent HIV/AIDS
            statistics, 176, 177
    breastfeeding, 220
    defined, 211
    elderly age factors, 206
    gay and bisexual men
            statistics, 184
    incarceration rates, 198
    mortality rates, 13, 229
    perinatal transmission, 15
    renal disease, 108

US HIV statistics, 10, 13–14
visually impaired
        statistics, 179
    See also African American
            community
Agenerase (Amprenavir),
        53, 369–381
Agnoli, Michelle, xxv
Agoraphobia, 168
Aid to Families with Dependent
        Children (AFDC), 195
AIDS
    in Africa, 2
    discovery and impact of, 2
    geographic factors, 13
    HIV origins of, 24–25
    minority statistics, 13–14
    naming the disease, 2
    prevalence statistics, 12
    responses to, 3
    See also Epidemiology of HIV
            infection and AIDS
AIDS Clinical Trial Unit (ACTU)
        Without Walls
AIDS Counseling and Education
        (ACE) program, 201
AIDS defining conditions in
        children with HIV infection.
    See Candidiasis, infant and
    child; Coccidioidomycosis,
    infant and child;
    Cryptococcosis, infant and
    child; Cryptosporidiosis,
    infant and child;
    Cytomegalovirus (CMV),
    infant and child;
    Histoplasmosis, infant and
    child; HIV-related
    encephalopathy, infant and
    child; HIV-related wasting
    syndrome, infant and child;
    Isosporiasis, infant and
    child; Malignancies, infant
    and child; Mycobacterial
    avium complex (MAC),
    infant and child;
    Mycobacterial tuberculosis,
    infant and child;
    Pneumocystis carinii
    pneumonia (PCP), infant
    and child; Progressive
    multifocal
    leukoencephalopathy (PML),
    infant and child; Recurrent
    bacterial infections, infant
    and child; Salmonellosis,
    infant and child;
    Toxoplasma gondii,
    infant and child
AIDS-defining illnesses
        (ADIs), 12

AIDS dementia complex (ADC)
    cognitive impairment, 126
    mobility impairment, 139
AIDS Drug Assistance Program
        (ADAP), 37, 195, 341
AIDS indicator diseases,
        adolescent and adult. See
        Bacterial pneumonia;
        Candidiasis, adolescent and
        adult; Coccidioidomycosis,
        adolescent and adult;
        Cryptococcosis, adolescent
        and adult;
        Cryptosporidiosis,
        adolescent and adult;
        Cytomegalovirus (CMV),
        adolescent and adult;
        Herpes simplex virus (HSV),
        adolescent and adult;
        Histoplasmosis, adolescent
        and adult; Isosporiasis,
        adolescent and adult;
        Mycobacterium avium
        complex (MAC), adolescent
        and adult; Mycobacterium
        tuberculosis (mTB),
        adolescent and adult;
        Pneumocystosis;
        Progressive multifocal
        leukoencephalopathy (PML),
        adolescent and adult;
        Salmonellosis, adolescent
        and adult; Toxoplasmosis,
        adolescent and adult
AIDS-related retrovirus (ARV), 2
AIDSVAX, 22
Al-Anon/Alateen, 225
Alcohol use, 37
    adolescent risk factor, 177, 178
    anxiety disorders, 169
    cognitive impairment, 126
    delirium, 171
    depression and, 164
    dyslipidemia and, 101–102
    gay and bisexual men, 184
    hepatitis B and C, 47
    Hepatitis C virus, 114
    homeless people, 194
    liver toxicity, 47
    medication adherence,
            decrease in, 47
    by transgender
            community, 227
    unsafe sex, 47
Alcoholics Anonymous (AA),
        224, 225
Alitretinoin, 380–381
American Sign Language
        (ASL), 189
Americans with Disabilities Act,
        187, 188, 222

Amitriptyline, 383, 402
Amphetamines, 221
Amphotericin B, 283, 284, 285, 383–384, 384
ANAC (Association of Nurses in AIDS Care), xvii
Anemia, adolescent and adult
  in African Americans, 212
  clinical presentation, 102
  diagnosis, 102
  etiology, Epidemiology, 102
  of HIV+ pregnant women, 216
  nursing implications, 102
  pathogenesis, 102
  prevention, treatment, 102
Anemia, infant and child
  clinical presentation, 268
  diagnosis
    hemoglobin decrease, 268
    physical signs, 268
  etiology, epidemiology, 268
  iron deficiency anemia, 298
  mycobacterial avium complex, 280
  nursing implications
    educate patients, 268
    iron supplementation, 268
    monitor lab work, 268
    nutrition counseling, 268
  pathogenesis
    bone marrow damage, 268
    chronic disease, 268
    iron deficiency anemia, 268
    parvovirus B19, 268
  prevention, treatment
    erythropoietin, 268
Angular chelitis, 46, 282
Anorexia, infant and child
  etiology
    medication side effects, 298
    oral candidiasis, 298
    psychological problems, 298
    upper GI disease, 298
  interventions, nonpharmacological
    fresh air, activity, 298
    highly flavored foods, 299
    mental health referral, 298
    nutrition assessment, 298
    social aspects of eating, 299
  interventions, pharmacological
    appetite stimulants, 299
    medication evaluation, 299
  loss of appetite, defined
    adolescent nutrient requirements, 298
    first year of life, importance of, 298
    iron deficiency anemia, 298
    nutrient requirements, 298

nursing assessment: objective, 298
nursing assessment: subjective, 298
nursing diagnosis, 298
  See also Weight loss, infant and child
Anorexia and weight loss, adolescent and adult
  etiology
    anorexia, defined, 124
    weight loss, defined, 124
  evaluation, 125
  goals, 124
  interventions, alternative, complementary, 125
  interventions, nonpharmacological
    daily records and checklists, 125
    enteral nutrition formulas, 125
    food safety, 124
    nutrition counseling, 124
    nutrition interventions, 124–125
    oral and dental care, 125
    parenteral nutrition, 125
    resistance-type exercise, 125
  interventions, pharmacological
    anabolic agents, 125
    appetite stimulants, 125
  nursing assessment, objective
    functional status, mood, cognition, 124
    laboratory studies, 124
    vitamin and mineral deficiencies, 124
  nursing assessment, subjective
    dietary patterns, 124
    medication review, 124
    nutrition-related symptoms, 124
    secondary infections, 124
  nursing diagnosis
    altered nutrition, 124
    related nursing diagnoses, 124
Anti-HCV EIA test, 360
Antiandrogens
  female sexual dysfunction, 147
  male sexual dysfunction, 149
Antiarrhythmic medication, 148
Anticholinergenics
  female sexual dysfunction, 147
  tricyclic antidepressants and, 167
Anticonvulsants
  female sexual dysfunction, 147
  male sexual dysfunction, 149
  pain therapy, 145, 297–298

Antidepressants
  anxiety disorders, 170
  depression therapy, 166, 167
  female sexual dysfunction, 147, 148
  folic acid and, 166
  pain therapy, 145
  sleep disturbances, 138
Antiestrogens, 147
Antifungal therapy, 283, 307, 308
Antihistamines
  male sexual dysfunction, 149
  pain therapy, 145, 298
  sleep disturbances, 138
Antihyperlipidemics, 148
Antihypertensive medication
  depression and, 164
  female sexual dysfunction, 147
  male sexual dysfunction, 148
Antimicrobial therapy
  infectious disease, 257
  norcardiosis, 275
  parotitis, 276
  sinusitis, infant and child, 277
  upper respiratory infection, 278
Antipsychotic medication
  female sexual dysfunction, 147
  male sexual dysfunction, 149
Antiretroviral therapy, adolescent and adult
  AIDS prevention, 12
  anxiety disorders, 168, 169
  diarrhea side effect, 141
  directly observed *vs.* keep on person, 200
  elderly age factors, 206
  gender factors, 232
  hormone therapy and, 228
  long-term consequences of, 18
  medications, 369–381 (*See also* *specific drug name*)
  for pregnant women, 215, 216–217, 217*table*, 218
  side effects, relief of, 49
  in women, 230, 232–233
  See also Adherence to medical regimens, infant and child; Antiretroviral therapy management, adolescent and adult; Antiretroviral therapy management, infant and child; specific medication name
Antiretroviral therapy, infant and child
  anemia, 268
  cardiomyopathy, 268
  diarrhea, 269–270

HIV-related
    encephalopathy, 290
MAC, 280–281
nephropathy, 274
neutropenia, 274–275
pain caused by, 294
parental guilt, 317
of perinatally transmitted HIV,
    242–247
    breast-feeding, 242
    classification system,
        children less than
        13 years, 244
    clinical categories, 244,
        246–247table
    clinical scenarios,
        recommendations
        for use, 243table
    diagnosis, evaluation of
        infant, 244
    HIV presentation
        patterns, 245
    immunologic categories,
        244, 245table
    infection status, 244
    prognosis, survival,
        245, 247
    zidovudine, 242
PML, 289
skin lesions, 305
thrombocytopenia, 277–278
Antiretroviral therapy
    management, adolescent
    and adult
    autoimmunization, 56
    fusion inhibitors, 53
    integrase inhibitors, 53
    non-nucleoside reverse
        transcriptase inhibitors
        (NNRTIs)
        function of, 52
        side effects of, 52
        in therapy for
            asymptomatic
            individuals, 54
    nucleoside reverse
        transcriptase inhibitors
        (NRTIs)
        function of, 52
        side effects of, 52
        in therapy for
            asymptomatic
            individuals, 54
    nucleotide reverse
        transcriptase inhibitor
        beneficial dosing
            schedule, 52
        function of, 52
    prescription guidelines
        acute infection
            treatment, 57

HIV infected adolescent
    focus, 57–58
HIV infected pregnant
    woman, 58
testing for resistance, 56–57
therapy changes, 56, 56table
therapy for initial
    treatment, 54, 55table
therapy goals, 53
therapy initiation in
    advanced disease, 55
therapy initiation in
    asymptomatic disease,
    54–55, 54table
therapy interruption, 55–56
therapy risks vs.
    benefits, 53–54
treatment readiness, 54
protease inhibitors (PIs)
    dosing schedule, 53
    drugs in class, 53
    function of, 52–53
    liver transmaminase
        elevation, 53
regimen adherence
    client challenges to, 58–59
    client trust, 59
    Freirean behavior change
        approach, 60–61
    harm reduction behavior
        change model, 60
    health care provider role, 59
    statistics regarding, 58
    strategies to enhance, 59
    team approach to, 59–60
    transtheoretical behavior
        change model, 60
    side effects of, 52, 53
    skill level requirement, 51–52
Antiretroviral therapy
    management, infant
    and child
    changing therapy guidelines
        alternative regimen
            indications, 259
        clinical failure
            evidence, 259
        immunologic failure
            evidence, 259
        toxicity, intolerance
            evidence, 259
        virologic failure evidence,
            259, 261
    contraindications, 257
    currently approved drugs,
        258table
    diagnostic issues, 261
    drug resistance testing
        HIV-resistance assays, 261
        phenotype, genotypic
            assays, 261

infectious disease treatment
    principles
    active decision making, 258
    ARV therapy to
        non-resistant virus
        strains, 257
    combination
        antimicrobial therapy
        recommended, 257
    early diagnosis,
        treatment, 257
    infectious agent
        eradication, 257
    viral load reduction, 257
initiating therapy guidelines,
    259, 260table
natural history differences, 261
pharmcokinetic issues, 261
prescribing guidelines,
    257–259
readiness to start treatment
    clinician, family
        collaboration, 259
    family readiness
        assessment, 258–259
risks and benefits of therapy
    combination therapy,
        benefits of, 258
    cross-resistance within
        classes of drugs, 258
    early aggressive treatment,
        benefits of, 258
    lack of adherence, effects
        of, 258
    subtherapeutic ARV levels,
        effects of, 258
    treatment before
        Category C, 258
    therapy goals, 257–258
Anxiety disorder
    of caregiver, 159
    caregiver decision making
        and, 314
    fatigue, 133
    female sexual dysfunction, 147
    of HIV infected infant,
        child, 316
    incarcerated persons, 197
    male sexual dysfunction, 148
    sleep disturbance, 137, 138
    substance abuse, 171
    See also Primary anxiety-
        spectrum disorders
Anxiolytic pain medication, 298
Aphthous ulcers
    nonpharmacological
        treatment, 306
    pharmacological
        treatment, 307
Apomorphine, 148
Appetite loss, defined, 298

Aphthous ulcers, 46
Aromatherapy, 298
Arthritis, Reiter's syndrome
    clinical presentation, 107
    diagnosis, 107
    etiology, epidemiology, 106
    Kaposi's sarcoma, 107
    nursing implications, 107
    pathogenesis, 106–107
    prevention, treatment, 107
    psoriasis and, 105, 107
ARV. *See* AIDS-related retrovirus
Ashwagandha, 151
Asian Americans
    heterosexual HIV
        transmission, 220
    immigration statistics, 219
ASL (American Sign
    Language), 189
Aspergillosis, 282
Aspirin, 296
Assessment. *See* Baseline
    assessment
Assisted suicide issue, 345
Asthma
    of HIV infected infant,
        child, 250
    mild opiate therapy, 145
    tobacco use, 222
Astragalus herbal therapy, 140
Atopic dermatitis, 269, 305, 308
Atovaquone, 384–385
Autonomic neuropathy, 74
Autonomy
    ethical concern for, 340–341
    See also Decision making and
        family autonomy
Avascular necrosis. *See*
    Osteopenia, osteoporosis,
    avascular necrosis
AVN. *See* Osteopenia,
    osteoporosis, avascular
    necrosis (AVN)
Aylovir, 307
Azithromycin, 385

B-cell lymphocytes, 25, 27
â-chemokines, 9
Bachanas, Pamela J., xxv
Bacterial infections, adolescent
    and adult, 125
    See also Bacterial pneumonia;
        Mycobacterium avium
        complex (MAC),
        adolescent and adult;
        Salmonellosis, adolescent
        and adult
Bacterial infections, infant and
    child. *See* Mycobacterial
    avium complex (MAC),
    infant and child;

Mycobacterial tuberculosis,
    infant and child;
    Salmonellosis, infant
    and child
Bacterial pneumonia
    clinical presentation, 75
    diagnosis
        blood cultures, 75
        CBC, 75
        chest radiography, 75
        sputum gram stain, 75
        TB test, 75
    dyspnea, 129
    etiology, epidemiology, 75
    nursing implications, 76
    pathogenesis, 75
    prevention, treatment
        cefotaxime, ceftriaxone,
            75–76
        vaccination, 75
Balt, Christine A., xxi–xxii, xxv
Barrett, Kathleen, xxv
Barroso, Julie, xxv
Bartonella henselae, 66
Bartonella quintana, 66
Bartonellosis, adolescent
    and adult
    clinical presentation, 66
    diagnosis, 66
    etiology, epidemiology, 66
    pathogenesis, 66
    prevention, treatment, 66
Baseline assessment
    health history
        family history, 36–37
        immunizations, 36
        medical history, 36
        medication history, 36
        STD history, 36
        surgical history, 36
    impact of HIV, 36
    laboratory and diagnostic
        evaluation
        immunology profile, 39
        tuberculin skin testing, 39
    patient coping mechanisms, 36
    patient knowledge, 36
    patient treatment history, 36
    physical examination, 39
    social history
        alcohol use, 37
        drug use, 37
        exercise and sleep, 37–38
        health insurance, 37
        needle and blood
            exposure, 37
        nutrition history, 38
        occupational history, 38
        pets, 38
        sexual history, 37
        tobacco use, 37

        travel, 37
        women's health, 38
    systems review, 38–39
Basophils, 25
Bataille, Catherine R., xxv
Beck Depression Scale, 126
Beneficence health care
    principle, 341
Bennett, Jo Anne, xxv
Benzodiazepine, 169
Berger, Barbara E., xxv
Bichloroacetic acid, 307
Bipolar disorders
    carbamazepine, 168
    lithium, 168
    valproate therapy, 167–168
Birth control pills, 147
Bisexual men. *See* Gay and
    bisexual men community
Bisexual woman, defined, 202
Bisexual women. *See* Lesbians and
    bisexual women community
Black, defined, 211
Bleomycin, 385–386
Blind and visually impaired
    community
    access to care, treatments
        or research
        employment, insurance
            coverage, 180
        transportation factors, 180
    community care
        approaches
        conference access, 181
        outreach efforts, 181
        sexuality education, 181
    community description
        blindness, defined, 179
        education statistics, 179
        employment, 179
        legal blindness,
            defined, 179
        low vision, defined, 179
        marital status, 179
        racial demographics, 179
        statistics regarding, 179
        visual impairment,
            defined, 179
    health issues
        knowledge, 179
        psychological, physical
            problems, 179–180
    individual care approaches
        guide dogs, 181
        immediately greet the
            person, 180
        indicate end of
            conversation, 180
        introduce yourself, 180
        physically guide people,
            180–181

precision in
descriptions, 180
speak directly to the
person, 180
use natural conversational
tone, 180
use the person's name, 180
use visually descriptive
language, 180
warnings of danger, 181
transmission, risk behaviors,
prevention issues, 180
visual impairment,
defined, 179
Blindness, defined, 179
Blood chemistry testing, 50
Body louse, 66
Branding, 46
Breast feeding, HIV transmitted
through, 11
immigrant customs, 242
oral and gastrointestinal tract
exposure, 242
safe substitute feeding, 242
statistics regarding, 242
Breathing, relaxation pain
intervention, 295
Bullous impetigo, 308
Burr, Carolyn Keith, xxv
Buspirone, 169

CAIDS (community acquired
immunodeficiency
syndrome), 2
Calypte HIV-1 urine test, 29, 356
Campylobacter bacterial infection,
142, 143, 299
Cancer
in African Americans, 211
parotitis differential
diagnosis, 276
See also Cervical neoplasia;
HIV encephalopathy,
adolescent and adult;
HIV-related wasting
syndrome, adolescent
and adult; HIV-related
wasting syndrome,
infant and child;
Human papillomavirus
(HPV) infection;
Kaposi's sarcoma;
Leiomyosarcoma, infant
and child; Malignancies;
Non-Hodgkin's
lymphoma
Candida albicans, 79, 129, 132,
282, 305
Candida esophagitis
in infants and children, 282
in women, 229

Candida glabrata, 79
Candida immitis, 81
Candida kruseii, 79
Candida parapsilosis, 79
Candida pneumoniae, 75
Candida tropicalis, 79
Candidiasis, adolescent and adult
Category B classification, 352
clinical presentation
disseminated infection, 80
esophageal candidiasis, 79
oropharyngeal
candidiasis, 79
vulvovaginal
candidiasis, 79–80
diagnosis
esophageal candidiasis, 80
oropharyngeal,
vulvovaginal
candidiasis, 80
dysphagia and
odynophagia, 130
etiology, epidemiology, 79
gastrointestinal pain, 143
nursing implications, 80
pathogenesis, 79
prevention, treatment
esophageal candidiasis, 80
oropharyngeal
candidiasis, 80
refractory cases, 80
vulvovaginal
candidiasis, 80
in women, 79–80, 230
Candidiasis, infant and child
clinical presentations
angular chelitis, 282
erythematous oral
lesions, 282
hypertrophic oral
lesions, 282
thrush, 282
diagnosis, 282
etiology, epidemiology
candida albicans, 282
esophageal candidiasis, 282
oral candidiasis, 282
other fungal infections, 282
nursing implications, 283
pathogenesis, 282
prevention, treatment, 282–283
wasting syndrome, 289
Capili, Bernadette, xxv
Carbamazepine, 168, 386
Cardiac tamponade, 269
Cardiomegaly, 269
Cardiomyopathy, adolescent
and adult
clinical presentation, 105
diagnosis, 105
etiology, epidemiology, 104

of HIV infected infant,
child, 250
nursing implications, 105
pathogenesis, 104–105
prevention, treatment, 105
Cardiomyopathy, infant and child
clinical presentation, 269
diagnosis, 269
etiology, epidemiology,
268–269
nursing implications, 269
pathogenesis, 269
prevention, treatment, 269
CARE (Comprehensive AIDS
Resources Emergency) Act, 4
Caregiver burden, strain
assessment, 160
caregiver variables
age, 159
gender, 159
life stressors, 159–160
socioeconomic status, 159
decision-making, 314
definitions, 159
etiology, 159–160
cantagion, fear of, 160
caregiver variables, 159–160
losses, 160
service organizations,
providers, 160
social isolation, 160
goals of care
illness prevention, 160, 231
quality of life
enhancement, 160
home care trends, 159
interventions
caregiver health, 161
community services, 161
coping options, 161
disease process
information, 161
institutionalization, 161
partnership with patent
and caregivers,
160–161
patient autonomy,
independence, 161
problem solving skills, 161
relationship difficulties, 161
social support assessment,
160, 160*table*
signs of, 159
See also Surrogate caregivers
Carroll, Doris, xxvi
Case management
access to care focus
definition, 339
issues related to, 339
continuity of care focus
definition, 339

interdisciplinary team
approach, 339–340
decreased fragmentation of
care focus
communication skills, 340
continual assessment, 340
definitions
case manager, defined, 338
collaborative process, 338
consumer support
process, 338
trusting and empowering
relationship, 338
education focus
on drug regimen
adherence, 340
empowerment, 340
on entitlement
programs, 340
on health care delivery
system, 340
on nutrition, 340
limitations of, 340
models of
community-based, public
health model, 338–339
diagnosis-related,
population-based
model, 339
medical model, 338
nursing model, 338
psychosocial model, 339
standards and protocols
for, 340
support group focus
follow-up importance, 340
holistic care approach, 340
Cats
feline immunodeficiency virus
(FIV), 23
feline leukemia virus
(FeLV), 22
Toxoplasma gondii, 22, 51, 87–88
Cause, defined, 5
CCR5-) 32 homozygous
mutation, 9
CD$_4$ cells, 27, 28, 29
arthritis and, 107
cell count, 357
gender differences in, 232–233
health care follow-up
monitoring, 49, 50, 51
of HIV infected infant,
child, 251
integrase inhibitors, 53
NRTIs therapy, 52
PIs therapy, 52
CD$_8$ cells, 27, 28
arthritis and, 107
health care follow-up
monitoring, 50

CD$_4$ lymphocyte categories, 352
CD$_4$ lymphocyte percentage,
357–358
CD$_8$ T-lymphocyte antiviral factor
(CAF), 9
CDC. *See* Centers for Disease
Control and Prevention
Cellulitis, 307
Center for Epidemiologic
Studies Depression Scale
(CES-D), 165
Centers for Disease Control and
Prevention (CDC)
AIDS
naming the disease, 2
prevalence statistics, 12
HIV incidence statistics, 12
tracking the disease, 2–4
Cervical carcinoma, 229
Cervical dysplasia, 230, 352
Cervical lymphadenitis, 280
Cervical neoplasia
clinical presentation, 93
diagnosis, 93
etiology, epidemiology, 93
nursing implications, 94
pathogenesis, 93
prevention, treatment, 93–94
CES-D (Center for Epidemiologic
Studies Depression
Scale), 165
CGHT (cross-gender hormone
therapy), 227–229
Chamomile, 131, 151
Chickenpox, 67
See also Varicella,
disseminated, infant
and child
Children. *See* Adherence to
medical regimens, infant
and child; Antiretroviral
therapy management, infant
and child; Clinical
manifestations and
management of the HIV
infected infant and child;
Symptom management of
the HIV infected infant and
child; specific symptomatic
conditions
Chinese herbs, 127
Chlorhexidine, 386
Choline magnesium
trisalicylate, 296
Christie, Beverly, xxvi
Cidofovir, 386–387
Circumcision, 20
Clarithromycin, 387–388
Clindamycin, 386
Clinical management of the HIV
infected adolescent and adult

long-term success, 35
See also Adolescent community;
Antiretroviral therapy
management; Baseline
assessment; Health
care follow-up;
Immunizations,
adolescent and adult;
Teaching for health
promotion, wellness and
transmission prevention
Clinical manifestations and
management of the HIV
infected infant and child
baseline assessment, 247–252
counseling, educating family
and child
ARV treatment and
guidelines, 255
Clinical trial
opportunities, 255
collaboration, primary
provider and HIV
specialist, 255–256
comprehensive
education, 255
confidentiality, disclosure
issues, 255
diet, nutrition, 256
frequent assessment, 255
follow-up visits
CBC with differential, 257
immunologic profiles,
256–257
laboratory, diagnostic
evaluation, 256
multichannel chemistry
panel, 257
nutrition assessment, 256
physical exam, 256
previous visit review,
diagnostic results, 256
systems review, 256
viral load testing, 257
general systems review, 248
cardiovascular, 249
ears, 249
eyes, 249
gastrointestinal, 249
genitourinary, 249
gynecologic, 249
head, 249
mouth and throat, 249
musculoskeletal, 249
neurologic, 249
nose and sinuses, 249
nutrition assessment, 250
psychiatric and
emotional, 250
respiratory, 249
skin, 249

health history
  birth history, 248
  childhood illnesses,
      immunizations, 248
  family history, 248
  medical history, 248
  medication history, 248
  nutrition history, 248
  social history, 248
  surgical history, 248
immunizations, 253–254*table*
  haemophilus
      influenza B, 252
  Hepatitis B, 252
  immune globulin
      preparations, 252
  inactivated polio
      vaccine, 252
  influenza, 252
  measles/mumps/
      rubella, 252
  pneumococcal
      vaccination, 252
  varicella vaccine, 252
interventions
  ARV therapy, 257
  counseling and
      education, 257
  nutrition intervention, 257
laboratory and diagnostic
      evaluation
  baseline triglycerides, 252
  CBC with differential, 251
  chest X-ray, 251
  cytomegalovirus
      serology, 251
  hepatitis profile, 252
  HIV RNA PCR (viral
      load), 251
  immunologic profile, 251
  multichannel chemistry
      panel, 251
  rapid plasma reagin
      test, 251
  syphilis screening, 251
  toxoplasmosis serologic
      test, 251
  tuberculin skin test, 251
  urinalysis, 251
  varicella serologic test, 251
physical examination
  abdominal exam, 250
  cardiovascular exam, 250
  general, 250
  growth and
      development, 250
  mouth and throat, 250
  musculoskeletal exam, 250
  neurological exam, 250
  respiratory exam, 250
  skin, 250–251

prophylaxis for opportunistic
      infections
  against pneumonia, 252,
      254–255, 255*table*,
      256*table*
  See also Adherence to medical
      regimens, infant and
      child; Antiretroviral
      therapy, infant and child;
      Perinatally acquired
      pediatric HIV
Clostridium difficile toxin, 142,
      143, 299
Clostridium tetani, 42
Clotrimazole, 307, 388
CMV. *See* Cytomegalovirus
      (CMV), adolescent and
      adult; Cytomegalovirus
      (CMV), infant and child
CMV chorioretinitis, 288
CMV colitis, 288
CMV esophagitis, 288
CMV pneumonitis, 288
CNS cryptococcosis, 83
Cocaine use, 20, 221
  See also Substance abuse and
      mental illness; Substance
      use; Substance users
      community
Coccidioides, 103
Coccidioides immitis, 283
Coccidioidomycosis, adolescent
      and adult
  candidiasis, 282
  clinical presentation, 81
  diagnosis, 81
  etiology, epidemiology, 81
  nursing implications
      educate about maintenance
          therapy, 82
      monitor for adverse effects
          of therapy, 81–82
  pathogenesis, 81
  prevention, treatment, 81
Coccidioidomycosis, infant
      and child
  clinical presentation, 283
  diagnosis, 283
  etiology, epidemiology, 283
  nursing implications, 284
  pathogenesis, 283
  prevention, treatment
      amphtericin, 284
      fluconazole maintenance
          therapy, 284
      lumbar punctures, 284
Cognitive Capacity Screening
      Exam, 140
Cognitive impairment, adolescent
      and adult
  depression and, 165

etiology
  bacterial infections, 125
  cerebrovascular disease,
      accident, 125
  CNS cancers, 125
  fungal infections, 125
  HIV or AIDS dementia, 126
  medications, 126
  metabolic imbalances, 126
  mycoplasmic
      infections, 125
  psychological, stress-related
      illnesses, 126
  systemic infections, 125
  viral infections, 125
evaluation, 128
goals, 126–127
interventions, alternative,
      complementary therapies
  Chinese herbs, 127
  energy work, healing, 127
  vitamins, 127
  Western herbs, 127
interventions,
      nonpharmacological
  advanced directives, 127
  HIV-related disease
      information, 127
  memory aids, 127
  safety assessment, 127
interventions, pharmacological
  agitation and anxiety
      drugs, 127
  antiretrovirals, 127
  depression drugs, 127
  mood and mania drugs, 127
  psychomotor drugs, 127
  psychoses drugs, 127
nursing assessment, objective
  cranial computerized
      tomography, 126
  lab work, 126
  lumbar puncture, 126
  neuroimaging, 126
  patient, family
      assessment, 126
  pharmacological
      history, 126
  physical exam, 126
  practitioner
      evaluation, 126
  psychological tests, 126
nursing assessment, subjective
  affective, 126
  behavioral, 126
  cognitive, 126
  early manifestations, 126
  late manifestations, 126
  motor, 126
nursing diagnosis, 126
See also Delirium

Cognitive impairment and
  developmental delay, infant
  and child, 316
  alternative, complementary
    therapy
    after-school programs, 303
    behavioral strategies, 303
  anemia, 268
  etiology
    CNS infection, 300–301
    comorbid factors, 301
    HIV progressive
      encephalopathy, 301
    opportunistic
      infections, 301
    statis encephalopathy, 301
  evaluation
    attention, behavior
      assessment, 303
    family advocacy
      assessment, 303
    improvement
      assessment, 303
    school assessment, 303
  goals
    evaluation consistency, 302
    family education, 302
    intervention services, 302
    mental health intervention
      services, 302
    pain evaluation, 302
    specialist evaluation, 302
  interventions:
    nonpharmacological
    intervention services, age
      appropriate, 302
    specialist referrals, 302
  interventions: pharmacological
    HAART, 303
    pain medication, 303
    psychostimulants, 303
  nursing assessment: objective
    global deficits or delays, 301
    milestone achievements,
      observable, 301–302
    physical growth
      assessments, 301
    specific deficits or
      delays, 301
    teacher and family
      assessments, 302
  nursing assessment:
    subjective
    milestone achievement
      delays, 301
    school difficulties, 301
  nursing diagnosis, 302
Colagreco, Joseph P., xxvi
Combivir (lamivudine), 370
Commercial sex workers'
  community

access to care, treatment and
  research
  addiction, mental illness, 182
  barriers to, 182
  health system stigma, 182
  poor treatment
    outcomes, 182
  self-care efficacy
    reduction, 182
community care approaches
  community-based
    services, 183
  condom distribution, 183
  health care provider
    education, 183
  health care services, 183
  holistic treatment
    approach, 183
  prison interventions, 183
  safer sex and substance use
    education, 183
  sex industry consumer
    education, 183
community description, 181
health issues
  living with violence,
    181–182
  psychological issues of, 181
  psychosocial issues of, 181
individual care approaches
  education and career
    counseling, 183
  establish trust, 182
  family, psychiatric, drug
    treatment services, 183
  financial support
    systems, 182
  foster hope,
    independence, 182
  healthy lifestyle
    knowledge, 182
  legal issues, 182
  peer group support, 183
  social assistance, 182
transgender community
  within, 227, 229
transmission, risk behaviors,
  prevention issues
  multidrug resistance to
    antiretrovirals, 182
  multiple contacts, 182
  multiple HIV subtypes, 182
  opportunistic infections
    transmission, 182
  STDs transmission, 182
  substance use risk
    factors, 182
Common cold, 278
Community acquired
  immunodeficiency
  syndrome (CAIDS), 2

Community-based, public health
  case management model,
  338–339
Community-based care issues
  barriers to
    caregiver substance
      use, 331
    domestic, environmental
      violence, 331–332
    state laws, 331
    stigma, discrimination
      fear, 331
  case management plan, 330
  child's family as community
    kinship groups, 330
    parent/caregiver, 329–330
    socioeconomic factors, 330
  community assessment, 331
  coordination of community
    care, 330
  cultural needs, 329
  existing resource referrals, 332
  MCHB bureau, 330
  residential locale, 330
  social welfare systems, 330
  spiritual referrals, 331–332
  state, county, city
    resources, 330
Comorbid complications,
  adolescent and adult. *See*
  Anemia, adolescent and
  adult; Arthritis, Reiter's
  syndrome; Cardiomyopathy,
  adolescent and adult;
  Dyslipidemia; Fat
  redistribution syndrome;
  Hepatitis A; Hepatitis B;
  Hepatitis C; Impaired glucose
  tolerance (IGT); Lactic
  acidosis; Leukopenia;
  Nephropathy (HIV-associated
  nephropathy, HIVAN),
  adolescent and adult;
  Osteopenia, osteoporosis,
  avascular necrosis; Psoriasis;
  Thrombocytopenia,
  adolescent and adult
Complete blood count (CBC)
  anemia, infant and child, 268
  bacterial pneumonia
    diagnosis, 75
  fever assessment, 304
  health care follow-up, 50
  of HIV infected infant, child,
    251, 257
  neutropenia, infant and
    child, 274
  thrombocytopenia, 277
Complicated Chickenpox. *See*
  Varicella, disseminated,
  infant and child

Comprehensive AIDS Resources Emergency (CARE) Act, 4
Condom use
  adolescents, 178
  by African Americans, 214
  commercial sex workers, 183
  erectile dysfunction, older men, 207
  female polyurethane condoms, 19, 43
  by Latin American immigrants, 220
  by lesbians and bisexual women, 203, 204
  oral and anal sex, 143
  in prison, 198
Condyloma acuminata, 305, 307
Congenital toxoplasmosis, 287
Congestive heart failure, 269
Continuity of care, defined, 339
Core Curriculum for HIV/AIDS Nursing, xv
Corticosteroids
  anxiety disorders, 168
  pain therapy, 145
Corynebacterium diptheriae, 42
Cough
  etiology, 128
  evaluation, 129
  goals, 128
  interventions, alternative, complementary, 129
  interventions, nonpharmacological
    energy conservation, 128
    fluid intake increase, 128
    oral hygiene, 128
    physical positioning, 128
    splinting techniques, 128
    suction secretions, 128
    throat-soothing remedies, 128
  interventions, pharmacological, 128–129
  nursing assessment, objective, 128
  nursing assessment, subjective, 128
  nursing diagnosis, 128
Coxsackievirus group B virus, 104
Crack cocaine use, 222
  See also Substance abuse and mental illness; Substance use; Substance users community
Crixivan, 370–371
Cross-gender hormone therapy (CGHT), 227–229
Cryotherapy, 307
Cryptoccoccus, 103
Cryptoccoccus neoformans, 82, 283

Cryptoccoccus neoforms, 47
Cryptococcosis, adolescent and adult
  candidiasis, 282
  clinical presentation, 82–83
  diagnosis
    CNS cryptococcosis, 83
    pulmonary cryptococcosis, 83
    toxoplasmosis, 88
  etiology, epidemiology, 82
  gastrointestinal pain, 143
  nursing implications, 83–84
  pathogenesis, 82
  prevention, treatment
    acute therapy, 83
    routine CRAG screening, 83
    suppressive maintenance therapy, 83
Cryptococcosis, infant and child
  clinical presentation, 283
  diagnosis, 284
  etiology, epidemiology, 283
  nursing implications, 284
  pathogenesis, 283
  prevention, treatment, 284
  skin lesions, 305
Cryptosporidiosis, adolescent and adult
  clinical presentations, 85
  diagnosis, 85
  etiology, epidemiology, 85
  gastrointestinal pain, 143
  nursing implications, 85
  pathogenesis, 85
  prevention, 85
  treatment, 85
Cryptosporidiosis, infant and child
  clinical presentation
    constitutional symptoms, 285
    diarrhea, 285
    GI symptoms, 285
  diagnosis, 285
  etiology, epidemiology, 285
  nursing implications, 285
  pathogenesis, 285
  prevention, treatment, 285
  wasting syndrome, 289
  weight loss, 299
Cryptosporidium, 85, 129, 269
Cunnilingus, 19
  See also Oral sex
Cutaneous stimulation pain, infant and child
  nonpharmacological interventions, 295
  pharmacological interventions, 296

Cutaneous stimulation pain intervention, 296
Cytarabine, 386
Cytokine activation, 99
Cytomegalovirus (CMV), adolescent and adult
  cardiomyopathy, 104
  clinical presentation, 89
  diagnosis, 89
  diarrhea, 142
  dysphagia and odynophagia, 130
  dyspnea, 129
  etiology, epidemiology, 89
  gastrointestinal pain, 143
  nursing implications, 90
  oral lesions, 132
  pathogenesis, 89
  prevention, treatment, 89–90
  screening for in infants, children, 251
Cytomegalovirus (CMV), infant and child
  clinical presentation
    CMV chorioretinitis, 288
    CMV colitis, 288
    CMV esophagitis, 288
    CMV pneumonitis, 288
  cognitive impairment, 301
  diagnosis
    CMV colitis, 288
    CMV esophagitis, 288
    CMV pneumonitis, 288
  diarrhea, 269
  etiology, epidemiology, 288
  lymphadenopathy, 273
  malignancies, 289
  nursing implications, 288
  pathogenesis, 288
  prevention, treatment, 288
  splenomegaly, 277
  wasting syndrome, 289
Cytomegalovirus (CMV) antibody test, 359
Cytotoxic T-lymphocyte, 9
Czarniecki, Lynn, xxvi

Dacarbazine, 389
Damiana life and herb, 148, 150
Dapsone, 389–390
Daunorubicin hydrachloride liposome, 389
Davis, Rachel, xxvi
Deaf and hearing-impaired community
  access to care, treatment, research
    barriers to, 190
    communication barriers, 190
    medication complications, 190

American Sign Language
(ASL), 189
communication modes
drawing, 188
lip reading, 188, 189
sign language, 188
community care approaches
cultural richness
appreciation, 191
develop targeted
services, 191
hire Deaf peer
counselors, 191
increase communication, 191
prevention planning, 191
community description
definitions regarding, 189
health care provider
distrust, 189
lack of knowledge, 189
richness of culture, 189
statistics regarding, 188
substance abuse, 189
health issues
access limitations, 189
family of origin
conflicts, 190
marginalization,
isolation, 189
stereotypes, misconceptions,
189–190
stigma, discrimination,
denial, 189
individual care approaches
deaf counselors, peer
educators, 190
empowerment, 191
grief expression, 191
health care system
support, 191
interpreting services, 190
telecommunication
devices, 190
visual aids, 190
transmission, risk behaviors,
prevention issues
children at risk,
abuse, 190
HIV positive rates, 190
isolation, 190
Death. *See* End of life issues
Decision making and family
autonomy
alternative treatment
issues, 313
antiretroviral therapy
decisions
burden healthy child, 313
explore medication
beliefs, 313
when to start, 312

autocratic management
style, 312
decision-making assitance
boundaries, family and
provider, 313–314
caregiver mental state, 314
case conference, 315
child protection
reporting, 314
child welfare system
issues, 314
communication
effectiveness, 314
cultural differences, 315
empowering families, 315
obstacles to, 314–315
rapport building, 315
resource provision, 315–316
substance abuse, 314–315
support system needs, 315
disclosure issues, 313
end of life issues, 313
family autonomy
independence from
others, 313
independent action, 313
inclusive management
style, 312
passive management style, 312
quality of life issues, 313
research protocol issues, 313
testing decisions, 312
treatment decisions, 312
Delavirdine (Rescriptor), 52
Delirium
assessment
anxiety indications, 171
clinical manifestations, 171
mental status changes, 171
sleep pattern changes, 171
description of, 171
etiology
infectious causes, 171
metabolic causes, 171
neurologic causes, 171
psychiatric causes, 171
toxic causes, 171
vascular causes, 171
goals of care, 171
interventions:
nonpharmacological,
171–172
interventions:
pharmacological, 172
prevalence of, 171
Denver Developmental
Screening Test, 250
Depression
anorexia and weight loss, 298
assessment, mental status
appearance, 165

cognition, 165
mood and affect, 165
perception, 165
thought processes, 165
assessment, suicidality,
165–166
assessment, tools of
Center for Epidemiologic
Studies Depression
Scale, 165
Folstein Mini Mental State
Examination, 165
Global Assessment of
Functioning, 165
Goldberg Depression
Scale, 165
Hamilton Depression
Rating Scale, 165
Johns Hopkins HIV
Dementia Scale, 165
PRIME-MD, 165
bereavement *vs.* depression, 164
of caregiver, 159
caregiver decision making
and, 314
cognitive impairment, 126
commercial sex workers, 181
delirium, 171
disease progression and, 164
etiology
biological, 164
chronic illness, 164
genetic, 164
medications, 164
psychobiological
syndrome, 164
social, psychological
factors, 164
substance abuse,
alcoholism, 164
fatigue, 133, 134
female sexual dysfunction,
147, 148
gender factors, 164
goals of care, 164–165
helplessness, hopelessness,
158, 163
incarcerated persons, 197
infant and child, 316
interventions:
nonpharmacological
alternative therapy, 166
coping and social skills
training, 166
cultural variations, 166
exercise, 167
grief counseling, 166
herbal therapy, 166
individual, group
support, 166
medication side effects, 166

nutrition, 166
psychotherapy, 166
self-harm risk
	determination, 166
significant others, support
	to, 166
interventions: pharmacological
atypical antidepressant
	medications, 167
mood stabilizers, 167–168
psychostimulants, 167
SSRIs, 167
tricyclics
	antidepressants, 167
male sexual dysfunction, 148
mobility impairment, 139
mood disorder,
	characteristics, 164
mood disorders, *DSM-IV*
	listing of, 164
sleep disturbance, 137, 138
statistics regarding, 164
substance abuse, 171, 222
suicide and, 164, 165–166
of visually impaired, 179
Depression Anxiety Stress
	Scale (DASS), 126
Dermatitis, infant and child
clinical presentation, 269
diagnosis, 269
etiology, epidemiology, 269
nursing implications, 269
pathogenesis, 269
prevention, treatment, 269
Desipramine, 390
Developmental delay. *See*
	Cognitive impairment and
	developmental delay, infant
	and child
Diabetes mellitus, 100
in African Americans, 211
HIV/AIDS in elderly, 206
Type 2, Hepatitis-C virus, 113
Diagnosis-related, population-
	based case management
	model, 339
Diarrhea, adolescent and adult
etiology
	bacterial infection, 142
	diet, 142
	invasive diseases, 142
	medication side effect, 142
	parasites, 142
evaluation, 143
goals, 143
interventions, alternative,
	complementary
	acupuncture, 143
	goldenseal alkaloids, 143
interventions,
	nonpharmacological

dietary changes, 143
electrolyte replacement, 143
food safety education, 143
fresh water safety, 143
hydration maintenance, 143
latex barrier condoms, 143
nutrient replacement, 143
skin integrity
	maintenance, 143
interventions, pharmacological
antibiotics, 143
antidiarrheal agents, 143
antispasmodics, 143
pancreatic digestive
	enzymes, 143
nursing assessment, objective
abdominal assessment, 142
dehydration signs, 142
laboratory analyses, 142
nursing assessment,
	subjective, 142
nursing diagnoses, 142
Diarrhea, infant and child
clinical presentation, 269–270
cryptosporidiosis, 285
diagnosis
	stool culture, 270
	symptoms, 270
etiology, epidemiology, 269
fever, 303
mycobacterial avium
	complex, 280
nursing implications
	ARV adjustment
		anticipation, 270
	caretaker education, 270
	social historic
		information, 270
pathogenesis, 269
prevention, treatment
	anti-diarrheal agents, 270
	antibiotics, infectious
		causes, 270
	ARV adjustments, 270
	nutrition changes, 270
	water supply evaluation, 270
wasting syndrome, 289
weight loss, 299
Didanosine (Videx, ddI), 52
Diphenoxylate/atropine, 389
Diptheria vaccine, 253*table*
Disclosure to the child
age-appropriate disclosure, 324
children's issues
	adaptation and functioning
		of child, 324
	experiential factor, 324
	health and illness
		concepts, 324
child's environment
	church factors, 325

community factors, 325
family factors, 324
school factors, 324–325
child's responses to, 325*fig*.
delayed disclosure,
	approaches to
	caregiver knowledge
		assessment, 326
	familial cultural
		assessment, 326
	interval interventions,
		325–326
	play therapy techniques, 326
family issues
	family reluctance, 324
	parental perspective, 324
	precipitating factors, 324
illness and disability
	perspective, 323–324
nursing implications, 326
process of, 323
Disseminated Mycobacterium
	avium complex (DMAC), 76
Distal symmetric polyneuropathy
	(DSP), 74
Distraction pain intervention, 295
DNA PCR assay, 356
DNR. *See* Do not resuscitate order
Do not resuscitate order (DNR),
	332, 343
Dole, Pamela, xxii, xxvi
Dolophine, 146
Domestic violence
	power imbalances, 230
	pregnant women and, 214
Donohoe, Marion, xxvi
D'Orlando, Dawn, xxvi
Doxepin, 391
Doxorubicin, 391
Doxorubicin hydrochloride
	liposome, 391–392
Dronabinol, 392
Drug use
	baseline assessment, 37
	cognitive impairment, 126
	disinhibited behavior, 48
	male sexual dysfunction, 148
	needle exchange, 48
	panic disorder and, 168
	risk factor of, 8, 11, 14–15,
		16, 18, 20
	thrombocytopenia, 103, 104
	See also Substance abuse and
		mental illness; Substance
		use; Substance users
		community
DSP. *See* Distal symmetric
	polyneuropathy
Dykeman, Margaret, xxvi
Dyslipidemia
	clinical presentation, 101

diagnosis, 101
etiology, epidemiology, 101
nursing implications, 102
pathogenesis, 101
prevention, treatment, 101–102
testosterone therapy and, 228
Dysphagia and odynophagia
etiology, 130
evaluation, 131–132
goals, 131
interventions, alternative,
complementary
capsaicin, 131
chamomile, 131
interventions,
nonpharmacological, 131
nutrition counseling, 131
oral care counseling, 131
swallowing retraining, 131
interventions, pharmacological
antifungal, antiviral
medication, 131
pain medication, 131
nursing assessment, objective
laboratory studies, 131
mental, cognitive status, 131
nutritional status, 131
physical inspection, 131
nursing assessment,
subjective, 131
nursing diagnosis, 131
Dyspnea
etiology, 129
evaluation, 130
goals, 129–130
interventions, alternative,
complementary, 130
interventions,
nonpharmacological
ADLs assistance, 130
bronchial hygiene, 130
exhalation breathing, 130
fluid intake increase, 130
irritant avoidance, 130
nutrition counseling, 130
oxygen therapy, 130
physical positioning, 130
smoking cessation, 130
interventions, pharmacological
antibiotics, 130
opioids, 130
nursing assessment,
objective, 129
nursing assessment, subjective
ADLs report, 129
medical, surgical
history, 129
patient-rating tools, 129
patient's report, 129
social assessment, 129
symptoms' history, 129

nursing diagnosis, 129
Dysrhythmia, 269

E. coli, 142
Eating disorders. *See* Anorexia,
infant and child; Anorexia
and weight loss, adolescent
and adult; Weight loss,
infant and child
EBV, 289
Eczema, 251, 269
Efavirenz (Sustiva), 52
EIA. *See* Enzyme-linked
immunosorbent assay
Ejaculation, 8
Elderly. *See* Older persons
community
Emancipated minor, defined, 176
Emanuele, Tom, xxvi
Encephalopathy, 298, 299, 301
End of life issues
comfort care
alternative therapies, 334
behavioral health
services, 334
pain management, 334
decision making
DNR *vs.* interventions, 332
ethics committee
intervention, 333
family autonomy, 313
hospice *vs.* institutional
care, 333
medical staff, disagreement
with, 333
parent and child,
disagreement
between, 333
definitions regarding, 332
HIV disclosure, 332
terminal status disclosure, 332
unfinished business
assessment, 332
Endocrinopathies, 105
Entameba histolytica, 143
Enzyme-linked immunosorbent
assay (EIA), 29
Eosinophilia, 268
Eosinophils, 25
Epidemiology of HIV infection
and AIDS
emerging and future
trends, 17–18
epidemiology, defined, 5
global characteristics
anti-HIV treatment access,
11–12
demographics, 10
incidence statistics, 9–10
mortality, 11
occupational risk, 11, 15–16

prevalence, 4, 10
transmission, 11
HIV in the United States
AIDS prevalence, 12
case surveillance,
categories, 16–17, 18
cohort studies, 17
demographics, 13–14
geography, 12–13
incidence, 12
mortality, 12–13, 18
registries, 17
risk factors, 16
transmission, 14–16, 17
measurements
absolute counts of
events, 5–6
attributable risk, 7
case-fatality rate, 6
changes in percentages, 6
cumulative numbers of
cases, deaths, 6
incidence rates, 7
mortality rates, 7
percentages or
proportions, 6
prevalence rates, 7
proportional mortality
rate, 6
rates, 6–7
relative risk ratio, 7
susceptibility to infection,
universality of, 9
systematic surveillance, 5
terminology definitions, 5
transmission cofactors
circumcision, 8
drug-injecting practices,
8, 11
mechanical contraception, 8
mucosal barrier
alterations, 8
sexual activity trauma, 8
spermicides, 8
STDs, 8
transmission routes
blood transmission, 8, 15
breast-feeding, 11
communicability period, 7
ejaculation, 8
female-to-female
transmission, 15
heterosexual
transmission, 15
host-to-host transmission,
7–8
injection drug use, 14–15, 16
men with male sexual
contact, 14
occupational exposure,
15–16

oral sex, 8
perinatal transmission, 15
relative efficiency of, 8–9
transmission mode, 7–8
vaginal and rectal entry
portals, 8
vaginal *vs.* Cesarean
delivery, 9
Epiglottitis, 278
Epivir, 371
Epoetin alfa, 392
Epstein-Barr virus, 73, 96
cardiomyopathy, 104
leiomyosarcoma, 272
lymphadenopathy, 273
malignancies, infant and
child, 289
oral lesions, 132
splenomegaly, 277
testing, hepatomegaly, 271
Erectile dysfunction, 148, 149
Erythrocytosis, 227
Erythropoiesis, 103
Erythropoietin, 268
Esophageal candidiasis, 79, 80,
282–283, 299, 352
Estrogen therapy, 227–228
Ethambutol, 392–393
Ethical and legal concerns
advance directive planning,
342, 343
assisted suicide issue, 345
beneficence principle, 339
clinical trials focus, 344
discrimination and worker
protection, 342
DNR order, 343
duty-based approach to ethical
decision making, 340
estate and will planning, 342
euthanasia issue, 345
fidelity and veracity
principle, 340
future care of dependent
children, 342–343
individual choice issue
accepting freely, without
coercion, 341
competence, 341
confidentiality, 341
disclosure, 341
informed consent, 341
privacy, 341
respect for autonomy, 341
right to accept, refuse
treatment, 341
inequitable access to care
issue
AIDS Drug Assistance
Programs, 341
ARV therapy expense, 341

developing countries,
inequities in, 341
experimental therapies, 341
managed care
complexity, 341
Medicaid, health insurance
coverage, 341
minority patient
inequality, 341
research participation, 341
justice principle, 340
medical system mistrust, 343
nonmaleficence principle, 339
obligation to provide care
issue, 344
privacy, confidentiality,
disclosure issues, 341–342
criteria to override
confidentiality, 342
duty to warn, 342
mandatory naming,
reporting, 342
mandatory testing, 342
partners' rights, 342
test results, 342
third-party notification
policies, 342
protecting health care workers
issue, 344–345
proxy decision maker, 343
public health focus, 343
patients continuing unsafe
behavior, 343
testing of pregnant women,
infants, 343–344
respect for autonomy
principle, 340
rights-based approach
to ethical decision
making, 340
suicide issue, 345
Etiology, defined, 5
Etoposide, 393–395
Euthanasia issue, 345
Exercise, 44

Famciclovir, 392
Family. *See* Caregiver burden,
strain; Decision making and
family autonomy; Surrogate
caregivers
Farmworker Health
Services, Inc., 206
Fat maldistribution, 53, 232
Fat redistribution syndrome
(lipodystrophy), 44–45, 49
clinical presentation, 99–100
diagnosis, 100
etiology, epidemiology, 99
dyslipidemia, 100
nursing implications, 100

pathogenesis, 99, 100
presentation, treatment, 100
Fatigue
anemia, infant and
child, 268
etiology
anxiety, 133
depression, 133
endocrinological
dysregulation, 133
nutritional deficiencies, 133
evaluation, 134
goals, 134
interventions, alternative,
complementary, 134
interventions,
nonpharmacological, 134
depression therapy, 134
energy conservation, 134
infection treatment, 134
napping, 134
physical therapy, 134
interventions,
pharmacological, 134
dextroamphetamine, 134
hyperbaric oxygen, 134
thyroid hormone
replacement, 134
nursing assessment,
objective, 134
nursing assessment, subjective,
133–134
drug use, 134
nutritional status, 134
sleep patterns, 134
nursing diagnosis, 134
Feline immunodeficiency virus
(FIV), 23
Feline leukemia virus (FeLV), 22
Female polyurethane condoms,
19, 43
Female sexual dysfunction
etiology
medication side effects, 147
organic causes, 146–147
psychiatric disorders, 147
evaluation, 148
interventions, alternative,
complementary
damiana leaf and herb, 148
Ginkgo biloba leaf
extract, 148
muira puama, 148
Yohimbine bark, 148
interventions,
nonpharmacological
anatomy and sexual
function education, 147
distraction techniques, 147
noncoital behavior
encouragement, 147

stimulation
enhancement, 147
interventions, pharmacological
apomorphine, 148
HRT, 147–148
l-arginine, 148
methyl testosterone, 148
phentolamine, 148
prostaglandin E1, 148
sildenafil, 148
nursing assessment,
objective
measurement tools, 147
physical exam, 147
nursing assessment,
subjective, 147
nursing diagnosis, 147
Female Sexual Function Index
(FSFI), 147
Ferri, Richard, xxvii
Fetanyl, 146
Fever, adolescent and adult
etiology, 135
evaluation, 136
goals, 136
interventions, alternative,
complementary
herbal extracts, 136
kava kava and valerian, 136
warm baths, 136
white willow bark, 136
interventions,
nonpharmacological, 136
interventions, pharmacological
antipyretic therapy, 136
NSAIDs, 136
nursing assessment,
objective, 135
nursing assessment,
subjective, 135
nursing diagnosis, 135–136
Fever, infant and child
alternative, complementary
therapy
Reiki therapy, 304
touch therapy, 304–305
etiology
antibodies, 303
fever, defined, 303
hypothermia, 303
infections, 303
evaluation
bone or joint pain, 305
dehydration, 305
diarrhea, 305
hospital admission
criteria, 305
meningeal signs, 305
oral thrush, 305
respiratory distress, 305
goals, 304

interventions:
nonpharmacological
cooling procedures, 304
discomfort relief, 304
lab tests, 304
parental guidelines, 304
interventions: pharmacological
acetaminophen, 304
antibiotics, 304
empirical treatments, 304
nursing assessment: objective
appearance assessment, 304
blood culture, 304
CBC with differential, 304
lab tests, 304
physical exam, 304
physical measurements, 304
nursing assessment: subjective
activity level, 303
eating habits, 303
elimination patterns, 303
exposure history, 303
immunizations, 303
medications, 303
systems review, 303
travel history, 303
nursing diagnosis, 304
Fleas, 66
Fluconazole, 283, 284, 307,
394–395
Flucytosine, 395
Follicle stimulating hormone
(FSH), 230
Follicular dendritic cells, 28
Folliculitis, 307
Follow-up. See Health care
follow-up
Folstein Mini Mental State
Examination (MMSE), 165
Folstein Mini-Mental Status
Exam, 140
Fomivirsen, 395
Food safety, 45–46
Fortovase, 372
Foster families, 322
Foxcarnet, 395
Freirean behavior change
approach, prescription
regimen adherence, 60–61
FSFI (Female Sexual Function
Index), 147
FSH (follicle stimulating
hormone), 230
FTM (female-to-male) sexual
transformation, 226
Fugate, Kelly, xxvii
Fungal infections, adolescent and
adult, 125
See also Candidiasis,
adolescent and adult;
Coccidioidomycosis,

adolescent and adult;
Cryptococcosis,
adolescent and adult;
Histoplasmosis,
adolescent and adult
Fungal infections, infant
and child. See Candidiasis,
infant and child;
Coccidioidomycosis, infant
and child; Cryptococcosis,
infant and child;
Histoplasmosis,
infant and child
Fusion inhibitors (T20), 53

G-CSF (granulocyte
colony-stimulating
factor), 274, 394
GAD (Generalized anxiety
disorder). See Primary
anxiety-spectrum disorders
GAF (Global Assessment of
Functioning), 165
Ganciclovir, 394
Garcia Jones, Sande, xxvii
Gardnerella vaginalis, 203
Gaskin, Susan, xxvii
Gastroesophageal reflux
disease, 130
Gay and bisexual men
community
access to care, treatment,
research
clinical trial
participation, 185
financial, social barriers, 185
treatment outcome
variables, 185
unethical research
practices, 185
community care approaches
community-based
organizations, 186
gay and bisexual media, 186
gay vs. HIV community
focus, 186
grief, bereavement support
groups, 186
HIV testing, name reporting
issues, 186
homophobia issues, 186
subtle inappropriateness, 186
community description
demographics, 184
gay identity
development, 183
health issues
alcohol, substance
use, 184
health care provider
attitudes, 184

mental health provider
issues, 184
STDs, HIV transmission, 184
individual care approaches
emotional issues, 185
marginalized
subpopulation
prevention
services, 185
traumatic outcomes
management, 185
older population, 207
transmission, risk behaviors,
prevention issues
gay bashing, 184
HIV/AIDS statistics, 184
legality issues, 184
social stigma, 184–185
Gay cancer, 2
Gay-related immunodeficiency
(GRID), 2
Geiger, Mary, xxvii
Generalized anxiety disorder
(GAD). *See* Primary
anxiety-spectrum disorders
Genital surgery, 226
Genotype assays for antiretroviral
resistance, 57, 358
Giardia lamblia, 143, 220
Ginkgo biloba, 148, 149–150
Ginseng, 140, 150
Global Assessment of Functioning
(GAF), 165
Glucose-6-phosphate
dehydrogenase test, 361
GM-CSF (granulocyte macrophage
colony-stimulating factor),
396–397
Goldberg Depression Scale, 165
Goodroad, Brian K., xxvii
Grage, Kristin, xxvii
Granulocyte colony-stimulating
factor (G-CSF), 274, 396
Granulocyte macrophage
colony-stimulating factor
(GM-CSF), 396–397
Granulocytes, 28
GRID (gay-related
immunodeficiency), 2
Grief
of caregiver, 159
depression, 166
spirituality and religious
interventions, 163
Gross, Elaine, xxiii
Growth hormone
deficiencies, 105
Guided imagery pain
intervention, 295
Guilt
depression, 164

initial diagnosis and, 158
of parent, 317
spiritual, religious
interventions, 162–163

HAART. *See* Highly Active
Anti-Retroviral Therapy
Haemophilus influenzae, 75, 276,
278, 279
Haemophilus influenzae type B
(Hib) vaccine, 40
Haiken, Heidi J., xxvii
Hairy-cell leukemia, 22
HAM-D (Hamilton Depression
Rating Scale), 165
Hamilton Depression Rating Scale
(HAM-D), 165
Harm reduction behavior change
model
prescription regimen
adherence, 60
substance abuse, 224
HAV. *See* Hepatitis A virus
HbsAB antibody test, 360
HBV. *See* Hepatitis B virus
HBV serology test, 360
HCV. *See* Hepatitis C virus
HCV genotype test, 361
HCV RIBA recombinant
immunoblot assay, 360
HCV serology test, 360
Health belief model, prescription
regimen adherence, 61
Health care follow-up
behavioral history, 51
blood chemistry testing, 50
CBC with differential, 50
CD_4 and CD_8 cell absolutes,
percentages, 50
dental exam, 51
diet and exercise, 51
eye exam, 51
food safety, 51
frequency of, 49
health history, 51
lipid profiles, 50
liver functions
monitoring, 50
Pap test, 50–51
patient teaching, 51
safer sex knowledge, 51
serology testing, 51
social history, 51
STD testing, 51
tuberculin skin testing, 50
viral lode (VL), 50
Health care workers. *See* HIV
infected health care workers
community
Health promotion. *See* Teaching
for health promotion,

wellness and transmission
prevention
Hearing impaired community. *See*
Deaf and hearing-impaired
community
Hemarthrosis, 192
Hematuria, 274
Hemophilia, 22
See also People with hemophilia
community
Hemotopoietic growth
factors, 274
Hepatic steatosis, 53
Hepatitis, infant and child
clinical presentation, 270
diagnosis
HCV nucleic acid in plasma
test, 270
plasmatic viral RNA
detection, 271
serum antibody
measurement, 270
etiology, epidemiology
Hepatitis C, 270
vaccination, 270
vertical transmission, 270
nursing implications
hepatitis A, B screen, 271
INF/ribaviran
treatment, 271
patient, family
education, 271
pathogenesis, 270
prevention, treatment
ARV, contraindication, 271
testing during
pregnancy, 271
See also Hepatitis A virus (HAV);
Hepatitis B virus (HBV);
Hepatitis C virus (HCV)
Hepatitis A virus (HAV)
clinical presentation, 110
diagnosis, 110
etiology, epidemiology, 110
nursing implications, 110
pathogenesis, 110
prevention, treatment, 110
vaccine for, 42, 253*table*
Hepatitis B virus (HBV)
clinical presentation, 111
diagnosis, 111
etiology, epidemiology, 111
malignancies, 289
nursing implications, 112
pathogenesis, 111
post exposure prophylaxis,
347–348
prevention, treatment, 111–112
vaccine for, 42, 252, 253*table*
Hepatitis C virus (HCV)
clinical presentation, 113

depressive disorders in, 164
diagnosis, 113
etiology, epidemiology,
    112–113
hemophilia, 193
impaired glucose
    tolerance, 100
infant and child, 270–271
intermenstrual bleeding, 230
nursing implications,
    113–114
pathogenesis, 113
post exposure prophylaxis, 348
treatment, 113
Hepatitis profile, 252
Hepatomegaly, infant and child
clinical presentation
    abdominal distention,
        pain, 271
    lymphoproliferation, 271
    physical exam, 271
diagnosis, 271
etiology, epidemiology, 271
lymphoid interstitial
    pneumonitis, 273
mycobacterial avium
    complex, 280
nursing implications, 271
pathogenesis, 271
treatment, 271
Hepatoxicity, 53, 167
Herbal therapy, 127
for cognitive impairment, 127
for depression, 166
for fever, 136
Kava, 140, 151
for mobility impairment,
    140, 151
for vision loss, 151
Heroin use, 221
    See also Substance abuse and
        mental illness; Substance
        use; Substance users
        community
Herpes simplex virus (HSV),
    adolescent and adult, 47
clinical presentation, 90
cognitive impairment, 125
diagnosis, 90–91
dysphagia and
    odynophagia, 130
etiology, epidemiology
    HSV-1, 90
    HSV-2, 90
gastrointestinal pain, 143
nursing implications, 91
oral lesions, 132
pathogenesis, 90
prevention, treatment, 91
woman to woman
    transmission, 203

Herpes simplex virus (HSV),
    infant and child
clinical presentations, 272
cognitive impairment, 301
diagnosis, 272
etiology, epidemiology
    herpes virus simplex, 271
    oral secretions, 271
nonpharmacological
    treatment, 306
nursing implications, 272
pathogenesis
    herpes labialis, 272
    latency, 271
prevention, treatment, 272
skin lesions, 305
See also Herpes simplex
    virus (HSV), adolescent
    and adult
Herpes zoster (varicella-zoster
    virus, VZV), adolescent
    and adult
Category B disease, 352
clinical presentation, 67
cognitive impairment, 125
diagnosis, 67
etiology, epidemiology, 66–67
of HIV infected infant,
    child, 251
pathogenesis, 67
    chicken pox, 67
    shingles, 67
prevention, treatment, 67
vaccine, 252
HHV-8. See Human herpes virus 8
    (HHV-8)
Hib vaccine. See Haemophilus
    influenzae type B (Hib)
    vaccine
Highly Active Anti-Retroviral
    Therapy (HAART)
for African Americans, 213
AIDS deaths, decrease in, 11
bacterial infection, infant and
    child, 280
cardiomyopathy and, 104
cognitive impairment, 303
dyslipidemia and, 101
fat redistribution syndrome, 100
HIV-associated
    nephropathy, 109
HIV concentrations in
    semen, 215
HIV encephalopathy therapy,
    98, 99
HPV infection, 69
Kaposi's sarcoma therapy, 95
LIP therapy, infant and
    child, 273
MAC, infant and child, 280
NHL therapy, 96, 97

PML, 92, 289
psoriasis, 106
quality of life issues vs., 313
therapy in advanced disease, 55
thrombocytopenia, 277
Highsmith, Connie, xxvii
Hispanic Americans
adolescent HIV/AIDS
    statistics, 176, 177
gay and bisexual men
    statistics, 184
incarceration rates, 198
mortality rates, 13
perinatal transmission, 15
rural population, 209
US HIV statistics, 10, 12,
    13–14, 229
visually impaired statistics, 179
See also Immigrants community;
    Migrant and seasonal
    farm workers community
Histoplasma capsulatum, 47, 84
Histoplasmosis, 103
Histoplasmosis, adolescent
    and adult
candidiasis, 282
clinical presentation, 84
diagnosis, 84
etiology, epidemiology, 84
gastrointestinal pain, 143
nursing implications, 85
pathogenesis, 84
prevention, treatment, 84–85
Histoplasmosis, infant and child
clinical presentation, 284
diagnosis
    antibody serology test, 284
    blood, tissue culture, 284
    bone marrow histopathic
        evaluation, 284
    histoplasma specific
        antigen, 284
    X-rays, 284
etiology, epidemiology, 284
nursing implications
    amphotericin B, 285
    itraconazole, 285
pathogenesis, 284
prevention, treatment, 284
Historical overview, 1
AIDS, discovery and impact
    of, 1, 2
AIDS, responses to, 3–4
behavioral risk factors, 3
CDC tracking the disease, 3–4
community mobilization, 3–4
government response, 4
naming the disease, 2
Ryan White Comprehensive
    AIDS Resources
    Emergency (CARE) Act, 4

searching for the cause, 3
stigmatizing those affected, 3
tracking the disease, 2–3
HIV-1
coreceptor affinities of, 23
lentivirus subgroup of, 23
primate to human lentivirus
transmission, 24
vs. HIV-2, 24
HIV-2, 2, 3
false negative test results, 30
lentivirus subgroup of, 23
primate to human lentivirus
transmission, 24
testing for, 29
vs. HIV-1, 24
HIV-1 enzyme immunoassay, 355
HIV-associated idiopathic
thrombocytopenic purpura
(HIV-ITP), 103
HIV-associated nephropathy
(HIVAN). *See* Nephropathy
(HIV-associated
nephropathy, HIVAN),
adolescent and adult
HIV Dementia Scale, 126
HIV encephalopathy, adolescent
and adult
clinical presentation, 98–99
diagnosis, 99
etiology, epidemiology, 98
nursing implications, 99
pathogenesis, 98
prevention, treatment, 99
HIV infected adolescent and adult
long-term success, 35
See also Adolescent community;
Antiretroviral therapy
management, adolescent
and adult; Baseline
assessment; Health
care follow-up;
Immunizations,
adolescent and adult;
Teaching for health
promotion, wellness and
transmission prevention
HIV infected health care workers
community
access to care, treatment,
research, 188
Americans with Disabilities
Act, 188
community care
approaches, 188
financial, legal concerns
confidentiality issues, 187
disability timing, 187
HIV status reporting, 187
insurance issues, 187
individual care approaches

Americans with Disabilities
Act, 188
confidentiality, 188
job expectations, 188
personal feelings, 188
physical concerns
HIV-related fatigue while
working, 186
job responsibilities, 186
opportunistic infections,
exposure to, 186
taking care of self, 187
psychosocial concerns
being the patient, 187
caregiver adjustment, 187
grief overload, 187
learning to ask, 187
overidentifying with
patients, 187
work *vs.* volunteering, 187
statistics regarding, 186
transmission, risk behaviors,
prevention issues
provider to patient
transmission risk,
187–88
right to work, 187
work issues
Americans with Disabilities
Act, 187
coworker issues, 187
safety guidelines, 187
whom to tell, 187
See also Preventing HIV
transmission in patient
care settings
HIV infection, transmission
and prevention. *See*
Epidemiology of HIV
infection and AIDS;
Historical overview; HIV
testing; Pathophysiology of
HIV infection; Preventing
HIV transmission in patient
care settings; Prevention of
HIV infection
HIV-related encephalopathy,
infant and child
clinical presentation, 290
diagnosis, 290
etiology, epidemiology, 290
nursing implications, 290
pathogenesis, 290
prevention, treatment, 290
HIV-related wasting syndrome,
adolescent and adult, 45
clinical presentation, 98
diagnosis, 98
etiology, epidemiology, 97–98
nursing implications, 98
pathogenesis, 98

prevention, treatment, 98
thalidomide therapy for, 125
HIV-related wasting syndrome,
infant and child
clinical presentation, 289
diagnosis, 289
etiology, epidemiology, 289
nursing implications, 290
pathogenesis, 289
prevention, treatment, 289–290
HIV RNA PCR, 356
See also Viral load (VL) tests
HIV testing
anonymous *vs.* confidential, 31
benefits of, 31
Calypte HIV-1 urine test, 29
disclosure of status issue,
31–32, 199
enzyme-linked immunosorbent
assay (EIA), 29
false negative results, 30
false positive results, 29, 30
Home Access Express test, 30
informed consent issue, 31
of inmates, 199
interpretations of
intermediate test results, 30
negative test results, 30
positive test results, 30
OraSure test system, 29
PBMC HIV culture, 30
polymerase chain reaction
(PCR) test, 30, 257
posttest counseling session,
32–33, 199
of pregnant women, 216,
343, 344
pretest counseling session,
32, 199
risks of, 30
Selected Laboratory Values,
355–361
Single Use Diagnostic System
(SUDS), 29
western blot, 29
HIVAN. *See* Nephropathy (HIV-
associated nephropathy,
HIVAN); Nephropathy
(HIV-associated nephropathy,
HIVAN), adolescent and
adult; Nephropathy
(HIV-associated nephropathy,
HIVAN), infant and child
Hivid, 372
Holmes and Rahe Stress Scale, 126
Holtzelaw, Barbara, xxvii
Home Access Express test, 30
Home Assessment Profile, 139
Homeless persons community
access to care, treatment,
research

financial distress, 195
health care incontinuity, 195
health care provider
    discrimination, 195
health care system
    complexities, 195
medication complexities, 195
community care approaches
collaboration, 196
community-based
    services, 196
culturally sensitive
    workers, 196
day programs, 196
flexibility, 196
mental health
    services, 196
mobil services, 196
one-stop health care, 196
perceptions, reported
    needs, 196
proven service models, 196
substance use programs, 196
workforce integration, 196
community description
abusive conditions, 193
alcohol and drug use, 194
comorbidity, 194
health care system
    discrimination, 194
HIV/AIDS statistics, 193
illegal immigrant status, 194
medical expenses, 193
mental illness, 194
stigmatization, 194
Stuart B. McKinney Homess
    Assistance Act, 193
unemployment, 193
health issues
comorbidities, 194
dropout tendency, 194
hygiene facilities
    inadequacies, 194
injuries, 194
nutrition deficiencies, 194
physical, sexual abuse, 194
sexual education
    limitations, 194
teen pregnancies, 194
incarceration, 197
individual care approaches
basic needs, 195
benefits eligibility
    assessment, 195
client-centered
    approach, 195
lifestyle realities, 195–196
listen carefully, 195
multidisciplinary team
    approach, 196
trust, 195

transmission, risk behaviors,
    prevention issues
diagnosis delay, 195
immune system trauma, 195
sexual, physical abuse, 194
substance use behavior, 194
teen condom use, 194
Homosexuality
risk assessments, 18–19
See also Gay and bisexual men
    community; Lesbians and
    bisexual women
    community
Hormone replacement therapy
antiretroviral therapy and, 232
cross-gender hormone therapy,
    227–228
female sexual dysfunction,
    147–148
HIV transmission, 231
Hospitalization. *See* Multiple
    hospitalizations
HPO (hypothalamic-pituitary-
    ovarian axis), 230
HPV. *See* Human papillomavirus
    (HPV) infection
HSV. *See* Herpes simplex virus
    (HSV), adolescent and adult
HTLV-III. *See* Human
    T-lymphotrophic virus type 3
Hughes, Valery, xxvii
Human growth hormone, 395
Human herpes virus 8 (HHV-8), 94
Human leukocyte antigen (HLA), 9
Human papillomavirus (HPV)
    infection
clinical presentation, 69
cognitive impairment, 125
diagnosis, 69
    colposcopy, 69
    Pap smear, 69
epidemiology
    cervical neoplasia, 93
    cofactors for, 68
    HPV and HIV
        relationship, 68
    HPV subtypes, 68
    HPV types in SIL disease, 68
    as major risk factor, 68
    sexual intercourse
        transmission mode, 68
    SIL rates increase, 68
malignancies, 289
nursing implications
    health maintenance
        behavior promotion,
        70–71
    psychosocial support, 71
    treatment modalities, 70–71
oral lesions, 132
pathogenesis, 68–69

prevention, treatment, 69–70
    5-FU antieoplastic cream, 70
    conization, 70
    cryotherapy, 70
    experimental treatments, 70
    HAART, 69
    hysterectomy, 70
    laser ablation, 70
    loop electrical excision
        procedure, 70
    safer sex, 69, 70–71
woman to woman
    transmission, 203
Human T-lymphotrophic virus-I
    (HTLV-I), 22, 289
Human T-lymphotrophic virus-II
    (HTLV-II), 22
Human T-lymphotrophic virus
    type 3 (HTLV-III), 2
Human T-lymphotrophic virus-V
    (HTLV-V), 22
Hydromorphone pain
    therapy, 146
Hypercholesterolemia, 100
Hyperglycemia, 53, 232
Hyperinsulinemia, 105
Hyperlactemia, 52, 109
Hyperlipidemia, 45, 49, 53,
    100, 206
Hypersomnia, 137
Hypertension, 206
Hypertriglyceridemia, 100
Hypoglycemia, 287
Hypothalamic-pituitary-ovarian
    axis (HPO), 230
Hypothermia, 303

Ibuprofen, 296
Ichthyosis, 306
IDAV. *See* Immunodeficiency-
    associated virus
Idiopathic thrombocytopenia
    purpura (ITP), adolescent
    and adult
Category B disease, 352
clinical presentation, 71
diagnosis, 71
etiology, epidemiology, 71
hemophilia, 192
nursing implications, 71–72
pathogenesis, 71
prevention, treatment, 71
    anti-RhO-(d) IgG, 71
    danazol, 71
    gamma globulin
        injections, 71
    HAART, 71
    immunosuppressive
        agents, 71
    platelet transfusions, 71
    splenectomy, 71

steroid therapy, 71
ziduvudine, 71
thrombocytopenia, 103
Idiopathic thrombocytopenia
purpura (ITP), infant and
child, 277
IDP. *See* Inflammatory
demyelinating
polyneuropathy
IDUs (injecting drug users),
221–222
IFA. *See* Immunofluorescent
assay (IFA) test
IgA antibodies, 9
IgG antibodies, 9
IGT. *See* Impaired glucose
tolerance
Imipramine, 395
Imiquimod, 307
IMMACT90 (Immigration Act
of 1990), 219
Immigrants community
access to care, treatment,
research
cultural stereotypes
regarding risks, 220
infectious diseases, 220
isolation, nondisclosure
trends, 220
poor health upon
arrival, 220
underreporting,
misclassification, 220
community care approaches
culturally appropriate
resource materials, 221
immigrants in prevention
planning, 221
interagency networking, 221
peer advocacy outreach, 221
community description
countries of origin, 219
immigrant, defined, 219
statistics regarding, 219
health issues
access issues, 219
employment factors, 219
health insurance status, 219
HIV status, deportation
fear, 219
immigration and the law,
219–220
mistrust of services, 219
illegal immigrant statistics,
219, 231
immigration and the law
HIV status, immigration
law, 219–220
individual care approaches
clinic hour flexibility, 221
cultural sensitivity, 220–221

nutritional assessment, 221
privacy issues, 221
traditional healing,
remedies, 221
translation services, 221
transmission, risk
behaviors, prevention
issues
blood products sale, 220
breastfeeding, 220
condom use resistance, 220
heterosexual
transmission, 220
mother-to-child
transmission, 220
MSM transmission, 220
needle sharing, 220
racial, ethnic minority
factors, 220
Immigration Act of 1990
(IMMACT90), 219
Immigration and Nationality
Act (INA), 219
Immune globulin, 397–398
Immune reconstruction, 99
Immune system. *See*
Pathophysiology of HIV
infection
Immunizations, adolescent
and adult
dosages, 40
live vaccine limitations, 40
preventable diseases
Haemophilus influenzae
(Hib), 40
hepatitis, 42
influenza, 40–41
measles, mumps and
rubella, 40
pneumococcal pneumonia,
41–42
tetanus-diptheria (td),
42–43
vaccinations
Hepatitis A vaccine, 110,
112, 113, 270
Hepatitis B vaccine, 111,
113, 270
inactivated vaccines, 43
live travel vaccines, 43
for travel, 43
Immunizations, infant and child,
248, 252, 253*table*
immune globulin
preparations, 252
influenza, 252
preventable diseases
measles, mumps, rubella,
252, 276
pneumococcal
pneumonia, 252

vaccinations
Hepatitis B vaccine, 252
herpes zoster, 252
inactivated polio
vaccine, 252
varicella vaccine, 252
Immunodeficiency-associated
virus (IDAV), 2
Immunofluorescent assay (IFA)
test, 29
Impaired glucose tolerance (IGT)
clinical presentation, 100
diagnosis, 101
etiology, epidemiology, 100
dyslipedmia, 101
HCV and, 100
protease inhibitors, 100
nursing implications, 101
pathogenesis, 100
prevention, treatment, 101
Impetigo, 306, 308
INA (Immigration and
Nationality Act), 219
Inactivated polio vaccination
(IPV), 43, 253*table*
Incarcerated persons community
access to care, treatment,
research
ART adherence, continuity
difficulty, 200
care standards, 200
clinical trial eligibility, 200
eighth amendment
rights, 200
informed consent,
confidentiality
issues, 200
Medicaid, Medicare benefits
ineligibility, 199
mortality statistics, 199
quality of HIV care, 199
researcher distrust, 200
treatment outcomes, 200
community care approaches
CO sexual assault
reduction, 202
community program
models, 201–202
HIV education, all
levels, 201
medication issues, 201
peer-led programs, 201
rehabilitation
advocacy, 202
community description
female gender
characteristics, 197
incarcerated, defined, 197
male gender
characteristics, 197
statistics regarding, 197

substance use, 197
violence exposure, 197
health issues
   literacy levels, 197
   overcrowded health
      hazards, 197
   predetention risk factor
      behaviors, 197
individual care approaches
   dependent children
      issues, 201
   literacy level assessment,
      200–201
   mental illness, substance
      abuse treatment, 201
   nutrition assessment, 201
   peer education classes, 200
   prerelease planning, 201
   preventive health behavior
      education, 201
   risk reduction
      education, 200
   stigmatizing avoidance, 201
transmission, risk behaviors,
      prevention issues
   condom distribution
      policy, 198
   educational materials,
      198–199
   gender factors, 198
   HIV acquisition while
      incarcerated, 198
   HIV/AIDS incidence
      rates, 198
   HIV testing, 199
   sexual abuse within
      prisons, 198
India, 10
Indinavir, 49
Indinavir mesylate (Crixivan), 53
Individual choice principle, 341
Infants
   HIV incidence rates, 12
   nutrient requirements, 298
   See also Antiretroviral therapy,
      infant and child; Clinical
      manifestations and
      management of the HIV
      infected infant and child;
      Community-based care
      issues; Decision making
      and family autonomy;
      Disclosure to the child;
      End of life issues;
      Multiple hospitalizations;
      Perinatally acquired
      pediatric HIV; Social
      isolation and stigma;
      Stress reduction and
      pediatric HIV infection;
      Surrogate caregivers;

Symptom management of
   the HIV infected infant
   and child; Symptomatic
   conditions in infants and
   children with advancing
   disease
Infection control. *See* Preventing
   HIV transmission in patient
   care settings
Inflammatory demyelinating
   polyneuropathy (IDP), 74
Influenza vaccine, 40–41, 252,
   253*table*
Injecting drug users (IDUs),
   221–222
Insulin resistance, 44, 100
Integrase inhibitors, 53
Interferon alfa 2a, 396
Interferon alfa 2b, 396
Interferon alfa n1, 396
Interleukin-2, 9, 168
Intravenous immune
   globulin (IVIG), 278
Invirase, 373
IPV. *See* Inactivated polio
   vaccination
Isoniazid, 396–397
Isospora belli, 86, 143
Isosporiasis, adolescent and adult
   clinical presentation, 86
   diagnosis, 86
   etiology, epidemiology, 86
   nursing implications, 86
   pathogenesis, 86
   prevention, treatment, 86
Isosporiasis, infant and child
   clinical presentation, 28
   diagnosis, 286
   etiology, epidemiology, 285
   nursing implications, 286
   pathogenesis, 286
   prevention, treatment, 286
ITP. *See* Idiopathic
   thrombocytopenia purpura
   (ITP), adolescent and adult
Itraconazole, 283, 285, 397–398

JCV genus *polyomavirus. See*
   Progressive multifocal
   leukoencephalopathy (PML),
   adolescent and adult
JCV (JC virus), 125, 288
Johns Hopkins HIV Dementia
   Scale, 165
Jones, Sande Garcia, xxii–xxiii

Kaletra, 373
Kaolin-pectin, 400
Kaposi's Sarcoma and
   Opportunistic Infections
   (KSOI) Task Force, 2

Kaposi's Sarcoma (KS), 2
   arthritis and, 107
   clinical presentation, 95
   cognitive impairment, 125
   diagnosis, 95
   diarrhea, 142
   etiology, epidemiology, 94–95
      thrombocytopenia, 103
   gastrointestinal pain, 143
   nursing implications, 96
   oral lesions, 132
   pathogenesis, 95
   prevention, treatment
      biologics, 96
      chemotherapy, 96
      cryotherapy, 95
      HAART, 95
      intralesional therapy, 95
      novel approaches, 96
      photodynamic therapy, 95
      radiation therapy, 95
      surgical excision, 95
      topical retinoic acid, 95
   registries, 17
   skin lesions, 305
   in women, 229
Karnofsky Performance Status
   Index, 139
Katz Index of Activities of Daily
   Living, 139
Kava herbal therapy, 140, 151
Keithley, Joyce, xxvii
Ketoconazole, 398–399
Kirton, Carl, xxi
Kirton, Carl A., xxvii
Klebsiella pneumoniae, 75
KS. *See* Kaposi's Sarcoma
KS/AIDS Task Force, 2

L-arginine medication, 148
Lactate test, 361
Lactic acidosis, 52, 53, 109
   ARV therapy in women, 232
   clinical presentation, 109
   etiology, epidemiology, 109
   nursing implications, 109–110
   pathogenesis, 109
   prevention, treatment, 109
Lamivudine (Epivir, 3TC), 52
Laryngotracheitis, 278
Latin Americans
   immigration statistics, 219
   needle sharing by, 220
   See also Hispanic
      Americans; Immigrants
      community
LAV. *See* Lymphadenopathy-
   associated virus
Leach, Eric G., xxviii
Lee, Young-Me, xxviii
Legal blindness, defined, 179

Legal issues. *See* Ethical and legal concerns
Leiomyosarcoma, infant and child, 289
  diagnosis, 272
  etiology, epidemiology
    Category B
      AIDS-definition, 272
    statistics on, 272
  nursing implications
    educate family, 273
    emotional support, 273
    rest, nutrition, 273
  pathogenesis, 272
  prevention, treatment
    chemotherapy, contraindication, 272–273
    local excision, 272
Lentivirus (*Lentiviridae*). *See* Pathophysiology of HIV infection
Leon, Wade, xxviii
Lesbians and bisexual women community
  community care approaches, 204–205
  community description
    bisexual woman, defined, 202
    lesbian, defined, 202
  health issues
    access to health care issues, 202
    health care provider stereotypes, 202
    sexual history, 202–203
    sexual orientation identity, 202
    social history, 202
    social retaliation, 202
  individual care approaches
    condom use, 204
    latex barriers, 204
    semen use precautions, 204
    sex toy and device cautions, 204
  transmission, risk behaviors, prevention
    douches, enemas, 204
    herpes simplex virus, 203
    human papillomavirus, 203
    sex toys, 204
    spermicides, 204
    statistics regarding, 202–203, 230
    STD transmission, 204
    transmission routes, 203–204
    women to women transmission, 203

Leucovorin, 399–400
Leukemia, 289
Leukocytes
  B-cell lymphocytes, 25
  basophils, 25
  eosinophils, 25
  monocytes, macrophages, 25
  natural killer (NK) lymphocytes, 26
  neutrophils, 25
  T-cell lymphocytes, 25–26
Leukopenia
  clinical presentation, 103
  diagnosis, 103
  etiology, epidemiology, 103
  nursing implications, 103
  pathogenesis, 103
  prevention, treatment, 103
Levorphanol, 146
Lewis, Martin, xxviii
LH (luteinizing hormone), 230
LIP. *See* Lymphoid interstitial pneumonitis (LIP), infant and child
Lipid profiles, 50
Lipodystrophy, 44
  See also Fat redistribution
Listeria monocytogenes, 72
Listeriosis
  Category B disease, 352
  clinical presentation, 72
  diagnosis, 72
  etiology, epidemiology, 72
  nursing implications, 73
  pathogenesis, 72
  prevention, treatment, 72–73
Lithium, 168
Liver function tests, 50
Loperamine, 400
Lopinavir/ritonavir (Kaletra), 53
Low vision, defined, 179
Luteinizing hormone (LH), 230
Lymphadenitis, 280
Lymphadenopathy, infant and child
  Category A symptom, 352
  clinical presentation, 273
  diagnosis, 273
  etiology, epidemiology, 273
  nursing implications, 273
  pathogenesis, 273
  prevention, treatment, 273
Lymphadenopathy-associated virus (LAV), 2
Lymphoid interstitial pneumonitis (LIP), infant and child
  clinical presentation, 273
  diagnosis, 273
  etiology, epidemiology
    AIDS-defining condition, 273

AIDS-defining condition, Category B, 273
  in children *vs.* adults, 273
  pathogenesis, 273
  prevention, treatment
    bronchodilators, diuretics, 274
    HAART viral replication control, 273
    prednisone, 273–274
Lymphoid organs, 28
Lymphopenia, 268
Lyon, Debra E., xxviii

MAC. *See* Mycobacterium avium complex (MAC), adolescent and adult
MacIntyre, Richard, xxviii
Macrophages, 25
Magnesium deficiency, 133
Male sexual dysfunction
  etiology
    iatrogenic causes, 149
    medication side effects, 148–149
    organic causes, 148
    premature ejaculation, 148
    psychiatric disorders, 148
  evaluation, 150
  goal, 149
  interventions, alternative, complementary
    damiana leaf and herb, 150
    Ginkgo biloba leaf extract, 149–150
    Ginseng root, 150
    Muira puama, 150
    Yohimbine bark, 149
  interventions, nonpharmacological
    couples counseling, 149
    psychotherapy, 149
  interventions, pharmacological
    oral agents, 149
    penile surgery, 149
    urethral therapies, 149
    vacuum or constriction devices, 149
  nursing assessment, objective, 149
  nursing assessment, subjective, 149
  nursing diagnosis, 149
Male-to-female (MTF) sexual transformation, 226
Malignancies, infant and child
  clinical presentation, 289
  diagnosis, 289
  etiology, epidemiology, 289
  nursing implications, 289

pathogenesis, 289
prevention, treatment, 289
Mallinson, R. Kevin, xxviii
Malnutrition, 45
Mantoux tuberculin test, 281
Marsco, Lawrence, xxviii
Mature minor, defined, 176
McNicholl, Ian R., xxviii
Measles vaccine, 40, 252, 253*table*
Medical case management
    model, 338
Medical regimens. *See* Adherence
    to medical regimens, infant
    and child
Medically emancipated minor,
    defined, 176
Megestrol acetate, 402
Menopause, 230
Mental illness. *See* Psychiatric
    disorders in HIV disease
Meperidine, 145, 146
Merriam, Nora, xxviii
Metformin, 403
Methadone, 223, 230, 402–403
Methotrexate, 403
Metronidazole, 403–404
Mexican Americans
    immigration statistics, 219
    See also Hispanic Americans;
        Migrant and seasonal
        farm workers community
Miconazole, 404
Microbicidal gels, 20, 43
Migrant and seasonal farm
    workers community
    access to care, treatment,
        research
        ability to work, 205
        community-based
            agencies, 205
        continuity of care, treatment
            regimens, 205
    community care approaches
        acculturation levels, 206
        Farmworker Health
            Services, Inc., 206
        generational differences, 206
        mobil services, 206
    community description, 205
    health issues
        cultural, language
            barriers, 205
        environmental stressors, 205
        knowledge deficiency, 205
        poverty, education, 205
    individual care approaches
        cultural and gender
            sensitivity, 205
        skills building, 205
    transmission, risk behaviors,
        prevention issues

condom use, 205
    gender role beliefs, 205
    knowledge deficiency, 205
    sex exchange for money, 205
    unprotected sex, 205
Mini-Mental Status Exam, 126
Minor, definitions
    regarding, 176
Mitochondrial dysfunction, 45
Mitoxantrone, 404
MM. *See* Monoeuritis multiplex
MMSE (Folstein Mini Mental
    State Examination), 165
Mobility impairment
    etiology
        AIDS dementia
            complex, 139
        infections, neoplasms, 139
        metabolic complications, 139
        movement limitation, 139
        musculoskeletal
            injury, 139
        neurological
            involvement, 139
        polyneuropathies, 139
        psychological
            complications, 139
    evaluation, 140
    goals, 140
    interventions, alternative,
        complementary
        diet and nutrition
            therapy, 140
        herbal therapies, 140
    interventions,
        nonpharmacological
        assistive devices, 140
        environmental
            adaptations, 140
        nutritional guidelines, 140
        pain control methods, 140
        physical activity, 140
        physical therapist
            consult, 140
        psychosocial
            interventions, 140
    interventions,
        pharmacological, 140
    nursing assessment, objective
        environmental, 139–140
        mental status, 140
        musculoskeletal, 139
        neurological, 139
    nursing assessment,
        subjective, 139
    nursing diagnosis, 140
Model of adherence factors,
    prescription regimen
    adherence, 61
Modified Hamilton Anxiety
    Rating Scale, 169

Molluscum contagiousum, 305
nonpharmacological
    treatment, 306
    pharmacological treatment, 307
Monocytes, macrophages, 25
Monoeuritis multiplex (MM), 74
Mononuclear phagocytes, 28
Mood disorders. *See* Delirium;
    Depression; Primary
    anxiety-spectrum disorders;
    Substance abuse and mental
    illness
Moran, Theresa, xxviii
Moraxella catarrhalis, 75, 276, 278
Morphine sulfate (MS) pain
    therapy, 145–146
Mouth care, 46–47
mTB. *See* Mycobacterium
    tuberculosis (mTB),
    adolescent and adult
MTF (male-to-female) sexual
    transformation, 226
Muira puama, 148, 150
Multichannel chemistry panel, 251
Multiple hospitalizations
    child concerns
        acting out, 328
        cue-controlled
            relaxation, 328
        depression assessment, 327
        discuss somatic
            complaints, 327
        fear of death, 327–328
        hypnotherapy, 328
        inadvertent disclosure, 327
        muscle relaxation, 328
        relaxation techniques, 328
        school-age child concerns,
            328–329
        tests and procedures, what
            to expect, 327
    empowering families
        service agency referral, 329
        support resources, 329
    family concerns
        child care, 329
        other children, 329
        sibling concerns, 329
        transportation, 329
    parental concerns, 327
    pediatric hospitalizations, 326
    religious beliefs, 329
    treatment decisions
        legal guardian factors,
            326–327
        parent responsibilities, 326
Mumps vaccine, 40, 252, 253*table*
Mycobacterial avium complex
    (MAC), infant and child
    clinical presentation, 280
    diagnosis, 280

diarrhea, 269
etiology, epidemiology, 280
nursing implications, 281
pathogenesis, 280
prevention, treatment
adverse effects, 281
ARV adjustments, 281
clarithromycin, 280
combination therapy, 280–281
skin lesions, 305
weight loss, 280
Mycobacterial infection, 277
Mycobacterial tuberculosis, infant and child
clinical presentation, 281
diagnosis
chest x-ray, 281
Mantoux test, 281
sputum sample, 281
tuberculin skin test, 281
etiology, epidemiology, 281
nursing implications, 281
pathogenesis, 281
prevention, treatment
four-drug regimen, 281
isoniazid therapy, 281
Mycobacterium avium, 47, 76, 142, 280
Mycobacterium avium complex (MAC), adolescent and adult
clinical presentation, 76
diagnosis, 76
dyspnea, 129
etiology, epidemiology, 76
thrombocytopenia, 103
gastrointestinal pain, 143
maintenance, 76–77
nausea, vomiting, 141
nursing implications, 77
pathogenesis, 76
prevention, 76
treatment, 76
Mycobacterium intracellulare, 47, 76
Mycobacterium marinum, 47
Mycobacterium tuberculosis, 75, 76, 77, 88, 129, 281
Mycobacterium tuberculosis (mTB), adolescent and adult
clinical presentation, 77
diagnosis, 77
etiology, epidemiology, 77
nursing implications, 77–78
pathogenesis, 77
prevention, treatment, 77
Mycoplasma pneumoniae, 75
Mycoplasmic infection, 125
Mycosis fungoides, 22
Myocarditis, 104

N. meningitidis, 75
NA. *See* Narcotics Anonymous
Nandrolone, 404
Naproxen, 296
Narcotics Anonymous (NA), 224, 225
National Clearinghouse for Alcohol and Drug Information, 225
National Commission on Correctional Health Care, 200
National Harm Reduction Coalition, 225
National Hemophilia Foundation
National Institute on Drug Abuse, 225
Native Americans, 209
Natural history of disease, defined, 5
Natural killer (NK) lymphocytes, 26, 27
Nausea and vomiting
etiology
antifungal therapy, 141
antineoplastic therapy, 141
antiparasitic therapy, 141
antiretroviral therapy side effect, 141
antiviral therapy, 141
HIV-related autonomic neuropathy, 141
mycobacterium avium complex therapy, 141
nausea, defined, 140–141
OI-induced endocrine dysfunction, 141
pneumocystis pneuma therapy side effect, 141
radiation therapy, 141
vomiting, defined, 141
evaluation, 142
goals, 141
interventions, alternative, complementary, 142
interventions, nonpharmacological, 141–142
interventions, pharmacological, 142
nursing assessment, objective, 141
nursing assessment, subjective, 141
nursing diagnosis, 141
Nelfinavir mesylate (Viracept), 53
Neoplasms, adolescent and adult, 227
See also Cervical neoplasia; HIV encephalopathy; HIV-related wasting syndrome, adolescent

and adult; Kaposi's sarcoma; Non-Hodgkin's lymphoma
Neoplasms, infant and child
cognitive impairment, 301
skin lesions, 305
thrombocytopenia, 277
See also HIV-related encephalopathy, infant and child; HIV-related wasting syndrome, infant and child; Malignancies, infant and child
Nephropathy (HIV-associated nephropathy, HIVAN), adolescent and adult
clinical presentation, 108
diagnosis, 108–109
etiology, epidemiology, 108
lithium and, 168
nursing implications, 109
pathogenesis, 108
prevention, treatment, 109
Nephropathy (HIV-associated nephropathy, HIVAN), infant and child
clinical presentation, 274
diagnosis, 274
etiology, epidemiology, 274
nursing implications, 274
pathogenesis, 274
PCP, 287
prevention, treatment, 274
Nervier, 373–376
Neutropenia, infant and child
anemia, 268
clinical presentation
fever, 274
respiratory tract symptoms, 274
urinary tract infection, 274
diagnosis, 274
etiology, epidemiology, 274
mycobacterial avium complex, 280
nursing implications, 275
pathogenesis
apoptosis of lymphocytes, 274
bone marrow cells inhibition, 274
myelosuppression, 274
prevention, treatment
ART interruption, 274–275
Granulocyte Colony Stimulating Factor, 274
Neutrophils, 25
Nevirapine (Viramune), 52
Newshan, Gayle, xxviii
NHL. *See* Non-Hodgkin's lymphoma

Nielsen, Craig E., xxix
NNRTIs. *See* Non-nucleoside reverse transcriptase inhibitors (NNRTIs)
Nokes, Kathleen M., xxix
Non-Hodgkin's lymphoma (NHL)
  clinical presentation, 96
  cognitive impairment, 125
  diagnosis, 97
  etiology, epidemiology, 96
    thrombocytopenia, 103
  infant and child, 289
  nursing implications, 97
  oral lesions, 132
  pathogenesis, 96
  prevention, treatment, 97
Non-nucleoside reverse transcriptase inhibitors (NNRTIs)
  depression and, 166
  dyslipidemia, 228
  function of, 52
  impaired glucose tolerance, 100
  side effects of, 52
  testosterone therapy and, 228
  in therapy for asymptomatic individuals, 52
  therapy in infants, children, 258*table*
  tricyclic antidepressants and, 167
Nonantiretroviral medications, 380–415
  See also specific medication name
Nonbacterial thrombotic endocarditis, 269
Nonbullous impetigo, 308
Nonmaleficence health care principle, 340
Nonoxynol-9, 43
Nonspecific immunity, 26
Nonsteroidal antiinflammatory (NSAIDs) pain relievers, 296
Norcardia asteroides, 275
Norcardia brasiliensis, 275
Norcardia caviae, 275
Norcardia otitidiscaviarum, 275
Norcardiosis, infant and child
  clinical presentation
    fever, 275
    lymphadenopathy, 275
    pulmonary infection, 275
    skin infections, 275
  diagnosis, 275
  etiology, epidemiology, 275
  nursing implications, 275
  pathogenesis, 275
  prevention, treatment
    antimicrobial therapy, 275
    multidrug regimens, 275
    sulfonamides, 275

Not Part of My Sentence: Violations of the Human Rights of Women in Custody (Amnesty International), 198
NRTIs. *See* Nucleoside reverse transcriptase inhibitors
NSAIDs. *See* Nonsteroidal antiinflammatory (NSAIDs) pain relievers
Nucleoside reverse transcriptase inhibitors (NRTIs)
  dyslipidemia and, 101, 228
  fat redistribution syndrome, 99
  function of, 52
  hyperlactatemia, 109
  side effects of, 52
  testosterone therapy and, 228
  in therapy for asymptomatic individuals, 54
  therapy in infants, children, 258*table*
Nucleotide reverse transcriptase inhibitor
  beneficial dosing schedule, 52
  function of, 52
Nursing case management model, 338
Nursing management issues. *See* Case management; Ethical and legal concerns; Preventing HIV transmission in patient care settings
Nutrition
  anemia, 268
  anorexia, weight loss, 124–125
  depression therapy, 166
  diarrhea, 270
  dysphagia, odynophagia, 131
  dyspnea, 130
  fat redistribution (lipodystrophy), 44
  fatigue, 133, 134
  HIV infected infant, child, 248, 250, 256, 257
  homeless persons, 194
  hyperlipidemia, 45
  of immigrants, 221
  incarcerated persons, 201
  insulin resistance, 44
  leiomyosarcoma, 273
  malnutrition, 45
  mitochondrial dysfunction, 45
  mobility impairment, 140
  pain management, 146
  pregnancy, 218
  skin lesions, 305, 306
  social history, baseline assessment, 38
  teaching for health promotion, wellness, 44–45
  wasting, defined, 45

  wasting syndrome, infant and child, 290
  See also Anorexia, infant and child; Anorexia and weight loss, adolescent and adult; Weight loss, infant and child
Nystatin, 307, 405

Obsessive-compulsive disorder (OCD), 168
OCD (obsessive-compulsive disorder), 168
Octreotide, 405
Odynophagia. *See* Dysphagia and odynophagia
O'Kane, Patti, xxix
Older persons community
  access to care, treatment, research
    health care provider reluctance, 208
    medication difficulties, 208
    menopause research, 208
  community care approaches
    extended family network, 208
    gay and lesbian community resources, 209
  community description, 206
  health issues
    antiretroviral interactions, 206
    chronic illness comorbidity, 206
    injection drug use complications, 206
    mortality rates, 206
    organ function decrease, 206
  individual care approaches
    ADL supports, 208
    respect, 208
  statistics regarding, 206
  transmission, risk behaviors, prevention
    condom use, 207
    drug use behavior, 207
    erectile dysfunction, 207
    gay community isolation, 207
    health care provider reluctance, 208
    male to male sex risk, 207
    menopause issues, 207–208
    older dating scene risks, 206–207
    prevention message target group, 206, 207
    stigmatization fears, 207
Oncovirus. *See* Pathophysiology of HIV infection

Ondansetron, 403
Onychomycosis, 305, 308
Opiates
    pain therapy, mild, 145
    pain therapy, strong, 145–146
Opioids
    addiction myth, 294–295, 298
    dose titration, 297–298
    equianalgesic conversion
        chart, 297*table*
    short *vs.* long acting
        preparation, 298
    side effects, 298
Oral candidiasis, 282–283
    anorexia, infant and child,
        298, 299
    nonpharmacological
        treatment, 306
    pharmacological treatment
        clortmazole oral troches, 306
        fluconazole, 307
        nystatin oral pastilles,
            306, 307
        nystatin oral suspension, 306
Oral hairy leukoplakia, 46, 132
    Category B disease, 352
    clinical presentation, 73
    diagnosis, 73
    etiology, epidemiology, 73
    nursing implications, 73
    pathogenesis, 73
    prevention, treatment, 73
Oral hygiene, 46
Oral Kaposi sarcoma, 47
Oral lesions
    etiology, 132
        behavioral factors, 132
        genetic factors, 132
        infectious causes, 132
        neoplasms, 132
        therapy related causes, 132
    evaluation, 133
    goals, 132
    interventions, alternative,
        complementary
        deglycyrrhizinated
            licorice, 133
        ethanol propolis extract, 133
        tea tree oil, 133
    interventions,
        nonpharmacologic, 132
    interventions,
        pharmacologic, 132
    nursing assessment,
        objective, 132
    nursing assessment,
        subjective, 132
    nursing diagnosis, 132
Oral sex, 8
OraQuick Rapid HIV-1 Test,
    355–356

Orasure Test, 356
OraSure test system, 29
Oropharyngeal candidiasis, 73,
    79, 80
Osteopenia, osteoporosis,
    avascular necrosis (AVN)
    clinical presentation, 108
    diagnosis, 108
    etiology, epidemiology, 107
    nursing implications, 108
    pathogenesis, 108
    prevention, treatment, 108
Osteoporosis. *See* Osteopenia,
    osteoporosis, avascular
    necrosis
Otitis media, recurrent, infant
    and child
    clinical presentation, 276
    diagnosis, 276
    etiology, epidemiology, 275
    nursing implications, 276
    pathogenesis, 275–276
    prevention, treatment, 276
Ownby, Kristin K., xxix
Oxandrolone, 405

P. aeruginosa, 278
Paclitaxel, 403
Pain, adolescent and adult
    etiology
        abdominal, 143–144
        anorectal, 144
        cardiovascular, 144
        dermatological, 144
        gastrointestinal, 143–144
        genito-urinary, 144
        musculoskeletal, 144
        neurological, 144
        oropharynx/esophageal, 143
        pulmonary, 144
    evaluation, 146
    goals, 144
    interventions, alternative,
        complementary
        aromatherapy, 146
        homeopathy, 146
        magnets, 146
        movement therapy, 146
        nutritional supplements, 146
    interventions,
        nonpharmacological
        individualized pain
            regimen, 144
        prayer, 144
        radiation therapy, 144
        relaxation techniques, 144
        rhythmic breathing, 144
        thermal modalities, 144
    interventions, pharmacological
        acetaminophen, 145
        adjuvants, 145

        anticonvulsants, 145
        antidepressants, 145
        antihistamines, 145
        corticosteroids, 145
        dolophone, 146
        fetanyl, 146
        hydromorphone, 146
        levorphanol, 146
        meperidine, 146
        morphine sulfate, 145–146
        nonopiate, 144–145
        NSAIDs, 145
        opiates, mild, 145
        opiates, strong, 145–146
        topicals, 145
        tramadol, 145
    nursing assessment,
        objective, 144
    nursing assessment,
        subjective, 144
    nursing diagnosis, 144
Pain, infant and child
    alternative therapies, 298
    etiology
        abdominal pain
            syndromes, 294
        biochemical effects, 294
        neurological pain, 294
        oral, throat esophageal pain
            syndromes, 294
        physiologic effects, 294
    evaluation, 298
    goals, 295
    interventions,
        nonpharmacological
        attender coping style, 295
        breathing, relaxation, 295
        cutaneous stimulation, 296
        distractor coping style, 295
        episodic, chronic,
            procedural pain, 295
        guided imagery, 295
        patient participation, 295
        with pharmacologic
            management, 295
    interventions, pharmacological
        adjuvants, 297–298
        cause, type, severity of
            pain, 296
        continuous
            administration, 296
        injection avoidance, 296
        local analgesia, 297
        medication dosage, 296
        mild pain indications, 296
        moderate pain
            indications, 296
        nonopioid use, 296
        opioid safety, 296
        opioid use, 294–295,
            296–297, 297*table*

principles of, 296
procedural pain
    indications, 296
severe pain indications, 296
side affects, 296
nursing assessment: objective
    behavioral signs of pain, 295
    pain medication trial, 295
nursing assessment: subjective
    ask about pain, 295
    teach use of pain assessment
        scale, 295
nursing diagnosis, 295
treatment sources of, 294
undertreatment of
    complexity of disease, 294
    knowledge deficiency, 294
    pain myths, 294–295
    virus control focus, 294
Pancreatitis, 287
Panic disorder
as anxiety disorder, 168
female sexual dysfunction, 147
male sexual dysfunction, 148
Pap test
cervical neoplasia, 93
health care follow-up, 50–51
HPV detection, 69
Para-amino-salicylate, 405–406
Parasomnia, 137
Paromomycin, 406
Parotitis, infant and child, 273
clinical presentation, 276
diagnosis
    malignancy differential
        diagnosis, 276
    physical exam, 276
etiology, epidemiology, 276
nursing implications, 276
pathogenesis, 276
prevention, treatment, 276
Parvovirus B19, 102, 268
Passion flower, 151
Pathophysiology of HIV infection
human immunodeficiency
    virus (HIV)
    AIDS, origin of, 24–25
    HIV-1 vs. HIV-2, 24
    life cycle phases of, 23–24
    primate to human
        lentivirus
        transmission, 25
    structure of, 23
immune system, normal
    cell-mediated immunity, 27
    humoral immunity, 26
    inflammatory response, 26
    leukocytes (white blood
        cells), 25
    NK cells, 27
    nonspecific immunity, 26

phagocytosis, 26
specific immunity, 26–27
immune system, response to
    HIV infection
    B lymphocytes, 28
    CD$_8$ CTLs and CD8
        suppressor cells, 27
    CD$_4$ T-helper/inducer
        cells, 27
    follicular dendritic cells, 28
    granulocytes, 28
    lymphoid organs, 28
    mononuclear phagocytes, 28
    NK cells, 27
natural history of HIV
    infection
    chronic infection, 28–29
    primary infection
        (time 0), 28
retroviruses
    lentivirus subgroup, 23
    oncovirus subgroup, 22–23
    properties of, 23
Patient care settings. See
    Preventing HIV
    transmission in patient care
    settings
Patient Self-Determination Act, 343
PBMC HIV culture, 30, 357
PCP. See Pneumocystis carinii
    pneumonia (PCP),
    adolescent and adult
PCR. See Polymerase chain
    reaction (PCR) test
Pediatric HIV Classification
    System: Clinical Categories,
    246–247table
Pediatric HIV Classification
    System, Immunologic
    categories, 244, 245table
Pelvic inflammatory disease,
    215, 230, 352
Pentamidine, 287, 404
People with hemophilia
    community
    access to care, treatment,
        research
        hepatitis C, 193
        research advocacy, 193
        stigma barriers, 192–193
    community care approaches
        public policy
            discussions, 193
    community description
        definition, 191
        Hemophilia A, 191
        Hemophilia B, 191
        incidence rates, 191
        plasma factor
            product transmission,
            191–192

self-infusion, 191
severity classifications, 191
health issues
    hemarthrosis, 192
    idiopathic
        thrombocytopenia
        purpura, 192
    procedures inducing
        bleeding, 192
    pseudohematomas, 192
    septic arthritis, 192
    thrombocytopenia, 192
individual care approaches
    safer sex education, 193
    viral transmission
        precautions, 193
transmission, risk behaviors,
    prevention
    safer sex, 192
Perinatally acquired pediatric
    HIV, 12, 15, 21, 43–44
antiretroviral therapy, 57
breast-feeding
    immigrant customs, 242
    oral and gastrointestinal
        tract exposure, 242
    safe substitute feeding, 242
    statistics regarding, 242
diagnosis, evaluation of
    HIV-exposed infant, 244
    classification system for
        HIV, 244–245, 245table,
        246–247table
    clinical categories, 244,
        246–247table
    clinical symptom
        diagnosis, 244
    HIV ELISA, Western blot
        diagnosis, 244
    HIV polymerase chain
        reaction diagnosis, 244
    immunologic categories,
        244, 245table
    infection status, 244
    transplacentally acquired
        HIV antibody, 244
    virologic assay
        diagnosis, 244
presentation patterns
    rapid symptom onset, rapid
        progression, poor
        prognosis, 244
    symptomatic after
        1 year, slower
        progression, 244
prevention of
    antiretroviral medication,
        242, 243table
    U.S. Public Health Service
        Perinatal HIV
        Guidelines, 242

zidovudine treatment, 242,
243*table*
zidovudine treatment,
breast feeding, 242
prognosis, survival
ARV therapy, slower
progression, 247
end organ failure, 245
moderate immune
suppression, 247
rapid progression in
untreated children,
245, 247
recurrent normal
infections, 247
severe immune
compromise, 245
registries, 17
Peripheral neuropathy (PN), 49
Category B disease, 352
clinical presentation
autonomic neuropathy, 74
distal symmetric
polyneuropathy, 74
inflammatory
demyelinating
polyneuropathy, 74
monoeuritis multiplex, 74
progressive
polyradiculopathy, 74
diagnosis, 74
epidemiology, 73–74
etiology, 74
nursing implications, 75
pathogenesis, 74
PCP, 287
prevention, treatment, 74–75
Perry, Lisa, xxix
Pet care, 47
Pharyngitis, 278
Phenotype assays for antiretroviral
resistance, 57, 358–359
Phentolamine, 148
Pidgin Signed English (PSE), 189
Piercing, 46
PIs. *See* Protease inhibitors
PML. *See* Progressive multifocal
leukoencephalopathy (PML),
adolescent and adult
PN. *See* Peripheral neuropathy
Pneumococcal pneumonia
vaccine, 41–42, 252, 253*table*
Pneumocystis carinii pneumonia
(PCP), adolescent and adult,
2, 75, 86, 87, 129
PCP prophylaxis, 252, 254–255,
255*table*, 256*table*
Pneumocystis carinii pneumonia
(PCP), infant and child, 287
clinical presentation, 286
diagnosis, 286

etiology, epidemiology
AIDS-defining illness, 286
HIV-infected women, 286
nursing implications, 287
pathogenesis, 286
prevention, treatment
pentamidine, 287
steroids, respiratory
support, 287
TMP-SMX, 286
Pneumocystosis
clinical presentation, 86–87
diagnosis, 87
etiology, epidemiology, 86
nursing implications, 87
pathogenesis, 86
prevention, treatment, 87, 141
Pneumonia
of HIV infected infant, child,
250, 279–280
See also Bacterial pneumonia
Podofilox, 307
Polio vaccination, 43, 252
Polycythemia, 227
Polymerase chain reaction (PCR)
test, 30, 244, 257
Polyneuropathy
mobility impairment, 139
See also Distal symmetric
polyneuropathy
(DSP); Peripheral
neuropathy (PN)
Porche, Demetrius, xxix
Posttraumatic stress disorder
(PTSD), 168, 181
PP. *See* Progressive
polyradiculopathy
Prednisone, 273–274
Pregnant women community
access to care, treatment,
research
ART, contraindications, 217
ART regimen, 216–217,
217*table*
chronic illness
stabilization, 216
early prenatal care, 216
knowledge assessment, 216
maternal risk factors, 217
mental illness factors, 217
obstetrical risk factors,
217–218
antiretroviral therapy, 58
community care approaches
community outreach, 219
early prenatal care
importance, 219
voluntary HIV testing, 218
community description
breast feeding
transmission, 214

vertical, perinatal
transmission,
defined, 214
vertical transmission
rates, 214
health issues
domestic violence, 214
economic dependency, 214
reproductive decisions, 214
unplanned pregnancies, 214
health promotion and
transmission prevention,
43–44
HIV-testing of, 343, 344
individual care approaches
cesarean section
counseling, 218
counseling, documentation
of, 218
economic stability
assessment, 218
fertility, ovulation
education, 218
guardianship issues, 218
mental health, substance
abuse referral, 218
nutrition assessment, 218
obstetrical history
assessment, 218
parenting skills
assessment, 218
partner assessment, 218
safer sex education, 218
tobacco use assessment, 218
in rural areas, 210
transmission, risk behaviors,
prevention issues
conception counseling, 215
HIV concentrations in
semen, 215
infertility issues, 215
insemination method
options, 215
pelvic inflammatory
disease, 215
preconception counseling
for men, 215
prenatal testing for
women, 216
self-insemination, 215
serodiscordant couples
issues, 215
sperm count, motility, 216
sperm donation, 215
substance use factors,
215–216
Premature ejaculation, 148, 149
Preventing HIV transmission in
patient care settings
HBV postexposure therapy,
347–348

HCV postexposure therapy, 348

infection control
- airborne precautions, 345–346
- contact precautions, 346
- droplet precautions, 345
- hand washing, 346
- safe environment for patients, workers, 345
- standard precautions, 345
- transmission-based precautions, 345–346

OSHA regulations
- biohazard labeling, 349
- cleaners, disinfectants restrictions, 349
- engineering controls, 348
- food delivery restrictions, 349
- laboratory specimen restrictions, 349
- linen procedures, 349
- medical emergency regulations, 349
- medical waste disposal, 349
- patient placement, 349
- sharp disposal unit, 348–349
- staff education, 349
- work practice controls, 348

postexposure prophylaxis
- determination factors, 346
- early ARV therapy, 346–347
- early ARV therapy, side effects, 347
- HIV, HBV, HCV, 346
- mucous membrane exposure, 346
- needle transmission, 346
- nonintact skin exposure, 346
- occupational injuries, 346
- pregnancy factors, 347
- rapid testing, 347

Prevention of HIV infection, 21
- blood and tissue transplantation, 21–22
- blood to blood transmission prevention
  - cessation of drug use, 20
  - harm reduction, 20–21
- cessation of drug use, 20

HIV vaccines
- AIDSVAX, 22
- humoral and CTL response, 22
- obstacles to development of, 22
- viral replication, suppression of, 22

perinatal transmission, 21

primary prevention
- abstinence, 19
- barrier protection, 19–20
- circumcision, 20
- safer sex, 20
- spermicides, microbicidal gels, 20

risk assessments
- of adolescents, 19
- of gay and bisexual adults, 18–19
- of heterosexuals, 18

See also Preventing HIV transmission in patient care settings

Primaquine, 405

Primary anxiety-spectrum disorders
- acute stress disorder, 168
- assessment
  - history, 169
  - physical signs, 169–170
  - psychological symptoms, 169–170
- etiology
  - biological factors, 169
  - drug and alcohol abuse, 169
  - genetic factors, 169
  - medication factors, 169
  - social and psychological factors, 169
- generalized anxiety disorder, 168
- interventions: nonpharmacological
  - aerobic exercise, 170
  - cognitive-behavioral therapy, 170
  - coping strategies, 170
  - cultural variations, 170
  - peer support groups, 170
  - support therapy, 170
- interventions: pharmacological
  - antidepressants, 170
  - benzodiazepines, 170
  - buspirone, 170
  - SSRIs, 170
- medical conditions, 168–169
- obsessive-compulsive disorder, 168
- panic disorder, agoraphobia, 168
- PTSD, 168
- social phobia, 168

Primary CNS lymphoma, 125

PRIME-MD depression assessment scale, 165

Prison inmates. *See* Incarcerated persons community

Probenecid, 405

Prochlorperzaine, 405

Progressive multifocal leukoencephalopathy (PML), adolescent and adult
- clinical presentation, 92
- diagnosis, 92
- etiology, epidemiology, 91–92
- nursing implications, 92
- pathogenesis, 92
- prevention, treatment, 92

Progressive multifocal leukoencephalopathy (PML), infant and child
- clinical presentation, 288
- diagnosis, 289
- etiology, epidemiology, 288
- nursing implications, 289
- pathogenesis, 288
- prevention, treatment, 289

Progressive polyradiculopathy (PP), 74

Propoxyphene, 145

Prostaglandin E1, 148

Prostitutes. *See* Commercial sex workers' community

Protease inhibitors (PIs)
- depression and, 166
- dosing schedule, 53
- drugs in class, 53
- dyslipidemia and, 101, 228
- fat redistribution, 44, 99
- function of, 52–53
- hyperlipidemia, 45
- IGT and, 100
- insulin resistance, 44
- liver transmaminase elevation, 53
- menstrual cycle impact of, 232
- oral lesions, 132
- SSRIs and, 167
- testosterone therapy and, 228
- therapy in infants, children, 258*table*
- tricyclic antidepressants and, 167

Proteinuria, 274

Protozoal infections, in adolescents and adults. *See* Cryptosporidiosis, adolescent and adult; Isosporiasis, adolescent and adult; Pneumocystosis; Toxoplasmosis, adolescent and adult

Protozoal infections, infant and child. *See* Cryptosporidiosis, infant and child; Isosporiasis, infant and child; Pneumocystis carinii pneumonia (PCP), infant

and child; Toxoplasma
gondii, infant and child
PSE (Pidgin Signed English), 189
Pseudo-Cushing's syndrome. *See*
Fat redistribution syndrome
(lipodystrophy)
Pseudohematomas, 192
Psittacosis, 47
Psoriasis
clinical presentation, 106
diagnosis, 106
etiology, epidemiology,
105–106
nursing implications, 106
pathogenesis, 106
prevention, treatment, 106
Psychiatric disorders in
HIV disease
in African Americans, 211–212
history of HIV infected infant,
child, 250
of pregnant women, 217
substance use and, 222
See also Delirium;
Depression; Primary
anxiety-spectrum
disorders; Substance
abuse and mental illness
Psychosocial case management
model, 339
Psychosocial concerns of the
HIV infected adolescent
and adult. *See* Adolescent
community; Caregiver
burden, strain; Delirium;
Depression; Primary
anxiety-spectrum disorders;
Responses to HIV diagnosis:
family and significant other;
Responses to HIV diagnosis:
infected person; Spiritual
and religious concerns, of
HIV infected persons;
Substance abuse and mental
illness
Psychosocial concerns of the HIV
infected infant and child.
See Community-based care
issues; Decision making
and family autonomy;
Disclosure to the child;
End of life issues; Multiple
hospitalizations; Social
isolation and stigma;
Stress reduction and
pediatric HIV infection;
Surrogate caregivers
Psychostimulants, 167
Psychotherapy
for anxiety disorders, 170
for depression, 134, 166

for guilt, 163
for male sexual
dysfunction, 149
for spiritual and religious
concerns, 162
PTSD (posttraumatic stress
disorder), 168
Public Health Service Revised
Classification System for
HIV Infection (Adolescents
and Adults), 351–353
Pulmonary cryptococcosis, 83
Pyrazinamide, 406
Pyridoxine, 405–406
Pyrimethamine, 406–407

Quality of life
of caregiver, 160
sleep disturbances, 137
substance use and, 224
of visually impaired, 180
Quantitative HCV PCR test, 361
Quantitative plasma
HIV RNA, 357

Rapid HIV test, 355
Rapid plasma reagin
test (RPR), 251
Recent immigrants. *See*
Immigrants community
Recombinant assays for
antiretroviral resistance, 57
Recurrent bacterial infections,
infant and child
clinical presentation
pneumonia, 279
recurrent, persistent
infection, 279
sinusitis, 279–280
diagnosis, 280
etiology, epidemiology
pneumonia, 279
sepsis, 279
sinusitis, 279
nursing implications, 280
prevention, treatment
HAART, 280
immunization, 280
site and source
dependence, 280
trimethoprimsulfamethoxa
zole, 280
Refractory disease, 80
Reiki therapy, 298, 304, 318
Reiter's syndrome. *See* Arthritis,
Reiter's syndrome
Religion. *See* Spiritual and
religious concerns
Renal disease, 108–109, 274
Renal tubular acidosis, 274
Rendiro, Susanne, xxix

Rescriptor, 376
Resistance testing, 358
Responses to HIV diagnosis. *See*
Caregiver burden, strain;
Responses to HIV diagnosis:
family and significant other;
Responses to HIV diagnosis:
infected person; Spiritual
and religious concerns, of
HIV infected persons
Responses to HIV diagnosis:
family and significant other
assessment, 159
etiology, 159
family function, alterations in,
158–159
family of origin, of choice, 158
goals of care, 159
interventions, 159
life transitions, alterations
in, 158
Responses to HIV diagnosis:
infected person
acceptance
focus on living, 158
health care participation, 158
relationships
reengagement, 158
returning to workforce, 158
sexual functioning, decision
making, 158
spiritual beliefs
evaluation, 158
initial reaction
anger, 158
blame, 158
denial, 158
guilt, 158
helplessness, hopelessness,
158, 163
shock, 158
transitional issues
fear of death, 158
losses, 158
relationship
restructuring, 158
Restless legs syndrome, 137
Retrovir, 377
Retroviruses. *See* Pathophysiology
of HIV infection
Ribavirin, 407–409
Ribavutin, 409–410
Rifampin, 410
Riley, Tracy A., xxix
Risk, defined, 5
Risk factor, defined, 5
Risk groups, defined, 5
Ritonavir (Norvir), 53, 54
RNA PCR. *See* Viral load (VL) tests
Robinson, Patrick, xxix
RPR (rapid plasma reagin test), 251

RT-PCR for HCV RNA test, 360
Rubella vaccine, 40, 252, 253*table*
Rural communities
  access to care, treatment,
      research
    health care provider
        shortage, 210
    resources, services
        shortage, 210
    treatment outcomes, 210
  common health issues
    chronic disease rates, 209
    health care providers, lack
        of, 209
    infant mortality rates, 209
    isolation, 209
    poverty, 209
    transportation factors, 209
  community care approaches
    continuing education
        network, 211
    county fairs, 211
    faith-based
        organizations, 211
    local law enforcement
        network, 211
    media prevention
        campaign, 211
    outreach intervention
        campaigns, 210
    professional
        partnerships, 211
    school networking, 210
    social gathering venues, 211
    state prevention network,
        210–211
    Web site identification, 210
  community description
    anonymity, lack of, 209
    employment factors, 209
    extended family factor, 209
    frontier area, defined, 209
    informal support
        resources, 209
    insiders *vs.* outsiders, 209
    nonmetropolitan area,
        defined, 209
    rural area, defined, 209
    self-reliance,
        independence, 209
    South *vs.* Northeast, 209
    subpopulations, 209
  individual care approaches
    cultural sensitivity, 210
    social isolation
        sensitivity, 210
    telephone outreach,
        services, 210
    transmission, risk behaviors,
        prevention issues
      confidentiality issue, 210

      educating adolescents
          issue, 210
      heterosexual
          transmission, 210
      low risk perception, 210
      minorities, women
          statistics, 209
      pregnant women
          factors, 210
      reporting rates, 209
      South, incidence, 209
      stigma issue, 210
      veterinary needle
          supply, 210
Ryan White Comprehensive AIDS
    Resources Emergency
    (CARE) Act, 4

S. pneumoniae, 75, 278
Safer sex
  health care-followup, 51
  health promotion, wellness
      and transmission
      prevention
    abstinence, 43
    condom use, 43
    defined, 43
    female polyurethane
        condom, 19, 43
    nonoxynol-9, 43
  for hemophiliacs, 192, 193
  HPV prevention, treatment, 69,
      70–71
  for pregnant women, 218
  primary HIV prevention, 20
  primary prevention, 29
  for transgender, transsexual
      persons, 229
  women negotiation skills, 230
Salivary Test, 356
Salmonella, 78, 142, 143, 279, 299
Salmonellosis, adolescent and
    adult
  clinical presentation
    bacteremia, 78
    enteric fever, 78
    enterocolitis, 78
  diagnosis
    blood cultures, 78
    bone marrow cultures, 78
    differential diagnoses, 79
    stool cultures, 78
  etiology, epidemiology, 78
  nursing implications, 79
  pathogenesis, 78
  prevention, treatment, 79
Salmonellosis, infant and child
  clinical presentation, 282
  diagnosis, 282
  etiology, epidemiology, 281
  nursing implications, 282

    pathogenesis, 281–282
    prevention, treatment, 282
Saquinavir (Invirase, Fortovase), 53
Sarcoptes scabiei, 305
Scabies, 306, 308
Schor, Leslie, xxix
Schulz, Jane, xxix
Seasonal farm workers. *See*
    Migrant and seasonal farm
    workers community
Seborrheic dermatitis, 269, 305
  nonpharmacological
      treatment, 306
  pharmacological treatment, 307
SEE (Signed Exact English), 189
Selective serotonin reuptake
    inhibitors (SSRIs)
  anxiety disorders, 168, 170
  depression therapy, 167
  female sexual dysfunction, 148
  sexual dysfunction, 167
Self-determination, 340–341
Self-insemination methods, 215
Sellers, Craig R., xxix
Septic arthritis, 192
Serology testing, 51
Sex workers. *See* Commercial sex
    workers' community
Sexual dysfunction. *See* Female
    sexual dysfunction; Male
    sexual dysfunction
Sexual reassignment
    surgery (SRS), 226
Sexually transmitted
    disease (STD), 8, 36, 51
  in African Americans, 212, 214
  of HIV+ pregnant women,
      216, 217
  HIV transmission, 231
  incarcerated persons, 197
  substance abuse, 222
  in women, 230
Shephard, Rebkah, xxx
Shigella bacterial infection, 142,
    143, 299
Shingles, 67
Short Portable Mental Status
    Questionnaire, 140
Signed Exact English (SEE), 189
Significant other. *See* Responses to
    HIV diagnosis: family and
    significant other
SIL. *See* Squamous intraepithelial
    lesions
Sildenafil medication, 148
Simian immunodeficiency virus
    (SIV), 23
Simian T-lymphotrophic virus
    (STLV), 22–23
Single use diagnostic system
    (SUDS), 29, 355

Sinus tacycardia, 269
Sinusitis, recurrent, infant
    and child
    bacterial infection, 279–280
    clinical presentation, 277
    diagnosis, 277
    etiology, epidemiology, 226
    nursing implications, 277
    pathogenesis, 276–277
    prevention, treatment, 277
    upper respiratory
        infection, 278
Skin abscesses, 307
Skin lesions, infant and child
    etiology
        bacterial infections, 305
        drug reactions, 305
        fungal infections, 305
        immune system
            deficiencies, 305
        neoplasm, 305
        nutrition deficiencies, 305
        vascular lesions, 305
        viral infections, 305
    evaluation
        diagnosis methods, 309
        document improvement, 309
        follow-up, 309
        previous conditions, 309
        systemic disease
            elimination, 309
    goals, 306
    interventions, alternative
        for atopic dermatitis, 308
        for skin irritation, diaper
            rash, 308
    interventions,
        nonpharmacological
        for aphthous ulcers, 306
        for herpes simplex, 306
        for ichthyosis, 306
        for impetigo, 306
        for molluscum
            contagiousum, 306
        for nutrition deficits, 306
        for oral candidiasis, 306
        for scabies, 306
        for seborrheic
            dermatitis, 306
        for tinea corporis, 306
        for varicella zoster, 306
        for xerosis, 306
    interventions, pharmacological
        for aphthous ulcers, 307
        for condyloma
            acuminata, 307
        for herpes simplex, 307
        for impetigo, 308
        for molluscum
            contagiosum, 307
        for onychomycosis, 308

    for oral candidiasis,
        306–307
    for scabies, 308
    for seborrheic
        dermatitis, 307
    for tinea corporis, 308
    for varicella-zoster virus, 307
    nursing assessment, objective,
        305–306
    nursing assessment,
        subjective, 305
    nursing diagnosis, 306
Sleep disturbances
    cognitive impairment, 126
    depression and, 164
    etiology
        decreased quality of life, 137
        hypersomnia, 137
        insomnia, 137
        parasomnia, 137
        restless legs syndrome, 137
    evaluation, 139
    goals, 137
    interventions, alternative,
        complementary
        acupuncture, 139
        biofeedback, 138
        melatonin, 138
        noise management, 139
        relaxation training, 138
        sleep restriction, 138
    interventions,
        nonpharmacological,
        137–138
    interventions, pharmacological
        antidepressants, 138
        antihistamines, 138
        benzodiazepines, 138
    nursing data, objective, 137
    nursing data, subjective, 137
    nursing diagnosis, 137
Slim disease, 2
Social isolation and stigma
    social isolation: consequences
        lifestyle disruptions, 318
        loneliness, 318
        self-concept, self-esteem
            development, 318
        social support resources, 318
        socialization development
            interruption, 318
    social isolation: factors
        social rejection fear, 318
        unpredictable course of
            illness, 318
    social isolation: family
        affected by
        adolescents, 318
        children, 318
        healthy siblings, 318
        parents, 318

stigma
    courtesy or associative
        stigma, 319
    intensity modulating
        factors, 319
stigma: assessment
    psychological results, 320
    questions regarding, 320
stigma: interventions
    counseling, 320
    disclosure issues, 320
    educate families,
        partners, 320
    referrals, 320
    strategies, 320
stigma: management of
    minimizing symptoms, 319
    social situation
        avoidance, 319
    undisclosed HIV status, 319
stigma: prevalence of
    decrease in, 319
    factors affecting, 319–320
    rejection, 319
stigma: results of
    limitations of
        opportunities, 319
    quality of life erosion, 319
    self-blame,
        disempowerment, 319
    shame, self-hatred, 319
    social identity, changes
        in, 318
    social rejection, 318
stigma: types of traits, 319
Social phobia, 168
South Africa, 9
Special populations. *See*
    Adolescent community;
    African American
    community; Blind and
    visually impaired
    community; Commercial
    sex workers' community;
    Deaf and hearing-impaired
    community; Gay and
    bisexual men community;
    HIV infected health care
    workers community;
    Homeless persons
    community; Immigrants
    community; Incarcerated
    persons community;
    Lesbians and bisexual
    women community; Migrant
    and seasonal farm workers
    community; Older persons
    community; People with
    hemophilia community;
    Pregnant women
    community; Rural

communities; Substance
users community;
Transgender/transsexual
persons community;
Women, community of
Specific immunity
cell-mediated immunity, 27
humoral immunity, 26
NK cells, 27
Sperm washing, 215
Spermicides, 8, 20
Spiritual and religious concerns,
of HIV infected persons
assessment
belief systems, practices,
community, 162
culture, family and
environment, 162
self-worth, self-esteem, 162
spiritual distress
indications, 162
at diagnosis, 158
etiology
spiritual wellness, issues
affecting, 162
spirituality, sources of,
161–162
goal of care, 162
interventions
assisted suicide
evaluation, 162
caring, supportive
presence, 162
grief, resolution of, 163
guilt or shame, dealing
with, 162–163
hope, despair, anger
assessment, 162
hope and acceptance,
instilling, 163
impending death
preparation, 163
nonjudgmental
listening, 162
pastoral counselors, 162
psychotherapy, 162
self-concept and illness, 162
self-esteem, reframing
of, 162
self-forgiveness, 162
spirituality, integrated
perspective on, 163*fig.*
spiritual distress,
defined, 161
spiritual wellness, defined, 161
spirituality, defined, 161
Splenomegaly, infant and child
clinical presentation, 277
diagnosis, 277
etiology, epidemiology, 277
nursing implications, 277

pathogenesis, 277
prevention, treatment, 277
Spramycin, 410–411
Squamous intraepithelial
lesions (SIL), 68
SRS (sexual reassignment
surgery), 226
St. John's Wort, 49, 140, 166
Stanley, Hopkins D., xxx
Staphyloccal infections
cellulitis, 307
folliculitis, 307
skin abscesses, 307
Staphylococcus aureus, 75, 276
State/Trait Anxiety Inventory, 126
Stavudine (Zerit, d4T), 52
STD. *See* Sexually transmitted
disease (STD)
Sterken, David J., xxx
Steven Johnson syndrome, 53
Stigmatization. *See* Social isolation
and stigma
Streptococcus pneumonia, 41,
276, 279
Streptococcus pyogenes, 75, 276
Streptomycin, 411
Stress management
alternative therapies, 49
health and wellness
promotion, 44
See also Stress reduction and
pediatric HIV infection
Stress reduction and pediatric
HIV infection
psychological, emotional
anxiety disorders, 316
behavioral responses, 316
cognitive responses, 316
emotional responses, 316
interpersonal, social
responses, 316
mood disorders, 316
stress management strategies
alternative therapy, 318
disclosure complexities, 317
education needs, 317–318
keeping family intact, 317
medication adherence
planning, 317
parental guilt
management, 317
permanency planning, 317
support system
assessment, 316
telling infected child,
316–317
telling siblings, 316
stress response,
developmental stage
infant, 316
preschooler, 316

preteen, 316
school age, 316
teenager, adolescent, 316
toddler, 316
stressors in children
chronic parent illness, 316
cognition, development
impairment, 316
increased instability, 316
Structured Clinical Interview
for *DSM-III-R* Non-Patient
Version-HIV (SCID-NP-
HIV), 169
Stuart B. McKinney Homeless
Assistance Act, 193
Substance Abuse and Mental
Health Services, 225
Substance abuse and mental
illness
anxiety disorders, 169
assessment, 173
delirium, 171
depression and, 164
depression therapy and, 167
dual diagnosis, defined, 172
etiology, 172–173
goals of care, 173
incarcerated persons, 201
interventions
nonpharmacologic, 173
pharmacologic, 173
See also Drug use; Substance
use; Substance users
community
Substance misuse, defined, 221
Substance use
adolescent risk factor,
177, 178
caregiver decision making,
314–315
commercial sex workers,
181, 182, 183
deaf and hearing-impaired
community, 189
elderly age factors, 206, 207
gay and bisexual men, 184
HIV-positive pregnant women,
215–216
homeless people, 194
incarcerated persons, 197, 201
by lesbians and bisexual
women, 202, 203, 230
by mother of HIV infected
child, 248
thrombocytopenia, 277
by transgender community,
227, 229
Substance users community
access to care, treatment,
research
distrust of authority, 223

drugs and prescribed meds, interaction, 223
lifestyle disorganization, 223, 231
mental illness factors, 223
methadone interactions, 223
pain management conflicts, 223
stereotyping myths, 223
common health issues
coping strategies, 222
distrust of authority, 222
infections, 222
mental illness, 222
nutrition deficiency, 222
organic syndromes, 222
race, gender, sexual preference factors, 222
self-medication problems, 222
sexual, physical abuse, 222
symptom relief, 222–223
treatment adherence problems, 222
community care approaches
child care services, 225
community-based care referrals, 224–225
community-based services, 225
day treatments, 225
detox focus, 225
harm-reduction services, 225
hospice, palliative care focus, 225
housing options, 225
mobil clinics, 225
multidisciplinary focus, 225
needle exchange centers, 225
outreach, case management programs, 225
outreach services, 225
prison alternatives, 225
resources list, 225–226
withdrawal, detox research, 225
community description
definitions, 221
injecting drug users (IDUs), 221–222
minimal to maximal use continuum, 221
non-IDUs, 222
individual care approaches
abstinence model, 224
communication focus, 225
comprehensive history taking, 224
coping mechanism, 224
discharge planning, 224

harm reduction model, 224
health care access difficulties, 224
home care agency referrals, 224
life style factors, 224
pain assessment, treatment, 225
patient advocacy, 225
patient manipulation and scamming, 224
patient's relationship with drugs, understanding, 224
peer programs, 224
person vs. effects of drug, 224
primary care referrals, 224–225
provide safer alternative, 224
recovery, not a requirement for care, 224
respect decision-making, 224
stress, fear, poor coping skills, 224
substance use culture knowledge, 223
support network assessment, 224
team approach, 225
trust establishment, 223
withdrawal symptom treatment, 224
transmission, risk behaviors, prevention issues, 223
See also Drug use; Substance abuse and mental illness; Substance use
SUDS. See Single Use Diagnostic System
SUDS (Single use diagnostic system), 355
Suicide
assisted suicide, 162, 345
depression and, 164, 165–166
substance abuse, 222
tricyclic antidepressant therapy and, 167
Sulfadiazine, 412
Surrogate caregivers
adoptive family
extended family, 322
HIV disclosure, 322
transracial, 322
biological parent contact, 323
concept of family
extended family, 321
nuclear family, 321
examples of, 321
extended family

cross-generational addiction history, 321–322
examples of, 321
preconceived feelings, 322
psychological, cultural benefits, 321
treatment, transmission education, 322
trust development, 322
voluntary vs. appointed, 321
family constellation
disease perspective, 323
include all caregivers, 323
fost-adopt, 322
foster families
diagnosis disclosure, 322
formalized relationship, 322
legal relationship, 322
specialized training, 322
need for
abandoned infants, 321
parental absence, 320–321
psychological, social well-being needs, 321
reunification vs. adoption focus, 321
single parent prevalence, 321
support for, 323
understanding family history
extended family medical history, 323
genogram, 323
Susceptibility to infection. See Epidemiology of HIV infection and AIDS
Sustiva, 375–376
Swanson, Barbara, xxiii–xxiv, xxx
Symptom management of the HIV infected adolescent and adult. See Adolescent community; Anorexia and weight loss, adolescent and adult; Cognitive impairment, adolescent and adult; Cough; Diarrhea, adolescent and adult; Dysphagia and odynophagia; Dyspnea; fatigue; Female sexual dysfunction; Fever; Male sexual dysfunction; Mobility impairment; Nausea and vomiting; Oral lesions; Pain, adolescent and adult; Sleep disturbances; Vision loss
Symptom management of the HIV infected infant and child. See Anorexia, infant and child; Cognitive impairment and developmental delay, infant

and child; Fever, infant and
child; Pain, infant and child;
Skin lesions, infant and child
Symptomatic conditions in
adolescents and adults,
with advancing disease.
See Bacterial infections;
Bartonellosis, adolescent
and adult; Comorbid
complications, adolescent
and adult; Fungal infections,
adolescent and adult; Herpes
zoster (varicella-zoster virus,
VZV), adolescent and adult;
Human papillomavirus
(HPV) infection; Idiopathic
thrombocytopenia purpura;
Listeriosis; Neoplasms,
adolescent and adult; Oral
hairy leukoplakia; Peripheral
neuropathy; Protozoal
infections; Viral infections
Symptomatic conditions in infants
and children with advancing
disease. *See* Anemia, infant
and child; Candidiasis, infant
and child; Cardiomyopathy,
infant and child;
Coccidioidomycosis, infant
and child; Cryptococcosis,
infant and child;
Cryptosporidiosis, infant and
child; Cytomegalovirus
(CMV), infant and child;
Dermatitis, infant and child;
Diarrhea, infant and child;
Hepatitis, infant and child;
Hepatomegaly, infant and
child; Herpes simplex virus
(HSV), infant and child;
Histoplasmosis, infant
and child; HIV-related
encephalopathy, infant and
child; HIV-related wasting
syndrome, infant and child;
Isosporiasis, infant and child;
Leiomyosarcoma, infant and
child; Lymphadenopathy,
infant and child; Lymphoid
interstitial pneumonitis
(LIP), infant and child;
Malignancies, infant and
child; Mycobacterial avium
complex (Mac), infant and
child; Mycobacterial
tuberculosis, infant and
child; Nephropathy (HIV-
associated nephropathy,
HIVAN), infant and child;
Neutropenia, infant and
child; Norcardiosis, infant

and child; Otitis media,
recurrent, infant and child;
Parotitis, infant and child;
Pneumocystis carinii
pneumonia (PCP), infant and
child; Progressive multifocal
leukoencephalopathy
(PML), infant and child;
Salmonellosis, infant
and child; Sinusitis,
recurrent, infant and child;
Splenomegaly, infant and
child; Thrombocytopenia,
infant and child; Toxoplasma
gondii, infant and child;
Upper respiratory infection,
infant and child; Varicella,
disseminated, infant and
child
Syphilis screening, 251, 359

T-cell lymphocytes,
25–26, 27
T-cutaneous lymphoma, 22
T-helper cells, 9
Taliaferro, Donna, xxx
Tattoos, 46
TD. *See* Tetanus-diptheria
Teaching for health promotion,
wellness and transmission
prevention
alcohol use, 47
alternative therapies
cost factors, 49
defined, 49
herbs, 49
increase in, 48–49
reliability, 49
symptom relief goal, 49
drug use, 47–48
exercise, 44
food and water safety, 45–46
hand washing, 45
mouth care
angular chelitis, 46
apthous ulcers, 46
herpes simplex virus, 47
oral hairy leukoplakia, 46
oral Kaposi sarcoma, 47
nutrition
fat redistribution
(lipodystrophy), 44
hyperlipidemia, 45
insulin resistance, 44
mitochondrial
dysfunction, 45
wasting, defined, 45
pet care
animal feces, 47
bird risk factors, 47
dog risk factors, 47

reptile risk factors, 47
toxoplasmosis (cats), 47
pregnancy, 43–44
safer sex
abstinence, 43
condom use, 43
defined, 43
female polyurethane
condom, 19, 43
nonoxynol-9, 43
skin and hair care, 46
stress management, 44
tobacco use, 47–48
travel factors, 48
See also Preventing HIV
transmission in patient
care settings
Tenofovir (Vread), 52
Terconazole, 414
Testosterone, 414
Tetanus-diptheria (TD), 42–43,
253*table*
Thalidomide, 414
Theory of planned behavior,
prescription regimen
adherence, 61
Therapeutic touch, 146, 298,
304–305
Thrombocytopenia, adolescent
and adult, 192
clinical presentation,
103–104
diagnosis, 104
etiology, epidemiology, 103
nursing implications, 104
pathogenesis, 103
prevention, treatment, 104
See also Idiopathic
thrombocytopenia
purpura (ITP), adolescent
and adult
Thrombocytopenia, infant
and child
advanced disease, 268
clinical presentation, 277
diagnosis, 277
etiology, epidemiology, 277
nursing implications
aspirin, NSAID
avoidance, 278
intramuscular injection
avoidance, 278
report physical, mental
status changes, 278
secondary bleeding
prevention, 278
stool softener use, 278
venipuncture pressure, 278
pathogenesis, 277
prevention, treatment,
277–278

Thrush, 282
Thyroid hormone
    deficiencies, 105
Ticks, 66
Tinea corporis, 306, 308
Tinea faciale, 305
Tinetti's Performance Oriented
    Mobility Test, 139
TMP-SMX (trimethoprim-
    sulfamethoxazole), 286
Tobacco use, 37, 47–48
    anxiety disorders, 169
    asthma, 222
    cocaine use, lung infection, 222
    dyspnea, 130
    of HIV+ pregnant women,
        217, 218
    male sexual dysfunction, 148
    oral lesions, 132
    osteopenia, osteoporosis, 108
Topham, Debra, xxx
Touch therapy, 146, 298, 304–305
Toxoplasma gondii, 22, 51, 87,
    88, 359
Toxoplasma gondii, infant and child
    clinical presentation, 287
    diagnosis
        cerebral spinal fluid
            changes, 287
        clinical presentation, 287
        MRI, CT scan, 287
        serologic screening, 287
    etiology, epidemiology, 287
    nursing implications, 288
    pathogenesis, 287
    prevention, treatment
        lifelong suppressive
            therapy, 287
        TMP-SMX, 287
Toxoplasmosis, adolescent and
    adult, 47
    clinical presentation, 88
    cognitive impairment, 125
    diagnosis, 88
    etiology, epidemiology, 87–88
    nursing implications, 89
    pathogenesis, 88
    prevention, treatment, 88–89
Toxoplasmosis, infant and
    child, 301
Toxoplasmosis serologic test, 251
Trans community. *See*
    Transgender/transsexual
    persons community
Transgender experience. *See*
    Transgender/transsexual
    persons community
Transgender/transsexual persons
    community
    access to care, treatment,
        research

distrust, 227
    hormone services
        search, 227
    public assistance legal
        issues, 227
community care approaches
    community-based
        organizations, 229
    cultural sensitivity, 229
    medical-legal issues, 229
    trans-community
        outreach, 229
    trans experience
        employment
        practices, 229
    trans experience media, 229
    trans-friendly health care
        services, 229
    transphobia issues, 229
community description
    female-to-male, 226
    gender-deviant
        presentations, 226
    heterosexual majority
        identity, 226
    HIV-positive stats
        regarding, 226
    legal documentation, 226
    male-to-female, 226
    sexual reassignment
        surgery, 226
health issues
    alcoholism, drug use, sex
        work, 227
    discrimination by
        marginalized
        communities, 226
    gender identity, hiding
        of, 226
    healthy care service
        stereotyping,
        226–227
    hormone use supervision
        access, 226
    information reliability, 226
    mental health care service
        insensitivity, 227
    social stigma, 226
individual care approaches
    antiretroviral therapy
        effects, 228
    cosmetic surgeries, effects
        of, 228
    cross-gender hormone
        therapy, 228, 229
    gender identity
        validation, 228
    internalized transphobia
        issues, 228
    legal counseling, 229
    life skills counseling, 229

marginalized group
    membership, 228
medical management, 227
mental health
    counseling, 229
safer sex counseling, 229
substance abuse
    counseling, 229
trans-sensitive specialist
    referral, 228
trust establishment, 227
transmission, risk behaviors,
    prevention issues
    behavior-change programs,
        deficiency, 227
    mandatory name reporting
        issues, 227
    vocabulary limitations, 227
Transmission prevention.
    See Preventing HIV
    transmission in patient care
    settings; Teaching for health
    promotion, wellness and
    transmission prevention
Transsexuals. *See* Transgender/
    transsexual persons
    community
Transtheoretical behavior change
    model, prescription regimen
    adherence, 60
Transvestites. *See* Transgender/
    transsexual persons
    community
Travel factors
    health and wellness
        promotion, 48
    social history assessment, 37
    vaccinations, 43
Trichloroacetic acid, 307
Trichomonas vaginalis, 203
Tricyclic antidepressants (TCAs)
    cautions with, 167
    pain therapy, 297
Triglyceride levels, 252
Trimethoprim, 414
Trimethoprim-sulfamethoxazole
    (TMP-SMX), 286, 415–416
Trimetrexate, 416
Trizivir, 376
TST (tuberculin skin test), 251
Tuberculin skin test (TST), 251,
    281, 359
Tuberculosis (TB)
    cognitive impairment, 125
    of HIV infected infant,
        child, 251
    immigrants, 220
    incarcerated persons, 197
    latent TB infection in HIV and
        general population, 6
    PCP and, 87

registries, 17
skin testing for, 50
substance abuse, 222 (*See also*
      Mycobacterium
      tuberculosis (mTB),
      adolescent and adult)
treatment strategies, 363*table*
   rifabutin-based regimen,
      high dose, 364*table*
   rifabutin-based regimen,
      low dose, 365*table*
   streptomycin-based
      regimen, 366*table*
   treatment information,
      366*table*

Upper respiratory infection,
      infant and child
   clinical presentation
      common cold
         symptoms, 278
      epiglottitis symptoms, 278
      laryngitis symptoms, 278
      pharyngitis symptoms, 278
      sinusitis symptoms, 278
   diagnosis, 278
   etiology, epidemiology, 278
   nursing implications, 279
   pathogenesis, 278
   prevention, treatment, 278
Urinalysis (UA), 251
Urine test, 356

Vaccines, vaccination
   AIDSVAX, 22
   humoral and CTL response, 22
   obstacles to, 22
   viral replication, suppression
      of, 22
   See also Immunizations,
      adolescent and adult;
      Immunizations, infant
      and child
Vagina
   transmission through, 8
   vs. Cesarean delivery, 9
Vaginal candidiasis
   in women, 230, 352
Valacyclovir, 416
Valerian herbal therapy, 140, 151
Valganciclovir, 416
Vanburen-Hay, Brooke, xxx
Vancomycin, 416
VanDemark, Rhys, xxx
Varicella, disseminated, infant
      and child
   clinical presentation, 279
   diagnosis, 279
   etiology, epidemiology, 279
   nonpharmacological
      treatment, 306

   nursing implications, 279
   pathogenesis, 279
   pharmacological treatment, 307
   prevention, treatment, 279
   skin lesions, 305
Varicella-zoster virus (VZV),
      adolescent and adult, 66–67
   oral lesions, 132
   screening for in infants,
      children, 66–67
   vaccine, 252, 253*table*
   See also Herpes zoster
      (varicella-zoster virus,
      VZV), adolescent and
      adult
Vertical transmission. *See*
      Perinatally acquired
      pediatric HIV; Pregnant
      women
Vesicular stomatitis virus (VSV), 74
Videx, 376–377
Videx EC, 377
Vinblastine, 415–416
Vincristine, 416
Viracept, 377–378
Viral infections, in adolescents
      and adults, 125
   See also Cytomegalovirus
      (CMV), adolescent
      and adult; Herpes
      simplex virus (HSV),
      adolescent and adult;
      Progressive multifocal
      leukoencephalopathy
      (PML), adolescent and
      adult
Viral infections, infant and
      child. *See* Cytomegalovirus
      (CMV), infant and child;
      Progressive multifocal
      leukoencephalopathy
      (PML), infant and child
Viral load (VL) tests, 50, 57
   of HIV infected infant, child,
      251, 257, 261
Viramune, 378
Viread, 378
Virologic assay diagnosis, 244
Vision loss
   etiology
      adnexa involvement, 150
      anterior involvement, 150
      infection, 150
      posterior involvement, 150
   evaluation, 151
   goals, 151
   interventions, alternative,
      complementary
      herbal therapies, 151
      stress reduction
         techniques, 151

   interventions,
      nonpharmacological
      education of patient,
         family, 151
      pain control techniques, 151
   interventions, pharmacological
      eye medications, 151
      intravenous
         medications, 151
      sideeffects, 151
   nursing assessment, objective
      decreased visual acuity, 150
      photosensitivity, 150
      unilateral or bilateral field
         loss, 150
      visual field testing, 150
   nursing assessment,
      subjective, 150
   nursing diagnosis, 150–151
   See also Blind and visually
      impaired community
Visually impaired. *See* Blind and
      visually impaired
      community
Vitamin therapy, 127
Vomiting. *See* Nausea and
      vomiting
Vulvovaginal candidiasis,
      79–80, 352
VZV. *See* Varicella-zoster virus
      (VZV), adolescent and adult

Water-borne illnesses, 46
WB. *See* Western blot test
Web of Addictions, 226
Weight loss. *See* Anorexia, infant
      and child; Anorexia and
      weight loss, adolescent and
      adult; Weight loss, infant
      and child
Weight loss, infant and child
   Class C aids-defining
      condition, 299
   etiology
      anorexia, 299
      endocrine abnormalities, 299
      fever, 299
      food supply inadequacy, 299
      HIV encephalopathy, 299
      medication side effects, 299
      opportunistic infections, 299
      organomeagaly, 299
      pain, 299
   evaluation, 300
   interventions,
      nonpharmacological
      dietitian referral, 300
      family diet recall, 300
      family involvement, 300
      malabsorption, rule out, 300
      nutritional support, 300

opportunistic infections, rule out, 300
weight gain decisions, 300
interventions, pharmacological
nasogastric feedings, 300
opportunistic infections, treatment, 300
nursing assessment: objective
anthropometric data, 299
esophagogastroduodeno-scopy, 300
height and weight measurements, 299
laboratory data, 299
opportunistic infections history, 299
physical exam, 300
nursing assessment: subjective, 299
nursing diagnosis, 300
wasting, defined, 299
Wellness. *See* Teaching for health promotion, wellness and transmission prevention
Western blot test, 29, 244, 355
Western herbs, 127
WIHS (Women's Interagency Health Study), 214
Williams, Gail B., xxx
Winson, S. K. Glenda, xxx
Women
African Americans, 212
African incidence rates, 10, 12
alcohol use, unsafe sex and, 47
breast feeding, 11
caregiver burden, 159
depressive disorders in, 164
female polyurethane condoms, 19, 43
female-to-female transmission, 15
health history, 38
Hispanic American incidence rates, 12, 13
incarcerated gender factors, 197, 198
incidence rates, 12
in India, 10
infected blood products, 207
injecting drug use, 16
menopausal factors, 207–208
minority HIV rates, 13–14
mortality rates, 13, 14
older HIV/AIDS factors, 206–207
Pap test, 50–51
of rural communities, 209, 210
susceptibility of, 9

vaginal candidiasis, 79–80
See also Adolescent community; Cervical neoplasia; Female sexual dysfunction; Human papillomavirus (HPV) infection; Incarcerated persons; Perinatally acquired pediatric HIV; Pregnant women; Women, community of
Women, community of
access to care, treatment, research
abusive partner factor, 231
caregiving factor, 231
clinical trial underrepresentation, 231–232
illegal immigrant status, 231
lifestyle factors, 231
psychosocial/cultural barriers, 231
community care approaches
clinical drug trials, 233
one-stop shopping focus, 233
community description
geographic variability, 229
mortality rates, 229
poverty rates, 229
statistics regarding, 229
health issues
amenorrhea, 230
anemia, 230
candida esophagitis, 229
follicle stimulating hormone, 230
hormone levels, 230
hypothalamic-pituitary-ovarian axis alterations, 230
intermenstrual bleeding, 230
luteinizing hormone, 230
menopause, 230
opportunistic infections, 229
STDs, 230
vaginal candidiasis, 230
individual care approaches
antiretroviral therapy response, 232
empowerment of women focus, 233
fat maldistribution, ARV therapy, 232
gender differences in ARV metabolism, 232
hormonal contraception interruption, 232

HRT interruption, 232
illness reframing, 233
life style alterations, 233
long-term planning for children, 233
PI, menstrual cycle changes, 232
survival rates, 232–233
transmission, risk behaviors, prevention issues
age, gender, cultural issues, 231
domestic violence, 230
douching effects, 231
drug dependence, 230
heterosexual acquisition rates, 230
heterosexual women involunerability issues, 230–231
hormonal therapy, 231
power imbalances, 230
safer sex negotiation, 230
STDs, 231
woman-to-woman transmission rates, 230
Women's Interagency Health Study (WIHS), 214
Working Group on Antiretroviral Therapy and Management of Children with HIV Infection, 259
World Health Organization, 226

Xerosis, 306

Years of potential life lost (YPLL)
HIV disease cause of, 13
of mortality rates, 7
Yohimbine bark, 148, 149
Young, Thomas P., xxx
Youth
incidence rates, 12
statistics regarding, 16
YPLL. *See* Years of potential life lost (YPLL)

Zalcitabine (Hivid, ddc), 52
Zeller, Janice M., xxxi
Zerit, 379
Zerit XR, 379
Ziagen, 379
Zidovudine ARV therapy
of perinatal transmission of HIV, 242, 243*table*
Zidovudine-induced myopathy, 133
Zidovudine (Retrovir, AZT), 52